Resources for Instructor Success—

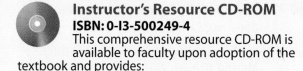

Instructor's Resource Manual
ISBN 0-13-503773-5
This manual contains a wealth of material to help faculty plan and manage their LPN/LVN nursing courses. It includes detailed learning outcomes, lecture outlines, teaching suggestions for the classroom and clinical settings, and more for each chapter. This supplement is available to faculty upon adoption of the textbook as an online download.

Instructor's Resource CD-ROM
ISBN: 0-I3-500249-4
This comprehensive resource CD-ROM is available to faculty upon adoption of the textbook and provides:

- *Instructor's Resource Manual.* This manual contains a wealth of material to help faculty plan and manage their LPN/LVN nursing courses. It includes detailed learning outcomes, lecture outlines, teaching suggestions for the classroom and clinical settings and more for each chapter.
- Animations and video library
- *Speaking Out* video library. A series of video clips of actual clients living with major mental health disorders
- Image Library
- Test Generator
- PowerPoint Lecture Slides

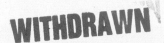
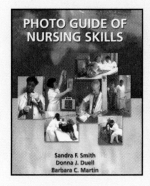

PHOTO GUIDE OF NURSING SKILLS

Sandra F. Smith
Donna J. Duell
Barbara C. Martin

Photo Guide of Nursing Skills
Provides a full-color atlas of all basic and intermediate skills. Its unique, easy-to-use format presents each procedure in logical steps—complete with appropriate illustrations, descriptions, and rationales. A critical thinking section focuses on unexpected outcomes.
ISBN: 0-8385-8174-9
Smith, Duell & Martin

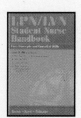

LPN/LVN Student Nurse Handbook
A bonus CD-ROM featuring an audio glossary of 800 terms and a flash-card maker accompany this "must-have" resource for practical and vocational nursing students.
ISBN: 0-13-094182-4
Brown, Boyd & Twiname

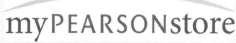

myPEARSONstore

For these and other resources visit
www.mypearsonstore.com

Brief Table of Contents

Mental Health

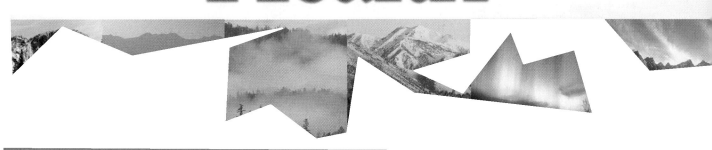

Nursing Care

Second Edition

Linda Eby, RN, MN
Instructor of Nursing
Coordinator of Nursing Student Success Program
Portland Community College
Portland, OR

Nancy J. Brown, RN, MSN
Adjunct Nursing Faculty/Former Director, Practical Nursing Program
San Juan Basin Technical College
Cortez, CO

PEARSON

Prentice
Hall

Upper Saddle River, NJ 07458

Library of Congress Cataloging-in-Publication Data

Eby, Linda.
    Mental health nursing care / Linda Eby, Nancy J. Brown.—2nd ed.
        p. ; cm.
    Includes bibliographical references and index.
    ISBN-13: 978-0-13-613692-7
    ISBN-10: 0-13-613692-3
    1. Psychiatric nursing. I. Brown, Nancy J. (Nancy Jo), RN. II. Title.
    [DNLM: 1. Mental Disorders—nursing. 2. Psychiatric
    Nursing—methods. 3. Psychological Theory. WY 160 E16m 2009]
    RC440.E29 2009
    616.89'0231—dc22   2007047121

Publisher: Julie Levin Alexander
Assistant to Publisher: Regina Bruno
Editor-in-Chief: Maura Connor
Senior Acquisitions Editor: Kelly Trakalo
Development Editor: Susan Geraghty
Editorial Assistant: Lauren Sweeney
Media Product Manager: John Jordan
Director of Marketing: Karen Allman
Senior Marketing Manager: Francisco Del Castillo
Marketing Specialist: Michael Sirinides
Managing Editor, Production: Patrick Walsh
Production Liaison: Yagnesh Jani
Production Editor: Trish Finley, GGS Book Services
Media Project Manager: Stephen Hartner
Manufacturing Manager/Buyer: Ilene Sanford
Composition: GGS Book Services
Printer/Binder: Courier Kendallville, Inc.
Senior Design Coordinator: Maria Guglielmo-Walsh
Cover Designer: Mary Siener
Cover Illustration: "Sunlight through Clouds at Biwa Lake, Japan" (background image), Photographer: Akira Kaede, Getty Images, Inc.–Photodisc; "Yosemite Falls in Winter," Photographer: Don Smith, Getty Images, Inc.–Photodisc; "Washer Woman Arch–Utah," Photographer: Richard Price, Getty Images, Inc.–Taxi; "Valley Fog between Mountain Ridges, California," Photographer: Mark E. Gibson, Creative Eye/Mira.com; "Winter by the Lake," Getty Images, Inc.; "View of a Colorful Aurora Borealis Display (Northern Lights)," Photographer: Pekka Parviainen, Photo Researchers, Inc.; "Cirrus Clouds over Moraine Lake, Alberta, Canada," Photographer: David Muench, Getty Images Inc.–Stone Allstock
Cover Printer: Phoenix Color Corporation

Pearson Education LTD.
Pearson Education Australia PTY, Limited
Pearson Education Singapore, Pte. Ltd
Pearson Education North Asia Ltd
Pearson Education Canada, Ltd.
Pearson Educación de Mexico, S.A. de C.V.
Pearson Education—Japan
Pearson Education Malaysia, Pte. Ltd
Pearson Education, Upper Saddle River, New Jersey

Notice: Care has been taken to confirm the accuracy of information presented in this book. The authors, editors, and the publisher, however, cannot accept any responsibility for errors or omissions or for consequences from application of the information in this book and make no warranty, express or implied, with respect to its contents.

The authors and publisher have exerted every effort to ensure that drug selections and dosages set forth in this text are in accord with current recommendations and practice at time of publication. However, in view of ongoing research, changes in government regulations, and the constant flow of information relating to drug therapy and reactions, the reader is urged to check the package inserts of all drugs for any change in indications or dosage and for added warning and precautions. This is particularly important when the recommended agent is a new and/or infrequently employed drug.

10 9 8 7 6 5 4 3 2

ISBN-13: 978-0-13-613692-7
ISBN: 0-13-613692-3

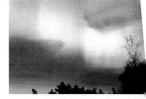

Student Success is built-in from the start...

Practical and vocational nurses from around the country told us that they needed two things to succeed as students in order to achieve their LPN/LVN licenses. First, they needed books that explain what the LPN/LVN needs to know and do. Second, they needed a variety of excellent review materials to reinforce their learning. *Mental Health Nursing Care* contains power-packed, built-in support to ensure your success throughout your LPN/LVN education.

As you start each chapter—

Brief Outlines preview what the chapter will cover for quick access and review.

Learning Outcomes identify what you can expect to learn from each chapter and help you focus your reading.

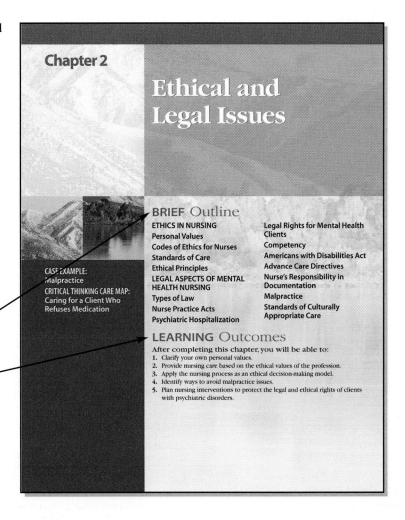

Chapter 2

Ethical and Legal Issues

CASE EXAMPLE:
Malpractice
CRITICAL THINKING CARE MAP:
Caring for a Client Who
Refuses Medication

BRIEF Outline
ETHICS IN NURSING
Personal Values
Codes of Ethics for Nurses
Standards of Care
Ethical Principles
LEGAL ASPECTS OF MENTAL HEALTH NURSING
Types of Law
Nurse Practice Acts
Psychiatric Hospitalization
Legal Rights for Mental Health Clients
Competency
Americans with Disabilities Act
Advance Care Directives
Nurse's Responsibility in Documentation
Malpractice
Standards of Culturally Appropriate Care

LEARNING Outcomes
After completing this chapter, you will be able to:
1. Clarify your own personal values.
2. Provide nursing care based on the ethical values of the profession.
3. Apply the nursing process as an ethical decision-making model.
4. Identify ways to avoid malpractice issues.
5. Plan nursing interventions to protect the legal and ethical rights of clients with psychiatric disorders.

Companion Website
- Learning Outcomes
- Chapter Outlines
- Audio Glossary
- NCLEX-PN® Review Questions
- Key Term Review—matching questions and crossword puzzles to help with new terminology and definitions.
- Case Studies—scenarios and critical-thinking questions
- Challenge Your Knowledge—visual critical thinking questions
- WebLinks—content-related hyperlinks
- Nursing Tools—handy reference materials

Makes need-to-know information easy to find and use!

Mental Health Nursing Care contains color-coded boxes and tables with important information for you to remember.

BOX 5-3	CULTURAL PULSE POINTS

Paralinguistic Cues

We are all speaking English; why don't we understand each other?

Verbal communication is composed of both what we say and how we say it. Our verbal messages are modified with the tone of our voice, rate of speech, pitch, loudness, and emotional expression. These *paralinguistic cues* (part of the spoken language that is in addition to the words) change the meaning of the spoken words. For example, imagine a European American nurse who has two clients (yes, this is a fantasy) and who is responding to their call lights. The first client is Vietnamese American and speaks English as a second language. She says, haltingly and quietly "I'm . . . in . . . pain." The second is a Persian American client (a native English speaker) in the same circumstances who says loudly, quickly, and choking back tears, "I'M IN PAIN!" The second client may not be feeling more pain than the first one. The loud, rapid speech may be how this client learned to express her feelings. The nurse may receive the second client's message more clearly because it is delivered more like the nurse expects it to be. People learn how to use their voices when they learn how to speak their native language, so the paralinguistic cues vary from one culture to the next. The nurse must be careful when interpreting these cues. The nurse can verify that s/he understands the client's message by **clarifying** what the client means. For example, communication would be improved if the nurse said: "You are in pain; would you like to have your pain medication?" instead of making assumptions about what the client might have meant.

Cultural Pulse Points boxes provide insight into populations and situations nurses may meet.

BOX 8-1	

Diagnostic Criteria for Schizophrenia

A. **Characteristic symptoms:**
   Two (or more) of the following symptoms must be present for a significant portion of the time during a 1-month period (or less if successfully treated):
   1. delusions
   2. hallucinations
   3. disorganized speech
   4. grossly disorganized or catatonic behavior
   5. negative symptoms (see text for description)

B. **Social/occupational dysfunction:**
   For a significant portion of the time sin disturbance, one or more major areas o as work, interpersonal relations, or self- below the level achieved prior to the o was in childhood or adolescence, failur expected level of interpersonal, acade tional achievement).

C. **Duration:**
   Continuous signs of the disturbance p months. This must include at least 1 m (or less if successfully treated) that me

D. **Exclusions:**
   The symptoms cannot be due to other ders, drugs or alcohol, or a general me

Note: Only one Criterion A symptom is required if or hallucinations consist of a voice conducting a c person's behavior or thoughts, or two voices conv

Source: Reprinted with permission from the *Diag Manual of Mental Disorders, Text Revision,* copyrigh Psychiatric Association.

Diagnostic Criteria boxes define mental health illnesses for the reader.

BOX 8-2	

Reality Check: Clients with Schizophrenia

What people with schizophrenia have said:

- "At first it just sounds like wind in the leaves, rustling and soft. Then it becomes voices, whispering then talking louder. If I concentrate I can hear them more clearly."
- "I am just here [psychiatric hospital] because I had a fight with my brother. There is nothing wrong with me. You are the one who is crazy!"
- "The witches are in my head and after me all the time. I'm never safe. It's OK, they won't get you."
- "An android named Bob told me that if I jumped off the bridge I could fly."
- "I am just afraid. I'm always afraid."
- "I talk to the animals, you know, through their bellies. I am a vegetarian. I could never hurt them. I know what it is like to be eaten alive."
- "I must work day and night to keep these demons at bay! It is exhausting."
- "If I listen to heavy metal [music] really loud through the headphones, it drowns out the voices sometimes."
- "The machine in my body was hungry, so I just injected some peanut butter and mayonnaise to feed him. That's how I got this" [indicating large necrotic arm wound].
- "The voices are talking to me all the time. They comment on everything, like 'You want that but it's too good for you, or you are so bad, or that man is going to kill you.'"
- "Sometimes I wonder: Is that a real memory, or not? Is that person trying to kill me? Will my thoughts hurt someone? My mother killed herself. I know why."
- "Please. Please, can you or one of your kind tell me what happened to me? Why are my thoughts like this? The last time I saw you, you were blue. Now you're red. I know you're an alien. Please tell me what is wrong with me!"
- "I don't remember much about my hospitalization. I do remember being afraid, terrified. I also remember a few people trying to help me, saying that I would be OK. Their reassurance could last me for days. It didn't happen very often."
- "Before the new medication, I spent all of my adult life in the hospital. Now that I'm being discharged I have some new problems I had never considered before, like 'How do I have fun?' And 'How do I prepare food?' These are not such bad problems to have."

Reality Check boxes express the reality of mental health disorders in the clients own words.

---

clinical ALERT

It is not the event itself that determines the severity of the stress response for the client, but the significance the event has for the client that gives it its meaning. The nurse must assess the client for personal attitudes related to health issues and treat all clients according to their individual needs.

Clinical Alerts call the student's attention to clinical roles and responsibilities for heightened awareness, monitoring, and/or reporting.

Critical Self-Check. What process does the therapeutic nurse-client relationship resemble? (*Hint:* In the nurse-client relationship you start by assessing the client's needs, then move to setting goals with the client, planning interventions, working to reach the client's goals, and finally evaluating the outcomes.)

CASE EXAMPLE

A person with Posttraumatic Stress Disorder said: "I was raped when I was 25 years old. For a long time, I spoke about the rape as though it was something that happened to someone else. I was very aware that it had happened to me, but there was just no feeling.

"Then I started having flashbacks. They kind of came over me like a splash of water. I would be terrified. Suddenly I was reliving the rape. Every instant was startling. I wasn't aware of anything around me; I was in a bubble, just kind of floating. And it was scary; having a flashback can wring you out.

"The rape happened the week before Thanksgiving, and I can't believe the anxiety and fear I feel every year around the anniversary date. It's as though I've seen a werewolf. I can't relax, can't sleep, don't want to be with anyone. I wonder whether I'll ever be free of this terrible problem."

Critical Self Checks encourage readers to clarify their own values and beliefs, and to think critically about mental health nursing.

Case Examples give you insight into actual clients.

Nursing Care Checklists provide students with a ready-reference summary of important nursing interventions.

TABLE 9-1

Antidepressant Agents

CLASSIFICATION/DRUG	ACTION AND USE	NURSING RESPONSIBILITIES	CLIENT TEACHING
Selective serotonin reuptake inhibitors (SSRIs) Citalopram (Celexa) Escitalopram (Lexapro) Fluoxetine (Prozac) Fluvoxamine (Luvox) Paroxetine (Paxil) Sertraline (Zoloft)	SSRIs ↑ 5-HT by blocking 5-HT reuptake in the presynaptic neuron. ↑ s neurotransmission of 5-HT. Primarily used for depression, but also used for obsessive-compulsive disorder, panic disorder, social anxiety disorder, posttraumatic stress disorder (PTSD), generalized anxiety disorder, bulimia nervosa, and premenstrual dysphoric disorder.	Assess for SEs: sedation or agitation, headache, dizziness, tremors, sexual dysfunction (↓ libido, anorgasmia, erectile dysfunction, delayed ejaculation), GI effects (↓ appetite, nausea, diarrhea, constipation), dry mouth, bruising. 　These tend to be the first choice for treatment of depression in elderly, who require lower doses.	Some clients may experience relief of anxiety or insomnia early after starting therapy, but it usually takes 2–4 weeks for antidepressant effects. Most side effects go away with time.
Serotonin and norepinephrine reuptake inhibitors (SNRIs) Duloxetine (Cymbalta) Venlafaxine (Effexor)	SNRIs ↑ 5-HT, NE, and DA. They block 5-HT and NE reuptake pumps, ↑ ing their neurotransmission. They ↑ DA neurotransmission in frontal cortex, especially at higher doses. 　Primarily used to treat depression. Also used for stress urinary incontinence, chronic and neuropathic pain, anxiety disorders.	Assess for SEs: ↑ BP (dose dependent), insomnia, sedation, headache, nausea, decreased appetite, sweating, sexual dysfunction (↓ libido, impotence, abnormal orgasm), seizures (rare).	Therapeutic action takes 2–4 weeks. Most side effects go away with time. 　Client should have regular BP monitoring.
Norepinephrine and dopamine reuptake inhibitor (NDRI) Bupropion (Wellbutrin)	↑ s NE and DA, by blocking NE and DA reuptake, and increasing their neurotransmission. 　Primarily used for depression and nicotine addiction, also used for bipolar depression, ADHD, and sexual dysfunction caused by other meds.	Assess client for SEs: dry mouth, constipation, nausea, anorexia, sweating, tremor, insomnia, agitation, and headache. Rarely causes seizures (dose-related risk). Evaluate drug effectiveness.	Takes 2–4 weeks to achieve desired effects. 　Teach client about constipation prevention. Most side effects go away with time.

Pharmacology Tables reinforce selected common medications nurses will encounter in practice.

Learn to prioritize nursing actions and deliver safe, effective nursing care as part of the healthcare team!

Nursing Care is presented in the five-step nursing process format, but emphasizing the scope of practice for the LPN/LVN. Rationales after each nursing intervention explain why the action is important and support evidence-based nursing process.

NURSING PROCESS CARE PLAN
Client with Neuroleptic Malignant Syndrome

You are a staff nurse on a medical-surgical unit where Roberto Valdez, a 56-year-old client, has been admitted with possible kidney stones (urolithiasis) and dehydration. You notice on his chart that he also has been diagnosed with schizophrenia and has been taking fluphenazine for 3 weeks.

Assessment. Mr. Valdez expresses anxiety about this hospitalization and his treatment. He is having severe pain all over his body and just wants medication for the pain. He loses his train of thought easily and sometimes does not respond to your questions. You assess that Mr. Valdez has an unstable BP from 100/50 to 180/104 and an irregular pulse of 120. His oral temperature is 103°F. He is very diaphoretic. He is stiff and pale. Based on your knowledge of fluphenazine and other antipsychotic medications, you realize that Mr. Valdez might be experiencing neuroleptic malignant syndrome brought on by the medical crisis of renal colic while trying to pass a kidney stone and the dehydration. You immediately notify the RN charge nurse who contacts the physician.

Nursing Process Care Plans illustrate nursing care in "real-life" scenarios and reinforce the progression from goals to interventions to evaluation.

Diagnosis. Several nursing diagnoses were identified for Mr. Valdez:

- Risk for Injury R/T adverse reaction to antipsychotic medication
- Pain R/T medication reaction and kidney stone
- Anxiety R/T not understanding his condition and treatment and possible reaction to antipsychotic medication

Expected Outcomes

- Client's physical condition will stabilize as evidenced by vital signs within normal limits within 24 hours.
- Client will state pain at a level of 3 or lower (on a 1–10 scale) within 1 hour of administration of pain medication.
- Client will state that he feels less anxious about his physical condition and treatment within 24 hours.

Planning and Implementation

- Monitor vital signs every 15 minutes.
- Monitor intake and output.
- Monitor mental status every 15 minutes.
- Prepare to transfer client to ICU.
- Explain all procedures to client simply and calmly.
- Discontinue fluphenazine as ordered by physician.
- Administer medication to reduce fever.

Evaluation. The client was transferred to the ICU. He was started on IV therapy and his vital signs stabilized. Within 24 hours, his BP returned to 130/86 and his pulse was 90 and regular. Temperature was 99° orally. Blood tests indicated no muscle or kidney damage. Mr. Valdez regained his alert mental sta[...] hallucinations or delusions. The phy[...] a psychiatric consultation to determ[...] chotic medication should replace th[...] was controlled with morphine, and [...] kidney stone. He stated a reduction[...] expressed his thanks to the staff.

Critical Thinking in the Nursing Process

1. What could have been the result if you had attributed the client's signs and symptoms to possible kidney stones and had not considered other options?
2. What other antipsychotic medications could precipitate NMS? Which category of antipsychotic medications is least likely to result in this syndrome?
3. What symptoms will you expect to occur as the fluphenazine is eliminated from his system?

Note: Discussion of Critical Thinking questions appears in Appendix I.

Critical Thinking questions allow you to apply your new knowledge to a specific client.

Comprehensive reviews at the end of the chapter...

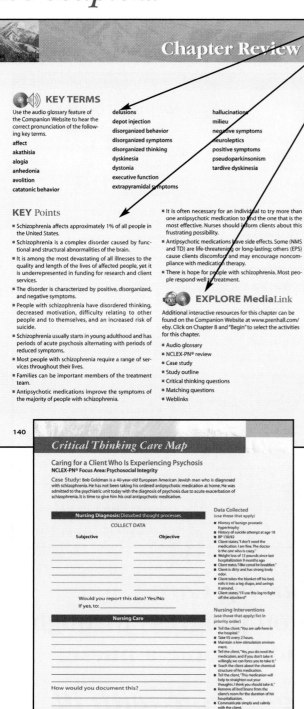

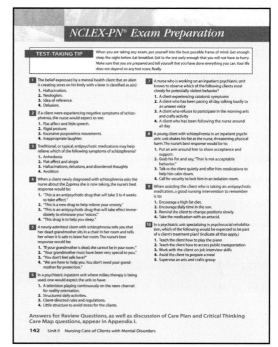

Key Terms list important new vocabulary

Key Points summarize need-to-know concepts from the chapter.

EXPLORE MediaLink encourages you to use the Companion Website for a multi-modal review, regardless of your learning style.

NCLEX-PN® Exam Preparation includes:
A Test-Taking Tip with a focused study hint.

- NCLEX-PN® style questions for review and test practice, with questions in both traditional and alternative formats. Answers are found in Appendix I.

Critical Thinking Care Map prepares you for success on NCLEX-PN®, in clinical, and on-the-job with a focused review of a client problem, including:
- NCLEX-PN® Focus Area
- Case Study
- Nursing Diagnosis
- Data Collection
- Reporting
- Nursing Care
- Documentation

Prepare for your career as an LPN/LVN...

After each unit in this book, you can use the **Learning About You!** pages as an opportunity to reflect on unit topics in terms of your own life experience and world view. This feature captures your interest and applies your learning to your own life.

Here are some activities you'll find for having fun and developing insight:

- Identifying your own personality traits
- Reviewing your mental health status
- Checking your coping mechanisms
- Looking at codependency tendencies
- Thinking about "strange" behavior
- Seeing where values play a part in your life
- Imagining the world of schizophrenia
- Practicing loose association
- Imagining your moods … intensified
- Identifying personality disorders
- Thinking about how you cope with anxiety
- Reviewing your developmental steps
- Considering your own self-concept

Learning About You!

CHAPTER 1 Understanding Mental Health and Mental Illness
Check out your own mental health status.

I feel good about myself.
☐ Yes ☐ No
I see things realistically.
☐ Yes ☐ No
I have satisfying personal relationships.
☐ Yes ☐ No
There is meaning in my life.
☐ Yes ☐ No
I am productive in my job and in school.
☐ Yes ☐ No
I enjoy opportunities where I can be creative.
☐ Yes ☐ No
I eat three well-balanced meals a day.
☐ Yes ☐ No
I feel that I am the only one responsible for my behavior.
☐ Yes ☐ No
I have a positive attitude most of the time.
☐ Yes ☐ No
I am flexible and adapt easily to change.
☐ Yes ☐ No
I sleep at least 6 hours every night.
☐ Yes ☐ No
I wake up feeling rested each morning.
☐ Yes ☐ No
I see conflict as a challenge and am not overwhelmed by it.
☐ Yes ☐ No

How did you do? Mostly yeses indicate you are in a relatively good state of mental health!

CHAPTER 2 Ethical and Legal Issues
Knowing that values and ethics intertwine to determine your behavior, think back over your week, and see where values clarification played a part in your response to different situations:

As a nursing student, I find that I value (*choosing*):
1.   2.
I was able to show how much my values meant to me this week by (*prizing*):
1.   2.
I demonstrated my values this week by (*acting*):
1.   2.

CHAPTER 3 Personality Theory
Decide on your own personality traits by checking the boxes below:

☐ Extrovert   ☐ Introvert
☐ Agreeable   ☐ Disagreeable
☐ Conscientious   ☐ Impulsive
☐ Emotionally stable   ☐ Emotionally unstable
☐ Open   ☐ Closed

What traits do you see in your friends?

Have you ever used a defense mechanism? Below are examples of some. Read the statement or situation, and decide which defense mechanism is being used.

Defense Mechanism
A. Suppression
B. Displacement
C. Compensation
D. Rationalization

Statement
1. "I didn't get an 'A' on my pharmacology paper because the instructor doesn't like me."
2. "I totally bombed at clinical today, but I just can't think about it now. I'll think about it tomorrow."
3. After being reprimanded by her Fundamentals instructor, the nursing student went home and yelled at her daughter, "Why is your room always so messy? I'm tired of picking up after you."
4. "I can't run as fast as my brother, so I'm joining the debate team instead of going out for track."

Answers to fun quiz
A (2)   B (3)   C (4)   D (1)

CHAPTER 4 Mentally Healthy Nursing
Check out your codependency tendencies with this questionnaire. (This is not an official research tool—just a fun exercise thought up by your authors.)

I have difficulty telling other people "no" when they ask me to do something for them.
☐ Yes ☐ No
I need everyone around me to like me.
☐ Yes ☐ No
I enjoy having my friends come to me to help them solve their problems.
☐ Yes ☐ No
I feel responsible for the feelings of those around me.
☐ Yes ☐ No

Chapter 7   Psychobiology and Psychopharmacology   **111**

Mental Health Nursing Care
will be a key resource as you progress through your nursing courses and become a nurse.

The nature of nursing—grow with it!

I dedicate this work to my family, especially to Monica and Kate.

■ *Linda Eby*

I dedicate this work to my husband, Herb, for his understanding, to Cindy, David, Cara, and Jana for their enthusiasm, and to my mother, Edith, an inspiration for my life.

■ *Nancy J. Brown*

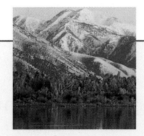

Preface

Mental Health Nursing Care was written to provide a broad fundamental knowledge base for LPN/LVN students that is interesting and engaging to read, and readily applicable to nursing practice. Our teaching philosophy is that learning is maximized when the teacher is enthusiastic about the subject; the material is presented in a clear and appealing style; and the concepts are relevant to real application. The learner must be willing to participate in the learning process. Learning is participative.

In this edition, we have added full color to make the book even more inviting, interesting, and reader friendly. The photographs are all clinically oriented and are included for the purpose of adding depth to the text. We have updated every chapter and changed the organization to improve the logical flow of information.

This book is written as psychosocial nursing is really practiced: with intelligence, empathy, caring, and based on evidence. It is above all practical, with strategies that students can actually use to promote the health, well-being, and empowerment of their clients.

The major curriculum concepts are:

- Mental health
- The biopsychosocial nature of mental disorders
- Insight development and mental health promotion for nursing students
- The nursing process (a part of which is critical thinking)
- Care of diverse clients (across ages, genders, and cultures)
- Client and nurse empowerment
- Collaborative care with other members of the healthcare team
- Psychosocial nursing as a component of general nursing practice, as well as in the psychiatric setting

The writing style is deliberately personal for the purpose of making this complicated and fascinating subject engaging and easy to understand. It is clear without oversimplification or disrespect to the subject or the student. The style, organization, and pedagogy are chosen with adult learning principles in mind.

We wrote this book with the knowledge that the majority of nurses do not practice in the mental health nursing specialty. Promoting mental health and working with clients with mental disorders and psychosocial issues are part of the nursing role in every practice setting. We teach students to practice psychosocial nursing with diverse clients in a variety of settings. We bring in case studies and quotes from clients in their own words to help students who do not have psychiatric nursing clinical opportunities to develop empathy for our clients. Photographs of clients add another dimension to help students see people who are affected.

The authors bring their enthusiasm and experience in teaching mental health nursing to this book. We teach the theory and practice of mental health nursing to diverse nursing students. The needs of students who speak English as a nonnative language, immigrant students, and other nontraditional students were considered in the writing of this book. Advocacy for people who have mental disorders and their families is an important aspect of the book as well. We are committed to mental health nursing education and to helping you teach your students.

Organization

UNIT I: *Foundations of Mental Health Nursing* provides a basis for understanding the fundamentals on which mental health nursing is built. The order of chapters in this unit has changed. We started this edition with the chapter on mental health and mental illness as a basis for the subsequent information. The stigma of mental illness remains as a societal factor that inhibits mental health care. Ethical and legal issues in mental health nursing follow. Personality theories are presented as the basis for the various therapeutic approaches to disorders of thinking, feeling, and behavior. Practical strategies for mental-health promotion are included.

This unit includes a chapter to encourage the mentally healthy practice of nursing. The critical care maps begin here as an interactive tool for students to practice the application of information presented in the chapter in a true-to-life case study. The nurse-client relationship is presented as the foundation of nursing practice. The importance of client advocacy is emphasized. The biological basis for mental disorders is discussed. Psychopharmacology is given its rightful place as a major cornerstone of mental health nursing, but not the only cornerstone.

UNIT II: *Nursing Care of Clients with Mental Disorders* covers specific biological and clinical information about the major mental illnesses included in the *DSM-IV-TR*. Client behavior, thoughts, and feelings are the basis for mental health nursing goals and interventions. The nursing process provides the format for nursing practice. Medication management, collaboration with other health professionals, and client empowerment are integral parts.

UNIT III: *Nursing Care of Clients with Disorders Related to Development* includes disorders of children, adolescents, and the elderly. Dementia and cognitive disorders are covered extensively because of their importance in nursing practice. Eating disorders are also presented here.

UNIT IV: *Special Topics in Mental Health Nursing* includes the timely topics of violence and abuse, as well as psychosocial issues for general client care. The final chapter takes psychosocial nursing to every client and presents realistic strategies for managing the care of "difficult" clients, clients with special mental health needs, and clients with spiritual needs in general nursing practice.

To the Student

This book was created to be a realistic and interesting resource for you as you learn about the fascinating subject of Mental Health Nursing. Whether you want to specialize in psychiatric nursing or you never see the inside of a psychiatric hospital, you can use the information you learn here to help clients with mental disorders and people with psychosocial needs in any nursing environment.

Keep an open mind, and enjoy the process. Before you read this book, think about what you already know about mentally ill people. Probably some of what you think you know is wrong (there are lots of misconceptions). We think you will learn some things that will help you see people with mental illnesses in a more positive and sympathetic light. Most important, we think you will learn some interesting things that you can use to improve people's lives, including your own.

Refer to the visual walkthrough at the beginning of this book for an overview of the features of the book.

Acknowledgments

First we want to acknowledge the people for whom this book was written: nursing students. We are humbled by the opportunity to help students gain knowledge and shape their attitudes about mental health nursing and their identity as nurses. We have a profound respect for people who live with mental disorders and hope this book will encourage the development of caring and competent nurses to empower and advocate for them.

Producing a textbook is like nursing: it requires teamwork. We extend our sincere gratitude and respect to the group of people who made this book possible. The original coach of our team was Barbara Krawiec, who inspired this project and brought us together. Barbara was followed by Kelly Trakalo, who possesses a contagious enthusiasm for practical/vocational nursing education. Kelly has been instrumental in developing the series of books for practical/technical nursing students, another team to which we are proud to belong. We are grateful for and indebted to the work of Susan Geraghty, our developmental editor, who has worked so closely with us in developing this book into a cohesive and articulate whole. She has gone above and beyond what we expected, working with us days, evenings, and weekends, and working around illnesses, weddings, and new grandbabies! Susan kept us on task as much as possible (which was something like herding cats).

We are thankful for Yagnesh Jani, the production editor, who has given us assistance with technical matters, such as providing us with access to a broad gallery of useful photographs.

Trish Finley, Production Editor for GGS Book Services, materialized our vision onto paper (this is a profound experience for us). Finally, we would like to thank all at Prentice Hall who flew us to Upper Saddle River, New Jersey, to visit the company, meet the staff, and participate in an unscheduled fire drill! We appreciate the time spent in explaining book production to us and giving us the impetus to begin this second edition and discuss ideas for future writing endeavors. Everyone was welcoming and encouraging!

Thanks to all of you!

Peace,

Linda Eby and Nancy J. Brown

About the Authors

Linda Eby, RN, MN

Linda Eby received her Bachelor of Science in Nursing and Master of Nursing degrees from the Oregon Health and Science University. Her work experience includes being a staff nurse and nurse manager in critical care, a home health/hospice nurse, case manager, Clinical Nurse Specialist in clinical genetics, and a psychiatric–mental health nurse. She has consulted and taught workshops on the topics of promoting student success and reducing culture bias in nursing education.

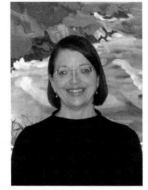

Linda currently teaches Psychiatric–Mental Health Nursing theory and clinical courses at Portland Community College. She is also Coordinator of the Nursing Student Success Program. This program promotes the success of nursing students who speak English as a nonnative language, immigrant students, students of color, academically disadvantaged students, and nontraditional students of nursing. Her greatest career accomplishment is contributing to the success of these inspiring students.

She is Secretary of AFT-Oregon, state affiliate of the American Federation of Teachers, and Vice President of the Portland Community College Faculty Federation. She has twin daughters, Kristine, who was recently married to Jens Schrader and is continuing her studies at Portland State University, and Monica, an artist, art teacher, and art student at Marylhurst University (she really likes art). Linda is a nature and arts and crafts enthusiast and a good friend to her dogs, Wendu and Charlie.

Nancy J. Brown, RN, MSN

Nancy J. Brown received her Bachelor of Science in Nursing from the University of Missouri and a Master of Science in Nursing from the University of Colorado. She has been actively involved in teaching practical nursing for the past 15 years. Other teaching experiences include staff development positions in long-term care and state institutions for 9 years, where she worked closely with LPNs in practice. Nancy had been involved in nursing administration as a Director of Nursing prior to going into nursing education. She received the "Teacher of the Year" award in 1998 from San Juan Basin Technical School later

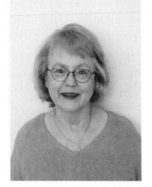

San Juan Basin Technical College. Nancy resigned from her administrative position at the school in 2005 to assume more family responsibilities. She remained as adjunct faculty, teaching mental health, geriatrics, leadership and management, and pharmacology to the part-time practical nursing students. In addition to teaching practical nursing, Nancy also coordinated and taught within the Certified Nursing Assistant program, creating an advanced level of certified nursing assistant that provided CNAs with more behavior management techniques for clients with dementia and mental health problems. Nancy has recently relocated to the state of Nebraska where her goal is to once again become involved in Practical Nursing and nursing assistant education. In her spare time, Nancy writes and performs puppet plays at her church. She has four children, Cindy, David, Cara, and Jana, who have presented her with eight grandchildren. Her husband, Herb, is retired and is a great support.

Contributor

Instructor Manual and PowerPoint Slide Contributor

Debra S. McKinney, MSN, MBA/HCM, BSN, RN
Nursing Education Consultant
Warrenton, VA

Reviewer Panel

Michele Blash, RN, MSN
Nursing Instructor
Hagerstown Community College
Hagerstown, MD

Jacquelyn Bryant, RN Med, MSN, FNP
Nursing Instructor
Lanier Technical College
Oakwood, GA

Kimberly S. Burgess, MSN, RN, APN, FNP
Nursing Instructor
Lake Land College
Mattoon, IL

Emily Cannon, RN, MSN
Associate Professor of Nursing
Ivy Tech Community College
Terre Haute, IN

Catherine M. Griswold, RN, MSN, CLNC
Assistant Professor of Nursing
Community College of Baltimore County
Baltimore, MD

Becki L. Quick, RN, BA, MAC
Director of Nursing, VN Program
Maric College San Diego
San Diego, CA

Sandra Monroe, RN, MSN
Department Chair, Practical Nursing
Fayetteville Technical Community College
Fayetteville, NC

Johnny J. Montemayor, RN, BSN
Nursing Instructor
McLennan Community College
Waco, TX

Kathleen L. Slyh, RN, MSN
Nursing Instructor
Technical College of the Lowcountry
Beaufort, SC

Jackie Sublett, MSN, RN
Director of Nursing
Frank Phillips College
Borger, TX

Nancy Turner, RN, C, MSN
Associate Professor of Nursing
West Kentucky Community and Technical College
Paducah, KY

Patricia C. Williams, RN, MSN
Associate Professor
Hagerstown Community College
Hagerstown, MD

Bobbie Williamson, BSN, RN
Nursing Instructor
San Jacinto College
Houston, TX

Contents

Appendices

Foundations of Mental Health Nursing

UNIT I

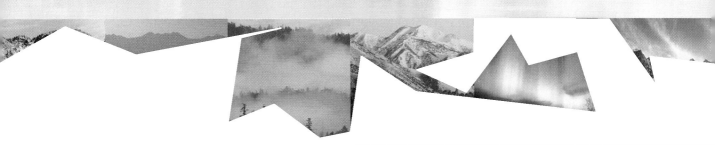

Chapter 1

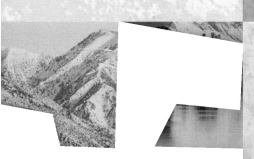

Understanding Mental Health and Mental Illness

BRIEF Outline

Mental Health

Mental Disorders

Stigma of Mental Illness

Historical Perspectives

Nurses' Role in Mental Health Promotion

Vulnerability of the Mentally Ill

LEARNING Outcomes

After completing this chapter, you will be able to:

1. Define mental health and mental illness in your own words.
2. Discuss the stigma of mental illness in our society.
3. Acknowledge the vulnerability of people with mental illnesses.

For many reasons, mental health and mental illness are difficult to define. People are unique and unpredictable. Each person has different life experiences. Acceptable behavior is not universal. Definitions of mental health and mental illness can change as culture and society change their attitudes and expectations.

Mental Health

There is no universally accepted definition of mental health. In fact, there are better standards for defining mental illness than there are for mental health. However, there is some agreement about what aspects of thinking, feeling, and behaving are considered healthy or unhealthy.

In general, there are seven important characteristics of mental health. Mentally healthy people:

- Interpret reality accurately
- Have a healthy self-concept
- Are able to relate to others
- Achieve a sense of meaning in life
- Demonstrate creativity/productivity
- Have control over their behavior
- Adapt to change and conflict

The ability to accurately determine **reality** (what really is or exists) is a basic component of mental health. It includes the abilities to differentiate between what really is and what might be, and to reasonably predict the consequences of one's behavior. (If I jump off the roof, I could be hurt.)

A healthy self-concept includes first a realistic appraisal of the self (abilities, function, and appearance). In addition, to have a healthy self-concept, people must accept themselves as they are. Figure 1-1 ■ shows a girl who challenges herself, is successful at sports at the level of her ability, and accepts herself as she is, including the fact that she has cerebral palsy. **Insight,** or self-understanding, is an important part of relating to oneself, because it allows people to see their own motivations or reasons behind their feelings and behavior. A person who lacks insight might refuse to take a medication because it causes his mouth to be dry. With insight, a person could decide that even though he does not like to take the medication, it helps his mental illness, so he will take it. Insight is critical for positive decision making about health issues. Without it people often do not realize that they have an illness.

Human beings are creatures that thrive best when they are with others. Love is the most important human emotion. Normal human development is not possible in

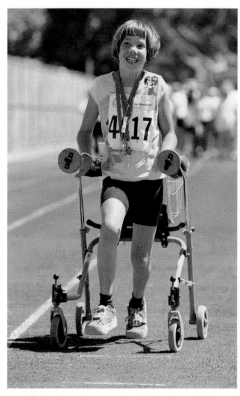

Figure 1-1. ■ A person with a healthy self-concept accepts herself as she is, including the fact that she has cerebral palsy. *Source:* PhotoEdit Inc.

isolation. People must be able to interact with and **relate to others** in order to flourish. Without the ability to relate to others in a satisfying way, a person cannot be healthy.

Humans seek reasons and **meaning in life**. Many people find a sense of meaning in the world through religion. Many others find meaning in nature, philosophy, ethics, or service to others (Figure 1-2 ■). This uniquely human sense of spirituality is an important part of what it means to be a person. A fully mentally healthy person will have a sense of what is important in life and what gives life meaning.

A person does not have to be an artist to be **creative**. Healthy people can solve problems creatively. They can interpret experiences abstractly. Some people think **concretely**, meaning literally or without creativity. For example, a concrete thinker may say that the proverb "A stitch in time saves nine" means that if you sew something up in time you will save nine stitches. A more abstract thinker might say it means that if you put a little bit of work into solving a problem early, you will save a lot of trouble in the long term. Another aspect of healthy creativity is a sense of productivity or contribution.

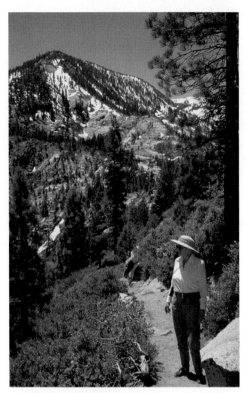

Figure 1-2. ■ Finding a sense of meaning in life is part of mental health. This hiker finds meaning in nature. *Source:* Omni-Photo Communications, Inc.

Healthy people want to feel like they make a difference to others or to the world.

Control of behavior means that mentally healthy people can balance conflicts with their instincts, conscience, and reality before they act. Healthy people do not act out violently just because they are frustrated in the moment, nor would they steal something just because it would be nice to have it. Mentally healthy people can delay gratification. They can act in a way that helps someone else, even if it is difficult for them. The healthiest people have the integrity to act on their values.

Adaptability is critical to success as a person. The one consistent thing around us is that everything is changing. Healthy people can compromise, plan, and be flexible. They can manage conflict successfully. Learning to change is not easy, but if people are healthy, they will manage it.

Mental health is really a range of behavior, thoughts, and feelings; it is a relative state instead of an absolute state. Nobody is at the ultimate level of health in every area all the time. Individuals can have anywhere from minimal to maximal mentally healthy behavior, whether they are diagnosed with a mental disorder or not. Just as all people are

developing throughout their lives, **all people have the potential for growth toward greater mental health**. Because nurses treat clients holistically, an important aspect of nursing is to promote the mental health of clients.

Critical Self-Check. Think of people you know who have no physical illnesses. Are some of them healthier than others? What makes them healthier? Does the same idea hold true for mental health?

People with chronic physical illnesses such as diabetes or heart disease can still be healthy (within the limits of their abilities) if they choose healthy behaviors and participate in treatment. Just as a person with a physical illness can be relatively healthy, people with mental illnesses can take their medications, choose healthy behaviors within their abilities, and be healthier also.

Mental Disorders

Mental disorders are illnesses with symptoms related to thinking, feeling, or behavior. They are due to genetic, biological, social, chemical, or psychological influences. These illnesses result in impairment of functioning and other symptoms.

The meaning of an illness to an individual is culturally related. Even the way a client describes the disorder is affected by culture. Box 1-1 ■ describes disorders as they are seen in the light of the client's culture.

Much research has been done on mental disorders. The definitive source for psychiatrists and other physicians to use for the diagnostic criteria for mental disorders is the *Diagnostic and Statistical Manual of Mental Disorders (DSM)*. It is revised as new knowledge is available (American Psychiatric Association, 2000). This book was written by international experts who created a standard terminology for mental disorders and a set of criteria for diagnosing them. Because of this, a physician in British Columbia and another in Florida will use the same list of criteria to diagnose their clients, and will call their disorders by the same names. This standardization is critical as a foundation for research and treatment of mental disorders.

The authors of the *DSM* have made a point to say that they are attempting to classify disorders, not people (American Psychiatric Association, 2000). People are not defined by their illnesses. A person with a disease is just that, a person first, not a diabetic, or a schizophrenic, or "the appendectomy in room 213."

The format for *DSM* diagnostic labeling is more thorough than traditional medical diagnosis because it includes psychiatric and physical disorders, current stressors in the

BOX 1-1	CULTURAL PULSE POINTS

This is the first in a series of Cultural Pulse Points boxes (look for one in each chapter) designed to prepare you to provide culturally competent nursing care.

Culture Assessment and Culture-Bound Syndromes

The functions of a culture include deciding who is sick, indicating how sick people should behave, and prescribing how they are treated. As a nurse, you will probably work with people from a variety of cultures. These people may describe their feelings or symptoms in ways that are unfamiliar to you. It will be important to consider the client's culture as an integral part of assessment. Culture assessment should include the following issues.

Cultural Identity of the Individual

European American is the dominant culture in the United States. Many clients are Americans but identify closely with the culture of their parents or their ethnic group (African American, Vietnamese American, Mexican American, etc.). Some clients who live in the United States are immigrants from other countries and have strong ties to their native culture. For example, they may consider themselves British, Nigerian, or Russian. Some indicators of cultural identity are clients' language, religion, whether most of their friends are members of the same cultural or ethnic group, the length of time in this country, and whether they went to school here (especially high school).

Cultural Factors Related to the Environment and Client Functioning

This area includes the *cultural meaning of stressors the client is experiencing*; for example, in a culture where mental illness has a severe stigma that extends to the entire family (some people may not want to marry into such a family), a client may feel a burden of guilt for affecting the whole family. The *availability of social support* is a culturally related issue, as shown in cultural groups that have little contact with their extended families after they marry, so they cannot expect that someone would be able to help them at home. *Religion* plays a role in the client's hospital experience when the client's religious needs (such as special dietary requirements, the need for certain religious practitioners, or specific circumstances for prayer) are not understood by the staff. Some cultural groups have *kin networks* (extended family and significant others that may be relied on for transportation, child care, financial support, or care for the sick) that can support the client's functioning.

Cultural Explanations of the Client's Illness

Europeans and North Americans have similar attitudes about mental illness, with local and individual variations. The *Diagnostic and Statistical Manual of Mental Disorders (DSM)* is based on these Western cultures. The nurse may encounter clients whose behavior is considered by their cultural group to be abnormal and troubling but is not listed in the *DSM*. These culture-bound syndromes are locality-specific patterns of abnormal behavior. Some examples from different cultures include:

- **Amok** is a dissociative episode. (The client's consciousness, memory, identity, and perception of the environment become disassociated with one another.) The client may have a period of brooding and feel persecuted, followed by violent behavior directed at people or objects. The client may not remember the episode and will return to usual functioning afterward. Amok was originally described in Malaysia. A similar condition with different names is found in the Philippines, Laos, Polynesia, and among the Navajo.

- **Bilis, colera, or muina** results in symptoms of acute nervous tension, headache, trembling, screaming, stomach disturbances, and possibly loss of consciousness caused by strongly experienced anger or rage. Anger is viewed among many Latino groups as a very powerful emotion that can have direct effects on the body. The major effect of anger is to disrupt the body's balance (between the material and spiritual or hot and cold aspects of a person).

- **Mal de ojo** is a concept widely found in Mediterranean cultures and elsewhere in the world. This Spanish phrase means "evil eye" in English. Symptoms include restless sleep, crying without apparent cause, diarrhea, vomiting, and a fever in a child or infant. Children are at higher risk, but adults (especially females) can have the condition.

- **Nervios** is an expression of distress among Latinos in the United States and Latin America. Several other ethnic groups have similar ideas about "nerves." It refers to a general state of vulnerability to stressful life experiences and to a range of symptoms of emotional distress brought on by difficult circumstances. Common symptoms include headaches that the client may describe as "brain aches," irritability, difficulty sleeping, easy tearfulness, stomach disturbances, trembling, and difficulty concentrating. Nervios tends to be an ongoing problem that has a wide range of expressions.

- **Falling out or blacking out** are episodes that occur mostly in the southern United States and in Caribbean groups. The client suddenly collapses, sometimes without warning, sometimes preceded by feelings of dizziness or "swimming" in the head. Clients report being unable to see, even though their eyes are open. They can hear what is happening around them, but are unable to move.

Source: Reprinted with permission from the *Diagnostic and Statistical Manual of Mental Disorders, Text Revision* © 2000. American Psychiatric Association.

person's life, and an assessment of how much their general functioning is affected. This type of thorough diagnostic process gives a much clearer picture of a whole person than just a diagnostic label such as "depression." The following is the *DSM*'s five-axis diagnosis system:

Axis I: Clinical Psychiatric Disorders

Axis II: Personality Disorders or Mental Retardation

Axis III: General Medical Conditions

Axis IV: Psychosocial and Environmental Problems

Axis V: Global Assessment of Functioning (see this assessment tool in Appendix I, "Mental Health Assessment Forms")

CASE EXAMPLE

A 50-year-old male client with a history of major depressive disorder was admitted to the hospital after he told his psychiatrist he was thinking of hurting himself. His wife left him 2 months ago and he lost his job about a month after because he was too depressed to go to work regularly. He has hypertension. He has no close friends. Our client's multiaxial diagnostic statement would be:

Axis I: Major Depressive Disorder

Axis II: None

Axis III: Hypertension

Axis IV: Separation from spouse, loss of job

Axis V: 50 (serious symptoms) on Global Assessment of Functioning Scale

Although nurses do not make these diagnoses, it is important for nurses to understand them. Nurses are part of the multidisciplinary treatment team that plans and provides care for the client. The client's mental and physical diseases, life stressors, and the effects on the person's ability to function are valuable data for planning client care.

Physicians look at mental disorders in terms of disease processes and medical management. Nurses concentrate more on how people are affected by these disorders. Nurses focus on clients' *response* to illnesses, both physical and mental. Look at the list of nursing diagnoses in Appendix II, "NANDA-Approved Nursing Diagnoses." Many of them diagnose psychosocial problems.

Mental disorders are a major problem for people all over the world. The incidence of mental disorders is often underestimated. One reason for this is probably that mental disorders are not recognized for the severe impact they have. In 1996, the Global Burden of Disease Study showed that mental illnesses make up 5 of the 15 leading

---

BOX 1-2

Five Most Common Mental Disorders in the World

- Major depressive disorder
- Alcohol abuse
- Schizophrenia
- Self-inflicted injuries
- Bipolar disorder

---

causes of disability in developed countries. Box 1-2 ■ lists the five most common mental disorders in the world.

Major depressive disorder is the leading cause of disability in developed countries. In the United States, almost half of all people will have a psychiatric or substance abuse disorder at some time in their lives (National Institute of Mental Health, 2006). Box 1-3 ■ provides more details about the incidence of mental illness in the United States.

BOX 1-3

Key Facts About the Incidence of Mental Illness in the United States

- In any given year, approximately 26.2% of the adult population (about 1 in every 4 adults) will be affected by a mental disorder.
- Mental illness is the leading cause of disability in the United States and Canada for ages 15–44.
- About 20% of children under age 18 have a mental illness severe enough to require treatment.
- 6% of Americans have a substance use disorder; 10.3 million of these people suffer from alcoholism.
- One-fourth of the nation's 700,000 homeless people have severe mental illnesses.
- At least two-thirds of the elderly in nursing homes have a mental disorder, such as major depressive illness.
- More than 25% of jail inmates have a mental disorder.
- Eleven out of every 100,000 people in the United States died by suicide in 2002. More than 90% of people who kill themselves have a mental or substance abuse disorder.
- The incidence of Alzheimer's disease (AD) has doubled since 1980. One in 10 people over 65 and 1 in 2 people over 85 have AD.
- Most private medical insurance either does not cover mental illness treatment or covers it at a lower level than general medical illness.

Source: Data from National Institute of Mental Health online at www.nimh.nih.gov/healthinformation/ (accessed 7/30/06) and Substance Abuse and Mental Health Services Administration, National Mental Health Information Center online at www.mentalhealth.samhsa.gov/cmhs/Homelessness/ (accessed 7/30/06).

Critical Self-Check. If a friend asked you "Do you have heart disease?" or "Are you mentally ill?" would you feel differently about the two questions? Why?

Stigma of Mental Illness

Try to list all the terms you have heard referring to people with mental illness. *Crazy, nuts, bonkers, one-brick-short-of-a-full-load, wacko, goofy,* and *mental* are a few. Can you list others? What do all these terms have in common? They are all negative, insulting, and demeaning. When we talk about physical illnesses, we do not use such insulting terms. We would never call a person with diabetes an "insulin junkie" or a "sugar fool." These labels are inaccurate, inappropriate, and unkind.

Simply talking about mental illness often causes people to laugh nervously because mental illness has a **stigma,** or "mark of disgrace," in our culture. It is very common for people to have negative attitudes that devalue people with mental illnesses.

People can feel so ashamed of having a mental illness that they refuse to seek treatment. People running for political office have dropped out of politics when it became known that they had been treated for mental illness. Even physicians sometimes hesitate to give their clients the diagnosis of a mental disorder for fear that the clients will be "labeled" and treated badly as a result.

It is true that people with mental disorders have symptoms and impairments in their functioning. However, these disorders are treatable. Affected people can be and are often successful at being politicians (including heads of state), artists, journalists, police officers, teachers (maybe your teacher), physicians, clergy, bus drivers, nurses, and nursing students. The stigma against the mentally ill is certainly not warranted. As client advocates, nurses should stop using negative labels about the mentally ill and discourage others from using them. They should educate the public that mental illness should be treated in the same way as physical illness. Nurses must avoid the tendency to explain mental illness according to their own fears and guesses. Nurses can take the lead by basing their practice on evidence, not assumptions or stereotypes.

Historical Perspectives

Mental illness came before psychiatrists and mental health nurses. In the earliest of recorded times, mental illness was thought to be due to supernatural forces. Mentally ill people were treated as though they were affected by either demons or divine influences.

In his "theory of disease" Hippocrates (460–375 B.C.) described the body "humors": blood, phlegm, yellow bile, and black bile. He believed that melancholia (depression) was caused by an excess of black bile. He also thought that bloodletting could relieve this excess (Frisch & Frisch, 2006).

In Europe in the Middle Ages and during the Renaissance (when art and science, but not treatment for the mentally ill, flourished) it was thought that people with mental illness were affected by the moon (the term *lunatic* comes from the Latin word for moon). Affected people were believed to be evil, witches, or heretics. They were feared, confined to institutions where they were treated as criminals, and punished for their behaviors. Mentally ill people were treated badly, restrained, beaten, and poorly fed and clothed (Frisch & Frisch, 2006).

In the 18th century, the mentally ill were still locked up in prisons where the employees were not trained and were more interested in punishment than treatment. A period of enlightenment slowly started to dawn on the treatment of the mentally ill in the 1790s. French physician Phillippe Pinel started "moral treatment" of the mentally ill. He released people from their chains and took a psychological treatment approach. He ordered that the basic needs for food and clothing of people with mental disorders be met. He studied them and their behavior, trying to understand their abnormal thinking. William Tukes applied the same ideas in England. He established the concept of the *asylum,* which was to be a safe haven for people who had been whipped, beaten, and starved because they were mentally ill. The Quakers (Friends) in the United States applied the tenets of the Quaker faith to the care of mentally ill people. They believed that treating people with kindness in a pleasant environment could bring recovery (Carson, 2000). The Quaker philosophy formed the foundation for *milieu therapy* (in which the environment is considered part of the therapy), which is still used today.

In the early 19th century, schoolteacher Dorothea Dix became aware of the horrible conditions of the mentally ill in the United States when she volunteered to teach Sunday school at the East Cambridge jail in Massachusetts. Figures 1-3 ■ and 1-4 ■ show devices used during this period to restrain people with mental disorders. She found the mentally ill and criminals crowded together in unheated cells. She spoke to legislatures and to community leaders. She crusaded for years to obtain

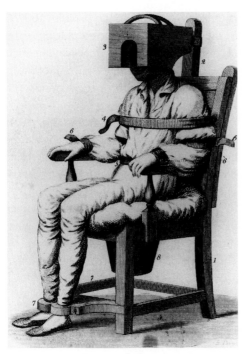

Figure 1-3. ■ The "tranquilizing chair" was used to control people with mental disorders in the 19th century. *Source:* National Library of Medicine.

facilities for treatment of the mentally ill. Her efforts eventually resulted in the establishment of hospitals in the United States, Canada, Scotland, and Japan (Carson, 2000).

Well into the 1800s, people who worked in the asylums had no training. It became clear that the new therapeutic model required caregivers who had training, compassion, and a willingness to care for others. In 1882 the McLean Asylum in Somerville, Massachusetts, opened the first training school in the world for mental health nurses. The plan was to "medicalize the care of the insane." They called their inmates "patients" and the attendants "nurses" (Frisch & Frisch, 2006). Also around the end of the 19th century, the Bellevue Training School in New York and the Connecticut Training School opened. They are important because they used the Nightingale model, in which nurses were educated by nurses, not by physicians.

In the 20th century mental health nursing made progress. In 1913 the Johns Hopkins Hospital School, under the leadership of Effie J. Taylor, started to include mental health nursing in the education of general nurses. This was the first time a hospital program offered mental health nursing to all of its students. Taylor's goal was to provide a standard knowledge base for all nurses so there would not be an artificial division of the mind and the body (Frisch & Frisch, 2006). This idea is the foundation of holistic nursing.

In the 1930s **somatic therapies** (physical therapies) were becoming popular. These therapies included deep sleep (coma) therapy, insulin shock, and electroshock therapy.

In 1946, the United States Congress passed the National Mental Health Act, establishing the National Institute of Mental Health (NIMH). This act provided federal funding for research and education in all areas of psychiatric care. Graduate education programs for mental health nurse specialists were established as a result of this act.

A revolution in psychiatric care occurred in the 1950s with the invention of **psychotropic drugs** (drugs that treat mental illness). Chlorpromazine (Thorazine) and lithium were the first to be widely used. Over the next decade, drugs were developed to treat anxiety and depression. For the first time there was an effective

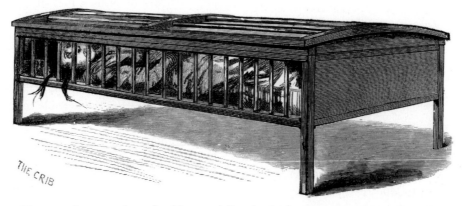

Figure 1-4. ■ "The crib" was used to control people with mental disorders in the 19th century. *Source:* Stock Montage, Inc./Historical Pictures Collection.

treatment for **psychosis** (loss of realistic thinking) for many people. People were discharged from psychiatric hospitals.

Deinstitutionalization of clients began in the 1950s. In this movement, people were discharged from psychiatric institutions and then the institutions were closed. Approximately 92% of the people who would have been living in public psychiatric hospitals in 1955 were not there in 1994 (Torrey, 1997). Two ideas were behind this movement:

1. People should be treated in the least restrictive environment possible.
2. It is cheaper to treat people in the community than in a state hospital.

Unfortunately, the result of this giant social experiment is that 2.2 million severely mentally ill people in the United States do not receive any psychiatric treatment. Community treatment needs are not being met. Many people are homeless, "where the 'least restrictive setting' turns out to be a cardboard box, a jail cell, or a terror-filled existence plagued by both real and imaginary enemies" (Torrey, 1997, p. 11). The deinstitutionalization experiment has been a failure.

Mentally ill people in the United States still suffer from the stigma of mental illness. There is housing discrimination and lack of insurance coverage due to insurance discrimination. Mental illness is often not covered as well as physical illness by medical insurance.

However, there still is hope. The 1990s were declared to be "the decade of the brain." Research developed new diagnostic studies and new drugs for mental illnesses. The most effective tools in history for the treatment of mental illnesses are currently available. Much more is known about the causes and treatments for mental disorders than ever before. The U.S. Department of Health and Human Services has made a list of goals for the people of the United States by the year 2010. Box 1-4 ■ lists the mental health objectives.

Nurses' Role in Mental Health Promotion

The evidence is clear: mental illness is a big problem. Many people are affected and the quality and length of their lives are diminished. What can nurses do? Box 1-5 ■ lists ways in which nurses can make a difference.

We will cover treatment and rehabilitation and recovery from mental illness in later chapters. The first step in

---

BOX 1-4

Healthy People 2010 Mental Health Objectives

- Reduce suicides to no more than 6 per 100,000 people
- Reduce the incidence of injurious suicide attempts by adolescents ages 14–17
- Reduce the proportion of homeless adults who have serious mental illness
- Increase the proportion of persons with serious mental illnesses who are employed to 51%
- Reduce the relapse rate for persons with eating disorders, including anorexia nervosa and bulimia nervosa
- Increase the number of persons seen in primary health care who receive mental health screening and assessment
- Increase the proportion of children and adults with mental health problems who receive treatment
- Increase the proportion of juvenile justice facilities that screen new admissions for mental health problems
- Increase the population of persons with concurrent substance abuse problems and mental disorders who receive treatment for both disorders
- Increase the proportion of local governments with community-based jail diversion programs for adults with serious mental illness
- Increase the number of states to 30 that track consumers' satisfaction with the mental health services they receive
- Increase the number of states with an operational mental health plan that addresses cultural competence, mental health crisis intervention, ongoing screening, and treatment for elderly persons

Source: Healthy People 2010: National Health Promotion and Disease Prevention Objectives. U.S. Department of Health and Human Services. © 2000. Washington, D.C.: Author.

---

prevention of mental illness is to recognize what the risk factors are and work to minimize them. Some factors, such as biological predisposition, cannot be changed. Others, such as inadequate resources or lack of knowledge, are modifiable risks. Figure 1-5 ■ depicts the factors that promote mental health or put people at risk for mental illness.

BOX 1-5

Nurses' Role in Mental Health Promotion

- **Prevention** of mental illness (primary, secondary, and tertiary)
- **Treatment** in the acute phase of illness
- **Rehabilitation** of clients after they have recovered from the acute phase of illness

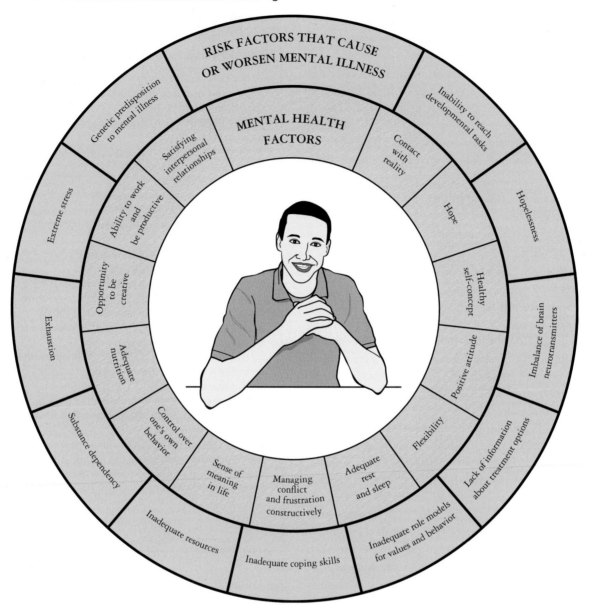

Figure 1-5. ■ Risks and prevention factors for mental illness.

PREVENTION

There are three types of prevention:

1. **Primary** prevention starts with healthy people and prevents them from being affected by a disorder. An example is drug abuse education with children. They learn to avoid drug use before they ever have a problem. Figure 1-6 ■ shows a drug abuse resistance class.

2. **Secondary** prevention involves people who are already affected by a disorder. They are identified and treated early to prevent the negative outcomes of the disorder. An example is depression screening, when

people are tested and cases of depression are identified early, before the people have experienced loss of jobs, despair, or even attempted suicide.

3. **Tertiary** prevention serves people who are already severely affected by a mental disorder. The goal is to help them recover and prevent further disability. An example of tertiary prevention is a community walk-in clinic where people with schizophrenia can come to learn socializing, independent living, and medication management skills that will help them stay out of institutions and in their homes.

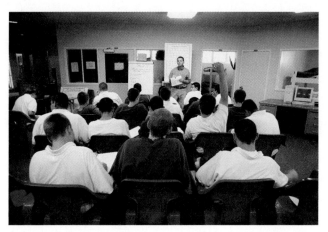

Figure 1-6. ■ Educating adolescents about avoiding drug abuse is a primary prevention strategy for mental illness. *Source:* PhotoEdit Inc.

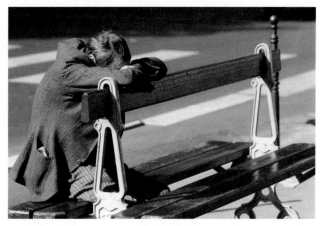

Figure 1-7. ■ There are more charitable donations to benefit homeless animals than for homeless people. *Source:* Photo Researchers, Inc.

Vulnerability of the Mentally Ill

People with mental illnesses are among the most vulnerable in our society. They are often too severely affected by their disease processes to be able to speak effectively for themselves. The disheveled homeless person stirs less sympathy from charitable contributors than children or even homeless animals (Figure 1-7 ■).

clinical ALERT

One of the most important roles of nurses in mental health care is client advocacy. Mentally ill people are very vulnerable and often have difficulty speaking for themselves.

The National Alliance for the Mentally Ill (NAMI) is a strong, yet underfunded organization that acts as an advocate for people with mental illness and their families. NAMI provides support, education, and political advocacy. There are also state affiliates of NAMI that help families cope with mental illness on a local level. The NAMI website, www.nami.org, has information for consumers and their families in English and Spanish.

Consumer, rather than *client* or *patient*, is the term used to describe a person in the community who uses mental health services.

Nurses everywhere are also client advocates. The mentally ill are especially in need of advocacy for access to diagnostic and treatment services, funding for services, and prioritization of research into new treatment modalities. Nurses can be advocates with the legislature for changes in law and health policy. They can encourage local agencies to make services and housing available. They can work alongside the mentally ill, who often need an advocate to meet the simplest of daily needs.

People with mental disorders often enter treatment for physical symptoms. Frequently, they are treated and discharged without concern for their continuing mental issues. With no diagnosis or knowledge of their mental disorders, these clients do not receive appropriate services. Asking for a mental health consultation for a hospitalized client is often an important act of client advocacy.

Note: The references and resources for this and all chapters have been compiled at the back of the book.

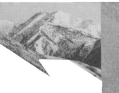

KEY TERMS

Use the audio glossary feature of the Companion Website to hear the correct pronunciation of the following key terms.

adaptability

deinstitutionalization

insight

psychotropic drugs

psychosis

reality

somatic therapies

stigma

KEY Points

- Mental health is a relative term: people can be slightly or very mentally healthy. They can be more or less mentally healthy whether they have a diagnosis of a mental disorder or not.
- All people have the potential for growth toward better mental health.
- Mental disorders are classified; people are not.
- Deinstitutionalization of the mentally ill resulted in many homeless and untreated mentally ill people.
- The stigma of mental illness prevents many people from obtaining the treatment they need.
- Nurses can promote the mental health of clients in any setting.
- Nurses have a role in all levels of prevention of mental illness.
- The mentally ill are a very vulnerable group.
- Asking for a mental health consultation is an important act of client advocacy by a nurse.

EXPLORE MediaLink

Additional interactive resources for this chapter can be found on the Companion Website at www.prenhall.com/eby. Click on Chapter 1 and "Begin" to select the activities for this chapter.

- Audio glossary
- NCLEX-PN® review
- Case study
- Study outline
- Critical thinking questions
- Matching questions
- Weblinks

1 Which of the following statements indicates that the speaker is missing an important aspect of a mentally healthy life?
1. "I am responsible for my reactions to situations; others have no control over my emotions."
2. "My goal in life is to always treat other people as I want to be treated."
3. "I am self-sufficient; I do not need personal relationships with other people."
4. "I see each problem as a challenge and a source of creative growth."

2 Which of the following is a false statement about mental health?
1. There are degrees of mental health.
2. There is no universally accepted definition of mental health.
3. All people have the potential for improving their own mental health.
4. A person with a diagnosed mental illness may not achieve a mentally healthier state.

3 Which of the following is a true statement about the current edition of the *DSM?*
1. It provides a holistic assessment of mental illness.
2. It is specific to mental health issues in the United States.
3. It is a classification of people with mental disorders.
4. It takes into consideration only clinical psychiatric and personality disorders.

4 According to the Global Assessment of Functioning Scale, a 40-year-old male with an antisocial personality disorder who has difficulty maintaining close personal relationships or holding a job for long is experiencing:
1. Minimal symptoms, good functioning in all areas.
2. Moderate symptoms or moderate difficulty in social, occupational, or school functioning.
3. Some mild symptoms, but generally functioning pretty well.
4. Serious symptoms or serious impairment in social, occupational, or school functioning.

5 Which of the following is the most common mental illness globally?
1. Alcohol abuse
2. Schizophrenia
3. Major depressive disorder
4. Bipolar disorder

6 A homeless person with schizophrenia has been admitted to a medical unit with pneumonia. The nurse would suspect that this client's living circumstance is a result of:
1. The experiment with deinstitutionalization.
2. Failure of psychotropic drugs to control the symptoms.
3. Not enough federal funding for housing.
4. The client not caring enough to obtain treatment.

7 Recommending that a client with schizophrenia be referred for a psychiatric consult to be considered for the community walk-in clinic and treatment program is an example of:
1. Primary prevention.
2. Secondary prevention.
3. Tertiary prevention.
4. Active intervention.

8 Why do people with a mental illness need the advocacy of nurses?
1. They are not very articulate.
2. They often cannot speak for themselves because of their illness.
3. They really do not understand their healthcare needs.
4. They are afraid to speak.

9 Where can families of people with mental illnesses go to find out about the illnesses and family support services?
1. National Alliance for the Mentally Ill
2. National Foundation for Mental Science
3. American Family Help Plan
4. Centers for Disease Control

10 Which of the following risk factors for the development of mental illness could be modified by the nurse as part of primary prevention? (Select all that apply.)
1. Lack of information about treatment options
2. Inadequate rest and sleep
3. Unhealthy self-concept
4. Genetic predisposition to mental illness
5. Inadequate coping skills

Answers for Review Questions appear in Appendix I.

Chapter 2

Ethical and Legal Issues

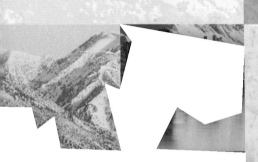

LEARNING Outcomes

After completing this chapter, you will be able to:

1. Clarify your own personal values.
2. Provide nursing care based on the ethical values of the profession.
3. Apply the nursing process as an ethical decision-making model.
4. Identify ways to avoid malpractice issues.
5. Plan nursing interventions to protect the legal and ethical rights of clients with psychiatric disorders.

The practice of professional nursing is based on the ethical principles of our profession and the laws of our society. Nursing has high standards. Our ethical and legal standards serve to protect our clients, our society, and ourselves. These standards change slowly over time as the values of our culture evolve. Laws vary among the states. You must be aware of the laws affecting nursing in the state where you will practice.

ETHICS IN NURSING

Ethics is the science relating to moral principles or standards that govern conduct. It is the body of knowledge that answers the question: "All things considered, what is the *right* thing to do in a given situation?" Nurses work with ethical issues every day. There are ethical issues involved when a neighbor asks for information about a famous person in the hospital; when a client does not understand his treatment; when a medication makes the client feel sick; or when a client is discharged before she is ready to be independent at home.

Personal Values

Nurses must understand their own values before they make decisions related to professional ethics. **Values** are personal beliefs about the worth of an idea, object, or behavior.

Values are an individual's decisions about what is right, what is wrong, and what is most important. People are often passionate on the subject of values. It is values (such as patriotism, freedom, justice, equality, religion) that make people go to war, or march against it. People are often willing to fight or even die for their values (Figure 2-1 ■). Why are personal values so important to nursing?

Personal values affect how humans (including nurses) interpret the world. Personal values can affect a nurse's behavior at work. A nurse who values self-sufficiency very highly may prioritize the care of an independent client over that of a client who has quadriplegia. A nurse who puts a high value on physical appearance may answer the call lights of attractive clients first. These nurses may not know why they behave this way unless they clarify their values for themselves.

Values clarification is a process of self-discovery in which people identify their own values and prioritize them. When nurses clearly understand their own attitudes about right and wrong, it is easier for them to decide on ethical professional behavior. The process of values clarification (Figure 2-2 ■) has three steps (Steele & Harmon, 1979):

1. **Choosing** from alternatives which values to hold
2. **Prizing** the chosen values, which means making a public commitment to the values (such as with bumper stickers, symbolic jewelry, tattoos, telling people, etc.)
3. **Acting** on the chosen values

Integrity means acting on one's values. If a person values honesty and acts consistently in an honest way, this person is said to have integrity. If this person says he values honesty, but acts in a consistently dishonest way, he is acting with *hypocrisy* (behavior contrary to stated values).

Nurses who understand their values are more able to act professionally with clients without allowing their personal issues to interfere with client care. Consider the case of a nurse who tends to act disrespectfully toward his clients who are overweight. If the nurse clarifies that he values physical fitness very highly, he will understand why he feels negatively toward people who are not physically fit. With some effort, this nurse can understand that a person's character is not measured on the bathroom scale. He can become less judgmental and more considerate of overweight clients. Without this self-discovery he may never modify his own behavior.

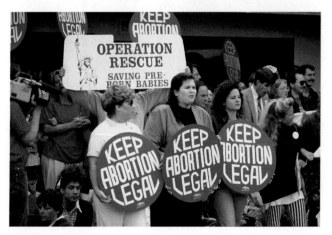

Figure 2-1. ■ People are often passionate about their values.
Source: PhotoEdit Inc.

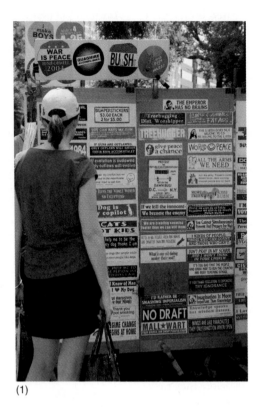

(1)

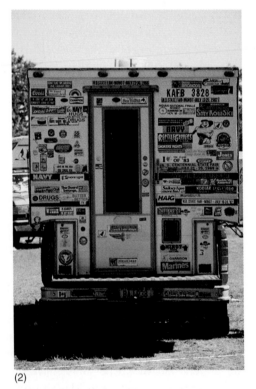

(2)

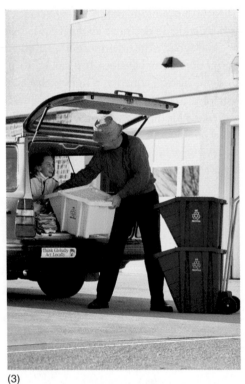

(3)

Figure 2-2. ■ Steps of the values clarification process. (1) Choosing freely from alternatives. *Source: Rough Guides.* Dorling Kindersley. (2) Prizing one's chosen values by making choices public. *Source:* The Stock Connection. (3) Acting on chosen values. *Source:* Photo Researchers, Inc.

Some personal values (such as racism) are not acceptable anywhere in the practice of nursing. Nursing students should learn about the standards and values of the nursing profession. Then they can decide whether to join the profession.

Sometimes the values of the profession (professional ethics) supersede the values of an individual nurse. Consider the nurse who is president of an antiabortion group. She is passionate about what she believes is the right to life for the unborn. She wants to work on an obstetrics unit. She would refuse to provide care for any person who had an abortion. However, the OB unit in her local hospital admits clients who have complications after abortions. In the nursing profession, the rights of all clients to nursing care are more important than an individual nurse's right to act according to her own values. This nurse will either need to work in a different area of the hospital or reexamine her decision to exclude certain clients from her care. A person who has personal values that require excluding groups of people from nursing care should consider other career options.

Nurses do not need to agree with the behavior or values of their clients. In fact, they often disagree. However, nurses must provide care to people with respect for their human dignity and regardless of their personal attributes.

In the psychiatric setting, nurses may care for clients who have engaged in predatory acts against other people (such as sexual assault) or other violent acts or abnormal behavior that nurses find offensive. No matter how difficult, it is necessary for nurses to separate the client's behavior from the client's need for nursing care.

You bring your individual values with you to the nursing profession. These values can mature and develop as you gain insight and experience in nursing.

BOX 2-1

American Nurses Association Code of Ethics for Nurses

1. The nurse, in all professional relationships, practices with compassion and respect for the inherent dignity, worth, and uniqueness of every individual, unrestricted by considerations of social or economic status, personal attributes, or the nature of health problems.
2. The nurse's primary commitment is to the patient, whether an individual, family, group, or community.
3. The nurse promotes, advocates for, and strives to protect the health, safety, and rights of the patient.
4. The nurse is responsible and accountable for individual nursing practice and determines the appropriate delegation of tasks consistent with the nurse's obligation to provide optimum patient care.
5. The nurse owes the same duties to self as to others, including the responsibility to preserve integrity and safety, to maintain competence, and to continue personal and professional growth.
6. The nurse participates in establishing, maintaining, and improving health care environments and conditions of employment conducive to the provision of quality health care and consistent with the values of the profession through individual and collective action.
7. The nurse participates in the advancement of the profession through contributions to practice, education, administration, and knowledge development.
8. The nurse collaborates with all other health professionals and the public in promoting community, national, and international efforts to meet health needs.
9. The profession of nursing, as represented by associations and their members, is responsible for articulating nursing values, for maintaining the integrity of the profession and its practice, and for shaping social policy.

Source: Reprinted with permission from American Nurses Association, *Code of Ethics for Nurses with Interpretive Statements,* © 2001 Nursesbooks.org, American Nurses Association, Washington, D.C.

Codes of Ethics for Nurses

The American Nurses Association (2001) has established an ethical guide for the entire nursing profession, the Code of Ethics for Nurses (Box 2-1 ■). Notice that the code provides principles and guidelines, but no specific directions for nursing interventions. Professional ethical codes must be general in order to cover the variety of situations in which they will be used.

The Code of Ethics for Nurses reflects the current ethical standards for nursing. The ethics of the profession evolve over time as societal attitudes and sociological circumstances change. The Code was first written in 1950.

It is periodically assessed and revised to keep it consistent with contemporary practice. The most recent revision emphasizes nurses' service to clients and duty to themselves as well. It also strengthens nurses' responsibility to improve healthcare environments through collective action and acknowledges the global responsibility of nursing.

The National Federation of Licensed Practical Nurses (NFLPN) is the professional organization representing Licensed Practical and Vocational Nurses (LPN/LVNs). In 2003 the NFLPN published the most current *Nursing Practice Standards for the Licensed Practical/Vocational Nurse.*

BOX 2-2

Legal/Ethical Standards for the Licensed Practical/Vocational Nurse

The Licensed Practical/Vocational Nurse:
1. Shall hold a current license to practice nursing as an LP/VN in accordance with the law of the state wherein employed.
2. Shall know the scope of nursing practice authorized by the Nursing Practice Act in the state wherein employed.
3. Shall have a personal commitment to fulfill the legal responsibilities inherent in good nursing practice.
4. Shall take responsible actions in situations wherein there is unprofessional conduct by a peer or other health care provider.
5. Shall recognize and have a commitment to meet the ethical and moral obligations of the practice of nursing.
6. Shall not accept or perform professional responsibilities which the individual knows (s)he is not competent to perform.

Source: Reprinted with permission: National Federation for Licensed Practical Nurses, Inc. (2003). www.nflpn.org/practice.

The organization has standards for education, legal/ethical status, practice, continuing education, and specialized nursing practice for Licensed Practical/Vocational Nurses. The standards for ethical/legal status are duplicated in Box 2-2 ■.

Standards of Care

Standards of nursing care are the ethical and legal expectations for practice; they are the level of work quality considered adequate by the profession. There are standard skills and knowledge commonly possessed by members of the nursing profession. Society expects that nurses will use at least ordinary and reasonable care to see that no unnecessary harm comes to the client. When there is a question about a nurse's care, the nurse's actions can be compared with professional standards (Guido, 2006).

Some standards are set by organizations that employ nurses. These *internal standards* often consist of written policies and procedures for doing nursing tasks. Nurses are held responsible for knowing and following the policies and procedures of their employer.

There are also *external standards*, which are set by state and national organizations. State boards of nursing, professional nursing organizations such as the ANA and the NFLPN, and the federal government all provide external standards (Guido, 2006). Nurses are expected to know about and adhere to these standards.

Ethical Principles

Ethical principles provide a basis for discussion and ethical decision making. These principles may be used alone, but are usually used in combination with each other (Guido, 2006). The seven ethical principles most pertinent to nursing are:

- **Justice.** Justice means that people have the right to be treated equally and fairly. All resources available for health care should be distributed equally to people.
- **Beneficence.** Beneficence means to do good for others. This is the foundation for most nursing actions: doing good.
- **Nonmaleficence.** Nonmaleficence means doing no harm. Health care providers should not harm their clients either intentionally or unintentionally (Aiken & Catalano, 1994).
- **Autonomy.** Autonomy involves personal freedom and self-determination. It is the right to choose what will happen to oneself.
- **Paternalism.** Paternalism allows someone to act "in the best interest" of other people, making decisions for others when they lack the full information or ability on which to base decisions (Aiken & Catalano, 1994).
- **Veracity.** Veracity means truth telling. This principle says that the whole truth should always be told.
- **Fidelity.** Fidelity means keeping promises. When you are loyal you keep your promises.

Critical Self-Check. Is the healthcare system in the United States based on the principle of justice? Why or why not?

Ethical principles may seem relatively simple at first, but they can be quite complex when they are applied in the real world. Sometimes several principles can be in conflict and sometimes one principle is more important than others. Consider the case of a person with a severe psychiatric disorder who does not want to take her medication. When she does not take her medication, she becomes agitated and may hurt herself or other people. The question is: Should this client be forced to take her prescribed medication? Based on the principle of autonomy, what should be done? Based on the principle of beneficence, what should be done? What action should be taken if the principle used is paternalism? Should this person be forced to take her medication? Ethical principles often conflict with each other, creating ethical dilemmas that cause decision making to be difficult.

ETHICAL DILEMMAS

Decisions about the right or wrong action in a given situation are complicated in part by which ethical principles are used (as in the previous example). Other complicating factors include the resources available, the culture and values of the people involved, who the decision maker is, and the possible consequences of actions (which may be different from each person's point of view).

An **ethical dilemma** exists when there are conflicting moral alternatives to consider for action. In an ethical dilemma, some evidence exists that a particular course of action may be right, and some evidence exists that it may be wrong.

ETHICAL DECISION MAKING

In the healthcare culture in the United States, the client's autonomy is highly valued. If a client is old enough to make legal decisions (the age varies by state), has not been declared legally incompetent by a court of law, or has not had a legal guardian appointed, the client is considered the decision maker in medical treatment situations. This sounds like a good idea in any medical care setting, but consider the following situations that can challenge nurses' ethical foundations:

1. A client on a Medical Surgical unit at a hospital is diagnosed with respiratory failure due to Chronic Obstructive Pulmonary Disease (COPD). This client smokes 1 to 2 packs of cigarettes per day. The nurses teach the client about the dangers of smoking every time he is in the hospital and every time he goes to the physician's office, but he still smokes. What should the nurses do?

2. A client on a psychiatric unit has schizophrenia. He has delusional thinking that makes him not want to take his antipsychotic medication. He thinks it causes his mental illness and he will not take it. What should the nurse do?

3. A client in long-term care is diagnosed with dementia. She does not like to take her medications, including the one that may improve her cognitive functioning.

Sometimes she will take them, but today she is refusing. What should the nurse do?

4. A woman with severe depression is admitted voluntarily to the psychiatric hospital. When she refuses to take the antidepressant medication that her psychiatrist ordered, her parents and her husband ask the psychiatrist if she can be forced to take the medication to make her feel better. What should the nurse do?

In all these cases it seems that the ethical principles of beneficence (doing good) and paternalism (knowing better for clients than they know for themselves) seem to indicate that something should be done to make the clients do what seems obviously to be in their best interests. But, the *more important* principle of autonomy indicates that the client should be allowed to decide in each of these cases. These legally competent adults have the right to choose whether to have surgery, if they will participate in group therapy, how much of their meals to eat, and whether to take their medications, among many daily decisions in a client's life. They also have the right to make their own decisions about their health-related behavior when they are at home. They can smoke, eat unhealthy food, work too hard without enough sleep, or engage in any number of other unhealthy behaviors, even if a nurse does not approve.

> **Critical Self-Check.** Is it ethically correct for a nurse in long-term care to trick a client into taking her medications by putting the client's crushed medications in food?

So, what good are nurses if we can't make clients do anything, you might ask. Clients don't need nurses to force them to act in a healthy way. Nurses create a relationship with their clients. In the nurse-client relationship we foster trust and we teach clients what they need to know so they can make informed decisions for themselves. We care for clients, teach them, and advocate for them. We do not have to approve of their behavior or ideas, we just care, teach, and advocate. The only behavior we can control is our own.

Of course the exception is when a client's behavior is dangerous. Every state has a law that allows for medical personnel to act to protect other people when a client is dangerous to them, or to protect clients when they are dangerous to themselves. Nurses should be aware of the pertinent laws in the states where they practice.

LEGAL ASPECTS OF MENTAL HEALTH NURSING

Although the ethical principles of nursing care protect the rights of clients, the law protects the needs of society. The legal context of care concerns the rights of clients and the quality of care they receive. The civil, criminal, and consumer rights of clients have been expressed and expanded through laws (Stuart & Laraia, 2005). Some laws affecting the mentally ill are federal; others are passed by the states and vary from one state to another. Nurses must be aware of the laws of the state in which they practice.

Types of Law

Two types of law apply most directly to nurses. They are statutory law, which is law that is passed by a legislative body, and common law, which is derived from previous court decisions. Both statutory and common laws have civil and criminal components. Civil law protects private and property rights. Torts are violations of civil law in which an individual has been wronged. Malpractice is a tort. Criminal law protects people from conduct injurious to the public welfare and provides for punishment of people who break these laws (Townsend, 2006). Figure 2-3 ■ shows the relationships among the types of laws that pertain to nursing practice.

Nurse Practice Acts

The legal definitions and scope of practice of registered and practical/vocational nurses are in each state's nurse practice act. These are statutory law (enacted by the state legislatures). It is important for nurses to understand the extent of their responsibilities when they practice

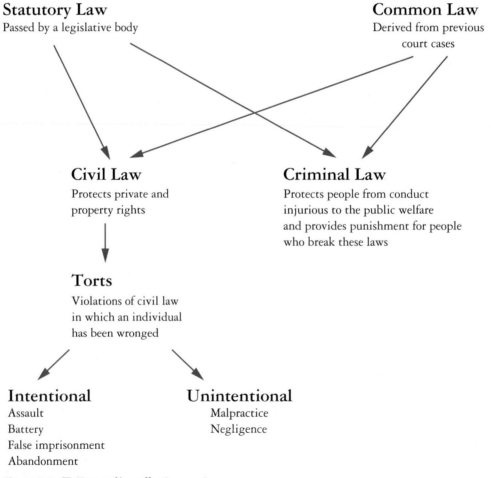

Statutory Law
Passed by a legislative body

Common Law
Derived from previous court cases

Civil Law
Protects private and property rights

Criminal Law
Protects people from conduct injurious to the public welfare and provides punishment for people who break these laws

Torts
Violations of civil law in which an individual has been wronged

Intentional
Assault
Battery
False imprisonment
Abandonment

Unintentional
Malpractice
Negligence

Figure 2-3. ■ Types of law affecting nursing.

nursing in their state. These laws vary from one state to another. They usually include:

- Definitions of nursing and the various types of nurses
- Requirements for educational preparation for each type of nursing
- Conditions for revoking a license
- A statement about the state agency (the State Board of Nursing) that has jurisdiction over nurses

Psychiatric Hospitalization

Voluntary admission for mental illness treatment is similar to medical hospitalization. The client signs a routine form requesting admission to the hospital and may leave at any time. Ideally, all treatment should be on a voluntary basis. However, mental illnesses are sometimes characterized by symptoms that make it impossible for affected clients to understand their condition or need for treatment.

Involuntary admission, or commitment, means that the client is hospitalized without the individual's consent. The rules regulating involuntary commitment are based on state laws and vary among the states. The basic criteria for involuntary commitment to psychiatric treatment facilities usually include that the client must be mentally ill and (as a result of this mental illness) be:

- Dangerous to self or others
- In need of treatment
- Unable to provide for own basic needs

People may be committed to psychiatric treatment through emergency hospitalization or *civil commitment*. An emergency psychiatric hospitalization is indicated when a person appears to be dangerous to self or others and refuses treatment. States can allow a brief (2- to 5-day) involuntary hospitalization for further evaluation and allow time for a court hearing on determining the need for a longer commitment. The states usually require that by the time the emergency hospitalization period has elapsed, mental health providers (usually psychiatrists) must petition the court for an extended commitment if they decide that the client needs further treatment. This extended involuntary hospitalization is called **civil commitment.** A court hearing is usually held to determine whether a person will be civilly committed. Civil commitments may vary in length of time, but may not last more than 1 year. If a client's condition improves during the commitment period, the client may be discharged.

OUTPATIENT COMMITMENT

Outpatient commitment is a court order requiring the mentally ill person to take medication and to comply with a treatment plan as a condition of release from the hospital. Outpatient commitment reduces rehospitalization, increases client compliance with medication, and decreases violence (Torrey, 1997). However, outpatient commitment is not available in all states.

CONDITIONAL RELEASE

Conditional release is another type of involuntary commitment available in some states. In this system, the committed client is released from the hospital on the condition that he or she participate in treatment in the community. This can be a day treatment or medication management program. A client who fails to comply with the conditions is rehospitalized.

Legal Rights for Mental Health Clients

People with mental illnesses are vulnerable to abuse and mistreatment. To protect the mentally ill, the U.S. Congress passed the Mental Health Systems Act of 1980, which passed into law the Universal Bill of Rights for Mental Health Patients. This bill of rights is summarized in Box 2-3 ■.

CIVIL RIGHTS

People who are voluntarily hospitalized for mental health treatment retain all their civil rights. Clients have the right to vote, hold office, conduct business, hold licenses, and practice their professions. States may abridge the rights of people who are committed. In some states, committed clients retain all their civil rights, including the right to refuse treatment.

Right to Least Restrictive Treatment Alternative

As stated in the Bill of Rights for Mental Health Patients, people have the right to the **least restrictive alternative** (treatment that restricts their personal freedom as little as possible). Treatment settings include community outpatient clinics, foster care homes, respite care, day treatment programs, home health care, and a variety of levels of inpatient care. In the inpatient setting, treatment decisions must consider the least restrictive alternative issue. When clients act out violently, whether to restrain, seclude, or medicate a client involuntarily is such an issue.

Restraint and Seclusion

In psychiatry, "restraints" refers to leather or other secure restraining devices on all extremities and around the body of the client to prevent the client from harming self or

Universal Bill of Rights for Mental Health Patients

The mental health patient has:

1. The right to appropriate treatment and related services in a setting that is most supportive of personal liberty, restricting liberty only as needed for treatment and legal requirements.
2. The right to an individualized written treatment plan; the right to treatment based on the plan; and the right to periodic review and revision of the plan, including a plan for treatment after discharge.
3. The right to ongoing participation in planning mental health services, consistent with the person's capabilities.
4. The right to receive an explanation that the patient can understand of the nature and risks of treatment, the reasons a treatment is considered, any alternative treatments, and reasons for limitation of certain visitors.
5. The right to informed, voluntary, written consent for treatment except in an emergency situation.
6. The right not to be involved in experimentation without informed, voluntary, written consent.
7. The right to freedom from restraint or seclusion except in an emergency situation.
8. The right to a humane treatment that provides reasonable protection from harm and appropriate privacy.
9. The right to access to own mental health care records.
10. The right, when admitted to an inpatient unit, to converse with others privately, to have access to telephone and mail, and to see visitors, unless contraindicated by the patient's condition.
11. The right to be informed promptly and in writing of these rights at the time of admission.
12. The right to assert grievances if these rights are infringed.
13. The right to exercise these rights without reprisal.
14. The right of referral to other providers.

Source: Adapted from *Restatement of Bill of Rights for Mental Health Patients* established by Mental Health Systems Act of 1980. Title II, Public Law 99-319.

is a type of restraint. A physician must order restraints and seclusion, except in an emergency situation. Even in an emergency the physician must be consulted and provide an order for the restraint as soon as possible (Joint Commission on Accreditation of Healthcare Organizations, 2005).

It can be a stressful, frightening, and powerless experience to be restrained. Clients who have experienced being controlled in leather restraints reported feeling vulnerable, helpless, coerced, and dehumanized (Johnson, 1998). In a study of clients' experiences with restraints in psychiatric emergency situations, clients were asked how they would prefer to be treated if they were unable to control their behavior. The vast majority (around 70%) said that they would prefer to be treated with medications, some would prefer seclusion (around 20%), and few would prefer restraint (around 10%) (Sheline & Nelson, 1993).

The current trend is toward using restraints less frequently than they were used in the past. Healthcare facilities are expected to avoid or minimize the use of restraints (Sailas, Wahlbeck, & Lie, 2005). After the client has recovered composure, explaining the need for restraint in terms of behavior management rather than punishment may help

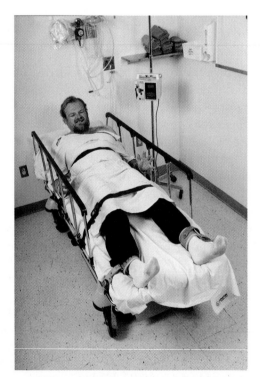

Figure 2-4. ■ Restraints are only used in behavioral emergencies when safety of the client or others is at risk. *Source:* Procision Video and Photography.

others (Figure 2-4 ■). Clients in psychiatric settings have been injured and even killed by restraints (Figure 2-5 ■). Restraints may never be used for the convenience of the staff or to punish the client. Other less restrictive alternatives must be attempted to decrease the client's agitation before restraints are considered. Less restrictive approaches include redirecting the client to his room or away from a stressful situation, talking with the client, and intervening with medications.

In psychiatry, **seclusion** means that the client is confined in a room alone. The seclusion room is usually furnished only with a bed or mattress for safety. Seclusion

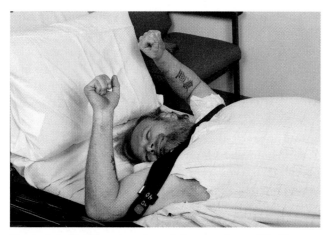

Figure 2-5. ■ Clients have been injured and even killed by restraints. *Source:* Procision Video and Photography.

the client understand the situation better. Talking with clients afterward about their feelings may help decrease the psychological impact of seclusion (Meehan, Bergen, & Fjeldsoe, 2004). Some psychiatric facilities are becoming "restraint-free" environments with the goal of protecting clients from the trauma of being restrained.

Nurses must be familiar with the restraint policies in the institutions where they work. Client behavior and the nurse's attempts at less restrictive alternatives to restraints must be carefully documented. Clients must be assessed every 15 minutes while they are restrained (Joint Commission, 2005).

Competency

Competency is a legal assessment that a person is able to make reasonable judgments and decisions. A person who is cognitively able to understand the information given in the consent process is considered *competent* for the purpose of medical care. Competency is an important concept because it is a foundation of the legal rights of people with mental illnesses. A competency verdict determines whether a person is capable of making informed decisions to consent or to refuse treatment. Clients who are committed to psychiatric hospitalization are assumed to be competent and therefore maintain their civil rights. **Incompetence** must be determined by a court. It refers to the inability to make judgments and be responsible for one's own decisions. A court ruling of incompetence deprives the person of some rights such as voting, entering into contracts, and driving.

Competency to stand trial is a different issue. This assessment determines whether the person is capable of understanding the significance and consequences of his/her actions, whether this person understands what is right and wrong, and if the person can assist a lawyer in his/her defense. State laws define competency.

RIGHT TO INFORMED CONSENT

Clients have the right to freedom from potentially hazardous treatment unless they give informed consent. **Informed consent** means that the physician has explained the treatment in terms the client fully understands (including the potential outcomes and the likely outcome without treatment) and that the client agrees and permits the treatment. Clients may also change their minds and stop a treatment that has already been started.

Before consenting to treatment, the client should understand:

■ The diagnosis
■ The description and purpose of the proposed treatment
■ The risks and benefits of the treatment
■ The alternatives to this treatment (including doing nothing) and their risks and benefits

It is the responsibility of the physician to give the client information for making treatment decisions. Nurses may witness the client's signature on a consent form. They may help to answer the client's questions. However, informed consent itself is the physician's responsibility.

Most mentally ill clients are competent and able to give informed consent, but those with severe mental health symptoms may lack the cognitive ability to understand consent. If the client has been deemed mentally incompetent, the legal guardian may give consent for treatment. If the client has severe symptoms (such as psychosis) and is unable to understand treatment but has no guardian, the client's nearest relative may be consulted. It is also possible for the physician to ask the court to appoint a guardian.

RIGHT TO REFUSE TREATMENT

Clients have the right to refuse to consent and to refuse treatment even if the physician thinks the treatment is in the client's best interest (Guido, 2006). A nurse can be charged with battery for touching a client in the process of treatment that the client refuses. Threatening to force treatment may constitute assault.

An important aspect of the right to refuse treatment is refusal of medication. This is an area of controversy. Sometimes a client does not want to take medication, but the client's disease process makes it impossible for him/her to understand the need for treatment. Add to this the fact that the client may become agitated and violent when not taking medication. The result is a situation in which the client's rights (autonomy) conflict with the rights of others (right to safety).

Ultimately, competent clients who are voluntarily admitted or committed involuntarily have the right to refuse medications. When an emergency occurs and the client is a danger to self or others, clients may be medicated against their will if professional judgment is used and due process guidelines are followed (Fortinash & Holoday Worret, 2004). A trusting nurse-client relationship may decrease the likelihood that forced medication will be necessary.

RIGHT TO CONFIDENTIALITY

Nurses are responsible for protecting clients' right to **confidentiality** (limits on access to information about a client). Even the fact that a person is a client in a mental health treatment facility is confidential. The stigma of mental illness is such that knowledge of a person's hospitalization may affect the individual's employment or professional standing. Clients must be able to trust that information about their diagnoses and treatment will remain among the people who need it for treatment purposes. Figure 2-6 ■ illustrates a patient's "circle of confidentiality." Only those within the inner circle of confidentiality may have access to treatment information about the client without the client's written consent.

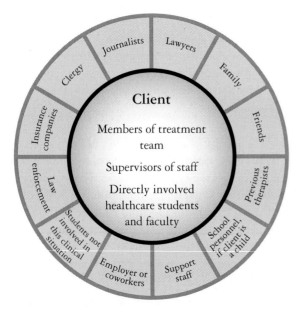

Figure 2-6. ■ Circle of confidentiality.

There are a few exceptions to the confidentiality rule. The most notable is those who fall within the Tarasoff rule. In the Tarasoff case, a client informed his psychologist that he planned to kill a young woman. The psychologist informed the police, but neither informed the woman, who was later murdered by the client. Her parents successfully sued the psychologist and others for failure to warn. The Tarasoff rule, or Tarasoff duty to warn, requires healthcare providers to assess the violence potential of their clients, and if specific victims are in imminent danger, to take some form of protective action. Other situations when a nurse may give client information to a third party without the client's consent are emergency situations for client care, court-ordered requests for information, child abuse proceedings, commitment proceedings, and reports required by law (such as communicable diseases, child abuse, or gunshot wounds) (Stuart & Laraia, 2005).

RIGHT TO KEEP PERSONAL ITEMS

People who are in a hospital, nursing home, foster care home, or other treatment facility retain the right to keep their personal possessions. Certain items of safety concern (such as guns, knives, scissors, glass bottles, or lighters) may be held in a secure place until the client's discharge, but they continue to be the property of the client.

Americans with Disabilities Act

The Americans with Disabilities Act of 1990 (ADA) makes it unlawful to discriminate in employment against a qualified person with a mental or physical disability. The ADA defines an individual with a disability as a person who has a physical or mental impairment that substantially limits one or more major life activities, has a record of such impairment, or is regarded as having such an impairment. Employers select the most qualified applicants for jobs, and if the most qualified applicant has a disability, the employer must accommodate that employee if reasonably possible. A history of mental illness cannot be used to deny a person employment.

Advance Care Directives

Advance directives are instructions from clients, documented when they are well, about what should be done in situations when they are unable to speak for themselves.

Advance directives include documents such as living wills or powers of attorney for health care. They relate to end-of-life decisions or healthcare decisions when a person is incapacitated. The opportunity for people with mental illnesses to designate a person to speak and decide for them when they are unable to do so is a more recent development. Some states are passing laws allowing mentally ill people to declare when they are well what treatment they would prefer or refuse if their decision-making capacity were impaired by a relapse of the mental disorder. The client and two witnesses must sign these directives.

Nurse's Responsibility in Documentation

In mental health care nursing there are some special concerns related to documentation. The first is documenting the administration of medications. When a nurse decides to administer a p.r.n. psychotropic medication (a drug affecting the mind), it is important to document the situation and the assessment findings that led to the decision to give the medication. This documentation should include the client behavior (including verbal statements) and less restrictive treatment alternatives tried before medication was given (such as talking to the client or redirecting the client to his/her room for a less stimulating environment). The client's response to all p.r.n. medications should be documented.

The nurse is also responsible for assessing the client's response to routine medications. The client's symptoms and how the client responds to the medication should be documented on a regular basis. The client's side effects and adverse drug reactions should also be documented. In the mental health care setting, clients often have difficulty explaining their side effects to the physician. Thus, it is especially important for the nurse to assess for and document these effects, to improve the quality of medication management.

Nurses should pay special concern to clients at risk for suicide. These clients require frequent assessment of mental status. These assessments should be carefully documented to show changes in status that might indicate a trend toward increased risk.

In the mental health care setting the client's behavior is especially important. Behavior indicates the severity of the client's disease process and response to treatment. The nurse must describe the behavior clearly, concisely, and specifically, without judgment. For example, it

is incorrect to chart: "The client is rude and unreasonable." It would be appropriate to chart: "The client was offered juice and refused. He was pacing and yelling and was asked to go to his room. He stated 'the demons are after me.'"

Nursing documentation in the mental healthcare setting and elsewhere should be:

- Clear
- Concise (keep it complete but simple)
- Accurate
- Specific
- Descriptive
- Legible (penmanship is a communication issue)

Malpractice

Malpractice is the failure of a professional person to act according to accepted professional standards, or failure to act as a reasonable member of the profession would act. In order for nursing malpractice to exist *all* of the following conditions must be present:

1. The nurse must have a *duty* to the client, which is established by the person being a client in a treatment facility where the nurse works.
2. There must be a *breach of duty*. A standard of care is not followed.
3. *Foreseeability*. The client's injury must be a reasonable expectation under the circumstances of the nurse's action.
4. *Injury*. The client must be injured or harmed.
5. *Causation*. The injury to the client must be caused by the nurse's breach of duty.

CASE EXAMPLE

A client in a mental healthcare setting was showing the following behavior: pacing, irritability, clenched fists, and loud talking. The nurse asked him how he was feeling and he yelled "None of your business!" The nurse looked at his chart and found a physician's order for a medication p.r.n. for agitation. The nurse asked the client if he was agitated and he said "*No!*" The nurse decided not to give the p.r.n. medication and went to work on charting. Meanwhile the client struck and injured another client. Was the injury to the second client the result of malpractice by the nurse? Review the tests for malpractice:

1. Did the nurse have a duty to the injured client? (Yes, even if he was not her assigned client.)
2. Did the nurse breach her duty? (Yes, protection from injury is a basic standard of care.)

3. Was the client's injury foreseeable? (Yes. The nurse did not need to be able to predict the future to see that the first client was becoming agitated. Agitated people are less able to control their impulses and are more likely to act out violently.)
4. Was the client injured? (Yes. He suffered a bruise on his head when the agitated client hit him with a book.)
5. Was the injury caused by the nurse's failure to intervene with the agitated client? (Yes. The nurse could have redirected the agitated client to his room. If that did not work she could have medicated him.)
6. Did malpractice occur? (Yes. The injured client may or may not take this case to court, but the nurse reasonably could have protected the injured client from harm.)

The best way for nurses to avoid malpractice is to know the standards of care and the scope of nursing practice for the states where they work and to adhere to those standards. Institutional policies and procedures are also standards for practice. The nurse must also maintain current knowledge in the nursing field, keep accurate and complete records, and maintain client confidentiality. Finally, and most important, the nurse should put the client's well-being first and develop a trusting nurse-client relationship.

Standards of Culturally Appropriate Care

As the population becomes more diverse, people in the healthcare system are becoming more aware of the need for services that meet the needs of clients from diverse cultures and those who have limited proficiency with the English language. Cultural Pulse Points Box 2-4 ■ lists the standards identified by the Office of Minority Health of the U.S. Department of Health and Human Services in 2001.

Note: The references and resources for this and all chapters have been compiled at the back of the book.

BOX 2-4	CULTURAL PULSE POINTS

National Standards for Culturally and Linguistically Appropriate Services in Health Care

Health care organizations should:

- Ensure that clients receive effective, understandable, and respectful care that is provided in a manner compatible with their cultural health beliefs and practices and preferred language.
- Recruit, retain, and promote a diverse staff and leadership that are representative of the people served by the organization.
- Provide ongoing education in culturally and linguistically appropriate service delivery to all staff.
- Provide language assistance including bilingual staff and interpreter service at no cost to all clients with limited English proficiency at all hours and points of contact.
- Provide written information in the client's native language about the right to receive language assistance services.

- Ensure the competence of language assistance. Family and friends should not be used to interpret, except on request by the client.
- Make written information and signs available in the commonly used languages of clients represented in the service area.
- Have a comprehensive plan for providing culturally and linguistically appropriate services.
- Collect information about clients' race, ethnicity, and spoken and written languages and keep it updated.
- Maintain a demographic, cultural, and epidemiological profile of the community served, as well as a needs profile.
- Involve the community in creating programs for culturally and linguistically appropriate services.
- Ensure that conflict and grievance procedures are sensitive to cultural and language issues, and capable of resolving cross-cultural conflicts or client complaints.
- Make information available to the public about their progress and innovations in implementing these standards.

Source: National Standards for Culturally and Linguistically Appropriate Services in Health Care. Final Report by Office of Minority Health, 2001. Washington, D.C.: Office of Public Health and Science, USDHSS.

Chapter Review

 KEY TERMS

Use the audio glossary feature of the Companion Website to hear the correct pronunciation of the following key terms.

autonomy

beneficence

civil commitment

competency

competency to stand trial

confidentiality

ethical dilemma

ethics

fidelity

incompetence

informed consent

integrity

justice

least restrictive alternative

malpractice

nonmaleficence

outpatient commitment

paternalism

seclusion

standards of nursing care

values

values clarification

veracity

KEY Points

- Through values clarification nurses can understand themselves better and avoid inflicting their personal biases on clients.

- Codes for nursing ethics form one of the standards by which competent nursing practice is judged.

- Clients make their own decisions about treatment options and health behavior; nurses support the client through the decision-making process.

- Clients can be treated voluntarily or committed involuntarily to mental health treatment.

- Mentally ill clients have a variety of rights. Hospitals and nurses must honor them.

- Mental health clients maintain their civil rights.

- For nursing malpractice to exist, the nurse must have a duty to the client, the nurse must breach that duty, the client must be harmed as a result, and the potential of the injury must have been foreseeable.

- The nurse may be charged with assault and battery for threatening to or actually forcing treatment on a client who refuses it.

- Documentation of the nursing process is important in mental health nursing.

 EXPLORE MediaLink

Additional interactive resources for this chapter can be found on the Companion Website at www.prenhall.com/eby. Click on Chapter 2 and "Begin" to select the activities for this chapter.

- Audio glossary
- NCLEX-PN® review
- Case study
- Study outline
- Critical thinking questions
- Matching questions
- Weblinks

Caring for a Client Who Refuses Medication
NCLEX-PN® Focus Area: Physiological Integrity

Case Study: Arthur Clay is a 47-year-old male European American client with schizophrenia. He is voluntarily admitted to the mental health care unit. He is experiencing psychotic symptoms and believes that his medication is poisoned. He is pacing back and forth in the hall talking to himself. Mr. Clay is obviously uncomfortable and afraid. He said that he would not take the poisoned medication.

> **Nursing Diagnosis:** Noncompliance with medication regimen R/T delusional thinking that medication is poisoned

COLLECT DATA

Subjective	Objective
_____	_____
_____	_____
_____	_____
_____	_____
_____	_____
_____	_____

Would you report this data? Yes/No

If yes, to: _____

> **Nursing Care**

_____
_____
_____
_____
_____
_____
_____
_____
_____
_____

How would you document this?_____
_____
_____
_____

Compare your documentation to the sample provided in Appendix I.

Data Collected
(use those that apply)

- History of type 2 diabetes, on no medication
- Blood glucose today is within normal limits
- Client asks, "Why do you want to kill me?"
- Client is having symptoms of delusional thinking (paranoid thoughts) about poisoned meds
- Oriented to person, place, and time
- Refuses to take his ordered antipsychotic medication
- Poor personal hygiene
- Lives in a monthly rental hotel
- Has lost contact with his family
- Client states, "You want me to take poison."
- Likes animals and gardening
- Has been off his meds for 3 weeks

Nursing Interventions
(use those that apply; list in priority order)

- Ask physician to order blood level of antipsychotic medication.
- Take vital signs immediately.
- Tell the client that he has to take the medication or you will have to restrain him.
- Establish trusting nurse-client relationship.
- Offer Mr. Clay a snack.
- Calmly explain that you are the nurse and you are here to help him.
- Ask the physician for a sedative order.
- Reassure the client that you will not hurt him.
- Tell him that this is his antipsychotic medication that will help him straighten out his thoughts. It is not poison. You would like him to take it.
- Carefully explain the chemical structure of the drug and its potential side effects. Include the mechanism of action, pharmacokinetics, and desired effects.
- Act in a cooperative, nonthreatening way.
- Thank him for his cooperation when he takes the medication.

1 Which of the following statements about ethical decision making is true for the nurse?

  1. Intuition is not an acceptable way for the novice nurse to make ethical decisions.
  2. The nurse's personal value system should not enter into ethical decision making.
  3. The client's personal value system should not enter into ethical decision making.
  4. Ethical decisions should be based strictly on the duty of the nurse with no other areas of concern considered.

2 Which principle of healthcare ethics is being violated in the following scenario? A client has told the nurse that he no longer wants to receive chemotherapy for his cancer and the nurse insists that he continue.

  1. Beneficence
  2. Justice
  3. Paternalism
  4. Autonomy

3 Making sure that the nurse follows good handwashing technique when caring for clients is following the ethical principle of:

  1. Nonmaleficence.
  2. Autonomy.
  3. Justice.
  4. Paternalism.

4 Family members of a depressed client asks the nurse whether or not they should go to court and have the client declared mentally incompetent. The best response by the nurse would be:

  1. "This is none of my concern. It's all up to you."
  2. "I think this is unfair to the client. She is not incompetent."
  3. "Let's talk about why you think this is the best option."
  4. "I don't think I'm the best person to ask."

5 Which of the following would be a legal reason for an involuntary admission or commitment of client to a psychiatric facility?

  1. The client has not been taking his antipsychotic medications as prescribed on an outpatient basis.
  2. The client has threatened suicide and describes his plan to the nurse.
  3. The client tells the nurse she has been hearing voices.
  4. The client cannot pay her rent and has no place to live.

6 A client is pacing the halls, muttering and shaking his fist at other clients. The best first response by the nurse would be to:

  1. Call his physician and get an immediate order to place the patient in leather restraints.
  2. Call for assistance from other staff to hold the client while the nurse administers an IM tranquilizer.
  3. Approach the client cautiously. Talk to him quietly and try to find the source of the behavior.
  4. Assist the client to a seclusion room until the behavior passes.

7 A nurse is caring for a severely psychotic client who is scheduled for electroshock therapy. The patient has not been declared legally incompetent but does not understand the treatment. The physician should:

  1. Consult with the client's nearest relative to obtain permission for the treatment.
  2. Not proceed with the treatment until the client is competent enough to agree.
  3. Proceed with the treatment regardless of permission.
  4. Explain the procedure to the client anyway making sure he covers the expected outcomes and possible complications.

8 A physician has ordered a Phospho-soda enema for a client prior to a diagnostic test and the client tells the nurse he does not want it. The nurse goes ahead and gives the enema. This can result in the nurse being charged with:

  1. Negligence.
  2. Battery.
  3. Assault.
  4. Malpractice.

9 The nurse has attempted to administer a PO antipsychotic medication to a client who is threatening to kill anyone who comes close. He refuses to take it and his behavior is escalating. The best action for the nurse to take next is to:

  1. Have several staff members overpower him and put him in restraints.
  2. Call for the hospital security guards to contact the local police to take him to jail until he "calms down."
  3. Call for staff assistance to restrain him while the nurse administers an IM antipsychotic medication.
  4. Do nothing. Avoid going close to the client, and keep other clients away from him as well.

10 A client's minister tells the nurse that he is representing the client's family who wants him to ask about the client's condition and when he might be getting released. The best response by the nurse would be:

  1. "I don't know when the client will be released. We will let the family know when that has been decided."
  2. "If his family wants to know that, they will have to ask themselves."
  3. "I am not at liberty to give out that information without the client's permission."
  4. "Why don't you call his physician and ask him?"

Answers for Review Questions, as well as discussion of Care Plan and Critical Thinking Care Map questions, appear in Appendix I.

Chapter 3

Personality Theory

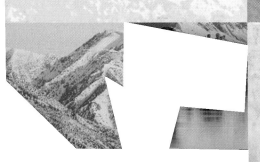

BRIEF Outline

Development of Personality
Psychoanalytic Theory
Ego Theories
Biological Theories
Trait Theories
Behaviorist and Learning
Theories

Cognitive Theories of
Personality
Existential and Humanistic
Theories
Interpersonal Theories

LEARNING Outcomes

After completing this chapter, you will be able to:

1. Explain how personality theories form a basis for psychotherapy.
2. Recognize the purpose and use of defense mechanisms in clients and yourself.
3. Plan nursing interventions to promote clients' psychosocial development.
4. Make decisions about client care priorities based on Maslow's hierarchy of needs.

What makes people human? What is normal behavior? What are mental health and mental illness? What should be done to treat a person with mental illness? Why do nurses need to study personality and psychology? The answers to these and many other important questions are to be found in your pursuit of mental health nursing.

Understanding the theories on the development of personality is a necessary prelude to the study of mental health nursing. Personality theories are attempts to explain human nature, what controls human behavior, and what it means to be human. Each personality theory presents an explanation of what causes behavior, and what treatment should be used for behavior that deviates from the norm. Each personality theory and treatment approach has implications for the practice of nursing.

This chapter summarizes how theories about personality and psychotherapy have evolved. It is intended to show how current nursing practice is built on a foundation of research in a variety of disciplines.

Development of Personality

Personality is the relatively stable way that a person thinks, feels, and behaves. Personality includes the psychosocial traits and characteristics (not physical qualities) that make a person an individual. For example, an extrovert is a person who enjoys being with people and is usually outgoing. People who are extroverts still have the trait of extroversion, even if they are quiet in certain situations. Extroversion describes the relatively consistent way they think, feel, or behave: a *personality trait*. Occasional shyness and quietness are exceptions to the usual behavior.

Eight key influences combine to form the personality of an individual (Friedman & Schustack, 1999):

- **Unconscious aspects** are parts of the personality not in the person's awareness.
- **Identity** is a sense of self (ego).
- The **biology** of personality is the unique genetic, physiological, and temperamental nature of the person.
- **Conditioning** shapes the personality through experiences that influence the person to react in certain ways.
- The **cognitive dimension** reflects how thinking about and interpreting the world shapes personality.
- **Specific traits, skills, and predispositions** are present in each individual.
- The **spiritual dimension** is the part of personality that prompts people to contemplate the meaning of their existence.
- **Interaction** between the individual and the environment is an ongoing process that affects personality.

Each aspect of the complete personality has theorists who have studied it and explained its effect on the human personality. These personality theories show how human behavior, thinking, and feeling can be explained from different points of view. Each theory has its own way of explaining the cause of the client's problems. Psychotherapists who adhere to each theory therefore have different approaches to the treatment of mental disorders. It is interesting to see how approaches to psychotherapy differ based on personality theory.

Personality theorists in the early part of the 20th century tended to interpret personality based on only one principle. For example, Freud stated that personality is shaped largely by early childhood experiences and that people have no free will to control their destiny. B. F. Skinner said that reinforcement of behavior is what shapes who humans are and who they become. In contrast, the more modern theories have an approach that is more holistic. **Holism** is a philosophy that considers the person as a total being with psychosocial, spiritual, and physical needs. Current theories state that many interacting parts and influences form the personality. Figure 3-1 ■ shows how current therapy is based on various personality theories.

Psychoanalytic Theory

One of the early personality theorists was Sigmund Freud of Austria. He developed his *psychoanalytic* theory in the early part of the 20th century. The focus of psychoanalysis is to find the root of unconscious thoughts and feelings that cause the client's anxiety. Freud had his clients "free associate" (talk freely about whatever came to their mind) about their early experiences. He believed that early experiences continue to influence people throughout their lives. He also analyzed clients' dreams. He theorized that dreams give clues to the person's unconscious mind, the part of the mind that is not accessible to conscious thoughts. Freud said that the mind is like an iceberg—it floats with only a small part above water (see Figure 3-2 ■). He divided the mind into three parts. He described the *id* as the part of the personality containing basic instincts and urges. The *ego*, according to Freud, is the "I." It is the part of the personality that develops to respond to the realities and problems of everyday life. The *superego* is a person's conscience and the internalized concept of the ideal self.

Freud's theory of development of personality is called *psychosexual development*. The child progresses through the oral stage, the anal stage, the phallic stage, the latency period, and

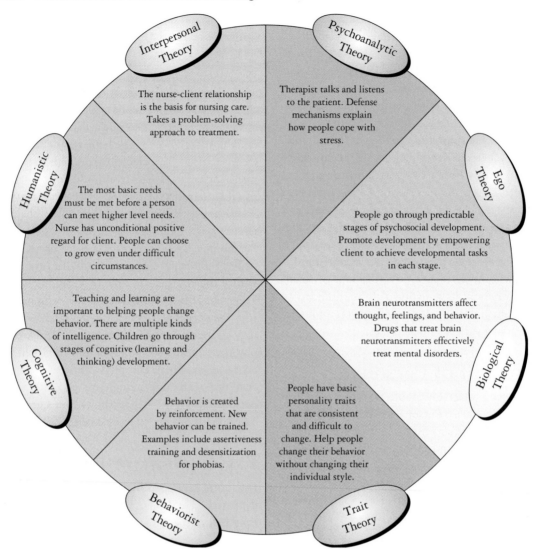

The nurse-client relationship is the basis for nursing care. Takes a problem-solving approach to treatment. *(Interpersonal Theory)*

Therapist talks and listens to the patient. Defense mechanisms explain how people cope with stress. *(Psychoanalytic Theory)*

The most basic needs must be met before a person can meet higher level needs. Nurse has unconditional positive regard for client. People can choose to grow even under difficult circumstances. *(Humanistic Theory)*

People go through predictable stages of psychosocial development. Promote development by empowering client to achieve developmental tasks in each stage. *(Ego Theory)*

Teaching and learning are important to helping people change behavior. There are multiple kinds of intelligence. Children go through stages of cognitive (learning and thinking) development. *(Cognitive Theory)*

Brain neurotransmitters affect thought, feelings, and behavior. Drugs that treat brain neurotransmitters effectively treat mental disorders. *(Biological Theory)*

Behavior is created by reinforcement. New behavior can be trained. Examples include assertiveness training and desensitization for phobias. *(Behaviorist Theory)*

People have basic personality traits that are consistent and difficult to change. Help people change their behavior without changing their individual style. *(Trait Theory)*

Figure 3-1. ■ Current psychotherapy includes principles from several personality theories.

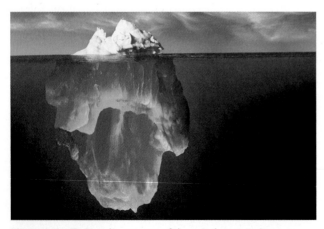

Figure 3-2. ■ Freud's concept of the mind as an iceberg.
Source: Corbis/Bettmann.

finally the genital stage. In his theory, human development is complete when the person reaches adulthood.

Much of Freud's psychosexual theory has been refuted by biological and sociological research and is no longer considered accurate. However, several points of Freud's research continue in current psychoanalytic thinking. One is that all behavior is *motivated* (not accidental), although the motivation is often not conscious. Another enduring concept is that of defense mechanisms (or ego defense mechanisms). **Defense mechanisms** are thoughts and behaviors that distort reality to protect the self (Friedman & Schustack, 1999). These processes are used to protect the ego from threatening impulses or the painful realities of life experiences. Table 3-1 ■ presents definitions and examples of defense mechanisms.

TABLE 3-1		
Defense Mechanisms		
DEFENSE MECHANISM	**DEFINITION**	**EXAMPLE**
Acting Out	Using actions instead of thoughts or feelings to respond to stress or emotional distress	A child who is afraid of being hospitalized kicks the nurse and knocks supplies off the hospital shelf.
Altruism	Dealing with emotional conflict by meeting the needs of others, receiving gratification either vicariously or from the reactions of others	A young man's fiancée leaves him, and he joins the Peace Corps.
Anticipation	Experiencing emotional reactions in advance of a stressful event	When first diagnosed with diabetes, a man begins to experience anticipatory grief for his eventual loss of function and health.
Compensation	Attempt (conscious or unconscious) to overcome perceived inadequacies	A girl who is disappointed in having little athletic skill works hard to excel in academics.
Denial	Refusal to acknowledge a painful reality	A person with alcoholism says: "I don't have a drinking problem; I can quit whenever I want."
Displacement	Transferring a feeling about one person or object to another usually safer one	A client is very angry with his doctor but yells at the nurse or his wife.
Dissociation	A breakdown in the usually integrated functions of consciousness, memory, or perception; detachment from emotional significance	A woman calmly describes her severe sexual abuse in childhood as though she was outside herself watching it happen.
Humor	Amusing or ironic aspects of a stressful experience are emphasized	After making a mistake in front of the class, the teacher makes a joke about it.
Intellectualization	Excessive use of abstract thinking or using generalizations to control disturbing feelings	A man analyzes and explains to a friend the interpersonal dynamics that led to his divorce.
Projection	Attributing one's own unacceptable feelings or thoughts to another	A person who does not like children says: "Children just don't like me."
Rationalization	Concealing the true motivations (even to ourselves) behind our actions with incorrect but acceptable motivations	Instead of admitting that he went to this college to be with his girlfriend, the student says that it is the best college in the state.
Reaction Formation	Substituting behavior or feelings that are the opposite of what one actually feels	A woman does not like her supervisor at work, yet she gives the supervisor gifts and compliments.
Regression	Return to an earlier, less stressful level of adjustment	A child returns to bedwetting after being hospitalized.
Repression	Removing unacceptable thoughts or wishes from consciousness	A woman has no memory of being raped but may feel anxious when she goes near the area where it happened.
Sublimation	Unacceptable feelings are diverted into socially acceptable behavior	A person is very angry and runs for hours on the track.
Suppression	Intentionally avoiding thinking about unacceptable or stressful feelings	A woman does not have enough money to pay her bills and keeps herself busy with housework to avoid thinking about money.

PSYCHOTHERAPY BY THE PSYCHOANALYSTS

The psychoanalyst uses dream analysis, free association, and interpretation of behavior. The idea is that if clients understand the reasons for their anxiety, their anxieties and conflicts will resolve. Freud thought that if clients were able to remember problematic situations they had repressed, and put the memories into words, these memories would lose their power (Carson, 2000).

Freud started the practice of talking with clients about their problems. This concept (that people are best understood when they talk with the therapist about their problems) continues today. Currently psychoanalysis is practiced only on a very limited basis.

NURSING IMPLICATIONS

Freud's concept of defense mechanisms is still well accepted and often used to explain behavior. These mechanisms can help nurses to understand their own behavior as well as the behavior of their clients.

The behavior associated with defense mechanisms can be either **adaptive behavior** (positive, health promoting, problem solving) or **maladaptive behavior** (unhealthy and does not promote problem solving). Whether the behavior is adaptive or not depends on the mechanism and how it is used. For example, the person with hypertension who rationalizes his high-sodium, high-fat diet to the nurse by saying, "It doesn't really matter what I eat, I'm taking medication," is using *rationalization* in an unhealthy or maladaptive way. The student who exercises after school to help manage the stress of college is using *sublimation* in an adaptive way (see Table 3-1 again for the definitions of these mechanisms).

When a client is using a defense mechanism maladaptively, the nurse should bring this process to the attention of the client. For example, the nurse should confront a person with alcohol dependency who continuously denies a problem despite negative consequences. Clear recognition of *denial* (or other maladaptive mechanisms) can give clients the insight they need to begin to work on changing behavior. The next step for the nurse is to discuss adaptive options for the client to use for stress reduction.

Critical Self-Check. Which of these defense mechanisms do you use? Are your defense mechanisms adaptive or maladaptive? Why?

Ego Theories

Carl Jung, Karen Horney, Erik Erikson, and others began with Freud's ideas and went on to create their own theories of personality. As a group these are called the *ego theories*.

CARL JUNG

Jung's theory (called *analytic psychology*) divided the mind into the conscious ego, the personal conscious, and the collective unconscious. He described the *collective unconscious* as psychic elements or memories inherited through generations via an unconscious channel and shared with all humans. He introduced the idea that culture plays an important role in personal development. Jung challenged parts of Freud's theory. Jung asserted that people's individual motives and goals were more important than sexual urges in determining the course of their lives.

ALFRED ADLER

Alfred Adler was interested in the need for a sense of autonomy and control. He was the first to use the term *inferiority complex* to describe people who are so frustrated in their attempts to succeed (or "strive for superiority" in his theory) that they give up trying. He was also the first to include social influences as important factors in development of personality.

Adler studied the effects of birth order on personality development. He found that first-born children strive to regain the status they once had as only children. They tend to be leaders, nurturers, and high achievers. Second-born children experience rivalry from the beginning, so they seek competition and strive for greater achievements. Last-born children, according to Adler, are more pampered than the other children. They have more sibling role models for comparison and may feel overly pressured to succeed in every area achieved by their siblings.

KAREN HORNEY

Karen Horney was a German theorist born near the end of the 19th century. In her time, femininity was associated with passivity, weakness, frailty, and inferiority. Masculinity was associated with strength, courage, competence, and freedom. One of her contributions to personality theory was to disprove Freud's concept of "penis envy." She found that women are not motivated by envy of having a penis, but from the desire to have the qualities associated with maleness.

Horney also proposed the concept of "basic anxiety," which she described as a child's fear of being helpless and alone. She connected the development of a "passive style," "aggressive style," or "withdrawn style" of personality to how children were treated and how they resolved their basic anxieties.

Her ideas form the foundation of modern child-rearing practices that emphasize a warm and respecting environment to promote healthy personality development

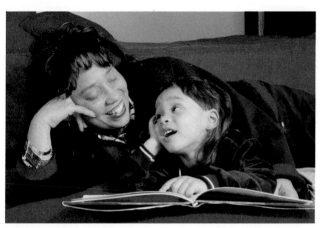

Figure 3-3. ■ Horney's theory states that to promote healthy development parents must treat a child with care, respect, gentleness, and generosity. *Source:* The Image Works.

(Figure 3-3 ■). Karen Horney's theory is at work when nurses teach parents that children "learn what they live" and that to raise a healthy adaptive child, parents must treat the child with care, respect, gentleness, and generosity.

ERIK ERIKSON

Erik Erikson was born in Germany in 1902. His formal education ended there in high school (Carson, 2000). He studied psychoanalysis, worked in a day-care center founded by Anna Freud (Sigmund's daughter), and later worked in the United States with Henry Murray, who was interested in personality development throughout life. Erikson created his own personality theory based on *psychosocial development*. In it he described how identity develops in a series of eight stages that are built on each other (Erikson, 1963, 1980). Figure 3-4 ■ shows Erikson's developmental stages. Each of Erikson's stages represents a conflict or core problem that the individual strives to overcome at a critical period of development. A person must successfully resolve each conflict in order to master the next one (Wong, Hockenberry-Eaton, Wilson, Winkelstein, & Schwartz, 2001). The activities required for mastery of each of the eight stages in Erikson's psychosocial development theory are called **developmental tasks.**

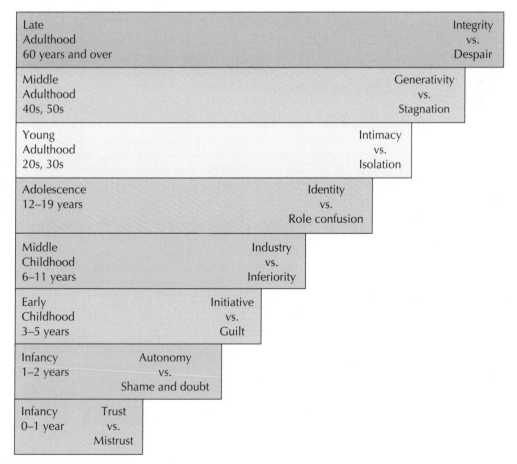

Figure 3-4. ■ Erikson's developmental stages. *Source: Human Development 4/E* by Rice F. Philips, © 2001. Reprinted by permission of Pearson Education, Inc., Upper Saddle River, NJ.

Each of Erikson's stages has two components: the successful and unsuccessful sides of the core conflict. At each developmental crisis point, the person either masters the developmental task successfully or fails to do so, with a negative outcome. For example, an adolescent either achieves the developmental task of identity or has the negative outcome of role confusion. Figure 3-5 ■ shows a group of adolescent boys who demonstrate their sense of identity with their peer group through their choice of clothing styles. Each step forward in development brings anxiety as the person moves out of old comfortable ways into new challenges and new ways of thinking about the self. Table 3-2 ■ provides a summary of Erikson's stages of psychosocial development.

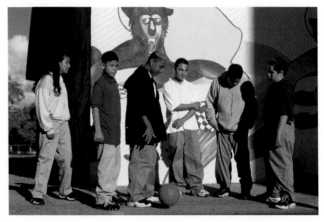

Figure 3-5. ■ Adolescents demonstrate peer group identity through clothing styles. *Source:* Will Hart.

TABLE 3-2			
Erikson's Stages of Psychosocial Development			
DEVELOPMENTAL CONFLICT	**AGE**	**CHARACTERISTICS**	**FAVORABLE OUTCOMES**
Trust versus Mistrust	Birth to 1 year	*Trust* is developed when the infant's needs are adequately and consistently met; parents are reliable. *Mistrust* happens when basic needs are inconsistently met.	Faith, hope, optimism
Autonomy versus Shame and Doubt	1–3 years	*Autonomy* is centered on children's ability to control their bodies and the environment. The use of their developing physical skills (toilet training, walking, manipulating objects) is important. *Shame and doubt* develop when the child is shamed or forced to be dependent in areas in which he or she is capable of independence.	Self-control, will
Initiative versus Guilt	3–6 years	Children at this stage are active and have powerful imagination. They develop a sense of *initiative* when they are able to pursue and reach their goals and to achieve a sense of purpose. They develop a conscience at this stage. *Guilt* develops when they are thwarted in their efforts or feel that their goals are bad.	Purpose, direction
Industry versus Inferiority	6–12 years	Interactions outside the family take on more importance. *Industry* happens when children are able to take on activities and projects that they can complete; achievement is important. They learn to cooperate and compete with others by the rules. *Inferiority* occurs when children fail to develop friendships or if they believe they cannot measure up to the expectations of others.	Competence
Identity versus Role Confusion	12–18 years	This is the stage associated with adolescence. *Identity* is characterized by integration of personal values with those of society, a clear sense of self in multiple roles, and by making choices about the future. *Role confusion* results from failure to establish an individual identity separate from the family and having no peer relationships or plans for an occupation.	Fidelity
Intimacy versus Isolation	Early adulthood	*Intimacy* develops when the person creates mature relationships, especially a love relationship with a partner. *Isolation* is the inability to create strong social ties without losing the self, or the inability to create intimate relationships at all.	Love

(continued)

TABLE 3-2			
Erikson's Stages of Psychosocial Development (continued)			
DEVELOPMENTAL CONFLICT	**AGE**	**CHARACTERISTICS**	**FAVORABLE OUTCOMES**
Generativity versus Stagnation	Adulthood	*Generativity* is a desire to improve society by one's own efforts. The person values work and helping others. This may take the form of raising children or community service with the goal of making the world a better place. *Stagnation* is characterized by the feeling that life is meaningless. The person in stagnation does not have concern for the flourishing of others.	Caring
Ego Integrity versus Despair	Maturity	When a person has developed wisdom over a lifetime of experiences and can look back to see a life of meaning and integrity they have achieved *integrity*, especially when they can pass this wisdom to younger generations. *Despair* is characterized by a sense of not accomplishing one's goals or maintaining one's values, and it is too late to do anything about it.	Wisdom

These conflicts are never solved completely but continue to be a challenge throughout life. For example, people who satisfactorily achieve a sense of trust (the first developmental task) will still be challenged to develop trust again in new situations, such as hospitalization. Initial success at trusting is a very important foundation for success in future challenging situations.

MARGARET MAHLER

Margaret Mahler proposed her ego theory in the 1970s. Her approach focuses on *separation-individuation* and is called an "object relations" theory. *Object relations* means that the person learns about the self through interaction with others. She believed that forming ties with the mother was critical for a child to develop psychological health.

Initially, an infant begins with total dependence on the mother and then matures to discover a sense of self and individual perspective on the world. During Mahler's ambivalence phase, the child begins the process of individuation-separation. In this phase the child has temper tantrums, moodiness, and strong reactions to separation from parents. The child is ambivalent, wanting both to be with the parent and to be separate. At 2 to 3 years of age, the child discovers that the parent is a separate individual or "object." With this revelation comes the ability to see others as separate individuals. Individuation allows the child to develop a sense of being a separate person who has empathy for the feelings of others. Mahler added the importance of mothering skills to the information known about healthy emotional development.

PSYCHOTHERAPY BY THE EGO THEORISTS

The goal of psychotherapy according to the ego theorists is to establish increasing levels of independence by assisting the ego or self to overcome developmental obstacles. The blocks to development in these theories often occur during the toddler period.

The therapeutic process includes the client talking with the therapist and working to develop insight into reasons for anxiety. The emphasis is on clients studying their own stories and understanding their own inner motivations and self-concept.

Play therapy is frequently used with children who are experiencing trauma or grief. Melanie Klein, a British psychiatrist, developed play therapy. In this therapy, toys or arts and crafts are used in the same way that dream analysis or free association are used by the ego theorists with adults. Children express their feelings and work out their conflicts in play.

NURSING IMPLICATIONS

Erikson's psychosocial development theory is perhaps the most commonly accepted theory of personality development. It is widely used in nursing as a basis for assessing clients' developmental level, for identifying developmental needs, and for planning nursing interventions to promote the development of clients. For example, if a pediatric client in the stage of Industry versus Inferiority is hospitalized, what kind of activities would the nurse provide for this client? The activity should promote the child's achievement of the developmental task of Industry. This developmental task requires the child to do projects that provide a sense of accomplishment. A puzzle or a craft project could promote this child's development. Remember, people of all ages are developing, so nurses can promote healthy development in clients of any age.

Erikson's psychosocial stages are also used in nursing to understand the client's priority concerns. Consider the case of two different clients with the same medical diagnosis: fractured femur. One is a 2-year-old boy and the other is a 40-year-old man. The child's developmental stage is Autonomy versus Shame and Doubt. His developmental task is to be independent of his parents. Without the fracture he would be walking or running all over the place. So, mobility is a priority for this child. He may benefit from a specially made walker or other mobility device that enables him to be mobile. In contrast, the 40-year-old is in the stage of Generativity versus Stagnation. His developmental task (Generativity) requires that he get back to work. If he has a "desk" job, maybe work can be brought home for him. If not, perhaps his job can be modified until he recovers (maybe he can answer the phone). The adult has different priorities than the child because of his developmental tasks.

Knowing the client's developmental priorities helps the nurse understand the client's motivation for learning. Clients will probably be most motivated to learn anything that helps them accomplish their developmental tasks. The 40-year-old man will probably be motivated to comply with any treatment that will help him get back to work. He may be less motivated to learn about other subjects, such as preventing future problems or starting general health promotion activities.

Critical Self-Check. When a nurse sits down with an elderly client and listens to the client's stories about her lessons from life, how is the nurse promoting the development of this client?

Biological Theories

The biological theorists believe that people are born with certain *predispositions* (tendencies) and abilities that affect personality. Unlike the other theorists who assert that the environment and life experiences shape personality, the biological theorists state that people are born with what makes them individuals. In other words, the forces that create personality are biological. The way people respond to stress, their susceptibility to developing mental disorders, even how they feel and act are caused by genetic, chemical, and physiological forces.

HANS EYSENCK

Hans Eysenck, a British psychologist, developed a biologically based personality theory. Eysenck's idea is that some people inherently have a relatively low level of brain arousal. These people seek stimulation and are termed *extroverts*. Other people have a higher level of central nervous system stimulation in general, so they tend to shy away from stimulating environments. These people are called *introverts*. Eysenck acknowledges the difficulty of measuring "brain arousal" but observes that there are physiological differences between introverts and extroverts, such as brain and skin electrical activity (Friedman & Schustack, 1999).

Eysenck is a biological theorist because he thinks that human personality is rooted in our genetics (our nature). Studies of twins are especially helpful in pursuit of answers to the **nature or nurture controversy** (debate about whether personality is due to biology or to environment and experiences). Identical twins raised apart have sometimes been found to have surprisingly similar attitudes and behaviors (such as the same career choices). This would suggest a strong genetic control of personality. Twins, whether *identical* (formed from one egg) or *fraternal* (formed from two eggs), have been found to be less alike in personality as they get older. This finding suggests that environment is important. However, some identical twins are not *concordant* (both affected) by genetic-predisposition diseases such as schizophrenia and depression. This suggests that genetics is not the only thing that determines how a person feels and behaves. The real answer to the nature or nurture controversy is that both biology and the environment, and the interaction between them, affect personality development.

There is a danger in accepting a purely biological explanation of personality. At its extreme, the biological theory negates personal responsibility for behavior. It claims that people have no control over their behavior. If people are truly biologically destined to act in certain ways and have no free will to affect their own destiny, then there is no hope for rehabilitation. Most biological theorists do not take this extreme view. Instead, they state that personality results from biological influences as well as environmental factors. Personality is shaped by an interaction between nature and nurture.

THERAPEUTIC PERSPECTIVE

The best evidence that biology affects thinking and behavior is found in psychopharmacology. Ever since the 1950s when antipsychotic drugs came into use, it has been clear that disorders of thought and mood (schizophrenia and the mood disorders) respond to medications. Because it is known that these drugs affect the functions of brain **neurotransmitters** (chemicals that transmit impulses from one neuron to the next in the brain), it is reasoned that thought and mood are controlled by these neurotransmitters (see Chapter 7, "Psychobiology and Psychopharmacology").

The effectiveness of medication therapy for mental disorders has been a great breakthrough in the quality of life for the people involved, but medications are not the only answer. The facts are that (1) drugs do not help everyone, (2) people are not completely cured by them, (3) individuals respond differently to drugs, and (4) other approaches to treatment are also effective. Therefore, mental illness and behavior are much more than a simple result of biochemistry.

NURSING IMPLICATIONS

Nurses are highly involved in biological treatment methods, especially psychopharmacology. Nurses collaborate with physicians who prescribe psychotropic drugs. Nurses administer medications, monitor the response of the client, and teach the client how to manage medications at home. Nurses are uniquely positioned to be key members of the healthcare team related to the client's medication therapy.

Nurses take a holistic approach to client care, whatever the client's diagnosis. Nursing theories recognize the client as a whole person made of mind, body, and spirit, who is influenced by internal (biological) and external (environmental) factors.

Trait Theories

Trait theories attempt to summarize and predict human behavior by identifying universal personality traits. Friedman and Schustack (1999) describe one well-accepted perspective on personality traits called the Big Five. In this theory there are five basic and *universal* (true across culture, gender, and age) personality traits:

- *Extroversion:* Extroverted people tend to be energetic, enthusiastic, dominant, sociable, and talkative. The other side of this dimension is **introversion.** Introverted people tend to be shy, retiring, submissive, and quiet.
- *Agreeableness:* Agreeable people tend to be friendly, cooperative, trusting, and warm. People low on this dimension, who are **disagreeable,** tend to be argumentative, cold, and unkind.

- *Conscientiousness:* Conscientious people are steady, cautious, dependable, organized, and responsive. **Impulsive** people tend to be undependable, careless, and disorderly.
- *Emotional stability:* Emotionally stable people are relaxed and contented. **Emotionally unstable** (formerly called *neurotic*) people tend to be nervous, anxious, high-strung, and worrisome.
- *Openness:* Open people tend to be imaginative, creative, and witty. People low in this dimension, **closed,** are simple, plain, or superficial.

PSYCHOTHERAPY BY TRAIT THEORISTS

Trait theory can be used to understand the client's abilities and uniqueness. Personality styles and skills can be tested. The therapist would determine which characteristics of the person are modifiable and which are not and would counsel the client how to act on the problematic traits that are subject to change. The principle is that goals and skills are subject to change, but basic temperaments are not.

NURSING IMPLICATIONS

If certain traits are innate to our basic disposition, and personal goals are modifiable, then nurses can use this knowledge to help people plan realistic goals. For example, consider a client who has been injured and must change careers. He asks the rehabilitation nurse for advice. The client is introverted, disagreeable, conscientious, emotionally stable, and closed. Since these traits are very difficult to change, the best advice for this client is not to pursue a career in child care, nursing, or retail sales because he does not enjoy or work well with people. He might be best suited for a job that requires skill with details (he is conscientious) but little contact with people, such as data processing, accounting, or computer applications.

Nurses may also use the knowledge that personality traits are constant as a basis for understanding individual client variations and learning needs. Clients may find it easier or harder to learn some new things (such as how to assertively tell the physician about their needs) or to change certain behaviors (such as poor planning for diet needs related to medication use) based on their personality traits.

Behaviorist and Learning Theories

The *behaviorist theories* are based on the idea that a behavior persists if it is positively reinforced. The behaviorists believe that personality is completely shaped by an individual's life experiences. Therapy intended to change a behavior includes planning and practicing a new behavior that will be reinforced so the desired behavior will continue.

IVAN PAVLOV

Ivan Pavlov was a Russian physiologist who studied *classical conditioning*. He regularly rang a bell when he gave food to hungry dogs, and they salivated. Eventually when he rang the bell the dogs would salivate even when there was no food. This is a classic experiment in learned behavior. Pavlov's research created the basis for *learning* or *behavioral* approaches to personality.

B. F. SKINNER

B. F. Skinner, an American born in 1904, was one of the most famous *behaviorists*. He rejected any idea of biological foundations for personality. His principle of *operant conditioning* stated that behavior is changed by its consequences. If a student is reinforced by receiving an "A" every time he writes with a blue pen, he will continue the blue-pen-using behavior even after a clear cause and effect have stopped. Skinner believed that people have no free will to determine their behavior: all behavior is the result of reinforcement. The value of a reinforcer comes from its meaning to an individual. One person might respond to praise, another to prizes, or grades, or privileges. Skinner found that an intermittent pattern of reinforcement was the most effective approach to making behavior continue. He also found that learned undesirable behaviors could be changed, again by reinforcement of desired behavior. This process of ending learned behavior is called *extinction*.

Much of the research on classical conditioning was done on rats and pigeons, demonstrating that there are universal rules affecting the behavior of animals. Some psychologists believe that the behavioral theories minimize the uniqueness of human potential.

BEHAVIORAL THERAPY

The behaviorists take a training approach to changing behavior. Each new desired behavior is rewarded with a reinforcement that is valuable to the client. Undesirable behavior is not reinforced.

Assertiveness training is a behavioral approach. Consider the case of a client who has a history of acting passively. Her need for information from her physician is not met, because she never asks questions. With her therapist or nurse, she plans to act assertively. When the assertive act is accomplished (telling the doctor that she does not understand some instructions and asking for an explanation), the client will receive reinforcement (the information she wants). Repeating the desired behavior (and the reinforcement) many times in different situations is required to establish the new behavior of assertiveness.

Desensitization is a behaviorist approach to treating *phobias* (persistent irrational fears). In this technique the client is exposed to the feared object in small stages, achieving success many times, until the fear is finally confronted fully. As an example, if a person has a phobia of snakes, the therapist may begin with a photograph of a snake. The client is reinforced with praise for looking at it and talking about it. They progress through seeing a toy snake, to seeing a real snake in a cage, and finally to actually touching a snake.

NURSING IMPLICATIONS

Nurses use a behaviorist approach whenever they give positive reinforcement to clients for desirable healthy behavior. Behavior modification with positive reinforcement is often used with children (the nurse may give a colorful sticker when the child is cooperative with a procedure).

Negative reinforcement is not commonly used. One example of behavior therapy with negative reinforcement is the drug disulfiram (Antabuse), which makes people violently ill when they drink alcohol.

Relaxation training is another example of the behaviorist approach. The client is taught to relax the muscles from one end of the body to the other. The client feels the calm and relaxing sensation progressing over the body, until the entire body feels loose and rested. The relaxation behavior is thus positively reinforced.

Cognitive Theories of Personality

Charles Darwin's theory of evolution stimulated thinking about the human mind as a biological entity instead of the unchangeable creation of a divine being. This new way of thinking inspired a great deal of discussion and research in cognitive psychology.

Cognition is the mental process by which knowledge is acquired and processed, including reasoning, judgment, memory, awareness, and perception. The cognitive theorists believe that it is human perception, thinking, and judgment that make us human.

GESTALT THEORY

Gestalt (which means *pattern* in German) psychology is a cognitive approach. The central idea in Gestalt psychology is that the complex pattern or arrangement of an experience is its essence. The essence of a complex experience is lost when it is taken apart for analysis of its parts. The main ideas in Gestalt theory are:

- Human beings seek meaning in their lives.
- People organize the stimuli they receive from the world around them into perceptions that have meaning to them.
- Complex experiences are more than the sum of their parts.

JEAN PIAGET

Jean Piaget, a Swiss biologist turned psychologist, developed a theory in the 1960s about the cognitive development of children. He described four stages (*schemas*) of intellectual development, with each stage building on the previous one. Piaget's stages of cognitive development are summarized as follows:

Sensorimotor Stage (Birth to 2 Years)

In this stage simple learning is governed by sensations. Children begin with reflex activity and then mature through simple repetitive behavior to imitative behavior. As they direct behavior toward objects, they develop a sense of "cause and effect" (when I turn the cup over, the water falls out). They are very curious; they enjoy new experiences; they experiment; they mainly solve problems by trial and error. They begin to develop a sense of themselves as different from their environment. They begin to understand *object permanence*, which means that an object continues to exist even when it is not visible. Children begin to use language and representational thought at the end of the sensorimotor period.

Preoperational Stage (2–7 Years)

In this stage children are *egocentric* (they are unable to imagine themselves in the place of another). They interpret events and objects in terms of their own relationship with or use for them. They can't understand another's point of view, and they can't see any reason to do so. Preoperational thinking is concrete and tangible. Children cannot reason beyond what they observe in this stage. They are not able to make deductions or generalizations. Their thoughts are largely about what they experience. They are increasingly able to use language to represent objects in their environment. Their reasoning becomes *intuitive* toward the end of this stage (The sun wakes up like I do). They begin to consider problems of time, weight, length, and size. Their reasoning is also *transductive*: because two events occur together they cause each other, or knowledge in one situation is transferred to another (e.g., "All men are daddies").

Concrete Operations Stage (7–11 Years)

Concrete operational thinking is more logical and coherent. Children are able to classify, sort, order, and organize facts and objects. They are able to organize facts for use in problem solving. They develop *conservation*, the concept that physical factors (volume, weight, and number) remain the same even though the outward appearance is changed. (The same amount of water is in an 8-ounce cup as in an 8-ounce bowl.) They are able to deal with different factors simultaneously. They are not able to think abstractly. They solve problems in a concrete, systematic way. Their reasoning is *inductive*: making a generalization from particular facts. Thoughts become less self-centered. They think in a more social way and can consider others' points of view.

Formal Operations Stage (11–15 Years)

This stage is characterized by adaptability and flexibility. In this stage people can use abstract thinking and symbols. They are able to do logical problem solving, considering multiple variables. They can make hypotheses and test them. They can consider theoretical and philosophical matters. They are able to resolve contradictions. They are able to imagine the thoughts of others. People who use formal operational thinking are no longer constrained by what is; they can consider what might be (Hockenberry, 2005).

HOWARD GARDNER

Part of cognitive personality theory is how people perceive the world around them and how they try to interpret and understand the world. Howard Gardner, an educational psychologist, proposed a theory of multiple intelligences. He says that the custom of measuring intelligence simply by IQ intelligence testing is much too limited. According to Gardner's theory, just as people vary in their traditional IQ-type intelligence, they vary in their abilities in the multiple ways of knowing about the world (intelligences). The different intelligences are:

- Language
- Logical-mathematical analysis
- Spatial representation
- Musical thinking
- Bodily-kinesthetic intelligence (body coordination and control of movement)
- Understanding self (intrapersonal)
- Understanding others (interpersonal)
- Naturalistic

Gardner's idea is that people have different strengths and potentials in each of the domains of intelligence (Gardner, 1999).

Critical Self-Check. Look at Gardner's multiple intelligences. Do you agree with Gardner that intelligence should be assessed more broadly to predict human potential than by traditional intelligence tests alone? Why? Do you have more intelligence in some of these areas than others?

ALBERT BANDURA

Albert Bandura is a social cognitive theorist who formulated what is known as *social learning theory*. Bandura found that not all behavior is explained in simple stimulus-response terms. He believed that human psychology is more complicated. His idea is that psychological functioning is the result of an interaction between personal attributes and environmental conditions.

Bandura proposed that people learn best by observing the performance of others and then by modeling the behavior (Carson, 2000). One of his most important contributions to personality psychology is his explanation of *observational learning*. He described situations in which people can learn without acting out a behavior themselves, but by watching others.

Bandura and his colleagues performed a famous study on how children learn aggressive behavior. In this study children were shown adults either acting neutrally or aggressively (hitting, kicking, punching) toward a large plastic clown doll. When they were allowed to play with the doll themselves, the children who saw the aggressive behavior were more likely to act aggressively. When the children saw the adult rewarded for the aggression, they were even more likely to act aggressively themselves. Children who saw the aggressive adult punished were less likely to behave aggressively than the other children. But seeing the aggressive behavior rewarded was not necessary to bring on increased aggression. The children who saw unrewarded aggression were more likely to act aggressively than children who saw the same adult act in a neutral manner (Friedman & Schustack, 1999). Bandura found that people are more likely to copy behavior that they believe will lead to a positive outcome. Television is considered by many to show situations to children in which violence is positively rewarded (Figure 3-6 ■).

Critical Self-Check. What does Bandura's observational learning research suggest about the effect of television violence on children?

Bandura's research on self-efficacy is important for nursing. **Self-efficacy** is the belief that a person is able to cause a desired outcome (reach a goal) by his or her own efforts. Positive self-efficacy is the attitude that one will be able to

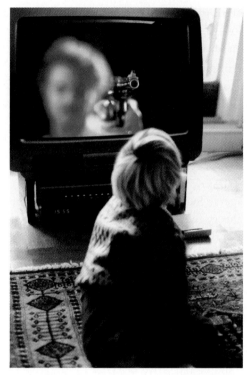

Figure 3-6. ■ Children who see violence positively reinforced are more likely to act aggressively. *Source:* Edourd Berne/Stone/Getty Images.

perform a task or behavior successfully. Without a sense of self-efficacy, clients believe that they are ineffective and that there is nothing they can do to change their lives. Bandura suggested that all psychotherapeutic treatment should have the goal of "strengthening expectations of personal efficacy" (Bandura, 1977, p. 193). He wrote that the more self-efficacy people feel, the more motivated and persistent they will be toward reaching a goal.

COGNITIVE PSYCHOTHERAPY

All the cognitive approaches share the view that human perception and human cognition (thinking) are at the center of what it means to be human. Cognitive therapists are not interested in unconscious or emotional motivations for behavior. Their goal is rational decision making through understanding thought processes.

Gestalt Therapy

Gestalt therapy focuses on the overall general meanings of client situations and behavior. These therapists do not look for unconscious or childhood meanings, but for the general significance of experiences to clients. Role-playing is sometimes used. For example, if a client feels bad because his mother died before he could tell her something, the Gestalt therapist may have the client tell his feelings to an empty chair, as though his mother were sitting there listening. This process allows the client to formulate thoughts and feelings into words, to express them, and to have a sense of closure about the issue.

Cognitive Therapy

Cognitive therapy seeks to change thought processes. The therapist is a teacher and a coach. The client learns new ways of thinking and problem solving. In current psychotherapy, cognitive and behavioral therapy techniques are combined in cognitive-behavioral therapy (CBT). CBT is one of the most effective psychotherapeutic approaches.

NURSING IMPLICATIONS

Nurses frequently engage in a cognitive approach while gaining clients' cooperation, while collaborating with the client to plan learning goals, and in client teaching. When teaching, nurses often emphasize how clients will use the information they are learning to promote their self-care. This is a critical part of empowering people to participate actively in their treatment.

When teaching clients, knowledge of cognitive development is especially important to nurses. Teaching must be consistent with a client's cognitive level. For example, diabetic teaching plans for 7-year-olds and 17-year-olds would have to be different based on the clients' different cognitive levels. Teaching for 7-year-olds would include concrete instruction about what they need to do in the short term, how to test blood glucose, and how to inject insulin. Teaching for 17-year-olds could also include the pathophysiology of the disease, consequences of nonadherence with the treatment plan, and planning how to do blood glucose checks while they are at school.

Cognitive therapy is used when the nurse corrects an error in the client's thinking. If a client believes that she is unable to follow her new treatment plan for arthritis management because it is too complicated, the nurse can show the client how to plan her activities and schedule her medications effectively. The client's perception of inadequacy in this situation was in error and the nurse helped her see her capability to follow her treatment plan.

Promoting a positive sense of self-efficacy is an important contribution of nurses. People who do not believe that they can perform health-promoting behaviors effectively are less likely to try them. In mental health nursing, where many of our clients have reduced energy and motivation, promoting self-efficacy is an especially

important part of client empowerment. We can promote self-efficacy in clients by:

- Being role models for healthy behavior
- Encouraging desirable behavior and discouraging undesirable behavior
- Allowing clients to talk about how they feel about behavior change
- Creating situations in which our clients can have positive experiences with health-promoting behavior

Existential and Humanistic Theories

Existential philosophy seeks the meaning of life or of human existence. The existentialists are more subjective than other theorists. One aspect of existential thought is *phenomenology*, the study of people's subjective experiences or perceptions. Existential theories claim that physical laws are not enough to explain the complexities of human behavior. The existentialists consider creativity, individual initiative, and self-fulfillment as important personality factors.

VIKTOR FRANKL

Viktor Frankl, who survived a Nazi concentration camp, was an existential-humanistic theorist. He emphasized the importance of personal choice. He stated that people can choose to grow, even when faced with terrible realities, and that existential struggle can result in triumph of the spirit. His theory is called *logotherapy* (the search for meaning). Frankl also emphasized the magnitude of love. He describes discovering "the truth—that love is the ultimate and the highest goal to which man can aspire—*the salvation of man is through love and in love*" (Frankl, 1963, pp. 58–59).

CARL ROGERS

The *humanistic* theories of personality focus on the personal worth of the individual and the essential role of human values. Carl Rogers, a humanistic psychologist, developed *client-centered therapy* in the 1950s. His theory marked a shift in theories about interpersonal development. One of the major contributions of Rogers was to offer a better understanding of the treatment of psychological problems. He emphasized the personal, subjective, and experiential aspects of human existence. He proposed that it is the client, not the therapist, who best understands what the problems are and what will help.

Like the existentialists, Rogers defined a person as a work in progress, a process of changing potentials, not a predetermined outcome or a finished product. His perspective is that people must come to terms with their own nature, their real selves. He urged his clients to experience and get in touch with their own feelings and to base their behavior on their ethical principles. He stressed personal responsibility and self-enhancement.

ABRAHAM MASLOW

Unlike many previous theorists who focused on pathology, Abraham Maslow focused on human needs and the most highly evolved state of human development. He and his colleagues identified human needs and placed them in five categories in a hierarchy, often represented by a pyramid (Figure 3-7 ■).

The base of the hierarchy is physiological needs. These needs must be met before the person may work to achieve the next level. Physiological needs at their most basic include air, food, and water. Other physiological needs include sleep, exercise, elimination, and sexual expression. Imagine a person living in severe poverty who has no access to food. This person must satisfy his need for food before he can focus on higher level needs, even the need to be safe. The hungry person will take risks to obtain food.

The next level is safety and security needs. These needs are characterized by avoiding harm, freedom from fear,

physical safety, and maintaining comfort. A person must feel safe from danger before being able to concentrate on higher needs. Love and belonging needs come next. These needs include companionship, interpersonal relationships, giving and receiving affection, and affiliation with groups. Religious needs are part of this level. Esteem needs have both internal and external components. From others, people need respect, recognition, attention, and appreciation. From ourselves, we need self-esteem, confidence, a sense of freedom, dignity, and self-respect (Maslow, 1968).

Maslow's ultimate level of human development is self-actualization. He describes self-actualized people as those who have realized their own potential, who prefer being themselves rather than being pretentious or artificial. They are self-directed, creative, and flexible. Self-actualized people can transcend themselves and connect with something beyond the self or help others find self-fulfillment and realize their potential (Maslow & Lowery, 1998).

Current evolutionary theorists reject Maslow's idea that humans are the most highly evolved animals. Many also disagree with his description of the highest level of human development. His self-centered, independent vision is not consistent with the attitudes of cultures outside Europe and the United States, or even with the

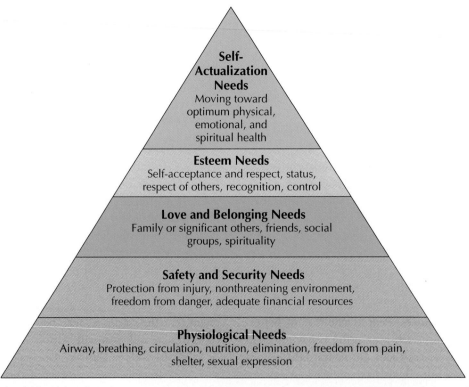

Figure 3-7. ■ Maslow's hierarchy of needs. *Source:* Craig, G. J. (2002). *Human development, 9e.* Upper Saddle River: Prentice Hall. p. 474, figure 14-2.

attitudes of many women. Current theorists reject the idea that a desire for relationships instead of independence is a weakness of women. However, Maslow's concept of prioritizing needs continues to be widely accepted.

HUMANISTIC PSYCHOTHERAPY

Carl Rogers's client-centered therapy is based on an open and accepting attitude by the therapist. The therapist is genuine, empathic, and offers unconditional positive regard.

Humanistic therapy encourages self-knowledge (insight) and authenticity in relationships. The goals of therapy are overcoming the crisis of discovering meaning in life and finding self-actualization, love, and dignity. Therapy is often conducted in groups. Humanistic therapists may encourage creative expression. They may encourage public service to combat alienation. Clients engaged in humanistic therapy are expected to take responsibility for their own behavior.

NURSING IMPLICATIONS

Humanism is an excellent foundation for nursing care. Nurses ideally provide holistic, nonjudgmental care to every client. Nurses provide clients with unconditional positive regard. We respect our clients' opinions about their problems and include clients in planning the goals for their care. We respect their diverse cultural backgrounds (Box 3-1 ■). Modern nurses in all settings consider clients to be active participants in their care when they take responsibility for and experience the consequences of their own behavior.

Maslow's hierarchy provides nurses with a basis for prioritizing client needs and nursing interventions. If a client has low self-esteem and also has inadequate nutrition, the nutritional needs must take priority because they are lower (more basic) on Maslow's hierarchy. These needs must be met before the client is able to focus on esteem, and before nursing plans for esteem-building are implemented.

BOX 3-1	CULTURAL PULSE POINTS

Transcultural Assessment Model

Culture is beliefs, values, and behaviors that have been learned and passed down from one generation to the next. The definition sounds tame, but people are willing to fight and die for these cultural issues. If you value your family, your religious beliefs, your political views and way of life, you understand the power of culture.

Every nurse must know about culture to make it possible to provide culturally appropriate and competent care. Culturally competent care is the adaptation of nursing care in a way that is compatible with the client's culture. To deliver this care, the nurse must know that each individual is unique and a product of past experiences and cultural learning. It is impossible for nurses to memorize specific information about the health beliefs and behaviors of every human culture (there are hundreds). Even if we could, we would be memorizing stereotypes and not allowing for individuals to vary from the most common attitudes of their culture. Fortunately, Giger and Davidhizar have formulated a model for assessment of culture that includes the six characteristics

affecting health behavior that are common to all cultures (see also Figure 3-8 ■):
1. **Communication** (verbal and nonverbal language, use of silence, pronunciation, voice quality)
2. **Space** (degree of comfort with closeness to others, body movement, perception of space)
3. **Social organization** (ethnicity, family and gender roles, work, leisure, religion, friends)
4. **Time** (use of time, measures of time, definition, social time, work time, time orientation: future, present, or past)
5. **Environmental control** (values, definition of health and illness, attitudes about who controls health such as physician, God, or client)
6. **Biological variations** (body structure, skin and hair color, physical characteristics, genetics, susceptibility to illness, nutritional preferences and tolerances, psychological characteristics)

Source: Reprinted from *Transcultural Nursing: Assessment and Intervention, 4/E*, J. N. Giger and R. E. Davidhizar, "Transcultural Assessment Model." © 2004 Mosby, with permission from Elsevier.

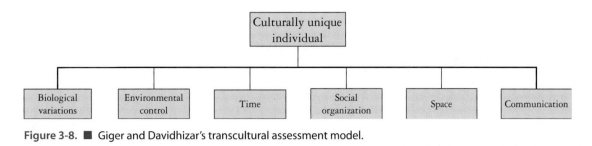

Figure 3-8. ■ Giger and Davidhizar's transcultural assessment model.

Interpersonal Theories

The *interpersonal theorists* believe that personality constantly changes as a result of interaction with others.

HARRY STACK SULLIVAN AND HILDEGARD PEPLAU

Harry Stack Sullivan studied people in the context of their relationships with other people. He theorized that personality is determined by interpersonal situations. He and his followers believed that society is the cause of people's problems. More recent interpersonal theorists have added the concept that people learn from their experiences with their environment and may change the way they react over time.

Hildegard Peplau, the mental health nurse theorist, is an interpersonal theorist. In the 1950s she was the first nurse to identify psychiatric-mental health nursing as an essential part of general nursing and as a specialty area. Peplau was the first nurse theorist to propose the nurse-client relationship as the foundation of nursing practice.

Hildegard Peplau is a powerful influence on current thinking about the profession of nursing. She proposed a shift in the *paradigm* (model or standard) that defined nursing in terms of the medical model to an interpersonal model of nursing (Peplau, 1989).

INTERPERSONAL PSYCHOTHERAPY

In the interpersonal approach the therapist helps the client develop trusting relationships, first with the therapist then with others. The client shares anxieties with the therapist. The therapist uses empathy to perceive the client's feelings and uses the relationship as a corrective interpersonal experience. The relationship between the client and therapist helps develop feelings of security and relieve feelings of anxiety.

NURSING IMPLICATIONS

Peplau's theory offers an explanation about how nurses can help clients make positive changes in their health and well-being. She suggests that nurses must become participant observers in therapeutic interactions with clients. Nurses collect assessment data by interacting directly with the client. Nurses must be aware of their own role in the therapeutic interaction and of the role the client may be expecting them to fulfill, such as friend, parent, love object, or participant in the client's problem. None of these roles is useful in providing nursing care to clients. Therefore, Peplau asserts that the social and personal needs of the nurse should not be a part of the nurse-client relationship (Carson, 2000).

Peplau outlined three phases of the nurse-client relationship:

- Orientation phase (expectations discussed and goals set)
- Working phase (identification of the problem and use of the process to enhance the client's personal growth)
- Resolution or termination phase (relationship is terminated, outcomes summarized)

She advocates a careful problem-solving approach to treatment. The nurse should first assist the client to identify and label current anxieties, encouraging self-understanding. The next step is for the nurse to help the client identify strategies to relieve the experience of anxiety. Third, the nurse assists the client to determine the causes of the anxiety. The fourth step involves helping the client gain personal insight (understanding of client's own role) into the cause of the anxiety (Carson, 2000).

Note: The references and resources for this and all chapters have been compiled at the back of the book.

Chapter Review

 KEY TERMS

Use the audio glossary feature of the Companion Website to hear the correct pronunciation of the following key terms.

adaptive behavior

cognition

culture

defense mechanisms

developmental tasks

dissociation

holism

maladaptive behavior

nature or nurture controversy

neurotransmitters

personality

self-efficacy

KEY Points

- People feel, think, and behave in ways that are determined by a variety of internal and external factors.

- There are several theories of personality development. Each theory has its own therapeutic strategies. Current psychotherapy integrates a variety of approaches from different theories for the benefit of the client.

- Defense mechanisms distort reality to protect the self. Everybody uses them, adaptively or maladaptively.

- People must accomplish developmental tasks before they can move on to the next developmental level.

- Psychopharmacology (study of medications that affect thinking and behavior) is an important part of the biological theory of personality.

- The five universal personality traits are extroversion, agreeableness, conscientiousness, emotional stability, and openness. Each individual has each of these traits to a greater or lesser degree.

- Feelings, emotions, and behavior can be learned and changed.

- The six aspects of culture that affect health behavior are communication, space, social organization, time, environmental control, and biological variations.

- Because of the process of cognitive development, people learn differently at different ages.

- It is human to search for meaning in life.

- People are affected by relationships and interactions with other people.

- The nurse-client relationship is the foundation of nursing care.

- Everyone continues developing throughout life. Nurses can promote personal growth in clients of any age.

- Nursing care is holistic: it is concerned with the body, mind, and spirit of the client.

- Nurses must prioritize their actions, providing for the client's most basic needs first.

 EXPLORE MediaLink

Additional interactive resources for this chapter can be found on the Companion Website at www.prenhall.com/eby. Click on Chapter 3 and "Begin" to select the activities for this chapter.

- Audio glossary
- NCLEX-PN® review
- Case study
- Study outline
- Critical thinking questions
- Matching questions
- Weblinks

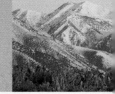

When a question asks you to prioritize assessments or interventions, use Maslow's hierarchy. The lower a need is on the pyramid, the higher its priority. Remember, physiological needs (breathing difficulties) are a higher priority than safety (falling out of bed).

1 As defined by Freud, the ego is that part of the mind that contains:

1. The basic instincts and urges.
2. The conscience.
3. The ability to respond to the realities of everyday life.
4. All elements of the holistic person.

2 A student who goes to the gym routinely after school to relieve the stress of studying is using the defense mechanism of:

1. Compensation.
2. Rationalization.
3. Sublimation.
4. Repression.

3 According to Erikson's theory of psychosocial development, children between the ages of 6 and 12 should be:

1. Beginning to develop consciences.
2. Disciplined for any incontinence episodes.
3. Competing with their peers following the rules of the game.
4. Integrating their personal values with those of society.

4 The successful use of antipsychotic medications indicates that there is validity to which theory of personality development?

1. Biological
2. Trait
3. Humanistic
4. Behaviorist

5 When a client who has a phobia against flying is shown videos of airplanes taking off and landing and photos taken from the windows of planes in flight, that client is being treated with which approach of the behaviorists?

1. Reality confrontation
2. Assertiveness
3. Desensitization
4. Reinforcement

6 Administering the drug disulfiram (Antabuse) to an alcoholic client to make him violently ill if he drinks alcohol while on the drug is an example of:

1. Reality confrontation.
2. Behavior modification.
3. Desensitization.
4. Positive reinforcement.

7 When nurses encourage desirable behavior in their clients and discourage undesirable behaviors, they are promoting _____ in their clients.

1. Self-efficacy
2. Assertiveness
3. Determinism
4. Dependence

8 A demanding client who is constantly putting the call light on for small, nonessential tasks, such as "fluffing" the pillow or straightening the covers, might be experiencing which human needs according to Maslow's hierarchy?

1. Physiological
2. Self-esteem
3. Love and belonging
4. Safety and security

9 A nurse who assists a client in discovering his own options for problem solving without telling him what to do is using which technique developed by Hildegard Peplau?

1. Interpersonal
2. Developmental
3. Behavior modification
4. Psychoanalytical

10 Based on Maslow's hierarchy of needs, number the following clients in the order of the priority of their needs, with 1 being the client whose need is the highest priority.

_____ A totally dependent client, whose side rails are lowered

_____ A client who requests the volunteer bring books from the hospital library

_____ A client who needs to be fed

_____ A client who has had a disfiguring accident

_____ A client who has had no visitors or phone calls since admission 3 days ago

Answers for Review Questions appear in Appendix I.

Chapter 4

Mentally Healthy Nursing

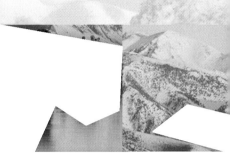

BRIEF Outline

Attributes of Caring
Burnout

LEARNING Outcomes

After completing this chapter, you will be able to:
1. Discuss ways to use caring in your nursing practice.
2. Identify factors that cause burnout in nurses.
3. Plan ways to prevent nursing burnout.
4. Plan strategies to promote your own mental health.

Caring is concern for the well-being of another. It is a universal human phenomenon that exists in all cultures. Each culture defines what caring behavior is and the meaning that caring conveys (Leininger, 1985).

Attributes of Caring

Caring forms the foundation of nursing practice (Watson, 1979). The attributes of caring are "the five Cs" (Roach, 1987). Figure 4-1 ■ illustrates the five Cs of caring. These attributes of caring include **commitment,** which is a personal pledge to a course of action, such as the choice to be a professional nurse or to provide the care necessary to meet each client's needs. **Compassion** involves sharing in the emotional state of another. It includes *empathy* (trying to understand how another feels) and acceptance of others as they are (not necessarily as we wish them to be). **Competence** is proficiency in understanding the principles underlying professional nursing practice and applying this knowledge to problem solving and decision making. It includes the ability to apply the nursing process. **Confidence** (belief in oneself) fosters a trusting relationship. A nurse must have self-confidence in order to foster the trust of clients. When clients trust that the nurse has the ability to help with their problems, they have confidence in the nurse. Finally, **conscience** is having an ethical conviction or belief about what is right and wrong and acting in accord with the ethics of the nursing profession.

Critical Self-Check. When a nurse is compassionate but incompetent, is this nurse caring for the clients? Why?

Caring is an important value in the nursing profession. Nursing standards require nurses to treat clients with respect, acceptance, competence, compassion, commitment, honesty, justice, support, and advocacy. All these add up to caring. If you are not capable of caring, you should not be a nurse.

NURSES UNDER STRESS

Nursing has a long history. Strong and visionary nurses came before us in our pursuit of caring for people. Although the idea that nurses care for other people has been around for a long time, the concept of nurses taking care of themselves is quite new.

Working as a nurse has always been challenging. Some of the challenges/stressors for nurses include the following:

■ *The work.* Nursing is hard work. Luckily we are not scrubbing floors anymore, but we work 8- to 12-hour shifts, around the clock (not to mention double shifts when we work overtime). The hospital is open and staffed by nurses 24 hours a day, 7 days a week. We lift, turn, and ambulate people who may be twice our size. As the healthcare delivery system changes, nurses are being expected to take responsibility for more clients who are more seriously ill and to delegate parts of their care to others. We also use more and more complex equipment to care for them (Figure 4-2 ■). The work is exhilarating and rewarding. It can also be exhausting.

■ *The profession.* As healthcare professionals, we expect ourselves not only to "be there" for our clients, but to do an excellent job of caring for them. Our nursing role involves caring, applying the nursing process, teaching, participating in the therapeutic environment, cooperating with others, promoting prevention activities, humanizing client care, and advocating for

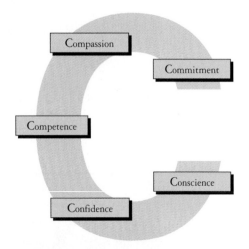

Figure 4-1. ■ The five Cs of caring.

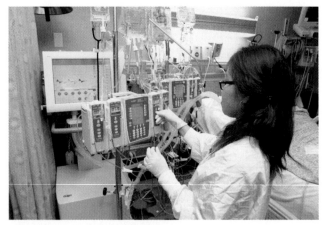

Figure 4-2. ■ The practice of nursing is becoming more focused on technology. *Source:* Phototake NYC.

clients. Meanwhile, our employer and our peers are evaluating us. They might say, "He is a really good nurse," or on a bad day they might say something else. Their opinions matter to us.

■ *The people.* Nurses love people, of course. They are why we went into nursing. But people can be challenging. Physicians and coworkers can be demanding, impatient, critical, and frustrating. Sick people can be all these things also and so can their families. Sometimes family members feel powerless to help the client. They may become demanding and critical of nurses in an attempt to exert some control over the situation (Lopez, 2007). Even when nurses know this, it is not easy to endure complaints and demands when we are working so hard to do our best. We know that we see clients at their worst, when they are in pain, anxious, or afraid. We try to make it easier for them, but they do not always recognize the contributions of nurses. Nurses are trying to please clients, families, coworkers, and supervisors. It is not easy (or possible) to keep everyone happy all the time.

■ *The feelings.* Nursing can be a heartbreaking profession. We see people die who should be alive and people for whom life itself seems a burden. Nurses work with people who are in the depths of suffering and grief. The clients see us, and we see ourselves, as the ones who come in to make a difficult or painful situation easier or more comfortable. Nurses ease human suffering, save lives, welcome babies into the world, and ease dying people out of it. Nurses really make a difference to people. What a great job! What a great responsibility!

Critical Self-Check. What does "nurses care from womb to tomb" mean?

Clearly, nursing is a powerful and satisfying job. There is no other quite like it. Just as nursing is an influential force to help people, it is also an incredible challenge for nurses themselves. Nurses give and give of themselves; it can be difficult to replenish the losses.

PERSONAL BOUNDARIES

The fact that nurses are caring people is not news. However, it is news that it is possible to "care too much." In their book *I'm Dying to Take Care of You* (what a great title!), Snow and Willard (1989) say that nurses often put the needs of others above their own needs. Nurses may allow themselves to be defined by others. Nurses may need the opinions of others to validate their

good intentions. We may also respond too sensitively to the stress created by those around us (clients, staff, and our own families).

We may lose our **personal boundaries,** the healthy limits people set on what is appropriate for them to do. Without healthy boundaries, nurses do things for people that they should do for themselves. An example is the nurse who calls in with an excuse for why her husband is sick when he really is drunk. Another is the nurse who works several double shifts in a row because the hospital asks him to, even though he is exhausted. Saying "no" to unreasonable requests from others requires boundaries.

Another reason that nurses need healthy personal boundaries is for the maintenance of professional relationships. Potential areas of boundary crossing with clients are as follows (Bunner & Yonge, 2006):

1. Touching
2. Gift giving
3. Self-disclosure

Touch can have many meanings, and the most important one is what the client thinks the touching means. An innocent hug by a nurse who feels sorry for a client can suggest to the client that the nurse loves him. When nurses accept gifts, they may be inadvertently communicating that they must be paid for their services. Most employers have a policy that prohibits individuals from accepting gifts from clients (for example, a box of candy may be accepted by the entire unit as a token of thanks from a client or family). Too much self-disclosure by the nurse moves the focus of the nurse-client relationship from the client, where it belongs, to the nurse, who is crossing personal boundaries by telling private things to clients. Maintaining healthy personal boundaries takes practice. It may help to talk with your peers or supervisor when you have doubts about the correct behavior in a certain situation.

CODEPENDENCY

Codependency, paraphrasing Beattie (1992), is letting another person's behavior affect you and becoming obsessed with controlling that person's behavior. Codependents make it possible for others to avoid the consequences of their own maladaptive behavior, thus encouraging the behavior to continue. Who are codependents? They are people who are in relationships with people who have substance abuse problems; they are people who love, care about, or work with troubled people. Many nurses are codependents. Melody Beattie (1992), who wrote *Codependent No More* and *Beyond Codependency*, warns that you may be in trouble with codependency:

- If concern has turned into obsession
- If compassion has turned into unhealthy care-taking
- If you are taking care of other people and not yourself

Acting in a codependent way means helping people avoid the consequences of their own actions. Codependents take on other people's responsibilities or enable people to avoid responsibility for their own behavior. In the classic example of codependency, a person worsens the substance dependency of a partner by making excuses, covering up problems, trying to control the partner, and allowing the habit to continue.

Codependency exists in the workplace as well. Nurses may ignore the erratic behavior that suggests that a colleague is impaired. We may allow physicians or supervisors to speak to us disrespectfully without pointing out their inappropriate behavior and encouraging them to change.

When a nurse tells a client with hypertension, "You're not doing so badly. Lots of people don't take their meds. I don't know what the doctor is so upset about," an opportunity is lost. Blaming the doctor, as the client blames his wife for cooking high-fat foods and for leaving the salt shaker on the table, takes the responsibility for the client's health away from him. He loses an opportunity to learn how to solve the problem adaptively. Box 4-1 ■ highlights the characteristics of codependency.

When a person interacts with a codependent, this individual may avoid the natural consequences of his or her behavior. As we learned in Chapter 3, behavior that is positively reinforced continues. When nurses allow the people in their lives to avoid natural consequences of their behavior, there is no opportunity for the individuals to change. Some people quit drinking when their children are disappointed in them and they lose their jobs. Others stop being verbally abusive when their behavior is not tolerated. Some clients begin to have healthy behav-

---

BOX 4-1

Characteristics of Codependency

Codependents may:
- feel responsible for other people's feelings, actions, well-being, and destiny.
- feel pity, anxiety, and guilt when other people have a problem.
- feel compelled to help other people solve their problems by giving unwanted advice, lots of suggestions, or "fixing their feelings."
- say yes when they mean no, do what they do not want to do, do more than their fair share of the work, and do things for other people that they can do for themselves.
- not know what they want or need or what their feelings are.
- try to please others instead of themselves.
- feel safest when giving and feel insecure and guilty when others give to them, rejecting compliments or praise.
- find themselves attracted to emotionally needy people and needy people attracted to them.
- feel bored or useless if they do not have a crisis or problem to solve.
- feel stressed, pressured, and overcommitted.
- feel angry, victimized, and used and blame others for their difficult position and their feelings.
- come from troubled or dysfunctional families.
- think they are not good enough and expect themselves to be perfect.
- fear rejection, especially if they show anger.

- have difficulty making decisions.
- get artificial feelings of self-worth from helping others.
- wish other people would like and love them and settle for being needed.
- focus all their energy on other people and their problems.
- wonder why they never get things done.
- feel controlled by events and people, especially other people's anger.
- ignore problems or pretend they are not happening.
- overeat, or cry a lot, get depressed, get sick, act hostile, or have temper outbursts.
- believe lies.
- not love or feel content with themselves.
- lie to protect and cover up for people they love.
- have difficulty asserting their rights and expressing their feelings honestly and openly.
- let others hurt them.
- not trust themselves or others.
- have difficulty having fun.
- not seek help because they tell themselves that the problem is not bad enough or they are not important enough.

These codependent characteristics contribute to problems with dependency, low self-esteem, unhealthy caregiving, obsessiveness, weak personal boundaries, poor communication, lack of trust, anger, and problems with intimacy, including sex.

How many of these characteristics do you have?

Source: Adapted from *Codependent No More. How to Stop Controlling Others and Start Controlling Yourself* by M. Beattie, 1992, New York: MJF Books. Adapted by permission.

TABLE 4-1	
Conquering Codependency	
CODEPENDENT STATEMENT	**HEALTHY STATEMENT**
"OK, I'll do it. I know you need someone to work a double shift. This is my third double this week."	"No, please find somebody else to work a double shift this time. I am really tired."
"Yes, dear. I'll call your boss and tell her you're sick. I know you don't want to get in trouble at work."	"No, dear. You will need to speak for yourself."
"It's OK, Mr. Smith, I know you try to take your meds, stay on your diabetic diet, and keep your appointments, but it is hard to do all that. I'd probably ignore it all, too."	"Mr. Smith, your diabetes is out of control. Let's work together to make a plan you can stick to."

ior when the nurse uses a mature problem-solving approach, giving the client responsibility for his or her own actions. None of these people would receive the feedback necessary to prompt change if a codependent shielded them from it. Table 4-1 ■ illustrates healthy versus codependent responses.

Critical Self-Check. Compare the healthy and codependent statements in Table 4-1. How is the nurse in the codependent statements helping people avoid the consequences of their own behavior? Can you think of real life examples of codependency?

The first step toward communicating and thinking in a healthy way is to recognize where the control is. Whose behavior can you control? Your child's? Your partner's? Your client's? The answer is none of these. **Each of us only has real control over our own behavior.**

SICK ORGANIZATIONS

Even the healthcare organizations that employ nurses sometimes support a distortion of the caring intentions of their nurse employees. Hospitals, long-term care facilities, managed care organizations, and home health agencies can be addictive in nature. Sick organizations undervalue the caregiver and emphasize financial and administrative functions. They demand more and more of nurses, who, because of their nature, give more and more. Codependency and weak personal boundaries set nurses up to be used and abused (Frisch & Frisch, 2006).

Employers must be concerned with the workload of nurses. Nurses' workload is directly associated with the mortality rate of clients. A 2002 study of surgical clients found that after a basic staffing ratio of four clients per nurse, each additional client per nurse increased the clients' likelihood of dying by 7%. Each additional client was also associated with a significant increase in nursing

burnout and job dissatisfaction (Aiken, Clarke, Sloane, Sochalski, & Silber, 2002). This study illustrated the importance of nurses in client outcomes and the fact that there is a limit to the number of clients for whom nurses can safely provide care.

Burnout

What do you get when you combine caregivers, codependency, weak personal boundaries, unhealthy organizations, and ever-increasing demands? The answer is burnout.

Burnout is a state of physical, emotional, and mental exhaustion caused by long-term involvement in situations that are emotionally demanding. It happens when people who started their caregiving careers with high hopes lose their spirit (Pines & Aronson, 1988).

People who become nurses expect to gain a sense of meaning from their profession. Nurses are idealistic, are highly motivated, and relate to their work as a calling. When nurses feel that their work is insignificant or that they make no difference in their clinical settings, they burn out (Malach-Pines, 2000).

Risk factors for nursing burnout include high workload, poor social or institutional support, a sense of putting in more than they receive back, perception of high stress, role conflict, and helplessness. Nurses have always worked hard. It is not the workload itself that makes nurses lose their spirit for nursing. It is a loss of hope that they can make a difference to clients or that they will have the time and resources to do the kind of nursing they hoped to do. Nurses struggle when they work in "toxic" environments where they are not able to practice according to their own personal philosophies of nursing care (Zerwekh & Claborn, 2006).

NURSING CARE

ASSESSING

How do you know if someone is burned out? The signs and symptoms of burnout are as follows (Malach-Pines, 2000):

- Decreased efficiency and productivity
- Perception that there is never enough time or staff to do the work right
- Dissatisfaction
- Increased illness and absenteeism
- Reduced sense of personal accomplishment

Zerwekh and Claborn (2006) describe the development of burnout: enthusiasm for the job, loss of enthusiasm, continuous deterioration, crisis, and finally devastation and inability to work effectively.

DIAGNOSING, PLANNING, AND IMPLEMENTING

The thought of nurses burning out is pretty depressing. However, there is hope for the nursing profession. There are many strategies for preventing burnout and promoting mentally healthy nursing. The concept of nurses taking care of themselves is relatively new, but nurses are good researchers and problem solvers, so good ideas abound. As a new nurse, you can begin your career with healthy habits, which is easier than breaking old self-defeating habits later.

We can diagnose clients and their families with Caregiver Role Strain and Ineffective Coping. If we look closely, sometimes we could apply these diagnoses to ourselves.

An old attitude in nursing is that "I am here to serve, period." Now we must add to this, "and my own needs must be met so I can meet the needs of my clients." Nurses must be their own advocates in the workplace. Look at Box 4-2 ■ for some ideas on how to care for yourself.

Develop Self-Understanding

Self-understanding (known as *insight*) is the best first step on the path to healthy nursing. Acknowledging your own feelings is important. Many people who become nurses have spent so much time responding to the feelings of others that they have trouble even recognizing or naming their own feelings.

It is healthy to recognize when you are feeling angry, frustrated, sad, guilty, lonely, or happy. Refer to Figure 4-3 ■ for a few of the many emotions that people feel.

| BOX 4-2 | NURSING CARE CHECKLIST |

Ways to Care for the Caregiver (Yourself)

- ☑ **Balance** is a key. Balance your work, family, and personal needs.
- ☑ Be as **healthy** as you can be. Nurture your body, mind, and spirit.
- ☑ Have **realistic** expectations for yourself.
- ☑ Recognize and **accept** your limitations, while striving for improvement.
- ☑ Every human makes mistakes. **Solving problems** is more important than blame.
- ☑ Be **flexible**. The only constant thing is change.
- ☑ Focus on the **accomplishments** of your work.
- ☑ Be **competent**. Be a lifelong learner. Keep up with changes.
- ☑ **Cooperate** with your coworkers. Everything goes better with teamwork.
- ☑ **Understand yourself** and your feelings.
- ☑ Recognize and **value each person** as an individual.
- ☑ Be **proud of yourself** and your work. Have a sense of self-efficacy.

A chart like this can also be used with clients to help them identify their feelings. It helps put names to feelings and also helps people see that there are lots of different feelings that will not last forever.

When negative feelings are not expressed or even acknowledged, they tend to build up. Built-up feelings can result in outbursts, or "emotional bingeing." An emotional binge might involve not expressing feelings at work, and then exploding in anger toward people at home, where you yell at your partner, kick the dog, burn the dinner, and send the kids to bed early. Sometimes unacknowledged feelings surface in physical disorders, such as headaches, anxiety, or gastrointestinal problems (Zerwekh & Claborn, 2006).

We all know that sometimes we feel generally good and sometimes we feel bad. Try to become more sensitive to your own feelings by putting a specific name on your sensations of happiness, sadness, and the more difficult feelings of frustration, fatigue, guilt, and anger. There are no wrong feelings. **It is healthy to have a wide range of genuine feelings, both positive and negative.**

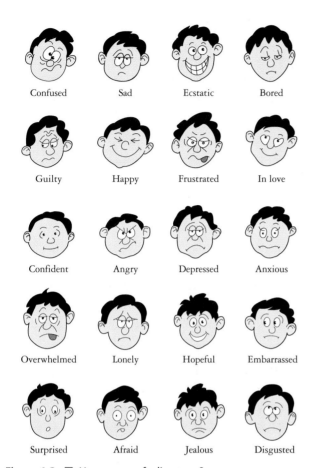

Confused   Sad   Ecstatic   Bored

Guilty   Happy   Frustrated   In love

Confident   Angry   Depressed   Anxious

Overwhelmed   Lonely   Hopeful   Embarrassed

Surprised   Afraid   Jealous   Disgusted

Figure 4-3. ■ How are you feeling now?

A personal feelings assessment might look like this: a nurse just left the room of a client who has diabetes. The nurse is feeling bad. He tries to name his feeling, which is frustration, because the client is having her foot amputated and she has not been following her treatment plan. When the nurse analyzes the situation, he sees that the client's behavior is not under his control (only the client can control her behavior). It is very important for nurses to recognize what they can and cannot control, beginning with the fact that the client's behavior is only under the client's control. He can help by making sure that the client has all the information and encouragement she needs, so the client can make informed decisions about her behavior. Then he can let his frustration go. The nurse will not go home from work with his usual headache today.

Use Teamwork

Acknowledge the hard work of your coworkers. A word of encouragement from you can go a long way to lift the spirits of your peers. After your good example, someone may give you encouragement someday too. The emotional tone in a work environment is an important part of everyone's job satisfaction. Help others with their work when you can, and equally important, **ask for help when you need it.** You are not in nursing alone. Most work is easier when people cooperate to get it done.

Use Healthy Professional Communication

When there are interpersonal problems at work, take a problem-solving approach to solutions. State the problem in a nonthreatening way. Make it clear that the problem is the behavior not the person. For example, when a coworker frequently comes to work late, you could say, "You are such a slacker," or you could say, "When you come to work late, I have to stay after my shift. I wish you would come on time." The latter example is much more professional and effective than calling the person names.

Don't gossip. Remember how codependents are obsessed with other people and their problems? Sometimes this encourages people to do a lot of gossiping in the healthcare workplace. People talk about each other's personal problems, which is unprofessional and unproductive. Try to avoid becoming involved in workplace gossip.

Use the chain of command appropriately. Talk directly to the person involved in a problem, and do not go to a higher level until you have tried a solution at lower levels first without success. Starting at lower levels promotes problem solving and decreases misunderstandings.

Look for a workplace that supports your values. Research shows that nurses become emotionally exhausted when they are unable to practice nursing according to their values. Interview potential employers before you take a job. Find out if an employer will be able to provide you with a work environment that allows you to be the nurse you want to be. Ask about the nurse-client ratio. If you will supervise the care of 40 clients with nursing assistants to do all the personal care, you will not be able to do much communicating with each client. If one-on-one communication is your goal, find a different job. Decide what is most important to you (insight again) and only take a job that can make it possible. Remember Bandura's idea of *self-efficacy* (a belief in your own ability) from Chapter 3? Nurses need a strong sense of self-efficacy to maintain job satisfaction. If it is not possible to do a job well, the nurse has no self-efficacy and no job satisfaction.

Many workplaces have health and safety committees. Nurses are members of these committees and as a member you will have the opportunity to have an effect on the health and safety of your coworkers and yourself. Physical injuries and stress-related risks can be reduced. Effective health and safety programs are directly correlated with both less illness and fewer injuries among nurses at work (Hess, 2005).

The values of the nursing profession change over time. Current trends in the culture of nursing include a trend toward more autonomy and empowerment for nurses. See the Cultural Pulse Points Box 4-3 ■ for information about current trends in the culture of nursing.

BOX 4-3	CULTURAL PULSE POINTS

The Culture of Nursing

Like other cultures that teach their young how to behave, how to dress, what is important, what is right and wrong, the meaning of cultural symbols, and what to believe, the profession of nursing has a culture of its own. Nursing has its patterned beliefs, values, norms, and behaviors that make up its culture. A few examples of nursing values in the United States are cleanliness, newness, timeliness, nursing uniforms as symbols of our role, orderliness, service, science, and the importance of the client's needs above all else.

Even though you are not a practicing nurse yet, you already know that if you came to your clinical course to care for clients in jeans, sandals, and a sleeveless T-shirt, this would be inappropriate. You know that if you leave your client's room in a mess, piled with used linens and old food, you might be flunked out of nursing school, even if you are very smart and write good nursing care plans, because you have already learned some of the values of nursing.

Leininger and McFarland (2002) described the following current trends in the culture of nursing:

- Transition from a patriarchal system (nurses serve physicians) to one of "female empowerment" with more autonomy for nurses.
- Male nurses are asserting their rights.
- Clients are served with high-tech skills, with less emphasis on interpersonal relationships. Nursing is becoming more "high-tech and low-touch."
- Nurses are more interested in financial, personal, and professional gains.
- Nurses have more knowledge and interest in politics and legal aspects of health care.
- There is a transition from nurses providing all client care to more emphasis on self-care by clients or client empowerment.
- More information is available about transcultural nursing. Nursing students are still not consistently prepared for the care of the multicultural clients they will be responsible for in the healthcare workplace.

Think Positively

Know what gives you satisfaction. If relieving a client's pain is what makes you feel like you make a difference in the world, choose a job that will include this intervention. Do not lose sight of the important and powerful things that nurses do to relieve the suffering of people. Even on a bad day, if you eased someone's suffering, the day was not wasted. Keep the successes in mind and try to learn from the failures. Set yourself up for success. Expect yourself to succeed.

Take Care of Yourself

There is a modern myth that it is possible to do it all: work as a nurse or go to nursing school; do homework or read nursing journals to keep up with changes; maintain a relationship; raise healthy children; support the children's activities (help with homework, go to soccer games); shop for and prepare three delicious and nutritious family meals daily; keep the house (cleaning, laundry, making the beds every day, etc.); maintain friendships with adults; attend religious services; care for pets; prepare holiday celebrations; keep in good physical shape; volunteer or participate in committees at school, work, or elsewhere; manage transportation to and from everything; and do it all with a smile. In reality, this is not possible. When we expect ourselves to meet these unrealistic expectations we feel inadequate. We say to ourselves, "Everybody else looks like they are doing it all. What is wrong with me?"

The following are some strategies for achieving balance and health in your life:

- *Start with realistic expectations.* Compromise. Schedule school and your life on the same calendar so you can see if you are double-scheduled. Learn to say "no." Know your limits. Set healthy boundaries. Develop your resources and use them (maybe Mom can pick the kids up from school). Decide on your priorities: the kids are more important than studying tonight. Tomorrow I'll study. Major house projects can wait until summer. Do your best on the important things. Nobody can do it all. Remember, Martha Stewart has a whole staff!
- *Plan fun into your schedule.* All fun activities do not cost too much time and money. Box 4-4 ■ lists some free fun ideas. Some nurses are so focused on service to others that they are unable to even answer the question "What do you like to do?" Think about it. If this is difficult for you, it is even more important that you do it. In a study of student nurses, those who regularly

BOX 4-4

Free Fun Things

- Go to a park.
- Play with a dog (or cat or hamster).
- Play with kids.
- Take your lunch and eat it outside on a blanket for a little picnic.
- Go for a walk (alone or with a friend; in your neighborhood or in an interesting new place).
- Sit on the porch and watch the neighborhood. Make up silly stories about where the people are going.
- Listen to music, maybe even some kind that is different for you.
- Call an old friend, or somebody you miss.
- Make a new friend (try to make some friends who are not nurses; it makes the conversations more interesting).
- Invite some friends over for a potluck dinner (not free, but you were going to eat anyway, and you only provide one dish).
- Take out your old basketball and shoot some hoops.
- Read, anything but nursing.
- Start writing a journal or short stories. Include all your nursing school stories. Maybe someday you can sell them for a soap opera TV show.
- Find that old hobby you started (painting, crocheting, or the rocket you never finished building) and work on it.
- Draw some pictures that don't have to be good. Patterns are fun.
- Play a game like cards or checkers.
- Just hang out and talk with your friends.
- Take a bath until your skin shrivels.
- Write a poem.
- Go for a bike ride if you have one (bring a friend if you want to). If you need to, borrow a bike.
- Sing. Do it in the shower or to your dog if you can't carry a tune, but sing anyway because it makes you feel good. Dogs like it.
- Do anything in nature. The sunsets and sunrises are a good show.
- Tell stories.
- Walk to a place where you usually drive.
- Put ice cubes in your glass of water; they are quite luxurious.
- Look through a cookbook for things you'd like to cook some day—no pressure to cook it tonight.
- Call someone to tell him or her a joke.
- Write a letter. Remember letters? People love to receive them.
- Go to the library when you have several hours to spend. Sit around and read magazines, or a novel, or children's books, or watch the people go by.
- Do anything that seems like it would be relaxing, amusing, or fun to you. Maybe write your own list of free fun things.

engaged in recreational activities were less depressed and scored lower on assessments of depression, burnout, and codependency (Zerwekh & Claborn, 2006). Find a hobby. Go outside (Figure 4-4 ■). Have you been to a museum lately? Talk to a friend or neighbor about nature, nectarines (have you ever had one?), or Nancy's new shoes, but not nursing (that is work, not fun).

- **Be physically healthy.** The behaviors that promote physical health can promote mental health as well. Exercise promotes a sense of well-being (Figure 4-5 ■). Does this advice sound familiar?
  1. Exercise regularly (aerobic exercise; do it on most days for 30 minutes).
  2. Eat right. (Eat a variety of foods and limit salt, sugar, refined foods, saturated and trans fats, and cholesterol; eat plenty of fiber, fresh fruit, and vegetables. Remember the food pyramid?)
  3. Limit your alcohol intake. Never use it to solve problems.
  4. Listen to your body. Eat when you are hungry. Drink when you are thirsty. Rest when you are tired. This sounds obvious, but many nurses ignore their body signals so often that they lose the ability to hear them any more.

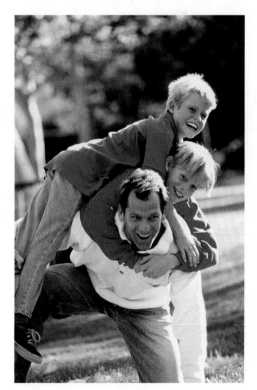

Figure 4-4. ■ Having fun promotes mental health.
Source: Photolibrary.com.

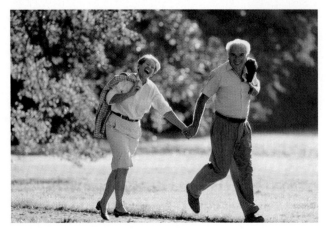

Figure 4-5. ■ Exercise promotes a sense of well-being. *Source:* Getty Images Inc.—Image Bank.

This advice sounds familiar because it is good common sense and because it is known that it works to make people healthier. Sometimes people believe that health comes naturally or happens accidentally. This is not true. Good health requires the hard work of developing good habits.

Critical Self-Check. Look at the self-care behaviors in this chapter. We tell our clients to do these things. Does that make nurses who do not engage in healthy behavior hypocrites?

■ *Nurture your spiritual self.* The holistic view of people says that we are made of body, mind, and spirit. The spirit is sometimes overlooked, but is necessary to a whole view of health. Spirituality includes religion, but is not limited to religious perspectives. Spirituality is really a broader idea that includes the meaning a person finds in life. Some ways you can nurture your spirituality are by appreciating nature (Figure 4-6 ■), reading poetry, thinking about meaning and purpose in life, meditating, helping other people, volunteering in an area that is important to

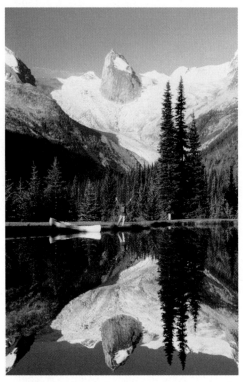

Figure 4-6. ■ Nature provides a spiritual experience for some people. *Source:* Getty Images Inc.—Stone Allstock.

you, reading religious or philosophical writings, or participating in religious services.

EVALUATING

Your goal is to have balance in your life: to live as well as work. Look back on the things you do to make this goal happen. Are you more satisfied at work and at home? Can you express your feelings? Does the exercise make you feel better? Do you feel challenged but not overwhelmed? Are you receiving as well as giving?

Note: The references and resources for this and all chapters have been compiled at the back of the book.

Chapter Review

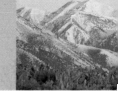

 KEY TERMS

Use the audio glossary feature of the Companion Website to hear the correct pronunciation of the following key terms.

burnout

caring

codependency

commitment

compassion

competence

confidence

conscience

personal boundaries

KEY Points

- Caring, regard for the well-being of others, is the foundation of nursing.
- Codependency is common in nursing. Nurses can recognize it, recover from it, and be healthy while they promote the health of their clients.
- Healthcare organizations may undervalue nurses and prioritize the financial and administrative aspects of the organization. Nurses must be their own advocates.
- When nurses are healthy, they can provide better client care.
- The only person you have control over is yourself.
- Burnout is physical, mental, and emotional exhaustion caused by prolonged exposure to certain stressors. It is an occupational hazard of nursing.
- Burnout is preventable and treatable.
- Nurses must decide on realistic expectations for functioning in the workplace.

- Nurses can plan strategies for their own good mental and physical health. Health does not occur accidentally; it responds to behavioral choices.

 EXPLORE MediaLink

Additional interactive resources for this chapter can be found on the Companion Website at www.prenhall .com/eby. Click on Chapter 4 and "Begin" to select the activities for this chapter.

- Audio glossary
- NCLEX-PN® review
- Case study
- Study outline
- Critical thinking questions
- Matching questions
- Weblinks

Caring for a Client with Ineffective Coping

NCLEX-PN® Focus Area: Psychosocial Integrity

Case Study: Alice M. is a 49-year-old European American nurse who is hospitalized for management of a diabetic emergency. Her blood glucose is currently within normal limits. The client has an adequate knowledge of diabetes management principles. She states that her life is so busy that she does not take time to eat regular meals. She states she is beginning to lose confidence in her ability to manage her diabetes.

Nursing Diagnosis: Ineffective coping

COLLECT DATA

Subjective	Objective
_____	_____
_____	_____
_____	_____
_____	_____
_____	_____
_____	_____
_____	_____

Would you report this data? Yes/No

If yes, to: _____

Nursing Care

_____

_____

_____

_____

_____

_____

_____

_____

_____

_____

_____

How would you document this? _____

_____

_____

Compare your documentation to the sample provided in Appendix I.

Data Collected
(use those that apply)

- Client states, "I don't even have time to drink water while I'm at work."
- BP 110/70, T 99 (oral), P 98, R 22
- Skin is warm and dry with normal red undertones.
- Client states, "It is really different being a client. I like being a nurse better."
- Height 5 ft (150 cm); Weight 160 lb. (72.7 kg.)
- Client's husband is unemployed.
- Client asks, "What can I do to get my life back?"
- 400 mL clear amber urine output this shift
- Client states, "I feel out of control of my life."
- Has 2 children, ages 14 and 16
- Lungs clear
- The client states she is beginning to lose confidence in her ability to manage her diabetes.
- Client is having difficulty sleeping while in the hospital.

Nursing Interventions
(use those that apply; list in priority order)

- Encourage the client to express her feelings about diabetes, her work, and her life stressors.
- Assess the coping methods the client has used in the past.
- Assess the client's parenting skills.
- Encourage the client to prioritize the demands on her time.
- Discuss ways the client can manage her diabetes, at home and at work.
- Discuss coping strategies.
- Give the client positive feedback when she has ideas about how to cope with her stressors in a healthy way.
- Teach the client basic information about the diabetes disease process.
- Support the client's positive attitudes about her ability to manage her life.
- Teach the client how to inject her own insulin.
- Tell the client, "If I were you, I would focus on the diabetes. If you don't control it, it will kill you."
- Tell the client, "I think you should tell your husband to get a job. He is putting too much pressure on you."

1 Which of the following is an example of a nurse who has lost her boundaries?

1. A nurse who insists that her husband call his employer for himself when he is going to be absent from work.
2. A nurse who apologizes to her son for forgetting to telephone him at home to wake him for his graduation practice.
3. A nurse who promises herself to work only one overtime shift per week.
4. A nurse who confronts a sexually aggressive client with his inappropriate behavior.

2 Which of the following is characteristic of the behavior of the codependent nurse?

1. He suspects a fellow nurse of substance abuse, so he finishes the nurse's tasks to prevent her getting into trouble.
2. He confronts a client about unhealthy practices and works with the client to develop an acceptable new lifestyle.
3. He does not offer advice to fellow employees but helps them to see their options.
4. He accepts praise graciously.

3 Which of the following is most likely to be a comment by a codependent nurse?

1. "I have plans to take my daughter to lunch tomorrow. I can't work extra."
2. "Fried chicken, mashed potatoes, and gravy are not on your low-fat diet."
3. "Having a chronic illness must get very tiresome. Let's look for some ways to make life a little easier for you."
4. "If I had to be on dialysis, I think I'd want to skip the diet, too. I understand why you want to enjoy the life you have left to its fullest."

4 Which of the following work scenarios is the most likely to cause burnout?

1. The manager speaks to the nurse about ways to improve work performance.
2. There is one nurse who consistently "calls in sick" only on weekends and suffers no disciplinary action.
3. The manager plans to change the tardiness policy and calls the staff together for suggestions.
4. The nurse consistently works in an environment where there is a nurse-client ratio of 1:4.

5 Which of the following could indicate burnout on the part of the nurse? The nurse:

1. Refuses to work more than one overtime shift a week.
2. Organizes a group of nurses to approach the unit manager concerning some time-saving approaches to care that might be initiated.
3. Gossips with other nurses about the poor working conditions on the unit and suggests that they all just call in sick until things change.
4. Receives a commendation for being "Employee of the Month."

6 Which of the following would be the best way to prevent professional burnout? The nurse should:

1. Quit and find another line of work.
2. Make a date with a spouse or significant other to go out to dinner and a movie once a week.
3. Treat self to ice cream after work each day as a reward for staying with the job.
4. Keep feelings about work inside, knowing it will make it worse to discuss them.

7 Which of the following is a good way to promote mentally healthy nursing? The nurse should:

1. Identify the client's feelings and respond to them above all else.
2. Work independently to enhance feelings of pride in the work.
3. Ask for help when it is needed.
4. Leave notes on the time cards of other coworkers who are doing their jobs poorly.

8 To solve a problem at work that is affecting staff morale, the nurse's best action would be to:

1. Take the problem straight to the Director of Nursing.
2. Go to the person directly involved in the problem and try to find a solution.
3. Gather the staff together and have them write anonymous complaints to be presented to the supervisor.
4. Meet with the rest of the staff and plan to refuse to work until the problems are solved.

9 Which of the following statements about spirituality is true?

1. It involves only the practice of an organized religion.
2. It is unimportant in one's total sense of well-being.
3. It is too abstract to be of much use to anyone's physical and emotional health.
4. It can be nurtured by nature walks and reading literature as well as by participating in religious services.

10 The nurse has a home health client who is seen once a week. Her daughter-in-law is the caregiver. Which of the following would indicate to the nurse that the daughter-in-law might be experiencing caregiver role strain? (Select all that apply.) The daughter-in-law:

1. Tells the nurse she's lost 10 lbs. this month because she has no appetite.
2. Has asked a neighbor to come in one afternoon a week, so she can go shopping.
3. Talks continuously about how her mother-in-law is ruining her marriage.
4. States proudly that she was able to get her mother-in-law to feed herself at least once a day.
5. Has the smell of alcohol on her breath at 10 A.M.

Answers for Review Questions, as well as discussion of Critical Thinking Care Map questions, appear in Appendix I.

Chapter 5

The Nurse-Client Relationship and Communication

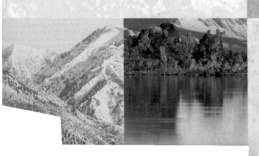

BRIEF Outline

Therapeutic Use of Self
Nurse-Client Relationship
Communication Process

Effective Communication Strategies
Barriers to Communication

LEARNING Outcomes

After completing this chapter, you will be able to:

1. Develop effective communication skills that will promote trusting nurse-client relationships.
2. Recognize and avoid communication barriers.
3. Conduct therapeutic communication as a nursing intervention with clients.

When nurses are asked what they do for clients they will usually make a list of tasks (dressing changes, medication administration, assessments, treatments, etc.). What about caring, client advocacy, teaching? What about holding the hand of a dying woman, letting her know that she is not alone? These powerful parts of nursing are sometimes forgotten in the rush to complete nursing tasks. Nursing is far more than the skilled tasks that we perform.

Therapeutic Use of Self

The **therapeutic use of self** is the ability to use the self, consciously and in full awareness, to structure nursing interventions (Travelbee, 1971). To be able to meet the needs of clients, nurses must understand themselves first. Nurses who are aware of their own real selves are in a better position to help their clients (Jourard, 1971). Nurses experience anxiety, anger, frustration, happiness, and joy when working with their clients. If nurses are to have open, authentic communication with clients, they must be able to examine their own feelings and appreciate how their feelings interact with those of clients (Eckroth-Bucher, 2001). You know that nurses use sphygmomanometers and syringes, but doesn't it make sense that nurses also use their interpersonal skills? *The* most important tools used by nurses to promote the health of their clients are the nurses themselves (Figure 5-1 ■ depicts the nurse using her interpersonal skills to help the client).

Remember in Chapter 3 when we talked about how nursing is *holistic*? Nurses need to learn about nurse-client relationships and therapeutic communication in order to meet their clients' needs related to mind and spirit, as well as body.

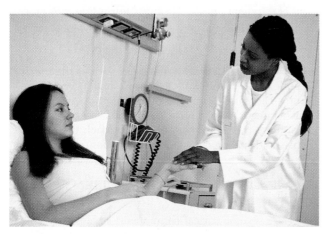

Figure 5-1. ■ Nurses use their interpersonal skills in the "therapeutic use of self" to help clients. *Source:* Phototake NYC.

Nurse-Client Relationship

Hildegard Peplau, a pioneer in psychiatric nursing, first described the nurse-client relationship in 1952. This relationship is used to help promote the client's growth, for problem solving, and for insight development. The professional nurse-client relationship differs from social relationships.

As a part of learning about their native culture, people learn from birth onward how to behave in social situations. By the time students enter nursing school they are very experienced with social relationships. You know how to act with people who are your friends, people who are strangers, and people who are older or younger than you are. In social relationships both people involved will benefit. You talk to a friend about your troubles and she talks about hers. There is mutual satisfaction. In a social relationship there is no goal except friendship or socializing. There is no time limit. Both parties freely express feelings and opinions.

The features of the professional therapeutic relationship are as follows:

- Client centered
- Goal directed
- Time limited

In the professional relationship, the nurse may take on different roles (such as socializing agent, advocate, counselor, or teacher), but the relationship always *focuses on the client's needs*. The professional relationship is also *goal directed*. The purpose of these relationships is to help the client meet adaptive (healthy) goals. Unlike the social relationship, the professional relationship is *time limited*. The nurse and client define how much time they are willing and able to spend. When the nurse is off work or the client is discharged from the facility, the relationship is over.

The appropriate degree of **objectivity** (detachment or neutrality, without emotion) is also important to the professional relationship. A common but erroneous assumption is that nurses must remain completely objective. If nurses were completely objective, they would be detached from concern about clients. Nurses should be open to and aware of their own feelings to be able to help clients. Nurses' feelings can be an important part of their assessment as well as intervention skills. For example, if a client says "I'm feeling fine, thanks," the nurse would use her or his own feelings to recognize a sense of despair or frustration that might be present in contrast to the spoken words, and to respond in a way that could help the client (Stuart & Laraia, 2005; Walker & Alligood, 2001).

BOX 5-1

Social Versus Professional Interaction

Note how these conversations are similar, yet only one is professional.

Social (feelings of both are expressed)

CLIENT: "I'm so sorry that I had to leave my children with a babysitter while I am in the hospital. Do you have kids?"

NURSE: "I know how you feel. I have two kids and I hate to leave them with my sister because her husband is impatient with them."

Professional (focus on client needs)

CLIENT: "I'm so sorry that I had to leave my children with a babysitter while I am in the hospital. Do you have kids?"

NURSE: "Yes, I have two kids. This must be hard for you. How are you feeling about it?"

Although nurses should not be completely objective, they should be free from personal bias and personal identification with clients' feelings. A subjective emphasis on the nurse's own feelings and opinions does not belong in the nurse-client interaction. With practice, nurses can balance their feelings with professional objectivity and become fully attentive to clients' needs (Fortinash & Holoday Worret, 2004). Box 5-1 ■ provides examples of how professional and social interactions differ, even when the content of the conversation is similar.

Sometimes what the client needs is a social conversation. People with chronic mental illnesses often have poor social skills and need practice. People in long-term care may have few social contacts. In these situations, the nurse uses social interaction with clients as a nursing intervention to meet client needs. This is not the time for nurses to discuss their own personal problems.

It is often difficult for nursing students to engage in professional relationships. Students have so much experience with social relationships, and sometimes this experience can get in the way. Your parents may have told you "If you don't have something good to say, don't say anything," or "Be nice!" or "Don't talk about going to the bathroom in public." But imagine a client who is hospitalized as a result of injuries he received while driving under the influence of alcohol. The nurse must tell the client that he was responsible for the injuries because he was driving drunk. This information is not "nice," but it is necessary to help the client connect the action with its consequences. It is not so

easy to ask someone about their bowel movements either. Professional communication can be difficult, especially when it requires the nurse to interact in a way that would be awkward if the interaction were social. Communicating like a professional can be challenging, but it can be learned with practice (like riding a bike or giving an injection). It is usually easier for a client to talk with a nurse about a potentially embarrassing topic (such as bowel movements, urine samples, and anything involving the perineum) when the nurse is confident and acts like this is just an everyday subject of conversation in the healthcare setting (which of course it is).

PHASES OF THE RELATIONSHIP

The nurse-client relationship has three phases: the orientation phase, the working phase, and the termination phase. In the **orientation phase,** the nurse and the client set the stage for the relationship to follow. They introduce themselves and set goals for the interaction. In the medical-surgical setting, a goal may be to learn about a new medication or treatment, or perhaps to discuss how the client feels about a surgical procedure. In the psychiatric setting, a goal may be to explore feelings or to develop problem-solving strategies. The time limit of the relationship is stated during this phase.

In the **working phase,** the nurse implements interventions to reach the goals set during the orientation phase. The nurse and client work together to achieve the client's optimal level of functioning and self-care, based on the client's strengths and challenges. One important possible nursing intervention in this phase is therapeutic communication (more on this later).

After the work of the working phase is done, the **termination phase** begins. In this phase the nurse and the client summarize their progress and evaluate the achievement of the client's goals. The nurse learns from this process about which interventions are effective and which are not. The client then moves on to other relationships.

Critical Self-Check. What process does the therapeutic nurse-client relationship resemble? (*Hint:* In the nurse-client relationship you start by assessing the client's needs, then move to setting goals with the client, planning interventions, working to reach the client's goals, and finally evaluating the outcomes.)

ELEMENTS OF THE NURSE-CLIENT RELATIONSHIP

There are several critical components to the nurse-client relationship, as shown in Box 5-2 ■. The art of this relationship lies in the nurse's ability to help the client participate

Elements of the Therapeutic Nurse-Client Relationship

Trustworthiness
Trustworthiness is behavior that is predictable, competent, and in the client's best interest. Trust is the foundation of the nurse-client relationship.

Caring
Caring is the concern for the well-being of another. It includes commitment, compassion, competence, confidence, and conscience. Caring is the basis for nursing itself.

Empathy
Empathy is the ability to understand a situation from the client's point of view and to communicate this understanding to the client. Empathy is necessary for the client to feel understood.

Genuineness
Genuineness is honesty, sincerity, openness, and congruence in verbal and nonverbal messages.

Respect
The nurse gives **respect** (unconditional positive regard without judgment, regardless of the client's situation or past behavior). This does not imply that the nurse condones inappropriate behavior, but assumes that the nurse will accept the client as a person, exactly as s/he is.

Concreteness
Concreteness is the use of realistic language, rather than jargon or medical terminology. The client is assisted to do realistic problem solving and to develop insight.

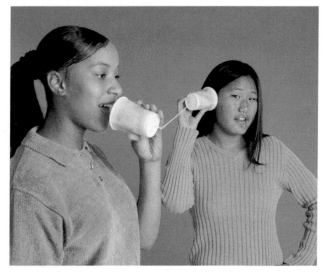

Figure 5-2. ■ The communication process appears to be simple but is really complex. *Source:* Pearson Learning Photo Studio.

Feedback is the response of the receiver to the message. The receiver's feedback alerts the sender to how the receiver perceived the message. Feedback may be verbal or nonverbal. Assessing the client's feedback is important for the nurse, because it allows the nurse to clarify misunderstandings or unclear messages as soon as possible.

Communication is vital to the practice of nursing. The clearest communication occurs when the receiver receives the same message that the sender intended to send. Nurses who are clear communicators and who understand the communication process are better able to help their clients understand information, learn, and improve their own communication skills.

in the self-care that will improve the client's health and well-being. The qualities of trustworthiness, caring, empathy, genuineness, respect, and concreteness empower the nurse to excel in the art of nursing.

Communication Process

Communication involves sending and receiving a message (Figure 5-2 ■). This seemingly simple process is really very complex. The sender of the message may express spoken or written words, body gestures or movements, music, art, or touch. The way the receiver accepts the message depends on the receiver's culture, language, gender, sensory function, cognitive abilities, experiences, and expectations. The sending and receiving of messages are affected by the environment and by the circumstances in which the message is sent (Figure 5-3 ■ depicts some of these influences). With all these variables, it is a wonder that people are ever able to understand each other at all!

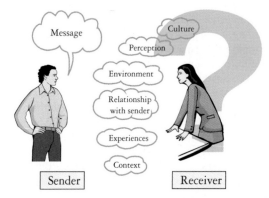

Figure 5-3. ■ Communication process: The sent message is affected by several factors before it is interpreted by the receiver.

TYPES OF COMMUNICATION

Written communication includes handwriting, typing, pictures, and inanimate messages, without interpersonal contact. The Internet has shown us how much can be communicated in this way.

Verbal communication includes spoken messages. It includes both what we say and how we say it. Cultural Pulse Points Box 5-3 ■ provides an explanation of how factors such as rate and loudness of speech can affect its meaning. Think about the limitation of messages transmitted by radio or what can be sent and received by telephone (Figure 5-4 ■).

Nonverbal communication refers to all of the messages that are sent without words and makes up the majority of the communication process. Yes, most communication is nonverbal. Nonverbal communication includes body movements, actions, posture, and gestures; body position and closeness; and facial expressions. Although it is

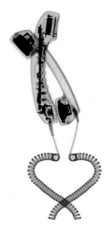

Figure 5-4. ■ Verbal communication can convey factual and emotional messages, but lacks nonverbal cues that are the most accurate communication information. *Source:* Photo Researchers, Inc.

relatively easy for people to say almost anything with their words (despite what they really feel), it is very difficult to lie with nonverbal messages. When you hear a person say: "I just love this hospital food!" but he is spitting a half-chewed bite of it into his napkin and making a very sick face, which message do you believe? Nonverbal communication is considered a more accurate expression of a person's true feelings.

Touch is an important aspect of nonverbal communication. Touch is frequently used by nurses to convey reassurance, support, and caring. Like other forms of communication, the meaning of touch lies not only in the sender's intentions but also in the receiver's perception. For this reason nurses must use touch carefully.

Touch can be professional/functional (client care), social/polite (a handshake), friendship/warmth (hugs between friends or a pat on the back), loving/intimate (kissing or hugging relatives or close friends), or sexual/arousing (between lovers) (Knapp, 1980). Considering all the potential errors in communication, it is possible that the sender could intend one meaning of touch and the receiver could perceive a different meaning.

In the professional environment it is the responsibility of the nurse to determine what is appropriate behavior. The nurse should assess the client for cues about whether touch is acceptable. If a nurse hugs a client and intends to show concern and the client thinks the nurse is attacking her, or in love with her, the nurse has made a mistake. When it comes to touching people, **the perception of the receiver is more important than the sender's intent.**

BOX 5-3	CULTURAL PULSE POINTS

Paralinguistic Cues

We are all speaking English; why don't we understand each other?

Verbal communication is composed of both what we say and how we say it. Our verbal messages are modified with the tone of our voice, rate of speech, pitch, loudness, and emotional expression. These *paralinguistic cues* (part of the spoken language that is in addition to the words) change the meaning of the spoken words. For example, imagine a European American nurse who has two clients (yes, this is a fantasy) and who is responding to their call lights. The first client is Vietnamese American and speaks English as a second language. She says, haltingly and quietly "I'm . . . in . . . pain." The second is a Persian American client (a native English speaker) in the same circumstances who says loudly, quickly, and choking back tears, "I'M IN PAIN!" The second client may not be feeling more pain than the first one. The loud, rapid speech may be how this client learned to express her feelings. The nurse may receive the second client's message more clearly because it is delivered more like the nurse expects it to be. People learn how to use their voices when they learn how to speak their native language, so the paralinguistic cues vary from one culture to the next. The nurse must be careful when interpreting these cues. The nurse can verify that s/he understands the client's message by **clarifying** what the client means. For example, communication would be improved if the nurse said: "You are in pain; would you like to have your pain medication?" instead of making assumptions about what the client might have meant.

Critical Self-Check. Can these ideas both be true? Why, or why not?

1. Touch is a critical part of the practice of nursing.
2. Nurses can distress people by touching them.

Psychiatric clients often have difficulty relating to other people. Distortions of reality can further complicate the meaning of communication, including touch. The usual standard of behavior for nurses in the psychiatric setting is to limit the amount of personal contact with patients to functional nursing needs and handshakes.

PERSONAL SPACE

The amount of space that people need in order to feel comfortable is determined by their culture and their personality. In the United States and Canada, which are generally low-touch cultures, there are generally four zones of personal space that represent the comfortable distance between people communicating with each other (Figure 5-5 ■ includes examples of nurses providing care in all the zones of personal space):

■ Public space (more than 10–12′): A comfortable distance between strangers, for example, between a teacher and a class.

■ Social space (4–12′): Comfortable distance for work, social, and business settings, for example, at a restaurant.

■ Personal space (18″–4′): Acceptable distance for people who have some connection with each other, such as students in a class.

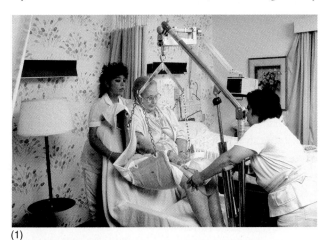

(1)

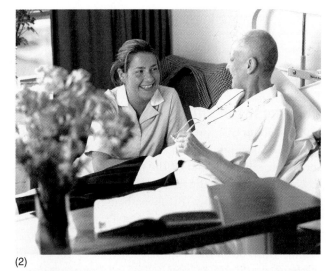

(2)

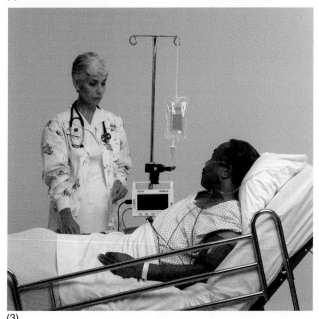

(4)

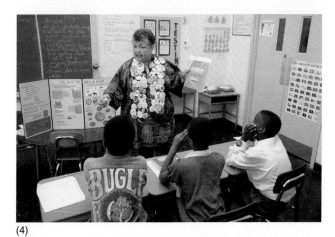

(3)

Figure 5-5. ■ Nurses provide care in clients' **(1)** intimate, **(2)** personal, **(3)** social , and **(4)** public zones of personal space.
Source: (1) Pearson Education/PH College; (2) Photo Researchers, Inc.; (3) Phototake NYC; (4) PhotoEdit Inc.

- Intimate space (less than 18"): Comfortable only for people with a close relationship, such as family and friends (Hall, cited in Frisch & Frisch, 2005).

Nurses are often expected to enter the intimate zones of clients, who are likely to feel anxious and threatened by the intrusion. The nurse should warn the client: "I'm going to take your blood pressure now," or "I need to lift up your gown to change your dressing." Be careful not to give the client choices if there is no real choice. If you must take the client's temperature, do not say "Is it OK for me to take your temperature now?" To give the client a sense of control, the nurse may offer a real choice: "Would you like to have your dressing changed now or after breakfast?"

Personal space attitudes are based on cultural expectations. When the nurse and the client are from different cultures with different standards for touching, misunderstandings can occur. The nurse must be sensitive to the client's feedback (which will often be nonverbal) about touching and personal space.

SELF-DISCLOSURE

Self-disclosure is any verbalization or behavior that reveals personal information about the self to another person. Some self-disclosure by the nurse can help clients to disclose their own feelings; however, the nurse must use self-disclosure carefully (Psychopathology Committee of the Group for the Advancement of Psychiatry, 2001). Ultimately, the nurse's motivation for disclosing personal feelings must be for the client's benefit, not for the benefit of the nurse (Stuart & Laraia, 2005). Table 5-1 ■ shows examples of nursing self-disclosure that are appropriate and some that are inappropriate. Imagine how the client might feel if a nurse said the inappropriate comments.

Effective Communication Strategies

ACTIVE LISTENING

There are several strategies for making communication more effective. One of the most important is **active listening,** which is careful attending to the sender's whole message, both the verbal and the nonverbal. The active listener also uses **attending behaviors,** which communicate the listener's attention and interest:

- Facing the other person (with body and face)
- Open posture (arms loose, not folded in front of chest)
- Leaning forward

- Giving verbal and nonverbal feedback to indicate interest and encouragement for the sender to continue

Have you seen two deaf people communicate with sign language? Ironically, because they face each other and attend to each other carefully while they sign, they may be better "listeners" than most hearing people. Active listening can even enhance the client's self-esteem, because in our fast-paced society it is rare to have the gift of someone's full nonjudgmental attention. It feels empowering to have this opportunity.

CONGRUENCE

Another important strategy for making communication effective is sending congruent messages. **Congruence** exists when the verbal and nonverbal messages are the same. Consider these two scenarios: The first nurse says to the client, "I would like to talk with you about how you are recovering from your hip surgery." While she says this, the nurse is picking up extra linens in the room, standing with her back to the client. When the client says nothing, she quickly walks out of the room. The second nurse sits in the client's bedside chair and says, "I would like to talk with you about how you are recovering from your hip surgery." This nurse looks at the client, leans forward, and waits quietly for a response. In the first scenario, the verbal and nonverbal messages are incongruent. What does this nurse really mean? Congruence really makes a difference.

CONCRETE MESSAGES

It can be challenging for clients to understand what is being said to them in the healthcare setting. They are often under stress and experiencing anxiety. Anxiety can impair *cognitive functioning* (the ability to learn, remember, and process new information). The nurse should use *concrete messages*. A concrete message is clear, realistic, and does not require interpretation. Many clients have special needs for concrete communication, such as people who have limited English language skills, cognitive impairment, anxiety, or severe mental illness. If the nurse says: "We'll deal with your Montgomery strap situation later," who knows what he meant? If he said: "I'll come back after lunch and change the dressing on your side. I'll also replace those ties that hold it on," the message would be a lot clearer.

All of the elements of the nurse-client relationship (see Box 5-2) are essential for effective communication between the nurse and the client. Get to know them: *trust worthiness, caring, empathy, genuineness, respect,* and *concreteness.* They will become an integral part of your professional life.

TABLE 5-1		
Nursing Self-Disclosure		
REASON FOR SELF-DISCLOSURE	**NURSE USING APPROPRIATE SELF-DISCLOSURE**	**NURSE USING INAPPROPRIATE SELF-DISCLOSURE**
Fostering the therapeutic relationship	**Client:** "Do you have time to talk to me?" **Nurse:** "Sure. I have 15 minutes, and I always enjoy talking with you."	**Nurse:** "Yes, it feels like a break. Most of the residents here are so mentally confused that I can't stand to be around them sometimes."
Assisting the client to express feelings	**Nurse:** "How do you feel when your husband says embarrassing things about you in public?" **Client:** "Not so good, I guess." **Nurse:** "I think many people would feel angry in a situation like that." **Client:** "Yes, I do feel angry! I feel so humiliated and powerless, too."	**Nurse:** "When my ex-husband embarrassed me by blaming me for our bankruptcy at a dinner party I was so mad!"
Modeling behavior change	**Client:** "When a clerk gives me the wrong change, I think she might get mad if I tell her about it, so I don't." **Nurse:** "I might say nicely, 'I gave you a five-dollar bill, and you gave me change for a one. Would you please give me the rest of my change?'"	**Nurse:** "I don't really care what people think of me."
Helping the client to see his or her own feelings as normal or rational	**Client:** "My cat died, and I don't know if I can go on. It seems stupid." **Nurse:** "I felt very bad when my dog died. Pets are very important to people. I felt better over time, though."	**Nurse:** "I know how you feel. When my champion racehorse died, I lost a million dollars."
Encouraging the client's autonomy	**Client:** "I don't know if I'm ready to be responsible for my own meds." **Nurse:** "You've told me how they work, and you've made a schedule for taking them. I think you're ready."	**Nurse:** "Taking meds is easy. If I can do it so can you."

EMPATHY

Empathy is the ability to enter into the life of others, perceive their feelings, and communicate this understanding. It requires the nurse to put aside personal values and judgments, become aware of the client's feelings, and confirm with the client the accuracy of the nurse's perceptions. The experience of empathy may give clients the feeling that they are not alone in the world, that they are understood by someone, and that their worth is increased because of this. Empathy is not the same as sympathy, which is feeling sorry for someone. The nurse is not expected to, and in fact should not, feel the same feelings as the client. The empathic nurse understands and appreciates the client's feelings, while maintaining the role of the professional nurse (Stuart & Laraia, 2005).

Barriers to Communication

GIVING ADVICE

There are several avoidable barriers to communication that must be recognized and eliminated from the nurse's communication tools. Table 5-2 ■ provides examples of communication barriers. The first barrier is giving advice. It may be easy for the nurse to say, "If I were you, I would . . ." but the nurse is not the client. The client is the decision maker, based on the ethical principle of autonomy. The

TABLE 5-2

Communication Barriers

COMMUNICATION BARRIER	EXAMPLES	WHY THIS IS A BARRIER
Giving Advice	"If I were you, I would have the radical mastectomy rather than the lumpectomy, just to be sure." "You should take your medications every day."	The client is the decision maker. The one who will experience the consequences must make the decision. This is based on the ethical principle of autonomy.
Agreeing	"I think you did the right thing to get a 'Do not Resuscitate' order for your mother." "You are right to go home early."	The client's goal is to do what is best for the client, not to seek the nurse's approval. Discourages further discussion.
Generalized Comments or Clichés	"I know exactly how you feel." "Don't worry; everything will be fine."	Clichés are used so often that they have no real meaning, except to allow the user to avoid expressing actual feelings.
Defensiveness	"Your mother only meant to help you." "He is a very good doctor and would never give you medicine that makes you sick on purpose."	Defensiveness stops discussion of feelings (which are the real point) and starts a need for excuses and competing comments.
Changing the Subject	**Client:** "I haven't felt so bad since my stepfather abused me." **Nurse:** "How about them Yankees?"	Diverts from real issue to avoid the discomfort of the nurse. Communicates that the subject is not acceptable.
Disrespecting	"It was only a dog, it's not like you lost a child or anything." "Your problem is not as big as you think it is."	Belittles the client's feelings. Discourages further discussion.

client will be the one to experience the consequences of any healthcare decision, therefore the client should be given information by the staff, and then allowed to make the final decision. The role of the nurse is to support clients' self-care, not to take away their control by making decisions for them.

AGREEING

Generally, it seems like a good idea to agree with people. However, in the therapeutic nurse-client relationship, the nurse's responsibility is not to decide whether the client is right or wrong. By agreeing with the client, the nurse suggests that the client should seek the nurse's approval. The client is trying to make the best decisions for the client's well-being, not for the nurse's approval.

Consider this situation: A woman has just been brought to a long-term care facility. Her tearful daughter is with her. Here are two possible conversations:

Conversation #1

NURSE: Why are you crying?

WOMAN: I feel so bad about putting my mom in a nursing home.

NURSE: It was the right thing to do. We will take good care of her here. You can visit any time.

Conversation #2

NURSE: You look sad.

WOMAN: I feel so bad about putting my mom in a nursing home.

NURSE: What brought you to this decision?

WOMAN: She has Alzheimer's disease. She has lived with me for years.

NURSE: Go on . . .

WOMAN: She has been getting so much worse. She turned on the stove and burned herself. Once she wandered outside and we couldn't find her for hours. She is not safe alone and I have to work.

NURSE: It sounds like you didn't have many other choices.

WOMAN: Right, I think it really was the best thing for her.

NURSE: We will take good care of her. You can visit any time.

WOMAN: Thank you. Now I can live with myself about this decision.

The nurse in the first situation did what nurses commonly do: she gave her approval to make the person feel better. The client will have the feeling that the nurse thinks she did the right thing. In the second situation the nurse allowed the woman to express her feelings, then she encouraged the woman to think through her decision. In this scenario the woman decides for herself that she had made the right decision. The nurse's opinion about admitting the woman to the long-term care facility was never the issue. The nurse in the second scenario did far more to help the daughter resolve her conflicted feelings.

GENERALIZED STATEMENTS OR CLICHÉS

It is so belittling to disclose some profound feeling and to have the nurse respond with some trite cliché. Some examples of these generalized statements are: "That's nice, dear," "Don't worry; everything will be all right," "God will not give you more than you can handle," and "Cheer up." Such generalized statements are used in any variety of situations. They are like the shredded paper in a box of new shoes: they just take up space. Avoid them—they are meaningless and encourage the receiver to feel that the nurse did not care enough to say something real.

DEFENSIVENESS

If the client has a problem and the nurse responds with excuses, communication becomes a contest. This is not good communication. Even if the client's problem is with the nurse, free expression of feelings is what opens communication. Allow the client to express both positive and negative feelings. This is what respect and acceptance are about.

CHANGING THE SUBJECT

If the client changes the subject, the nurse says: "Let's get back to what we were talking about," because we know that clients often do not want to talk about challenging or threatening issues. Examples of threatening or difficult issues are the client's behavior, embarrassing bodily functions, and serious disease processes. Sometimes these issues must be addressed. We should not turn away when the subject becomes stressful for us either. Changing the subject when the client presents a legitimate concern communicates that the nurse is not willing to talk about the client's problem. The topic often is stressful when significant or threatening issues are being discussed. To meet the client's need, nurses must keep their objectivity and continue the conversation.

DISRESPECTING

Nurses usually do not intentionally disrespect a client, but when the nurse belittles a client's concerns, it is disrespectful. Even if the issue seems small to the nurse, the nurse should respect that it is a significant concern to the client and treat it as important.

The European American culture may have the least formal social behavior in the world. You might expect the staff to call you by your first name if you were a client in a healthcare setting. Many people would find this disrespectful. Especially if clients are older than you or are from other countries, address them by their title, such as Mr. X or Ms. Y, and let them tell you if they prefer to be addressed by their first names.

TRANSFERENCE

Another potential block to communication is **transference.** In transference the client feels emotions from the past and applies (or transfers) them to the therapeutic relationship. A client may have feared for years that he would develop diabetes because a family member suffered from diabetes complications. He may transfer his considerable fear and anger onto the nurse who tries to help him learn to test his blood glucose.

Transference can cause the client to have strong positive or negative feelings for the nurse or to overvalue or ignore the nurse's expertise. The client may transfer negative feelings that originated toward an abusive parent to the nurse who tries to ask the client to change behavior. The client may react by resisting all authority figures, or may have some other reaction that originated long before the client ever met the nurse.

Nurses must learn to recognize transference. It explains why a client may have an exaggerated reaction to a nurse when he or she has no clear reason to react this way. Calling attention to the client's behavior and the nurse's perception may help. For example, if a client said "You make me sick! You are always telling me what to do!" The nurse might respond calmly, "I just met you today. I haven't told you what to do. I am trying to help you understand your new medication schedule. You seem angry. Is there a problem?" This may help the client see that he is not reacting to the current situation. It is also important for the nurse not to take a client's transference reactions personally. If a client is exaggerating about how much trouble the nurse is, the nurse is probably not the real problem.

When it is the nurse who has feelings toward the client based on the nurse's previous experiences, the process is called **countertransference.** Some nurses experience countertransference when they care for specific kinds of clients. For example, a nurse whose father died of lung cancer may have automatic strong protective or even negative feelings about people who smoke. A nurse may feel comfortable being overly responsible for people with alcoholism because the nurse learned this role in childhood. A nurse who had a manipulative partner may have exaggerated feelings about clients who manipulate the staff to get their needs met. Countertransference is common, and it can get in the way of objective client care. Nurses must make their decisions based on the facts and not on feelings transferred from another situation.

The best preventive strategy for countertransference is for nurses to develop self-understanding (insight). Recognizing countertransference when it occurs and talking with a trusted colleague can often put these feelings into perspective (Varcarolis, Carson, & Shoemaker, 2006). If you instantly have negative or uneasy feelings about a client, it is probably not the individual who is initiating these feelings, but countertransference. Box 5-4 ■ lists signs of countertransference.

BOX 5-4

Recognizing Countertransference

The following feelings by the nurse may suggest counter-transference (transferring feelings from previous experiences onto the client):

- The client reminds you of yourself or someone else you know.
- You think about the client frequently outside the work setting.
- You feel uneasy about the relationship with this client.
- You feel angry about the client's behavior.
- You feel proud of the client.
- You believe that you are the only one who really understands this client.
- You have personal feelings toward the client.

NURSING CARE

The nursing process can be used as a framework for determing client needs. Communication is used in all aspects of the nursing process.

ASSESSING

The nurse-client relationship provides the foundation for all other nursing actions involving the client. The relationship establishes the duty of the nurse to care for the client and the responsibility of the nurse to apply the nursing process to help the client. In the nursing process, the nurse will first collect data for assessing the client's needs. Because of the trust in the nurse-client relationship, the client is usually able to give information about personal feelings, lifestyle behaviors, and needs to the nurse.

In gathering data for assessment about the psychosocial needs of clients, it is helpful to ask questions about areas of functioning.

If you want to determine the *client's understanding* of the current medical condition and reason for hospitalization, you could ask:

- "What brought you to the hospital this time?"
- "What do you know about your condition?" (You might find the client has Deficient Knowledge.)

If you want to know if needs for *socialization* are being met, you can ask:

- "Who visits you while you are in the hospital?"
- "Who lives with you?"
- "What kinds of things do you do with your friends?" (The person whose needs aren't being met might be given a nursing diagnosis of Social Isolation, Loneliness, or Impaired Social Interaction.)

If you want to learn about *coping* skills, you may ask:

- "How do you usually solve problems like this?"
- "What do you usually do when this happens?"
- "Who can help you with this?"
- "How do you manage this at home?" (A person with difficulties in this area may have Ineffective Coping.)

If you want to explore the client's feelings of *self-efficacy*, you can ask:

- "Who is responsible for your health?"
- "If you have a health problem, how do you manage it?"
- "Can you make a difference by your own actions to improve your life?"
- "Do you think you will feel better?" (Answers in the negative may be described as Powerlessness or Hopelessness.)

To determine the client's level of *anxiety*, you can ask:

- "How are you feeling now?"
- "Do you feel nervous, scared, or anxious?" (Responses might indicate a nursing diagnosis of Anxiety or Fear.)

To explore the client's attitudes and feelings about *self* and *self-concept*, you may ask:

- "How do you feel about yourself?"
- "How do you feel about your body?" (Answers from the client might lead to a nursing diagnosis of Situational Low Self-Esteem or Chronic Low Self-Esteem.)

If you need to learn whether the illness or injury affects the client's development or *role performance*, you might ask:

- "What things could you do before this illness/injury that you cannot do now?"
- "What do you want to do that you can't do because of this illness?" (Responses might indicate a nursing diagnosis of Ineffective Role Performance.)

DIAGNOSING, PLANNING, AND IMPLEMENTING

Many of clients' psychosocial problems can be treated within the nurse-client relationship using therapeutic communication. The following nursing diagnoses often respond well to psychosocial nursing interventions:

- Deficient Knowledge
- Social Isolation *or* Loneliness *or* Impaired Social Interaction
- Ineffective Coping
- Powerlessness *or* Hopelessness
- Anxiety
- Situational Low Self-Esteem *or* Chronic Low Self-Esteem
- Ineffective Role Performance

Therapeutic Communication

In addition to all the other uses of communication (socializing, connecting with others, giving or receiving information), **therapeutic communication** can be used as a nursing intervention, and is shown when the nurse uses communication techniques to help the client achieve desired outcomes. Desired outcomes that may be achieved through therapeutic communication are that the client will:

- Develop insight into self.
- Engage in problem solving.
- Build self-esteem.
- Plan adaptive coping skills.
- Express and examine feelings.

Therapeutic communication is an effective tool. Like anything new and challenging, it takes practice to learn and do well. Students tend to find therapeutic communication unnatural, because it is unnatural. This is not the kind of communication you learned at home. It is a professional nursing intervention. Table 5-3 ■ describes different therapeutic communication techniques.

TABLE 5-3		
Therapeutic Communication Techniques		
TECHNIQUE	**DEFINITION AND GOAL OF THIS TECHNIQUE**	**EXAMPLES**
Broad Opening	A general statement that allows the client to select the topic of discussion.	"How has life been treating you?" "What are you up to?" "How are you dealing with being in the hospital?" "What's new?"
Clarifying	The nurse may restate the client's message in the nurse's own words, or ask about the client's message for the purpose of ensuring that sender and receiver understand the same message.	"What do you mean by that?" "Did you say that you are uncomfortable?" "I think you said that you are afraid of alligators, is that right?"
Encouraging Evaluation	The nurse encourages clients to evaluate their feelings and experiences for the purpose of insight development.	"How were you feeling when your mother called the police?" "What happened after you quit taking your meds?" "What did you learn from your experience with . . .?"

(continued)

TABLE 5-3

Therapeutic Communication Techniques (continued)

TECHNIQUE	DEFINITION AND GOAL OF THIS TECHNIQUE	EXAMPLES
Focusing	This includes making generalizations specific. Focusing requires the client to consider the truth behind generalized statements.	**Client:** "Everybody hates me." **Nurse:** "Give me an example of someone who said they hate you."
General Leads	This is a brief statement intended to indicate that the nurse is listening and to encourage the client to continue talking on the same subject.	"Go on . . ." "Tell me more about that. . . ." "And then . . .?"
Offering Self	Introduction of self and role or relationship. This clarifies what the nurse's position and intentions are. It also offers the company of the nurse.	"My name is Monica. I'm a student nurse, and I'll be working with you today." "I'll stay with you during the procedure."
Open-Ended Question	The nurse asks a question that requires an explanation or extended response by the client. This question does not lend itself to a yes/no or one-word answer. It is intended to allow clients to organize and express their thoughts.	"What is it like for you to be in the hospital?" "What happened that brought you to the hospital this time?"
Planning for Coping	The nurse encourages the client to plan adaptive responses to future stressful situations to improve coping skills.	"The next time you disagree with Dan, how can you resolve it without hitting him?" "How else could you ask somebody to turn down the TV?" "If they don't give you the correct change, what can you do?"
Reflection	The nurse repeats part of what the client says (like reflecting in a mirror) for the purpose of encouraging the client to explore these feelings further.	**Client:** "When everything is really stressful I can get so overwhelmed." **Nurse:** "You get so overwhelmed."
Sharing Observations	The nurse expresses client behavior in words to call attention to implied meanings or to bring awareness of incongruence between client words and actions.	"When you cover your head with the sheets, it looks like you don't want to talk." "You say you feel fine, but you are crying."
Silence	A period of quiet can allow the nurse and/or the client to collect their thoughts.	
Validation	The nurse recognizes and acknowledges the client's feelings verbally to show that the nurse understands that the client is experiencing a challenge or accepts the client's feelings. Shows empathy.	"This must be very hard for you." "Being in the hospital away from your family can be lonely."

Because it is a nursing intervention, therapeutic communication is used as a part of the nursing process. The nurse identifies the client's need and plans a therapeutic communication goal to help the client achieve outcomes. The nurse plans the interaction at a point when there will be adequate time for a conversation. During the interaction, the nurse will use therapeutic communication techniques to help the client express feelings, solve problems, develop coping skills, or to reach whatever the goal is for the interaction. Finally, the nurse will evaluate how effectively the goal was reached.

Process Recordings

A **process recording** is a written record of a conversation between a nursing student and a client. The verbal communication is written from the student's memory. Using tape recorders or taking notes tends to make people nervous, so they should be avoided. Both verbal and nonverbal cues are noted. The record includes which therapeutic communication techniques are used and the student's analysis of the communication.

Yes, therapeutic communication is an unnatural way to communicate, but when nurses are good at it, they can help clients make real progress. Even when you are really new at it, clients often respond positively. It seems more natural to the receiver than it does to the sender. Learning something complex like therapeutic communication is easier when students think about what they are trying to accomplish with the communication techniques. This is why process recordings are used.

Table 5-4 ■ is an example of a process recording. It may be a relief to know that nurses do not document

---

TABLE 5-4

Sample Process Recording

Setting and situation: We were in the client's room. She was in bed. I was in the chair. When we started she was looking sad. We agreed earlier to have a talk after breakfast.
Medical diagnosis: Cancer of the Lung (8 cm. tumor in right lung)
Therapeutic communication goal: Client will express her feelings about having cancer.

CLIENT (VERBAL AND NONVERBAL)	NURSE (VERBAL AND NONVERBAL)	TECHNIQUE USED	ANALYSIS (ANALYZE WHETHER EACH TECHNIQUE WORKED AS YOU PLANNED)
	"Good morning again, Mrs. King. I am Kate and I'm the student nurse who was going to talk with you." [I'm smiling.]	Offering Self	I was so nervous! I feel like I am impersonating a nurse! I hoped she would talk to me.
"Hi, Kate. What did you want to talk about?" [She looks sad.]	"I heard that you got the diagnosis of lung cancer yesterday. How are you handling it so far?"	Broad Opening	I was hoping to start with a broad opening so she could take whatever direction she wanted. I was scared to mention the cancer, but the nurse said she hasn't talked much about it yet.
"Yes. I think I knew it was cancer, but I am still shocked."	"You're shocked?"	Reflection	I thought maybe she would talk more about her feelings if I could keep her talking.
"Sure. This is a hard thing to hear."	"Do you mean that it's hard to find out that you have cancer?"	Clarifying	Duh! This felt like a stupid question, but I got an unexpected answer.
"Yes, but I think it really hit home when the doctor said that I have only 6 to 12 months left to live." [There is a tear in her eye. She looks out the window.]	"Oh! That must be so hard." [I am blinking a lot to keep from crying, too.]	Validation	What can you say when somebody is dying? All I could do is show that I know it must be so hard for her.
"I can't really talk with my daughters and sons about this."	"You can't talk to them?"	Reflection	It is funny how when you say back what somebody said they talk more about it. This works.
"I can't share this burden with them. How can they handle it? They have their own lives and problems."	"Have you ever shared bad news with them before?"	Planning for Coping	I was trying to get her to find a way she could talk to the people I thought would be her support system. Maybe they have had some success before that they can draw on.

(continued)

TABLE 5-4

Sample Process Recording (continued)

CLIENT (VERBAL AND NONVERBAL)	NURSE (VERBAL AND NONVERBAL)	TECHNIQUE USED	ANALYSIS (ANALYZE WHETHER EACH TECHNIQUE WORKED AS YOU PLANNED)
"Well, [long pause] we did get through my husband's cancer and death OK."	"What helped you get through that?"	Planning for Coping	I hope she will find an answer for what can help her.
"We talked a lot. We looked at old pictures and we spent a lot of time together and we all talked a lot. You know the doctor told me that if there is anything I've always wanted to do, I should do it. I think all I really want is to be with my kids and grandkids as much as I can."	"Will you be able to talk to them, do you think?"	I was trying to do Planning for Coping.	I was glad she was talking to me. It seems like she lightened up, became calmer.
"Yes, I'll call my daughter tonight." [She made a tiny smile.]	"It will be good to talk to her." [Smiling].	I was trying for Validation.	I felt really relieved at this moment.
[She is looking out the window again.]	"Thanks for talking to me, Mrs. King." [I got up to leave and squeezed her hand.]	Showing the end of the conversation and I wanted her to know I care about her.	
"Thank you for talking to *me*, Kate."			

Evaluation: Was the goal met? How did you feel during the interaction? How would you do it differently if you could?
I think my goal was reached. I wanted her to talk about her feelings. The outcome was that she worked through her idea that she couldn't talk to her children and decided in the end to call them, which is good because she needs some support now.
I felt anxious during this, but I felt good about it in the end.
If I could do it again, I would have a better summary at the end. I could have restated that she decided to call her daughter and that that was good.

their therapeutic conversations on process recordings (they are only a learning tool). It may also be good to know that the therapeutic communication techniques are not expected in all your professional conversations, only the therapeutic ones. You are not expected to go around restating, using general leads, and focusing in every conversation. What a relief!

Promoting Healthy Professional Boundaries

It is very rewarding for people to have a caring, nonjudgmental listener. Sometimes, though, clients misinterpret the nurse's attention and caring as social interest. The nurse may need to clarify that s/he is doing a job and not trying to start a friendship. There are a few measures nurses can take to promote clear boundaries and to make it clear that the nurse's role is professional. There are four areas that create problems with personal boundaries:

- Touch
- Self-disclosure
- Gifts
- Contact with clients outside work

Nurses should use common sense about touching clients. Be especially careful about using touch in the psychiatric setting. Psychiatric clients may have a distorted reality or a history of abuse that gives touch other meanings. Be careful with self-disclosure. Although some disclosure relevant to the client's situation may be indicated to demonstrate empathy, remember to keep the focus on the client.

Do not accept gifts from clients. Some clients believe that the nurse expects a gift in return for care, or that care will be improved if a gift is given. Others may hope to continue their relationship with the nurse after their discharge. Use common sense in this area also. If a client's family member brings a box of candy for the entire staff, this would be acceptable. If an individual gives the nurse a gift of jewelry or money, it is not appropriate for the nurse to accept it.

Clients may ask for your telephone number or your address. Maybe they just want to call with some medical questions, or to send a card to express their thanks. Do not give this information about yourself or other nurses to clients or families. It is not appropriate for the nurse to maintain contact with clients outside the work setting. You might say, "I can't give you that information, but you could send a card for the nurses to the hospital," or "There is an advice nurse you can call for help when you are home. I will give you the number." The nurse has a professional relationship with clients, which ends when the client is discharged from the facility. This distinction between professional and personal relationship can be difficult, especially when the client has been hospitalized for a long time. Clients may be invited back to share their progress with the staff, but not to the homes of the nurses. If a client needs home care, a referral should be made through the client's physician or the agency's social services department.

Nurses must be aware of the power that is present in their helping role. The therapeutic nurse-client relationship is built on the foundation of trust, respect, and the appropriate use of power. Nurses must understand the power differential in the nurse-client relationship in order to establish and maintain professional boundaries. Clients are only able to safely explore treatment issues when the nurse conducts the professional relationship using appropriate boundaries.

Recognizing Communication Barriers

- Become familiar with communication barriers. *As with anything else, you learn to improve your communication skills as you practice. Do not expect yourself to be perfect. Learn from your mistakes and improvement will come over time.*
- Avoid the temptation to agree with the client's decisions or to disrespect her or his concerns, however small they may seem to you. Do not answer real concerns with pat generalized phrases. *Your job is to focus on the client's concerns. Agreeing with a client's choice shifts the focus away from the client's thinking and encourages the client to make decisions that meet with your approval. At the other extreme, dismissing a client's concerns means that you judge them to be unimportant. In both instances, that makes the nurse more important than the client.*

Using Therapeutic Communication Skills

- Plan therapeutic interactions and follow through on them. *For example, decide that during a bed bath you will talk with the woman waiting to have surgery for ovarian cancer. Plan a time when you can listen and allow her to express her feelings. You may share your experience to a limited degree to show understanding, but keep the focus of the interaction on the client.*
- Use active listening techniques. Resist the temptation to end stressful conversations to get away. *Listening carefully and allowing the client to express feelings can be scary, especially if the feelings are negative. If the client is transferring feelings to you, do not take the feelings as a personal attack. If the client has a legitimate complaint, you may be able to identify some ways to solve the problem.*
- Show respect for personal boundaries. *You will build trust by being sensitive to verbal and nonverbal feedback from the client about personal space. Tell the client when you must come into her or his personal space and why.*

EVALUATING

As with any other nursing actions, the nurse must review the effectiveness of interventions used in therapeutic communication. Strategies that were effective can be remembered and used again in similar situations. Strategies that were ineffective should be reviewed to identify the barrier they created.

Sometimes a nurse knows exactly when he or she has said the wrong thing. It can be very useful in those situations to say immediately, "That's not what I meant to say. I meant . . ." Prompt attention to the client's feedback can be valuable in maintaining a trusting nurse-client relationship.

NURSING PROCESS CARE PLAN
Communicating Effectively with Client

Clara Barefoot is an 86-year-old Native American client who is in the hospital for treatment of an injury to her shoulder as a result of a fall at home. She is a delightful, intelligent, and interesting woman who is a retired elementary school teacher. She still works, teaching quilting and children's art classes. Discharge is ordered in 2 days. She asked the nurse to visit her home to enjoy some of the vegetables from her garden and to help her with "a few little things, like washing my hair and going to the grocery store." She has many friends and relatives visiting her at the hospital each day.

Assessment. T 97.6, P 110, R 16, BP 140/80. Client is left-handed. She is eating 50–100% of her meals. Skin is dry and intact. Large purple ecchymosis with slight swelling over left shoulder. Circulation, movement, and sensation of hand distal to injured shoulder are within normal limits. Range of motion in injured shoulder is limited. She is unable to raise her left arm above shoulder level, or above her head. Client states: "What will I do? I can't go home. I'm all alone."

Diagnosis. The following nursing diagnoses are identified for Ms. Barefoot:

- Self-Care Deficit: bathing/hygiene R/T limited ROM of left shoulder
- Ineffective Coping R/T inability to formulate plan for help with care after discharge

Expected Outcomes. The expected outcomes for Ms. Barefoot are:

- Client will demonstrate bathing and hair washing using right arm by tomorrow.
- Client will form a list of resources for help with instrumental activities of daily living (such as transportation, laundry, and shopping) by discharge.

Planning and Implementation. The following nursing interventions are implemented for Ms. Barefoot:

- Establish a trusting nurse-client relationship.
- Encourage client to express her feelings about her injury and her temporary disability (use therapeutic communication).

- Assist client to bathe self and wash hair using right arm. Help her learn to set up supplies in advance.
- Teach client safety issues related to bathing when she is off-balance due to left arm in sling.
- Help the client develop a list of activities with which she will need help and a list of people who could help her.
- Involve daughter in planning for discharge and in identifying resources.

Evaluation. By the day of discharge, Ms. Barefoot had a list of friends and relatives and their phone numbers who were willing to help her with a variety of tasks (transportation, shopping, yard work). Her daughter will help her wash her hair. Members of her church volunteered to visit her daily.

Critical Thinking in the Nursing Process

1. What could the nurse say to Ms. Barefoot when she asked for help at home?
2. If she did not have so many friends and family to help her, should the nurse have volunteered to visit Ms. Barefoot at home? Why or why not?
3. If this was the client's third fall and she stated that she is afraid to go home alone, which member of the healthcare team should be involved to help with discharge planning?

Note: Discussion of Critical Thinking questions appears in Appendix I.

Note: The references and resources for this and all chapters have been compiled at the back of the book.

Chapter Review

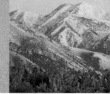

KEY TERMS

Use the audio glossary feature of the Companion Website to hear the correct pronunciation of the following key terms.

active listening

attending behaviors

clarifying

communication

concreteness

congruence

countertransference

empathy

focusing

general leads

genuineness

objectivity

open-ended question

orientation phase

process recording

reflection

respect

self-disclosure

sharing observations

termination phase

therapeutic communication

therapeutic use of self

transference

trustworthiness

validation

working phase

KEY Points

- Professional and social relationships are different. A professional relationship focuses on client needs, is goal directed, and is time limited.
- The phases of the nurse-client relationship are orientation, working, and termination.
- The essential elements of the nurse-client relationship are trustworthiness, caring, empathy, genuineness, respect, and concreteness.
- When clients base their responses to the nurse on their previous experiences, it is called *transference*.
- It is called *countertransference* when the nurse reacts to a client because of the nurse's previous experiences, not because of this client.
- Nurses need to recognize what factors make communication effective and what factors are barriers to communication.
- Therapeutic communication is a nursing intervention used to reach client goals such as exploration of feelings, insight development, problem solving, and planning for adaptive coping.

- Issues that can affect the personal boundaries of professional nurses are touching clients, self-disclosure, accepting gifts, and continuing relationships with clients outside work.
- Self-disclosure by the nurse is only appropriate when it is for the purpose of helping the client.

EXPLORE MediaLink

Additional interactive resources for this chapter can be found on the Companion Website at www.prenhall.com/eby. Click on Chapter 5 and "Begin" to select the activities for this chapter.

- Audio glossary
- NCLEX-PN® review
- Case study
- Study outline
- Critical thinking questions
- Matching questions
- Weblinks

Caring for a Client with Chronic Low Self-Esteem

NCLEX-PN® Focus Area: Psychosocial Integrity

Case Study: Dorothy Ortiz is a 50-year-old European American woman who is hospitalized for a bowel resection for diverticulitis. She works full time and has a 6-week medical leave for recovery from the surgery. Her incision is well approximated, without exudate. She is reluctant to ask for pain medication, which is ordered p.r.n. She has never used her call light. She is reluctant to ambulate. She has raised four children as a single parent, and they come to visit her in the hospital regularly. One of her daughters has an 18-month-old baby.

Nursing Diagnosis: Chronic low self-esteem

COLLECT DATA

Subjective	Objective
_____	_____
_____	_____
_____	_____
_____	_____
_____	_____
_____	_____
_____	_____

Would you report this data? Yes/No

If yes, to: _____

Nursing Care

_____

_____

_____

_____

_____

_____

_____

_____

_____

How would you document this? _____

_____

_____

Compare your documentation to the sample provided in Appendix I.

Data Collected
(use those that apply)

- Alert, oriented X3
- History of hypertension
- Vegetarian
- T 99.0, P 98, R 16
- BP 138/84
- Client states, "I don't want to bother anyone."
- Works as a nursing assistant
- Client states, "I just hate myself. I don't know why you want to take care of me."
- Lack of eye contact
- When told that she has a beautiful robe, she stated, "This ugly old thing?"
- Client states that she feels tired.
- When her daughter brought Dorothy's grandson in to visit, she stated, "Why would he want to see me?"

Nursing Interventions
(use those that apply; list in priority order)

- Establish trusting nurse-client relationship.
- Take vital signs more frequently.
- Encourage client to express her feelings.
- Teach client how to have adequate protein in her diet.
- Spend time with the client each shift to show acceptance.
- Discuss the use of positive self-talk (changing the automatic negative thoughts about self to positive affirmations of client's positive qualities).
- Offer pain medication to client every 4 hours.
- Help the client identify her own strengths.
- Discourage negative comments about self.
- Help client practice asking for what she needs.

When a question asks for a sequence of nursing actions, think about the nursing process. Questions will often ask for the first or initial action by the nurse in a situation. The choices might be four correct nursing actions, but only one is the best thing to do *first*. Of course, nurses always *assess* first, before they take action.

1 Which of the following statements about a therapeutic interaction is false?

1. A therapeutic interaction facilitates growth, developmental maturity, improved functioning, and improved coping.
2. A therapeutic interaction requires that there be a sender, message, and receiver.
3. It is unnecessary to validate the receiver's perception of the message for a therapeutic interaction to occur.
4. The receiver may have to restate the message to the sender to ensure understanding.

2 Which of the following comments by the nurse indicates that the nurse is being empathetic?

1. "Oh, I feel so sorry for you!"
2. "I can't understand how you can handle so much pain and still be cheerful."
3. "How can you tolerate your roommate?"
4. "I know how it feels to lose someone you love. Would you like to talk about it?"

3 Which of the following statements about active listening is false?

1. It is difficult to listen actively when you do not value what the other person is saying.
2. Active listening requires practice.
3. It is possible to listen actively and still plan what you will say in response.
4. You can let the "sender" know you are listening by nodding your head and maintaining eye contact.

4 To communicate a willingness to discuss a topic with a client who is in bed, the best body position for the nurse is:

1. Sitting in a chair pulled up close to the client's bedside, so the nurse is at eye level.
2. Standing at the foot of the bed.
3. Standing at the bedside but leaning on the table over the bed.
4. Sitting in a chair about 4 feet away from the client with the nurse's arms folded.

5 Which of the following is a true statement about nonverbal communication?

1. Nonverbal communication is interpreted the same by all observers.
2. A client who avoids eye contact with you has something to hide.
3. Touch is not always associated with comforting and caring by all clients.
4. The hands are the most expressive part of the body.

6 A female client is crying quietly in her room. When the nurse asks what is wrong, she does not answer. The best response by the nurse in this situation would be:

1. "I can see you're in no mood for company now. I'll come back later."
2. "I can see you're upset about something. I would really like to help you, but I can't do anything for you if you won't talk to me. When you're ready, put on your call light, and I'll come back."
3. "I see you're sad. You know every cloud has a silver lining, so I'm sure things will get better for you too."
4. "I see that you're sad. I'll sit right here by your bed just to be with you. If you feel like talking, that's okay; if not, that's okay too. I just want you to know I care."

7 Which of the following is an open-ended question?

1. "How do you feel about being in traction for a month?"
2. "Is the traction comfortable?"
3. "Will you lose your job while you're in traction for a month?"
4. "Can you brush your teeth while you're in traction?"

8 If a client says to the nurse, "I feel like I'm going to die," and the nurse wants to use the reflecting technique to respond, s/he might say:

1. "You're not feeling well today?"
2. "Tell me about that feeling."
3. "You feel like you're going to die."
4. "I can see you're depressed today."

9 A client is having difficulty deciding what to do after leaving the hospital and asks the opinion of the nurse. The nurse's best response would be:

1. "I know exactly what you should do. Have your doctor order home health for you and get your daughter to move in with you for a little while."
2. "What do you see as your options when you go home? Let's talk about those."
3. "I don't have a clue what you should do."
4. "Oh, I don't get involved with discharge stuff. My job stops here at the hospital."

10 A client says to the nurse, "I have nobody any more. I wish I could just die." Which response by the nurse would block further communication?

1. "Oh, don't think about that. It's just too depressing."
2. "You would like to die?"
3. "Tell me more about those feelings."
4. "You have no one?"

Answers for Review Questions, as well as discussion of Care Plan and Critical Thinking Care Map questions, appear in Appendix I.

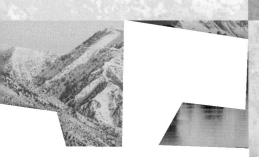

Chapter 6

Stress and Coping

BRIEF Outline

Homeostasis   Adaptation to Stress
The Stress Response

LEARNING Outcomes

After completing this chapter, you will be able to:

1. Explain how stress affects an individual acutely and chronically.
2. Differentiate between adaptive and maladaptive coping methods.
3. Assess clients' stress levels.
4. Promote clients' adaptive coping abilities.

Like all living organisms, people are exposed to stress from physical challenges, but unlike the others we are also stressed by psychological issues. Other animals can experience grief, fear, and other feelings (in response to actual events), but only humans experience stress from worry about things that have not happened. People are increasingly exposed to chronic psychological stressors, and this is changing the pattern of human disease. Stress-related disease is on the rise (Sapolsky, 2004). The good news is that nurses can help people learn to cope with stress in a more healthy way.

Homeostasis

The study of stress begins with the concept of homeostasis. **Homeostasis** is the state of dynamic balance of the human body's internal environment, which is always adjusting in response to internal and external changes. This stable internal environment is necessary for survival. The ability of the body to maintain homeostasis depends on thousands of physiologic control systems. Homeostatic mechanisms within our bodies include the systems that maintain fluid and electrolyte balance, oxygen levels, and even the neuroendocrine systems that influence behavior (Porth, 2007).

A stressor can throw off the homeostatic balance, as surely as if one child were to get off a seesaw (Figure 6-1 ■). A **stressor** is anything that puts the individual out of homeostasis. The brain has evolved to seek homeostasis, so it initiates the **stress response,** which is the reaction of the body in an attempt to restore homeostasis (Sapolsky, 2004).

The Stress Response

In the animal kingdom in general, stressors are physiological events. For example, an alligator (Figure 6-2 ■) may experience stress from hunger. The alligator will

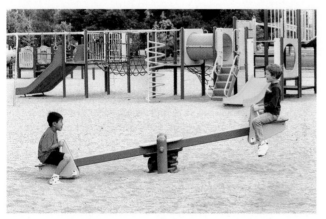

Figure 6-1. ■ A stressor can offset homeostasis just like one child getting off a seesaw. *Source:* PhotoEdit Inc.

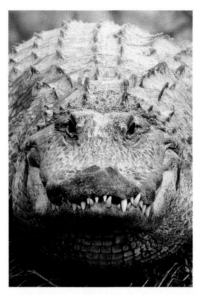

Figure 6-2. ■ The alligator only experiences physiological stressors. *Source:* Getty Images Inc.

not, however, experience psychological stressors, such as distress about whether her mate will be disappointed over her choice of a meal. Humans, however, frequently experience such psychological stressors ("Will my husband like the meatloaf?" "Does this outfit make me look fat?" "How will I make the rent payment?").

Theorist Hans Selye (1976) described stress as the physiological response to changes experienced by a biological organism. He found that the stress response is a general body reaction. Whether a person is being chased by a hungry alligator or has to walk up on a stage to accept an important award, the physiological reaction will be the same. This physiological reaction to a stressor is called the **fight or flight response.** Epinephrine stimulates the sympathetic nervous system to prepare the body to fight the source of danger or to run away. This stress response is only adaptive when the stressor is a physical threat. Figure 6-3 ■ illustrates how the various organ systems are affected by the fight or flight response.

When you look closely at the physiological reactions to stress in Figure 6-3, you can see how these responses would be very helpful to a person who had to face physical danger such as coming in contact with an alligator. In such an emergency, it would help people survive if they could see better in low light (dilated pupils), could run faster (blood diverted away from GI tract to skeletal muscle), and had more energy to run longer (increased glucose availability).

Unfortunately, most modern stressors are not from people being chased by alligators. Nursing stressors are usually more like the pressure to care for groups of clients

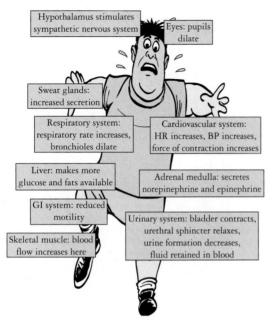

Figure 6-3. ■ The fight or flight response.

without enough help, the concern that the client may suffer if we forget something, or the pressure to give all the medications by an exact schedule despite many interruptions. Because the human body responds with the same stress reaction whether the stressor is an alligator or heavy traffic keeping us from getting to work on time, the fight or flight syndrome bombards people frequently.

Chronic exposure to sympathetic nervous system stimulation is not healthy. Although increased blood glucose is great in an emergency, prolonged hyperglycemia causes early fatigue and increased risk of type 2 diabetes. The stress response inhibits the release of growth hormone. Over time this can reduce growth in children and hinder the repair of tissues in adults. A chronically elevated blood pressure can increase risks of stroke, heart attack, and kidney disease. Inhibition of the immune system increases the risk of infection in the short term and inhibits tumor immunity in the long term (Sapolsky, 2004). Even the reproductive system is affected. Menstrual and premenstrual symptoms become more severe and testosterone levels and sperm count decrease under chronic stress. Fertility decreases as well (Hertig, 2004).

INDIVIDUAL VARIATION

The stress response can become damaging, especially when it is frequent and severe. The stressors themselves, however, do not cause disease directly. Individuals vary in their response to specific stressors. The same potential stressor can cause different responses in different people (Porth, 2007).

Lazarus and Folkman (1984) described stress as a relationship between the person and the environment. People may judge an experience as challenging their resources or threatening their well-being, which would make the event stressful. It is the person's *perception* of an event that makes it stressful. One person receiving an immunization who has had several before with no problems may not be concerned about it (and experience no stress response). Another person, whose father died from anaphylactic shock after an immunization, may be terrified (and will experience a severe stress response). Figure 6-4 ■ shows some potential stressors. The ability of each situation to cause the stress response depends on how an individual perceives it. Which ones would cause you the most stress?

clinical ALERT

It is not the event itself that determines the severity of the stress response for the client, but the significance the event has for the client that gives it its meaning. The nurse must assess the client for personal attitudes related to health issues and treat all clients according to their individual needs.

A variety of factors influence how a person perceives and reacts to a stressor. The predisposing factors include age, maturity, culture, life experiences, and personality traits.

EFFECT OF CULTURE ON STRESS RESPONSE

Culture is the learned pattern of values, attitudes, roles, communication, and behavior that is passed from one generation to the next. A person's cultural origin affects how the person perceives events in the world. Culture affects a person's behavior and the meanings of various life events (and therefore how stressful certain events are perceived to be). See Cultural Pulse Points Box 6-1 ■. For

BOX 6-1   CULTURAL PULSE POINTS

Cultural Effects on Signs and Symptoms of Stress
Western European and North American cultures generally expect that emotional stress will be expressed emotionally and physical stress will be expressed physically. In contrast, the majority of African, Asian, and Central American cultures expect people to express emotional distress in physical terms (Gonzales, Griffith, & Ruiz, 2001). For example, a client from Mexico, Nigeria, or Vietnam may have abdominal pain or a headache when they are worried or under psychological stress. To be culturally sensitive, nurses must recognize that a client's physical discomfort may have emotional causes and must include this possibility in nursing assessments.

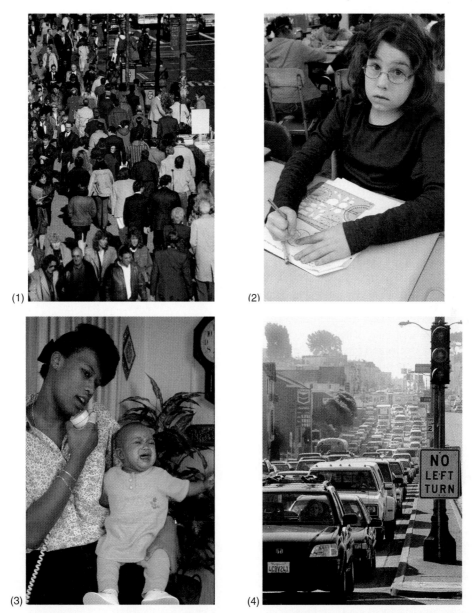

Figure 6-4. ■ Potential stressors include **(1)** crowds, **(2)** testing, **(3)** parenting challenges, and **(4)** traffic. Individual factors influence how much of a stress response a person may feel in each of these situations. Which situation causes you the most stress? *Sources:* (1) Corbis/Bettman; (2) Ellen Senisi; (3) PhotoEdit Inc.; (4) AP Worldwide Photos.

example, a fracture of a right-handed client's right hand requiring a cast may be especially stressful if the client is from the Middle East where the left hand is considered unclean. This client would not be able to touch people politely, gesture, or even pass food or other items to another person with her left hand, so she would be under more stress and would feel more disabled than a European American client with the same injury who only sees it as an inconvenience to function with her nondominant hand.

Adaptation to Stress

We all experience stress in our daily lives. People can respond in either a healthy way that promotes or sustains their development or in a way that disintegrates their health. These responses (**coping mechanisms**) are part of our pattern of behavior in reaction to stress. **Adaptation** is behavior that maintains the integrity of the individual. It is a healthy response to stress or life events. **Maladaptation** is unhealthy behavior that disrupts the integrity of the

TABLE 6-1		
Factors Affecting the Ability to Adapt to a Stressor		
FACTOR	**EXPLANATION**	**EXAMPLE**
Age	The capacity to adapt is decreased in the very young and the old.	A baby or an elder is more likely to suffer dehydration when spending prolonged time in the sun.
Genetics	A family history of psychological or physical conditions, intelligence, or physical strength or weakness may affect ability to cope with stressors.	A person who has always been strong and healthy may recover quickly from surgery.
Health status	Severe or chronic illness can decrease a client's reserves of energy and healing capacity when confronted with a new stressor. Good nutrition and adequate sleep can improve the ability to adapt.	A client with cancer may have more difficulty adapting to moving into a new home or recovering from a fall.
Past experiences	The individual's prior experience in a similar situation may help (by learning strategies for success) or hinder (by causing the anticipation of a bad result) the ability to adapt this time.	Because he was stung by a bee at camp last summer, a child cries when his parents prepare for him to go this year.
Resources	The availability of financial, personal (such as maturity), social, and coping skills improve the individual's ability to adapt.	A person with no job, unsafe living conditions, no friends, and few coping skills has difficulty adapting to diabetes.

individual (Roy, 1976). If a nurse had a difficult day at work, adaptive ways to relieve the stress would be to talk to someone about what happened, to go for a walk, or to take a warm bath. Maladaptive responses would be to kick the dog, to sit alone and worry, or to drink alcohol.

There are positive and negative ways that people behave when managing or coping with stress (Lazarus & Folkman, 1984; Roy, 1976).

POSITIVE (ADAPTIVE) STRESS RESPONSES

- *Problem solving.* Identify the problem, plan a response, and actively work on it.
- *Using social support.* Request and accept help from caring others.
- *Reframing.* Redefine the situation to see positive as well as negative sides and how to use the situation to your advantage.

NEGATIVE (MALADAPTIVE) STRESS RESPONSES

- *Avoidance.* Choosing not to deal with the situation. Negative feelings may become chronic.
- *Self-blame.* Blaming self takes the focus off working toward resolution of the problem. Feelings are about the self and not the problem.

- *Wishful thinking.* Thinking that "everything will be fine" to the exclusion of doing anything to make this happen. This is a form of denial.

The ability of an individual to adapt to a stressor is affected by several factors (Table 6-1 ■). Nurses should take these issues into consideration when planning care. Promoting a client's ability to adapt to stressors is an important part of health promotion.

NURSING CARE

Every living organism experiences stress. The goal of nursing is not to remove all stress, because it is a part of life. The stress response can become unhealthy, however, and that is when nurses can help through health promotion. Health promotion must include strategies for stress reduction and management. Nurses can apply the nursing process to stress management. The nursing process seems to work everywhere.

ASSESSING

A part of the admission nursing assessment of every client should be the current stressors of the client. If a client is admitted to the emergency department with a fracture, it is useful to know that this person just lost his job, his wife left him, and his dog is sick. He may need coping strategies as much as he needs treatment of his fracture.

Along with asking about a client's stressors, the nurse must also assess the client's coping patterns. Some examples of questions to assess a client's stress and coping are:

- "How is this affecting you?" (*to assess the severity of the stressor for the client*)
- "How do you feel about this?" (*to see how it affects the client's emotional state*)
- "What do you usually do when something like this happens?"(*to assess usual coping behavior*)
- "Can you think of anything you can do about this?" (*to assess coping strategies*)
- "Whom can you call on to help you with this?" (*to assess the client's social support resources*)

DIAGNOSING, PLANNING, AND IMPLEMENTING

Ineffective Coping is a common nursing diagnosis for people under stress who are unable to form a valid appraisal of the stressors and have inadequate choices of positive responses and/or inability to use available resources. Possible *etiologies* (causes) for this problem are situational crisis, personal vulnerability, inadequate support system, inadequate coping skills, and fear of failure.

There are several strategies for dealing with stress. The most effective approach to controlling stress in everyday life is the cognitive-behavioral approach. See Chapter 3 for a description of the theories of *cognitive* (thinking and teaching) and *behavioral* (practicing) therapy.

The *cognitive approach* focuses on teaching the client or helping the client think about the problem. Keeping a journal is an effective cognitive therapy. Keeping an informational diary of daily events, activities, and feelings can reveal much about stressors in a person's life. After identifying the stressors in the journal, the client can examine priorities and goals. If the stress-producing activities are not meeting the client's own goals, can they be dropped? The next step is making the change from stress-producing to stress-relieving activities (Varcarolis, Carson, & Shoemaker, 2005).

Cognitive reframing, as described by Lazarus and Folkman (1984), suggests restructuring irrational or self-defeating beliefs. The irrational beliefs are replaced with positive adaptive statements. Examples are replacing "I never do well in school" with "If I study hard, I have a better chance to do well in school" or replacing "I am afraid to talk to clients" with "I can talk to clients like I talk to other people" (Varcarolis et al., 2005). The nurse might explain cognitive reframing to a client like this: "When people regularly say negative things to themselves, they begin to believe them. To change the negative thinking, you need to change those negative statements. Convert them to positive ones like: "I *can* control my diabetes if I focus on it."

Problem solving is an excellent adaptive coping strategy. After an objective assessment of the situation, the problem-solving/decision-making model can be used (Townsend, 2005):

1. Assess the facts of the situation.
2. Formulate goals for resolving the problem.
3. Study the alternative choices for dealing with the situation.
4. Determine the risks and benefits of each alternative.
5. Select an alternative.
6. Implement the chosen alternative.
7. Evaluate the outcome of the alternative implemented.
8. If the first choice is not effective, select and implement another alternative.

Behavioral approaches include having the client try new stress-reducing behavior. The behavior will be reinforced by causing a reduction in stress and will then be more likely to be repeated. Assertiveness training, in which the client practices acting assertively, is an effective behavioral therapy. Table 6-2 ■ provides examples of the different levels of assertiveness.

One approach that helps with stress in relationships is to practice assertively asking others to change their behavior (asking for own needs to be met, treating the other person respectfully).

The nurse can teach the client to use a three-part method of assertively asking for behavior change. Nurses can also use this technique themselves.

1. When you _____ (fill in the blank in a nonaccusing and nonthreatening way, describing the behavior you want to change, for example, When you give me so much homework)
2. I feel _____ (fill in the blank with your feelings, not opinions, for example, I feel overwhelmed)
3. I wish you would _____ (fill in the blank with what you want changed; keep this about the behavior, not the person, for example, I wish you would give us fewer reading assignments in everything except that mental health nursing book that I love)

TABLE 6-2		
Levels of Assertiveness		
LEVELS OF ASSERTIVENESS	DEFINITION OF BEHAVIOR	EXAMPLE
Passive	The *passive* person meets the needs of others, without asking for own needs to be met.	"OK, you can have my ice cream cone. I didn't want it anyway."
Assertive	The *assertive* person asks for own needs to be met, with respectful concern for the needs of others.	"Sure, I'll drive you to work today. Will you drive me on Tuesday when my sister needs to use my car?"
Aggressive	The *aggressive* person demands for own needs to be met, without regard for the needs of others.	"I want to play now. I don't care if you think it's your turn."

Some other behavioral strategies are progressive muscle relaxation and biofeedback (which requires special training).

Critical Self-Check. There are many drugs that treat the stress response, such as the benzodiazepines (Valium and Ativan). Why are the nursing approaches suggested in this book a healthier first strategy for stress management than medication?

Other stress management strategies include:

- Listening to music (must be selected by the client because music tastes are very individual).
- Interpersonal communication with a caring other. Talking about the problem with a friend can stop the escalation of stress (Townsend, 2005).
- Pets. Pets, especially dogs and cats, give unconditional love. They provide an outlet for our own expression of affection. They can help with socialization in cognitively impaired people. Pets can even decrease the blood pressure of people with mental stress (Allen, Shykoff, & Izzo, 2001).
- Meditation trains the mind to develop greater calm and then to use that calm to bring about greater insight. It has been shown to reduce blood pressure. Meditation can also help people develop stress reduction strategies, make adaptive choices under pressure, and feel more engaged in life (Kabat-Zinn, 1993).
- Breathing exercises have helped people to manage the discomfort of labor and to reduce stress in more everyday situations. It works partly by helping clients to interrupt stressful thoughts, to quiet mental confusion, and partly by distraction.
- Aerobic exercise increases endorphin release, which causes a sense of well-being. It improves mood. Aerobic exercise reduces anxiety, depression, and sensitivity to stressful events (Salmon, 2000).

Critical Self-Check. Which of these stress management strategies do you use? Are you willing to try others?

EVALUATING

The nurse can ask the following questions to evaluate whether the client has achieved the desired outcomes for Ineffective Coping:

- Can the client identify the source of stress?
- Is the client able to identify which behaviors are maladaptive?
- Is the client using effective coping or problem-solving skills?
- Is the client able to ask for help?
- Can the client identify resources for help with problem solving?
- Is the client willing and able to initiate the lifestyle change necessary to cope with stressors in an adaptive (healthy) way?

NURSING PROCESS CARE PLAN
Client with Ineffective Coping

A 19-year-old college student, Casey James, has been admitted to a surgical unit following emergency surgery to remove a ruptured appendix. Casey appears very angry, criticizing the staff and demanding that someone "fix" his PCA pump so that it delivers more medication. He rates his pain at an "11" on a scale of 1 to 10. He constantly turns on his call light and refuses to follow the doctor's orders to ambulate. He tells the nurse that he is in too much pain to even move. He is uncooperative with offers to assist him with bathing. He insists on using the bedpan or urinal rather than getting up to use the bathroom.

Assessment. In talking to Casey, the nurse discovers that his appendicitis symptoms began during his first final, not giving him the opportunity to complete the final or take the other three finals for which he was scheduled. He is sure that his instructors will fail him, and he really wants to succeed. He is the first person in his family to attend college. In addition, Casey has no car and had arranged a ride home for the holidays with a friend who also lives in the same small town 300 miles from the college. His friend had to leave without him. He has no family here but has a mother and a sister back home. He admits his anger and frustration and tells the nurse that he doesn't know what he's going to do. He was looking forward to the month break from school. He doesn't know how he will finish up his class work, and he doesn't know how he will get home. He says, "I just hate it here."

Diagnosis. Three nursing diagnoses were identified for this client:

- Ineffective coping R/T situational crisis and lack of immediate support system
- Powerlessness R/T perceived lack of control over situation
- Noncompliance, therapeutic regimen R/T anger over situation

Expected Outcomes. The client's expected outcomes for the plan of care are:

- The client will verbalize 2 choices of coping behaviors that will be appropriate for his situation.
- The client will identify 2 areas in his situation in which he can demonstrate control.
- The client will ambulate around the surgical unit at least 3 times a day as prescribed in the physician orders.

Planning and Implementation. The nurse will implement the following interventions:

- Spend time talking with the client. Encourage him to express his feelings about his situation (not completing finals and not going home for the school break). The client is expressing anger, but not his feelings, which are likely to be sadness, frustration, fear, and loss. *The client can begin coping with his feelings when he recognizes what they are.*
- Discuss the resources for problem solving that the client has. Does he have an academic advisor? Can he contact his instructors? Is there a dean of students?

When a client is stuck in anger, he may not be able to consider problem-solving strategies. After he has identified his real feelings, he will probably be able to move on to problem solving. Suggestions by the nurse of possible resources may get him started on recognizing that he does have resources, and setting priorities on which he will use first. Moving from anger to problem solving is likely to make the client feel in more control.

- The client was planning to visit his family for the holidays. Arrange for him to be able to talk with them on the phone. Refer the client to social work. They or the chaplain may be able to arrange for transportation of his mother and sister by bus to the hospital to see him if he will not be able to get home. Allow him to be involved in any planning or decision making. *Powerlessness can result from being in a new situation without knowing the possibilities or alternatives. Including clients in decision making, even about small nursing care issues, can impart a sense of control in a situation where the client feels like he has no control.*

- Once the client is expressing his real feelings instead of anger, he is likely to be better able to cooperate with the treatment plan. Teach him why ambulation is important and expect him to participate in his treatment. *Angry clients must usually cope with the anger as a priority before other activities. Clients who understand their treatment plan are more likely to comply with it.*

Evaluation. Casey responded well to treatment and was discharged five days after his surgery. He was able to take a bus home to be with his family for the holidays. He contacted each of his instructors and they were all willing to allow him to make up their final exams due to the medical circumstances.

Critical Thinking in the Nursing Process

1. What is the likely outcome if Casey did not take the active coping approach of contacting the instructors about missing the final exams?
2. Why was Casey less cooperative when he was angry?
3. Was the sudden onset of appendicitis any different than if Casey had experienced symptoms for a week before he became ill?

Note: Discussion of Critical Thinking questions appears in Appendix I.

Note: The references and resources for this and all chapters have been compiled at the back of the book.

KEY TERMS

Use the audio glossary feature of the Companion Website to hear the correct pronunciation of the following key terms.

adaptation

cognitive reframing

coping mechanisms

fight or flight response

homeostasis

maladaptation

stressor

stress response

KEY Points

- Stress has become an epidemic in our society.
- The stress response functions to alert the individual to a threat and to return the body to homeostasis. When it lasts after the stressor is resolved or is activated too frequently, some diseases are more likely to occur.
- People can respond to stress adaptively or maladaptively.
- The stress response begins with the fight or flight response.
- The stress response is nonspecific, meaning that the body responds the same no matter what the stressor is.
- The degree of stress caused by an event depends on how the individual perceives it. Two people experiencing the same event can feel different amounts of stress related to it.
- Culture affects how people perceive and react to stressful events.
- There are many approaches to stress management.
- Nurses experience many job-related stressors and must engage in self-care.

 ## EXPLORE MediaLink

Additional interactive resources for this chapter can be found on the Companion Website at www.prenhall.com/eby. Click on Chapter 6 and "Begin" to select the activities for this chapter.

- Audio glossary
- NCLEX-PN® review
- Case study
- Study outline
- Critical thinking questions
- Matching questions
- Weblinks

Caring for a Client with Difficulty Coping
NCLEX-PN® Focus Area: Psychosocial Integrity

Case Study: Julio Hernandez is a 37-year-old male client who was admitted to the hospital with a fractured pelvis. He sustained the fracture in a motor vehicle wreck in which he was the passenger. He works as an engineer. Mr. Hernandez has been hospitalized for 3 days and his pain is under control. Bed rest is his ordered activity. He is restless, moves around the bed a lot, and has difficulty sleeping. He has an indwelling urinary catheter and an IV infusion. His wife, Elena, states that he is not usually so anxious. When their children come to visit, the nurse notices that one of them walks with a brace on her leg.

Nursing Diagnosis: Ineffective coping

COLLECT DATA

Subjective	Objective
_____	_____
_____	_____
_____	_____
_____	_____
_____	_____
_____	_____
_____	_____

Would you report this data? Yes/No

If yes, to: _____

Nursing Care

_____
_____
_____
_____
_____
_____
_____
_____
_____

How would you document this? _____
_____
_____
_____

Compare your documentation to the sample provided in Appendix I.

Data Collected
(use those that apply)

- Weight 176 lbs/80 kg
- BP 160/96
- Temperature 98.8°F, tympanic
- Pulse 100; respiratory rate 22
- Client states: "I can't handle all of this stress. It is killing me."
- 725 ml of clear yellow urine output this shift
- Lungs clear, no respiratory distress
- Client's wife states, "He is not usually so anxious."
- Client's wife states, "His father died last month in a hospital in Mexico."
- The client clutches the bedspread or pulls away when anyone touches the catheter or the IV.
- Sometimes the client rocks his upper body back and forth.
- Client's wife states: "He is having trouble at work."
- Skin is intact, without lesions, with normal red undertones.

Nursing Interventions
(use those that apply; list in priority order)

- Check vital signs every hour.
- Monitor urine output every hour.
- Say to the client, "What do you mean when you say 'the stress is killing me'?"
- Ask the client, "Besides the fractured pelvis, what other things are stressful for you now?"
- Assess the client's social support by asking, "Who can help you with these problems?"
- Assess the client's coping strategies by asking, "What will you do to manage these problems?"
- Tell the client, "Don't worry, everything will work out fine."
- Say to the client, "You seem anxious when I touch the catheter or the IV. Would you tell me about this?"
- Say to the client, "Your wife told me that your father died recently. That must be hard for you."
- Offer urinal frequently.
- Say to the client, "You look like you are under a lot of stress. I will ask the doctor to give you a sedative medication."

1 A nurse is caring for a client who was admitted to the hospital with pneumonia. The client is constantly clenching his fists, refusing to eat, and having difficulty sleeping. He may be experiencing stress from more than his current illness. If all of the following events had recently occurred for this client, which would be the most likely source of his obvious stress?

  1. Promotion at work
  2. Recognition for 25 years of service at his firm
  3. Divorce
  4. Ticket for minor traffic violation

2 According to Hans Selye's theory of a general body reaction to any stressor, which of the following symptoms might be experienced by a client concerned about his X-ray results?

  1. Hypoglycemia
  2. Increased heart rate
  3. Increased urine output
  4. Constricted pupils

3 Which of the following physical conditions can be caused by continuous stimulation of the sympathetic nervous system?

  1. Hypoglycemia
  2. Glaucoma
  3. Cardiovascular disease
  4. Chronic obstructive pulmonary disease

4 As a nurse, you would be more concerned about the stress response of a client being admitted into the hospital if you knew that:

  1. His wife died in the same hospital recently.
  2. This was his first hospitalization.
  3. This was his first serious illness.
  4. He is concerned about missing his son's first soccer game.

5 Which of the following clients is likely to be more susceptible to the negative aspects of stress?

  1. A teenager living at home with a single parent
  2. A poor, elderly widow suffering from chronic back pain due to osteoporosis
  3. A young married woman with her first pregnancy
  4. A successful businessman with a broken hip

6 Which of the following clients is handling stress in an adaptive way?

  1. The client assesses a situation to see why he is responding in such a stressed way.
  2. The client avoids dealing with the stressor, assuming it will disappear soon.

  3. The client assumes he is responsible for the situation and therefore has things under control.
  4. The client takes an "every cloud has a silver lining" attitude to all stress-provoking events.

7 A newly admitted client has an accidental gunshot wound to her thigh. She states that she is concerned that she might lose her job if she has to be in the hospital for a long time. Choose the best response by the nurse.

  1. "It's too soon to worry about that right now."
  2. "You have a great physician. I'm sure you won't be in here a long time."
  3. "I can see this is really a concern to you. Let's talk about this."
  4. "Do you have a history of attendance problems at work?"

8 The nursing diagnosis of Ineffective Coping is appropriate for a client who:

  1. Discusses her stress openly and frequently with family and friends.
  2. Chooses not to discuss the source of her stress.
  3. Writes about her feelings daily in a private journal.
  4. Requests to see the hospital chaplain for prayer.

9 Select the best stress management technique that you might suggest to a client confined to bed:

  1. Drink herb tea.
  2. Practice progressive muscle relaxation.
  3. Practice being aggressive with those who have been a source of stress in the past.
  4. Get a cat or dog.

10 The client has expressed extreme stress about his current health situation of chronic renal disease. He is recently widowed and his wife had done all the driving due to his poor vision.

   He has now been told that he must begin renal dialysis. The nurse and the client agree that a nursing diagnosis of "Ineffective Coping related to a situational crisis" is appropriate. Select the appropriate early nursing interventions from the following choices.

  1. Ask the client to list all perceived sources of his stress.
  2. Reassure the client that everything will work out.
  3. Review community resources for alternate transportation sources to dialysis.
  4. Educate him on the methods of dialysis available.
  5. Ask him if he is sure that dialysis is necessary at this point.
  6. Advocate with his physician for a stress-relieving medication for him.

Answers for Review Questions, as well as discussion of Care Plan and Critical Thinking Care Map questions, appear in Appendix I.

Chapter 7

Psychobiology and Psychopharmacology

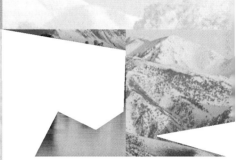

BRIEF Outline

PSYCHOBIOLOGY
Mental Disorders
Brain Anatomy and Function
Genetics of Mental Illness

Neuroendocrine System
PSYCHOPHARMACOLOGY
Pharmacokinetics
Pharmacodynamics

LEARNING Outcomes

After completing this chapter, you will be able to:

1. Teach clients about the biological basis of the major mental disorders.
2. Reinforce client teaching about the desired effects and adverse effects of psychotropic medications.
3. Safely and effectively administer psychotropic medications.
4. Apply the nursing process to clients receiving psychotropic medications.

There is a common misconception that mental disorders are under the client's control, that people can just "cheer up" or "get over it." Friends and family members may say, "What do you have to be depressed about?" or "get a grip on yourself!" or "I would never take drugs that affect my mind." Because of the stigma associated with mental illness, families often want to blame drug use, a life event, or clients themselves for mental disorders. Making the reality of brain disorders clear to families and clients is a job for the mental health team, including nurses.

PSYCHOBIOLOGY

The major mental disorders—schizophrenia, major depressive disorder, and bipolar disorder—are caused by disorders of brain structure and function. The onset, signs, and symptoms of these disorders can vary among individuals due to individual differences, life experiences, and cultural factors, but the disorders themselves are caused by physiological brain abnormalities. The major mental disorders have some symptoms that are similar to problems caused by life experiences. This fact makes diagnosis of mental disorders more challenging, and it can make family members confused about what caused the behavior of their loved one. A person who has experienced a loss may feel very sad, almost like a person with depression. A person who had many life stressors may have poor social skills like a person with schizophrenia. These people, however, are not mentally ill. They have a symptom, but not a brain disorder.

Mental Disorders

Mental disorders cause abnormalities of cognition (thinking), feeling, and behavior. Anatomical and physiological abnormalities in the brain are major causative factors of mental disorders. However, people with mental disorders clearly respond best to treatment that includes a holistic approach. Mental health treatment is most effective when it includes active involvement of the client, *psychotropic medications* (medications affecting the mind), a trusting therapeutic relationship, and cognitive and behavioral therapies.

Diagnostic criteria for mental disorders are included in *The Diagnostic and Statistical Manual of Mental Disorders* (American Psychiatric Association, 2000). The *Diagnostic and Statistical Manual (DSM-IV-TR)* describes specific behavioral, mood, and cognitive signs and symptoms for each mental disorder. Excerpts from the *DSM* will be included in the chapters about specific mental disorders.

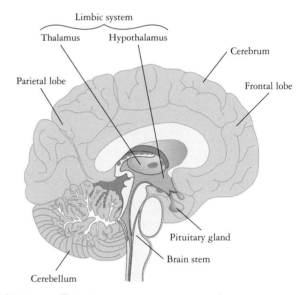

Figure 7-1. ■ Brain anatomy.

Brain Anatomy and Function

The brain is divided into the cerebrum, the limbic system, the brain stem, and the cerebellum. Figure 7-1 ■ shows the brain's anatomy. Table 7-1 ■ provides a summary of brain structures and functions, including the psychiatric implications of abnormalities in specific areas of the brain.

The work of the human brain is performed by approximately 100 billion neurons. The neurons are all interconnected, with an average neuron receiving input from 1,000 to 10,000 neighboring neurons. Figure 7-2 ■ depicts an electron micrograph of actual brain neurons. The complexities of the connections in the human brain are currently incomprehensible (Torrey, 2001). Research is seeking the answers to questions about the exact causes of brain disorders such as schizophrenia, depression, and bipolar disorder, and what treats these disorders specifically and effectively. Although new information is rapidly becoming available, some types of treatment are used because they are effective

TABLE 7-1		
Brain Anatomy and Function		
BRAIN STRUCTURE	FUNCTION	IMPLICATIONS FOR MENTAL DISORDERS
Cerebral Cortex		The frontal lobes are affected in schizophrenia, which causes disordered thought processes, lack of motivation.
Frontal Lobes		
Prefrontal Area	*Prefrontal area* controls thought, inhibition, goal-oriented behavior.	
Motor Cortex	*Motor cortex* controls voluntary movement.	Abnormalities in the motor area (for example, Parkinson's disease) cause movement disorders: rigidity, resting tremor, slow movement, shuffling gait, sudden jerky movement, and athetosis (meaningless unintentional motions). These movement disorders can also be medication side effects (called *extrapyramidal side effects*).
Pyramidal System	*Pyramidal system* or corticospinal tract affects voluntary movement.	
Extrapyramidal System	*Extrapyramidal system* affects movement patterns, automatic motor functioning of walking, and inhibits lower motor neurons from overactivity (involuntary movement).	
Basal Ganglia	In the *basal ganglia*, complex motor skills (driving a car, activities of daily living [ADLs]) become so memorized that the ability to perform them persists even after damage to memory in the frontal lobes.	
Temporal Lobes	Auditory receptive and auditory association areas, olfactory function, language expression and interpretation	Aphasia (receptive or expressive) is caused by damage in the temporal lobes.
Parietal Lobes	Sensory association	
Occipital Lobes	Visual reception and visual association	Damage to occipital lobes can cause blindness.
Limbic System		
Refers to limbic lobe and structures that function with it: hippocampus, amygdala, thalamus, hypothalamus, brainstem nuclei, autonomic system	Controls feeling pleasure, feeding and drinking behavior, the fight or flight response, aggression, submission, memory, body temperature, sexual behavior, emotions, and motivation for behavior. It is responsible for physical reactions to emotions. Limbic system also interprets olfactory sensations. Hippocampus converts short-term memories to long term. Thalamus also has sensory relaying and stimulus filtering functions.	Schizophrenia decreases limbic system function (anhedonia, **polydipsia** [an abnormal, persistent increase in thirst], loss of motivation). Cocaine may stimulate limbic system to provide pleasure. Thiamine deficiency in alcoholics (Korsakoff's syndrome) affects limbic function and causes loss of short-term memory. Hippocampus degenerates in Alzheimer's disease.
Brainstem		
Midbrain	Most of brain dopamine is synthesized here.	Reduced dopamine activity causes the extrapyramidal movement disorders of Parkinsonism. Increased dopamine activity in schizophrenia.

(continued)

TABLE 7-1

Brain Anatomy and Function (continued)

BRAIN STRUCTURE	FUNCTION	IMPLICATIONS FOR MENTAL DISORDERS
Pons	Conducts motor and posture information to cerebellum. Controls reflexes. Norepinephrine is made in the pons.	Norepinephrine activity is decreased in depression and increased in schizophrenia.
Medulla Oblongata	The medulla controls respiration, regulation of blood pressure, partial regulation of heart rate, vomiting, and swallowing. Cerebral motor fibers collect here in the shape of *pyramids*. Here the motor fibers that begin in the cerebral cortex cross to the opposite side of the corticospinal motor pathway.	Damage to the medulla can stop spontaneous breathing. The fact that motor fibers cross at the medulla explains why a stroke affects the movement of the opposite side of the body from where the brain damage occurred.
Reticular Formation Reticular Activating System (RAS)	Sensory input is integrated in the reticular formation and conducted to other brain areas. It affects sensory, motor, and visceral functions. The RAS allows screening/filtering of stimuli so the brain does not have to react to all stimuli. RAS controls the sleep-wake cycle.	Reticular formation may be involved in attention deficit disorder (may be due to an inability to filter sensory stimuli normally). If the RAS is disrupted and a person cannot sleep, psychosis can result.
Cerebellum	Cerebellum mainly coordinates muscle activity and function, and maintains equilibrium. It may be involved in cognitive and behavioral functions because of its connections to other brain areas.	Cerebellar disorders cause ataxia (awkward gait and uncoordinated intentional movement), intention tremor, decreased reflexes, and nystagmus. Cerebellar ataxia may be caused by malnutrition in severe, prolonged alcoholism.

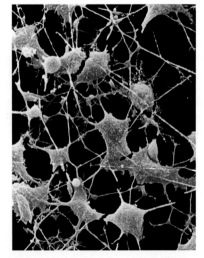

Figure 7-2. ■ Electron micrograph of brain neurons. *Source:* Photo Researchers, Inc.

at relieving client symptoms, and not because their mechanism of action is fully understood.

NEUROTRANSMITTERS

Neurotransmitters are chemical messengers that conduct impulses from one neuron to the next. Figure 7-3 ■ illustrates neurotransmitter function. Review it carefully because it is the basis for understanding treatment of mental disorders with psychotropic drugs.

Human consciousness, behavior, learning, memory, emotion, and creativity are all the result of physiological brain functions. Neurotransmission is the communication between neurons conducted by neurotransmitter chemicals. Neurotransmission must occur for the brain to perform normally (Keltner, 2000).

The building materials for neurotransmitters are brought into the body in food. The intake of adequate

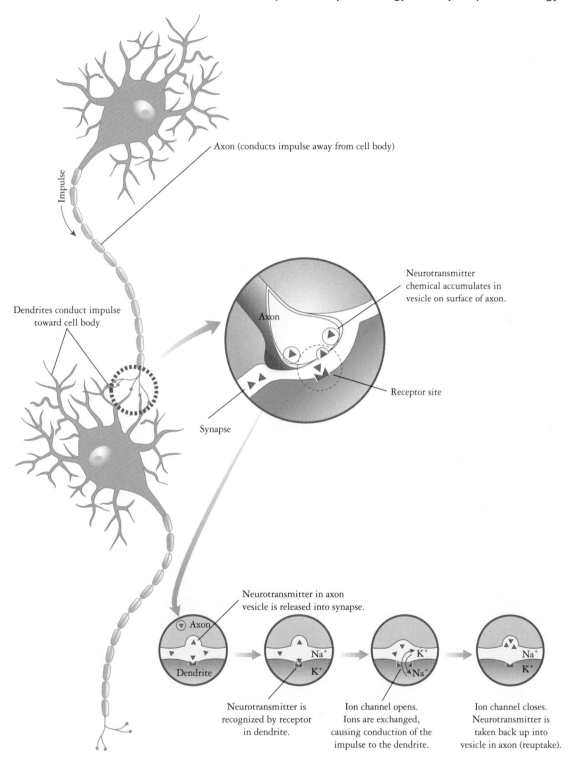

Figure 7-3. ■ Neurotransmission. First inset shows axon-dendrite interface. Second inset illustrates neurotransmission step-by-step.

dietary protein, carbohydrates, fats, vitamins, and minerals is necessary for normal brain function.

Neurotransmitters are manufactured in the *neuron* (nerve cell). They are released from the *axon* (the part of the nerve cell that carries an impulse away from the cell body) into the **synapse** (space between the axon and its target cell's dendrite). The neurotransmitter chemical stimulates the *dendrite* (the part of the neuron that picks up the impulse from the synapse) and conducts it toward the cell body (see Figure 7-3).

The neurotransmitter must fit into a specific receptor site on the surface of the dendrite. When the receptor site is stimulated, it opens an *ion channel* into the dendrite. The ion channel allows for interchange of ions (sodium, potassium, and calcium), which changes the electrical charge of the cell (*depolarization*). Thus, the electrical impulse passes from one neuron to the next.

After the neurotransmitter is released into the synapse, it either excites or inhibits the next neuron (depending on the neurotransmitter). Then one of two things happens (this is important because it is the basis for the activity of some important drugs). The neurotransmitter may be taken back into the axon to be stored for later use (this process is called **reuptake**). Or the neurotransmitter may be inactivated and metabolized by enzymes, most commonly by the enzyme monoamine oxidase.

Approximately 100 neurotransmitters have been identified. Some of them are of special interest in the study of mental illness. Table 7-2 ■ provides information about these neurotransmitters, their functions, and their implications for mental illness.

BRAIN IMAGING

Brain imaging technology has made it possible to study the brain structure and function of people affected with major mental disorders. Preliminary findings suggest that structural and functional brain abnormalities are associated with some mental disorders. Structural imag-

TABLE 7-2

Neurotransmitters

NEUROTRANSMITTER	TYPE	PHYSIOLOGIC EFFECTS	RELATIONSHIP TO MENTAL DISORDERS
Acetylcholine (ACh)	Monoamine	Affects sleep-wake cycle, coordination of muscle movement, pain perception, memory acquisition and retention.	↓ in Alzheimer's and Parkinson's diseases.
Dopamine (DA)	Monoamine	Controls complex movements, cognition, motivation, pleasure; regulates emotional responses.	↑ in schizophrenia and mania. ↓ in depression and Parkinson's disease. Some drugs of abuse stimulate dopamine release (cocaine and amphetamines).
Norepinephrine (NE)	Monoamine	Affects attention, learning, memory; regulates mood, sleep, and wakefulness.	↓ in depression. ↑ in schizophrenia, mania, and anxiety.
Serotonin (5-HT)	Monoamine	Affects sleep and wakefulness, especially falling asleep. Affects mood and thought processes.	Probably plays a role in the thought disorders of schizophrenia (hallucinations, delusions, and social withdrawal). ↓ in depression. Possibly decreased in anxiety and obsessive compulsive disorders.
Gamma-aminobutyric acid (GABA)	Amino acid	Modulates other neurotransmitters.	↓ in anxiety and in schizophrenia.
Glutamate	Amino acid	Controls opening of ion channels for calcium, affecting neurotransmission.	Implicated in schizophrenia. Neurotoxicity results from overexposure to glutamate (as in Huntington's disease) ↑ in Alzheimer's.

Note: ↓ = decreased; ↑ = increased.

ing is possible with CT (computed tomography) scanning and MRI (magnetic resonance imaging). Functional imaging is available with PET (positron emission tomography) and SPECT (single photon emission computed tomography). Table 7-3 ■ compares the various brain imaging techniques.

TABLE 7-3

Brain Imaging Techniques

TECHNIQUE	HOW IT WORKS	USES AND COMPARISON WITH OTHER METHODS	SAMPLE NORMAL BRAIN IMAGES
Computerized Tomography (CT or CAT Scan)	CT scanning relies on the way different tissues deflect X-ray beams that are passed through the subject from numerous points around the circular scanner. CT produces images that represent a "slice" through the body. Done with and without contrast media.	Typical applications are related to the structure of soft tissues, such as locating tumors or bleeding in the brain. CT technology is more readily available and less expensive than MRI.	
Magnetic Resonance Imaging (MRI)	MRI scanners also produce "slice" images. MRI employs a cylindrical magnet that produces a powerful magnetic field. Radio wave pulses emitted by the scanner interact with atoms in the body affected by the magnetic field, and radio signals rebounding are picked up by the detector.	Used for studying the structure of soft tissues, such as the brain and other organs. MRI produces the most detailed images of soft tissue structures. MRI uses no ionizing radiation. Contraindicated in clients with metal implants due to strong magnet and those who fear enclosed spaces (see Figure 7-4 ■).	
Positron Emission Tomography (PET Scan)	PET scanning relies on a radioactive tracer, injected into the bloodstream, to reveal metabolic activity in the brain. As seen here, normal brain metabolic activity produces a roughly symmetrical pattern in the yellow areas of left and right cerebral hemispheres.	PET scanning is used to study metabolic activity in the brain. It can map such functions as glucose uptake in the brain, blood flow, and neurotransmitter activity. The color-coded scan in the example shows brain activity from low (blue) to high (yellow). PET is the most expensive of these scans.	
Single Photon Emission Computed Tomography (SPECT) Scan	SPECT uses injected isotopes (radionuclides) that emit photons. SPECT creates visual images of brain activity similar to those of PET using a gamma camera that rotates around the head. A computer assembles the image.	Use is similar to PET, but SPECT is more widely available and less expensive because it does not require a cyclotron.	

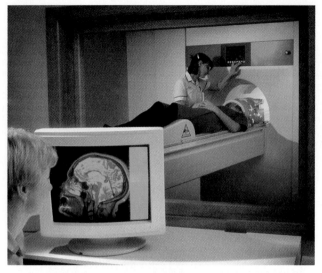

Figure 7-4. ■ MRI brain scanning. Some clients experience fear of the enclosed space in this model of MRI scanner. *Source:* Photo Researchers, Inc.

CT and MRI scans have shown structure abnormalities in schizophrenia, bipolar disorder, multi-infarct dementia, and Alzheimer's disease. PET scanning was a major advance in brain imaging because it can demonstrate aspects of brain function. PET and SPECT confirm that brain activities do cause mental processes and that these processes occur in specific areas in the cerebral cortex. Figure 7-5 ■ compares the PET scans of the brain of a healthy person with one with schizophrenia. PET and SPECT have demonstrated increased dopamine receptors and abnormalities in the limbic system in clients with schizophrenia and abnormalities in the temporal lobes in people with mood disorders.

These scans are not commonly used for diagnostic or treatment purposes for clients with mental disorders. Diagnoses are usually made on the basis of clinical signs and symptoms according to the *DSM-IV-TR* criteria. The scans are more likely to be used in research on the structure and function of the brain as it relates to brain disorders.

Genetics of Mental Illness

Scientists have known for many years that mental disorders are more likely to occur in some families. For example, if one identical twin has schizophrenia, the other twin is more likely to also have it than another sibling is. Identical twins do not always both have (or not have) schizophrenia, though. There is a genetic component to the major mental illnesses, but they do not follow the pattern of single gene inheritance.

The Human Genome Project is attempting to discover the complete set of human genetic instructions, including the genetic nature of mental illness. As they work on the genetics of mental illness, geneticists face several issues that make their work more challenging. Several genes may be necessary to cause psychiatric disorders. The system of psychiatric diagnosis periodically changes the definitions of mental disorders. Factors that are not genetic contribute to mental disorders also (Collins, 1999). Currently, genetic counseling about most mental disorders is based largely on statistical risks.

The latest developments in the genetics of mental illness include the identification of specific genes that reliably increase a person's risk of mental illnesses such as schizophrenia, depression, and bipolar disorder. Researchers found that when people have a variant of the gene that codes for a transporter for serotonin (a neurotransmitter) and they experience stress, they are more likely to have depression (Caspi et al., 2003). A version of a gene in the prefrontal cortex associated with schizophrenia was shown to impair planning and problem-solving skills (Egan et al., 2001). Further genetics research is likely to lead to new understanding and new treatments for mental illness.

Neuroendocrine System

The neuroendocrine system involves the interaction between the nervous system and the endocrine system. It includes the hormones that react to stimulation from nerve cells. Table 7-4 ■ summarizes neuroendocrine and other biological changes related to major mental disorders.

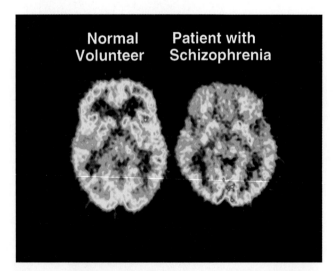

Figure 7-5. ■ PET scans comparing brain of healthy subject with one who has schizophrenia. *Source:* Monte S. Buchsbaum, M.D.

TABLE 7-4			
Psychobiology of Mental Disorders			
MENTAL DISORDER	**BRAIN STRUCTURE**	**NEUROTRANSMITTERS**	**HORMONES**
Schizophrenia	Enlargement of brain ventricles (from brain atrophy). Decreased size of temporal lobes. Changes in the limbic system, thalamus, basal ganglia, hippocampus, and frontal cortex.	Excess of dopamine activity in brain. May be due to increased amount of dopamine, increased sensitivity, or decreased ability to metabolize dopamine. May also have abnormalities in norepinephrine, serotonin, GABA, and acetylcholine.	Decreased prolactin.
Mood Disorders (Depression and Mania)	Abnormalities of the limbic system, basal ganglia, hypothalamus.	Serotonin is decreased in mood disorders. Decreased activity of norepinephrine and dopamine in depression, with increase of these in mania.	Elevated cortisol in depression. Hypothyroidism can cause depression. Hyperthyroidism has been associated with mania. Increased melatonin in seasonal affective disorder (SAD).
Anxiety Disorders	There may be limbic system abnormalities, especially in obsessive-compulsive disorder (OCD).	Elevated norepinephrine in panic disorder. Decreased serotonin in OCD. There may be a decrease in GABA function in anxiety.	In anxiety disorders there may be increased thyroid stimulating hormone (TSH) and prolactin. May be increase in cortisol. Neuroendocrine causes of anxiety are not well understood.

To fully understand the mental disorders and psychotropic drugs, nurses should understand that abnormalities in brain function cause abnormalities in hormone and neurotransmitter levels, which then cause abnormalities in thinking, feeling, and behavior. The drugs that treat mental disorders affect the levels of brain neurotransmitters to bring brain function back into balance and to decrease the signs and symptoms of mental illness.

PSYCHOPHARMACOLOGY

Psychotropic medications can improve or stabilize mood, normalize thinking, reduce anxiety, or allow a person to sleep. Psychotropic medications are a critical part of effective treatment, yet they do not "cure" mental disorders. Psychotropic drugs work best in conjunction with psychosocial treatment and rehabilitation.

Clients have the best outcomes when they have:

- An understanding of their disease process and treatment plan
- An active, participative role in their treatment
- A social support system
- A safe and healthy place to live, where all their basic human needs are met
- Healthy coping and problem-solving skills
- Appropriate psychotropic medications

- A therapeutic relationship with healthcare providers who cooperate with them to find the most effective treatments for their mental disorder

Pharmacokinetics

Pharmacokinetics describes the effects a drug has on the body (Keltner, Schwecke, & Bostrom, 2007). Figure 7-6 ■ shows a diagram of the process. Pharmacokinetics includes four parts:

1. **Absorption.** Absorption involves the drug entering the bloodstream. It takes place in the GI tract with oral meds, or in the mucous membranes, muscle, skin, or subcutaneous tissue, depending on the route used to give the drug. Drugs given intravenously do

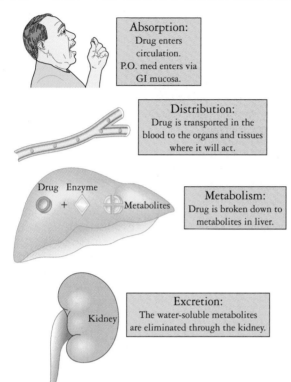

Absorption:
Drug enters circulation.
P.O. med enters via GI mucosa.

Distribution:
Drug is transported in the blood to the organs and tissues where it will act.

Metabolism:
Drug is broken down to metabolites in liver.

Excretion:
The water-soluble metabolites are eliminated through the kidney.

Figure 7-6. ■ Pharmacokinetics.

not need to be absorbed because they are already in the blood; they go directly into distribution.

2. **Distribution.** When the drug is in the bloodstream it is distributed or transported to the tissues and organs where it will act or be stored.

3. **Metabolism.** Metabolism is the breakdown of drug molecules. It happens most often in the liver, but can also occur in the kidneys, lungs, plasma, and GI tract. The original drug is usually broken down into metabolites that are more water soluble. Enzymes facilitate the breakdown process.

4. **Excretion.** Excretion happens when the drug or its metabolites are moved from the target tissues back into the circulation and then to the organs of elimination, usually the kidneys. The skin, GI tract, and breast milk can also be involved in excretion.

Pharmacodynamics

Pharmacodynamics are the actions and outcomes on the body caused by drugs (Keltner et al., 2007). The mechanism of action of each drug results from the way the drug interacts with the target cells in the body. Some drugs stimulate cellular functions (these are **agonists**). Other drugs prevent or inhibit cell functions (these are **antagonists**). The drug's effect is reflected in changes in the client's physical or psychological state. The primary consequence of a drug is the *desired effect*. Drugs usually act only on specific body tissues. For example, antidepressant drugs act on specific brain neurotransmitters. They do not affect hearing, digestion, or other functions. However, the target body tissues may have several functions and the client may experience effects other than the desired effects. Antidepressant drugs have anticholinergic effects (constipation, increased heart rate, dry mouth) that are not related to depression. These undesirable secondary outcomes are **side effects**. Side effects are usually predictable, based on knowledge of drug function.

Adverse effects are less predictable and are serious undesired effects. **Toxic effects** result from excessive drug levels or drug interactions. The occurrence of adverse effects can be related to the metabolic rate of the client. See the Cultural Pulse Points Box 7-1 ■ for more information.

The degree to which a drug can cause the desired response is its *efficacy*. The number of receptor sites and the drug's attraction for binding to the receptor sites affects the magnitude of the response.

PHASES OF MEDICATION TREATMENT

The period of time between when the client begins taking a medication and when the desired effects are achieved is the *stabilization phase* of medication treatment. During the

---

BOX 7-1	CULTURAL PULSE POINTS

Variations In Metabolic Rate

Ethnically distinct groups tend to have different rates of metabolizing drugs. The rate of drug metabolism affects the duration of drug action, the side effects, and potential toxicity. Slow metabolism would clear a drug slowly from the body and increase the risk of side effects. As a group, Asian people have a relatively slower rate of metabolism, so they are likely to respond to lower doses of medications. Asians are also very likely to experience extrapyramidal symptoms (EPS) with antipsychotic drugs. African and European Americans have a relatively higher rate of metabolism and have EPS less frequently. The therapeutic range of lithium is also affected by metabolic rate (Kneisl, Wilson, & Trigoboff, 2004).

Source: Data from *Contemporary Psychiatric Mental Health Nursing* by Kneisl/Wilson/Trigoboff, © Pearson Education, Inc., Upper Saddle River, NJ.

stabilization phase, nursing responsibilities include the following:

- Assessing client's symptoms
- Assessing client's response to the drug
- Observing for adverse effects
- Obtaining lab tests, as ordered, to monitor drug levels, liver function, or potential adverse effects
- Educating client

The *maintenance phase* begins when the client's target symptoms are treated and the therapeutic effect is achieved. The medical treatment goal during the maintenance phase of psychotropic drug treatment is symptom management, using the lowest possible drug dose with the least possible adverse effects. The nursing goal is for the client to achieve optimal functioning and quality of life. Nursing responsibilities in the maintenance phase include the following:

- Ongoing assessment of drug effects
- Assessment for long-term side effects

- Continued client education, focusing on medication management at home, treating side effects, and the importance of continuing therapy after the symptoms are relieved

TARGET SYMPTOMS

Before administering psychotropic medications to clients, nurses must know what the desired effects are. We need to know what specific symptoms the medications are expected to treat: the **target symptoms** (Trigoboff, Wilson, Shannon, & Stang, 2005) (Figure 7-7 ■). If nurses only know the name of the disease each drug is treating, they may not know if the drug is causing the desired effect. For example, imagine a client with schizophrenia who is experiencing hallucinations and takes an antipsychotic drug. If the nurse is wondering whether the drug is effective, the nurse must look for hallucinations (one of the target symptoms), not schizophrenia (the disorder). The client will still have schizophrenia, but if his hallucinations are relieved, the drug is effective.

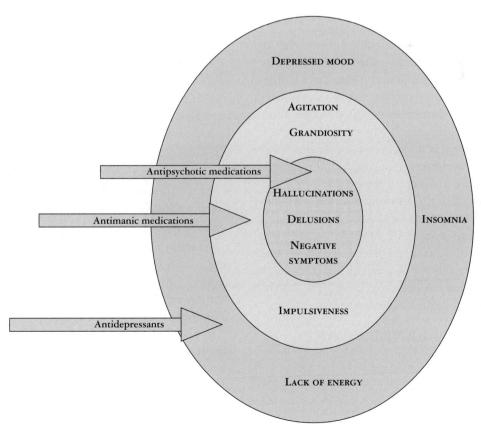

Figure 7-7. ■ Target symptoms.

NURSING CARE

ASSESSING

The nurse collects data from several sources while applying the nursing process to clients taking psychotropic medications. The primary sources of data are the direct objective and subjective findings from the client. What is the client's mental status? Her feelings? His behavior? Vital signs? A good secondary source is the medical record. It is helpful for the nurse to read the physician's history and physical exam to provide a baseline of information about the client's condition on admission. The treatment plan will show the desired outcomes and map the planned course of treatment to reach them. The family is an often-ignored fund of information and source of assistance.

Because of stringent confidentiality regulations, it is necessary for the facility to obtain written permission from clients to discuss their condition with family members. This permission should be sought for any family members who are actively involved in the care of the client on an outpatient basis. Family members can be great allies in the treatment process if they are included. They can ignorantly and innocently undermine the treatment process if they are not informed about it.

An important nursing responsibility is monitoring the client for side effects of medications. The nurse's observations must be based on current information about psychotropic and other medications (their actions, target symptoms, and possible side effects). Know what side effects to expect and watch for them. Although the "5 Rights" (giving the right drug, at the right time, in the right dose, by the right route, to the right client) are important nursing functions, they are only the beginning of the licensed nursing role.

If the nurse gives the lithium that the physician ordered to the right client in the right dose, but the client was having symptoms of ataxic gait, fever, hypotension, and mental confusion and died from lithium toxicity, it will not be a defense for the nurse to say, "But I did what the doctor ordered." The nursing process says: "Assess before you intervene."

DIAGNOSING, PLANNING, AND IMPLEMENTING

The nursing issues related to psychotropic drug therapy include the following:

- Safe medication administration
- Client empowerment through practical knowledge
- Client compliance with treatment
- Client advocacy
- Documentation
- Keeping current with knowledge about psychiatric drugs

Some common nursing diagnoses for clients receiving psychotropic medications are as follows:

- Deficient Knowledge, Medication Management
- Ineffective Therapeutic Regimen Management

Desired outcomes for clients receiving psychotropic medications might be as follows:

- By discharge, client will be able to state the name of her/his mental disorder.
- Client will list the names of the medications taken for that condition before discharge.
- Client will state the basic target effects of the medications taken for the mental disorder before discharge.
- Before discharge, the client will list possible side effects of psychotropic medication and whether to notify the provider or even whether to continue medication if they occur.
- Client will express feelings about taking psychotropic medications.
- Client will list resources for help or information about medications before discharge.

Basic client education includes how and when to take each medication safely. If this basic knowledge is power, then full participation by the client in her/his own care is superpower. Client empowerment requires that the client have the following:

- Knowledge
- Ability to communicate his or her own needs
- Participation in the treatment plan
- The support he or she needs to reach treatment goals

When clients can do these things, they have the superpower they need to be in control of their own future. The treatment team must ask the client questions like: "How does this drug affect you? What do you think about this? Are you willing to try this medication for 2 months? What side effects are you having?"

If the nurse and others prepare clients appropriately, clients will be able to discuss their medications with the provider, describing their side effects as well as the status of the target symptoms. Imagine two clients with bipolar disorder. One says, "Yes, Doctor, whatever you want me to do is fine." The second one says, "I would rather not continue taking lithium because the side effects are too

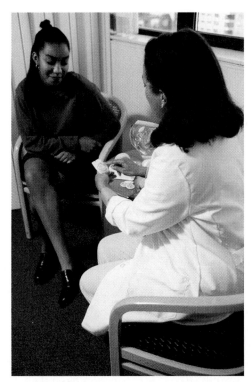

Figure 7-8. ■ Nurses empower clients by giving them the knowledge they need to manage their own health. *Source:* Getty Images, Inc.— Photodisc.

bad. Can we try another medication?" The second one is the empowered client. By the way, which of these clients is likely to go home and be noncompliant with his or her meds? Figure 7-8 ■ shows a nurse empowering a client.

Deficient Knowledge, Medication Management, R/T Lack of Information

■ Determine the client's current knowledge level about disorders, medications, and treatment. The LPN/LVN may be reinforcing teaching that was previously done by the RN or the physician. *Teaching should include what the client needs to learn, which varies among individuals. The nurse should respect the expertise the client already has. Clients are the experts on how the disease and drugs affect them. However, do not assume that clients are knowledgeable just because they have had a disorder for years. Many clients benefit from reinforcement of teaching. People learn best when they are ready to learn.*

■ Teach the client and significant others what the medications are expected to do and what side effects might arise. For example, "This is risperidone. It is an antipsychotic, so it is supposed to straighten out your thoughts and make the voices go away. Let me know if your

muscles feel tight, especially your jaws. This is a side effect and we have a medicine for it if it happens." *Clients are empowered when their active participation in treatment is expected. Empowerment requires usable knowledge.*

■ Teach clients in clear, simple terms, avoiding medical jargon and excessive technical information. *Clients must be able to understand information in order to use it.*

■ Reinforce teaching with printed information when possible. Keep the written information as clear and brief as possible. Printed information should be available in the client's preferred language. *People learn best with a variety of teaching approaches. The best approach is to allow the client actually to practice the material you are teaching. Including both verbal and written instructions promotes understanding. Written instructions can aid the client's memory. People often forget details over time.*

■ Encourage the client and family to ask questions. Ask them questions to evaluate their understanding. *People will often hesitate to ask questions for fear of appearing stupid. The nurse can promote a safe learning environment where it is acceptable to ask. Asking the client a practical question, such as "What will you do if you forget to take your morning med and it is lunch time?" will give the nurse much more information than "Do you understand?"*

■ Give the client several opportunities to learn and discuss the new information. *Mastery and skill can be improved with practice.*

■ Plan to teach when the client can concentrate and cooperate. *If clients are confused, agitated, anxious, depressed, or psychotic, they will be unable to learn or remember very much. At these times, provide simple instructions for clients to follow. Learning is most effective when clients are ready.*

Ineffective Therapeutic Regimen Management

■ Ask clients to describe how they take their medications at home. *A question about how the client applies treatment recommendations gives the nurse information about how much the client understands, and helps the nurse decide what to teach.*

■ Teach the client the skills needed for cooperation with a treatment plan. *Clients may be noncompliant with treatment recommendations because they do not understand them or because they do not know what to do.*

■ Help the client to develop a personalized medication management plan. It should include the times that the client will actually take the meds and any special instructions for this individual. *A generic plan is not as useful as a real practical plan that the client can take home and use. Having a specific personal plan improves the chance for compliance.*

- Discuss problem-solving issues. *Practical information is most useful. Discuss real issues such as what to do when a prescription runs out, who could drive to the pharmacy, whom to call when the client has symptoms of toxicity, how to remember the morning meds, and other realistic medication management issues. This helps the client be prepared to solve problems as they arise. A written list of resources (people and their phone numbers), strategies, and instructions will help the client remember what was taught.*

EVALUATING

The nurse evaluates client outcomes related to the effects of drug therapy. The client's response to drug therapy will be documented and reported to the provider (physician or nurse practitioner). Because psychotropic medications often have late onset (especially drugs that treat mood disorders and psychosis), it may not be possible for the nurse in an acute-care setting to evaluate the full effects of these medications. If a client is discharged before the full drug effect is achieved, careful teaching about what to expect is necessary. It is very important to teach clients when full drug effects are expected. If clients do not know this, they may discontinue the medications, thinking that they are not effective (Stuart & Laraia, 2005). It can be disappointing to clients who finally begin treatment to have to wait even longer for the medications to work. The nurse can help keep hope alive.

Nurses in long-term or subacute settings are often able to evaluate medication outcomes, such as:

- To what extent the client achieves the desired target effects
- Presence of side effects and adverse effects
- Toxicity

Discharge Considerations

The nurse provides the client and family with a list of resources to call from home for problem solving. It is best to plan in advance for times when the client and family might have problems rather than to wait for problems to occur. Outpatient appointment phone number, pharmacy phone number, emergency advice hotline, family or friends who could discuss whether the client should go to see the provider, and the Alliance for the Mentally Ill are resources that can be provided in written form for future need.

Emphasize that the medications should be taken regularly for an extended period because they treat brain neurotransmitters. The meds should not be discontinued when the client feels better. Improvement in the client's symptoms means that the drug is working. Teach the client about what side effects are expected, what can be done to relieve them, and when to call the provider.

Two of the most common reasons for medication noncompliance are side effects and stopping when the symptoms are relieved. Clear understanding of appropriate drug use enhances compliance.

NURSING PROCESS CARE PLAN
Client with Readiness for Enhanced Knowledge

Juan Sanchez is a 38-year-old Latino with a diagnosis of bipolar disorder. He is hospitalized now for an unrelated cholecystectomy. He was hospitalized in the psychiatric unit 4 months ago during a manic episode. He is alert, oriented, and cooperative with his care. Since his psychiatric hospitalization, Mr. Sanchez has taken his prescribed valproic acid daily to stabilize his mood. The client states that he was so manic when he was in the hospital that he was unable to ask questions or to remember clearly what happened. He has seen his psychiatrist as an outpatient and has learned more about his bipolar disorder.

Assessment. Client states that he is interested in learning more about his medication. He does not like taking it because it "slows his thinking." It also makes him nauseated occasionally. He states that he is ashamed for anyone to know he takes this medication. He says that taking this medication makes him feel like he is different from other people, "like I am crazy."

Diagnosis. The following nursing diagnoses are established for Mr. Sanchez:

- Readiness for Enhanced Knowledge: prescribed medication R/T new clarity in thinking
- Situational Low Self-Esteem R/T taking psychotropic medication

Expected Outcomes. The client will:

- List desired target symptoms of valproic acid.
- List common side effects of valproic acid, including the ones he experiences.
- Express his feelings about taking psychotropic medication.

- Discuss the consequences of noncompliance with medication.

Planning and Implementation.   The nurse will:

- Reinforce teaching about desired effects and side effects of valproic acid.
- Discuss the client's side effects.
- Discuss the consequences of not taking this medication.
- Have a therapeutic conversation with Mr. Sanchez to encourage him to express his feelings about taking a psychotropic medication.
- Encourage him to restructure his thinking (cognitive restructuring) about bipolar disorder as an illness, not a negative reflection on his character.

Evaluation.   Mr. Sanchez states that he is still not happy about the need to take medication. He will continue to take it because he wants to prevent the negative consequences he has experienced during manic episodes in the past (including the breakup of his marriage and the loss of his business). He will think about changing the way he perceives taking a psychotropic drug.

Critical Thinking in the Nursing Process

1. Why is Mr. Sanchez embarrassed to tell anyone that he takes a psychotropic medication?
2. Is it ethical for the nurse to encourage this client to take a medication knowing that it causes side effects?
3. Did this client's nurse during his psychiatric hospitalization do an adequate job of medication teaching?

Note: Discussion of Critical Thinking questions appears in Appendix I.

Note: The references and resources for this and all chapters have been compiled at the back of the book.

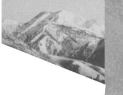
 KEY TERMS

Use the audio glossary feature of the Companion Website to hear the correct pronunciation of the following key terms.

adverse effects

agonists

antagonists

polydipsia

reuptake

side effects

synapse

target symptoms

toxic effects

KEY Points

- Mental disorders can be caused by abnormalities of brain anatomy (structure), neurotransmitter function, or neuroendocrine (hormone) function.

- There is a genetic component to the cause of mental disorders, but a single gene alone does not cause them. These disorders are probably multifactorial (caused by a combination of biological and social factors).

- Neurotransmitters go from the axon of one neuron, pass through the synapse, and stimulate the dendrite of the next neuron to transmit signals through the nervous system.

- Psychotropic drugs treat the symptoms of mental disorders by acting on brain neurotransmitters.

- People with mental disorders clearly respond best to treatment that includes a holistic approach (psychotropic medications, a trusting therapeutic relationship, and cognitive and behavioral therapies).

- Client empowerment requires that the client have knowledge, ability to communicate his or her own needs, resources to meet those needs, and participation in the treatment plan.

- Teach the client skills needed for cooperation with treatment plan.

- Two of the most common reasons for medication noncompliance are side effects and stopping the meds when the symptoms are relieved.

 EXPLORE MediaLink

Additional interactive resources for this chapter can be found on the Companion Website at www.prenhall.com/eby. Click on Chapter 7 and "Begin" to select the activities for this chapter.

- Audio glossary
- NCLEX-PN® review
- Case study
- Study outline
- Critical thinking questions
- Matching questions
- Weblinks

Caring for a Client Taking Psychotropic Drugs
NCLEX-PN® Focus Area: Health Promotion and Maintenance

Case Study: Ann Lee is a 57-year-old client who has multiple sclerosis and has been admitted to a long-term care facility for management of skin breakdown. Her wound is healing, her caregiver has been educated about skin care, and she is planning to be discharged home in 2 days. Ms. Lee has been experiencing symptoms of depression intermittently for over a year. She was diagnosed with depression 4 days ago. The physician ordered fluoxetine (Prozac) 20 mg PO daily, and explained the therapy to her at that time. Fluoxetine is an antidepressant.

Nursing Diagnosis: Deficient Knowledge about new medication

COLLECT DATA

Subjective	Objective
_____	_____
_____	_____
_____	_____
_____	_____
_____	_____
_____	_____
_____	_____

Would you report this data? Yes/No

If yes, to: _____

Nursing Care

_____

_____

_____

_____

_____

_____

_____

_____

_____

_____

How would you document this? _____

_____

_____

_____

Compare your documentation to the sample provided in Appendix I.

Data Collected
(use those that apply)

- Weight 150 lbs
- Retired Spanish teacher
- Decubitus ulcer on coccyx is healing well.
- Appetite fair, eats 25–50% of meals
- Client asks, "Do I have to take this medication because I am crazy?"
- Client states, "I hope I will feel less depressed by the time I go home."
- Client complains of sadness and low energy.
- Last BM was yesterday.
- Client states, "My legs are too weak to walk."
- Client states, "I will be able to quit taking this medication in a few weeks when I feel better."
- Client is unable to state the potential side effects of fluoxetine.
- Client is unable to state the target effects of fluoxetine.
- Lives alone, with caregiver for 8 hours each day

Nursing Interventions
(use those that apply; list in priority order)

- Turn every 2 hours. Keep skin clean and dry.
- Teach the client that depression is a biological illness caused by low levels of neurotransmitters in the brain.
- Teach the client that the target effects of fluoxetine are more energy, an improved mood, and improved mental concentration.
- Teach the client that the side effects of fluoxetine are dry mouth, constipation, and increased heart rate. It may cause some people to feel anxious.
- Schedule fluoxetine (Prozac) for every AM because it can make clients anxious and may affect sleep if taken at bedtime.
- Teach the caregiver to weigh the client daily.
- Instruct client to take fluoxetine in the morning at home.
- Teach client that the medication may take several weeks to be effective.
- Instruct client that she should continue taking the medication even when she feels better.
- Ask MD for an order for a sleeping pill.
- Ask the client if she has any questions.
- Instruct the family that she will need a 24-hour caregiver now that she has a psychiatric diagnosis.

1 The spouse of a client with schizophrenia asks about the probable source of the disorder. The best response by the nurse would be, "It is probably due to . . ."
1. "Parental neglect during childhood."
2. "Physical and mental abuse as a teenager."
3. "A brain disorder involving the structure and function of your spouse's brain."
4. "Illicit drug use during young adulthood."

2 The main function of neurotransmitters within the nervous system is to:
1. Conduct impulses from one neuron to the next.
2. Nourish the neurons.
3. Create nerve pathways between the nerve cells.
4. Manufacture the enzymes that facilitate communication within the nervous system.

3 Which diagnostic tool would be inappropriate for a schizophrenic client who has a fear of enclosed spaces?
1. PET scan
2. SPECT scan
3. MRI
4. CT scan

4 If a client who has an identical twin with schizophrenia asks about chances for her developing the disorder herself, the best response by the nurse would be:
1. "There is no genetic component to schizophrenia."
2. "Your risk for developing schizophrenia is greater than your siblings."
3. "Your risk factors are no greater than the general public."
4. "I would not worry about that if I were you."

5 A client diagnosed with seasonal affective disorder is most likely to be experiencing:
1. Excess cortisol.
2. Excess melatonin.
3. Decreased cortisol.
4. Decreased melatonin.

6 A depressed client asks how his antidepressant works. The best response by the nurse would be, "Antidepressants . . ."
1. "Change the anatomical structures of the temporal lobe of the brain."
2. "Increase the brain's utilization of glucose."
3. "May increase the availability of some of the neurotransmitters involved in mood control."
4. "Alter a person's genetic makeup."

7 A client asks the nurse to further explain a CT scan. The nurse's best response would be, "A CT scan is . . ."
1. "A computer-assisted X-ray that allows the doctor to look at a cross-section of your brain."
2. "A closed tube that uses powerful electromagnetic energy to produce a visual image of your brain without using radiation."
3. "A test involving the injection of a radioactive tracer that will allow the doctor to reconstruct images of brain sections, including utilization of glucose and oxygen. It requires a machine called a cyclotron."
4. "A test involving the injection of a radioactive tracer without the use of a cyclotron to allow the doctor to create visual images of brain activity."

8 The mother of a clinically depressed client asks what she did wrong to cause the illness. The best response by the nurse would be:
1. "Don't worry about the past. We must deal with what is going on today."
2. "Although there could be multiple causes, an imbalance of certain neurotransmitters has probably affected your daughter's mood."
3. "The most likely cause is a structural defect in your daughter's brain."
4. "I'm sure you did nothing wrong."

9 A new client in an outpatient mental health clinic asks the nurse about the benefit of taking psychotropic medications. The best response would be, "Psychotropic medications . . ."
1. "May be used as the only treatment for a mental disorder."
2. "Can cure any mental disorder."
3. "May improve a client's condition enough to make other treatment modalities more effective."
4. "Work well and have few serious side effects."

10 During the stabilization phase of medication treatment, nursing responsibilities include (select all that apply):
1. Observing for adverse effects
2. Assessing client's current symptoms
3. Ongoing review of client's medical history
4. Assessing the client's response to the medication
5. Educating the client about the medication

Answers for Review Questions, as well as discussion of Care Plan and Critical Thinking Care Map questions, appear in Appendix I.

Learning About You!

CHAPTER 1 Understanding Mental Health and Mental Illness
Check out your own mental health status.

I feel good about myself.
☐ Yes   ☐ No

I see things realistically.
☐ Yes   ☐ No

I have satisfying personal relationships.
☐ Yes   ☐ No

There is meaning in my life.
☐ Yes   ☐ No

I am productive in my job and in school.
☐ Yes   ☐ No

I enjoy opportunities where I can be creative.
☐ Yes   ☐ No

I eat three well-balanced meals a day.
☐ Yes   ☐ No

I feel that I am the only one responsible for my behavior.
☐ Yes   ☐ No

I have a positive attitude most of the time.
☐ Yes   ☐ No

I am flexible and adapt easily to change.
☐ Yes   ☐ No

I sleep at least 6 hours every night.
☐ Yes   ☐ No

I wake up feeling rested each morning.
☐ Yes   ☐ No

I see conflict as a challenge and am not overwhelmed by it.
☐ Yes   ☐ No

How did you do? Mostly yeses indicate you are in a relatively good state of mental health!

CHAPTER 2 Ethical and Legal Issues
Knowing that values and ethics intertwine to determine your behavior, think back over your week, and see where values clarification played a part in your response to different situations:

As a nursing student, I find that I value (*choosing*):
1.   2.

I was able to show how much my values meant to me this week by (*prizing*):
1.   2.

I demonstrated my values this week by (*acting*):
1.   2.

CHAPTER 3 Personality Theory
Decide on your own personality traits by checking the boxes below:

☐ Extrovert   ☐ Introvert
☐ Agreeable   ☐ Disagreeable
☐ Conscientious   ☐ Impulsive
☐ Emotionally stable   ☐ Emotionally unstable
☐ Open   ☐ Closed

What traits do you see in your friends?

Have you ever used a defense mechanism? Below are examples of some. Read the statement or situation, and decide which defense mechanism is being used.

Defense Mechanism
A. Suppression
B. Displacement
C. Compensation
D. Rationalization

Statement
1. "I didn't get an 'A' on my pharmacology paper because the instructor doesn't like me."
2. "I totally bombed at clinical today, but I just can't think about it now. I'll think about it tomorrow."
3. After being reprimanded by her Fundamentals instructor, the nursing student went home and yelled at her daughter, "Why is your room always so messy? I'm tired of picking up after you."
4. "I can't run as fast as my brother, so I'm joining the debate team instead of going out for track."

Answers to fun quiz
A (2)   B (3)   C (4)   D (1)

CHAPTER 4 Mentally Healthy Nursing
Check out your codependency tendencies with this questionnaire. (This is not an official research tool—just a fun exercise thought up by your authors.)

I have difficulty telling other people "no" when they ask me to do something for them.
☐ Yes   ☐ No

I need everyone around me to like me.
☐ Yes   ☐ No

I enjoy having my friends come to me to help them solve their problems.
☐ Yes   ☐ No

I feel responsible for the feelings of those around me.
☐ Yes   ☐ No

I am more interested in pleasing other people than in pleasing myself.
☐ Yes ☐ No

I am uncomfortable when others praise me.
☐ Yes ☐ No

I find myself volunteering for projects that I don't really have the time and energy to do.
☐ Yes ☐ No

I have difficulty relaxing.
☐ Yes ☐ No

I have difficulty making decisions concerning myself and my own problems.
☐ Yes ☐ No

I mentally "beat myself up" for weeks after I make a mistake.
☐ Yes ☐ No

"Yes" answers indicate a tendency toward codependency. This chapter should have provided you with helpful hints to begin your journey toward mentally healthy nursing.

CHAPTER 5 The Nurse-Client Relationship and Communication

In the past 24 hours, my interaction experiences looked like this:

1. Of my interactions with others today, _____ were social and _____ were professional (connected to work or school).
2. Examples of nonverbal communication I used:
   _____
3. Examples of nonverbal communication I observed others using: _____
4. My messages were *always* clearly understood by the receiver of the message. ☐ Yes ☐ No
5. I understood completely all of the messages that were sent to me. ☐ Yes ☐ No
6. I physically touched most of the people I had interactions with today. ☐ Yes ☐ No
7. I asked permission to touch the people I touched today. ☐ Never ☐ Sometimes ☐ Always
8. I listened attentively to all the verbal and nonverbal messages sent to me. ☐ Yes ☐ No

This exercise will give you a pretty good idea as to how you communicate as well as how well you use your communication skills.

CHAPTER 6 Stress and Coping

Check out your own coping mechanisms for dealing with stress.

When I feel myself getting stressed, I immediately try to identify the source of the discomfort.
☐ Yes ☐ No

I feel that I am the only one with control over my stress level.
☐ Yes ☐ No

When I feel stressed, I seek out friends and/or family members to discuss my feelings.
☐ Yes ☐ No

I try to look at all sides of a stressful situation.
☐ Yes ☐ No

I feel that stress can at times be a positive experience.
☐ Yes ☐ No

I can say "no" when I feel myself becoming overwhelmed by the demands placed on me by others.
☐ Yes ☐ No

How did you do? Mostly yeses indicate you cope with stress in a mentally healthy manner.

CHAPTER 7 Psychobiology and Psychopharmacology

Think of people you have known who "act strangely." Then answer the following questions.

1. What kind of behavior do you classify as "strange"?
2. Before you read this chapter, what reasons did you think there were for "strange" behaviors?
   ☐ Physiological ☐ Patient's past experiences
3. Describe your past reactions to people who acted "strangely."
   ☐ Avoidance ☐ Fear
   ☐ Tried to include in conversation and activities
   ☐ Amusement ☐ Other
4. Now that you know about the psychobiology of mental illness, will your reaction to "strange" people be different? In what way?

Match the psychotropic medications and the specific mental health disorder for which they are used (drugs may be used for more than one condition):

Medication	Mental Health Condition
1. Risperdal (risperidone)	A. Depression
2. Cogentin (benztropine)	B. Bipolar disorder
3. Ativan (lorazepam)	C. Anxiety
4. Abilitat (aripiprazole)	D. Obsessive-compulsive disorder
5. Haldol (haloperidol)	
6. Elavil (amitriptyline)	E. Insomnia
7. Prozac (fluoxetine)	F. Schizophrenia
8. Wellbutrin (bupropion)	G. Pseudoparkinsonism
9. BuSpar (buspirone)	H. Panic disorder
10. Prolixin (fluphenazine)	I. Premenstrual dysphoric disorder
11. Effexor (venlafaxine)	
12. Lithium	J. Posttraumatic stress
	K. Bulimia nervosa

Answers

1 (F) 2 (G) 3 (C, E) 4 (F) 5 (F) 6 (A) 7 (A, D, I, J, K)
8 (A) 9 (C) 10 (F) 11 (A) 12 (B)

Nursing Care of Clients with Mental Disorders

UNIT II

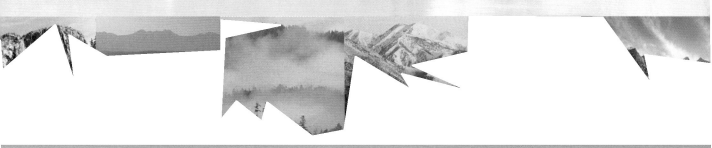

Chapter 8

Schizophrenia

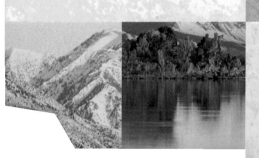

BRIEF Outline

Schizophrenia

Causes of Schizophrenia

Diagnosis and Clinical Features

Course of the Disease

Recovery

Collaborative Care

Advocating for Clients

LEARNING Outcomes

After completing this chapter, you will be able to:

1. Provide basic information to the client or family about the cause, clinical features, and treatment of schizophrenia.
2. Monitor the mental status of a client.
3. Safely administer antipsychotic medications.
4. Apply the nursing process to the care of a client with schizophrenia.

Schizophrenia is a complex disorder of the brain. It has significant short-term and long-term consequences for affected individuals, their families, and society. Approximately 1 out of every 100 people will experience schizophrenia during his or her lifetime. People with schizophrenia often experience considerable distress in their personal and work lives. They are also likely to suffer from prejudice and discrimination in the workplace, in society, and even in the healthcare system. Nurses can help affected people recover and live better lives by using the correct information about schizophrenia and keeping hope alive.

Schizophrenia

Schizophrenia is a major brain disorder that alters the affected person's perception, thoughts, feelings, and behavior. The symptoms are usually divided into **positive symptoms** (also called **psychosis**) including hallucinations, delusions, and disorganized thinking; **negative symptoms** such as emotional apathy, lack of motivation, social withdrawal, and self-neglect; and **disorganized symptoms** such as purposeless behavior, evidence that the client's thoughts are disorganized, and flat or inappropriate expression of emotions.

There are several subtypes of schizophrenia that are defined by their predominant symptoms at the time of evaluation. The *catatonic* type is diagnosed whenever catatonic symptoms are present. The presentation of catatonia may be a client who is awake but unresponsive and remains in a fixed position for extended periods of time with the inability to move or talk. The client may have agitated catatonia in which she has strange repetitive movements. Clients may repeat what other people say (echolalia) or copy the movements of others (echopraxia).

The *disorganized* type is diagnosed if the client does not have catatonia and has disorganized speech and behavior, and inappropriate expression of emotions (such as laughing that is not related to the content of the person's speech or a flat affect in which no emotions are expressed at all).

Schizophrenia of the *paranoid* type is diagnosed when clients have frequent auditory hallucinations or prominent delusional thinking (delusions are false beliefs—more on this later) and the clients' thinking is still functioning. The delusions are usually persecutory or grandiose. Some clients with schizophrenia have a combination of symptoms from more than one subtype and are diagnosed with the *undifferentiated* type.

There is limited value in diagnosing the schizophrenia subtypes for clinical treatment or research purposes.

Alternative subtyping ideas are being investigated (American Psychiatric Association, 2000). The subtypes are included here because you may see them used in the diagnoses of your clients, but we will present schizophrenia in general terms to prepare you for care of clients with any type of the disorder.

There are other disorders that cause psychosis, which include schizoaffective disorder (a combination of schizophrenia with a mood disorder), bipolar mania, and depression with psychotic features, but this chapter will focus on schizophrenia as a prototype for the nursing approach to care of people with thought disorders.

There are approximately 2.2 million people in the United States with schizophrenia (Torrey, 2001). It affects women, men, people of all races and nationalities, and people of all socioeconomic classes.

Although schizophrenia is a relatively common and devastating illness, it is underrepresented in research funding and in services for clients and their families. Only 60% of people with schizophrenia are receiving treatment at any given time. There are more people with schizophrenia in jail than in the hospital. People with schizophrenia are often homeless and often are victims of crime. Untreated people with the disorder are more likely to be violent (especially if they are abusing drugs), and this is the biggest cause of the stigma against the entire group of affected people. Public psychiatric treatment services, housing, and rehabilitation services for people with schizophrenia are grossly inadequate (Torrey, 2001). Schizophrenia is a major public health issue, yet inadequate resources are available to those who suffer from it, their families, and communities.

Causes of Schizophrenia

Current thought is that schizophrenia is caused by a combination of genetics and environmental influences. There are many genes involved in the genetic code for structure and function of the brain. Recent research demonstrates that some genes start out working normally but may become abnormal under stress.

E. Fuller Torrey has researched and written extensively on schizophrenia. He describes 10 findings related to the potential causes and consequences of the disorder (Torrey, 2001):

1. **The disease is familial.** Schizophrenia "runs in families." It is more likely to recur in a family that already has a family member with schizophrenia, but it is not a purely genetic disorder. Identical

twins are not always concordant (the same) for schizophrenia. If it were purely genetic, identical twins would always both have it or both not have it, but this is not true. Siblings of a person with the disorder are nine times more likely to have schizophrenia than the general population. There is a genetic component, but genetics is not the whole story.

2. **Neurochemical changes.** There are almost certainly neurochemical differences in the brains of people with schizophrenia, especially in the hippocampus and frontal lobe. The major neurochemicals that have been studied are neurotransmitters and their receptors, especially dopamine, norepinephrine, serotonin, GABA (gamma-aminobutyric acid), and glutamate (Goff & Coyle, 2001). The effectiveness of antipsychotic drugs is probably due to the fact that they affect the function and availability of neurotransmitters.

3. **Changes in brain structure and function.** Structural changes in the brains of people with schizophrenia have been repeatedly found by imaging studies. The structural abnormalities include enlargement of the brain ventricles, decrease in the size of the limbic system, and changes in the cell structure in the hippocampus, amygdala, parahippocampal gyrus, entorhinal cortex, and cingulate.

4. **Cognitive impairments.** Four types of *cognitive* (thinking) function are affected by schizophrenia: attention, **executive function** (abstract thinking and problem solving), awareness of the illness (insight), and short-term memory. These thinking impairments are part of schizophrenia. They occur even in people who have not taken medication, so they are not due to medication side effects. It is important to note that while the disease does affect some aspects of thinking, other aspects of thinking are intact, such as language skills, knowledge of information, and visual-spatial abilities.

5. **Neurological abnormalities.** The disease can cause abnormal reflexes (such as the grasp reflex found normally only in infants). It can cause confusion between right and left and an inability to perceive two simultaneous touches on the body. Abnormal eye movements (rapid eye movement and blinking too frequently or not often enough) have been associated with the disease. It is also important to note that abnormal body movements can be caused by the disease itself, as well as by medications used to treat it.

6. **Brain electrical abnormalities.** Electroencephalograms (EEGs) have shown that people with

schizophrenia are more likely to have abnormal electrical activity in the brain.

7. **Immunological and inflammatory abnormalities.** Reduced immune function and an increase in cytokines (interleukin-6) have been documented in people with schizophrenia. There have also been reports of abnormalities in leukocytes and immunoglobulins. The difficulty with studying this aspect of the disease is that antipsychotic medications can also affect immune function, so it is difficult to determine what the disease causes and what the medication causes.

8. **Season of birth.** People with schizophrenia are born more frequently in the winter and spring than in the summer or fall. More than 100 studies in 34 countries have shown an increase in the birth rate of people with schizophrenia of 5–8% during the months of December through April. The reason for this seasonality is not known. Some researchers have theorized that a maternal viral infection, especially during the second trimester of pregnancy, may be a causative factor. In support of this idea is the fact that influenza infection is most common in the winter and in crowded areas.

9. **Urban living.** People born or raised in an urban area have a greater risk for having schizophrenia. The birth rate of affected people in the city is twice the rate in rural areas. The suburbs have a rate between the other two. Also, people with the disorder tend to move to cities.

10. **Other abnormalities.** Pregnancy and birth complications, minor physical anomalies, and an absence of rheumatoid arthritis are associated with schizophrenia.

A great deal of research has been done to find the cause of this debilitating disorder. The current answer is that schizophrenia is a disorder caused by abnormalities in brain structure and function. Schizophrenia is probably more than one distinct disorder. People may have similar symptoms with different causes. There are many different genes that code for brain functions, some of which may only cause abnormal function under stress. Some risk factors are known, but the final word has not yet been written.

Diagnosis and Clinical Features

The standard for diagnosis of mental disorders is the *Diagnostic and Statistical Manual of Mental Disorders* (4th ed., text revision, 2000). The diagnostic criteria for schizophrenia are in Box 8-1 ■. The diagnosis is based on the client's signs and symptoms.

BOX 8-1

Diagnostic Criteria for Schizophrenia

A. Characteristic symptoms:

Two (or more) of the following symptoms must be present for a significant portion of the time during a 1-month period (or less if successfully treated):

1. delusions
2. hallucinations
3. disorganized speech
4. grossly disorganized or catatonic behavior
5. negative symptoms (see text for description)

B. Social/occupational dysfunction:

For a significant portion of the time since the onset of the disturbance, one or more major areas of functioning, such as work, interpersonal relations, or self-care, are markedly below the level achieved prior to the onset (or if onset was in childhood or adolescence, failure to achieve expected level of interpersonal, academic, or occupational achievement).

C. Duration:

Continuous signs of the disturbance persist for at least 6 months. This must include at least 1 month of symptoms (or less if successfully treated) that meet Criterion A.

D. Exclusions:

The symptoms cannot be due to other psychotic disorders, drugs or alcohol, or a general medical condition.

Note: Only one Criterion A symptom is required if delusions are bizarre or hallucinations consist of a voice conducting a commentary on the person's behavior or thoughts, or two voices conversing with each other.

Source: Reprinted with permission from the *Diagnostic and Statistical Manual of Mental Disorders, Text Revision,* copyright 2000, American Psychiatric Association.

BOX 8-2

Reality Check: Clients with Schizophrenia

What people with schizophrenia have said:

- "At first it just sounds like wind in the leaves, rustling and soft. Then it becomes voices, whispering then talking louder. If I concentrate I can hear them more clearly."
- "I am just here [psychiatric hospital] because I had a fight with my brother. There is nothing wrong with me. You are the one who is crazy!"
- "The witches are in my head and after me all the time. I'm never safe. It's OK, they won't get you."
- "An android named Bob told me that if I jumped off the bridge I could fly."
- "I am just afraid. I'm always afraid."
- "I talk to the animals, you know, through their bellies. I am a vegetarian. I could never hurt them. I know what it is like to be eaten alive."
- "I must work day and night to keep these demons at bay! It is exhausting."
- "If I listen to heavy metal [music] really loud through the headphones, it drowns out the voices sometimes."
- "The machine in my body was hungry, so I just injected some peanut butter and mayonnaise to feed him. That's how I got this" [indicating large necrotic arm wound].
- "The voices are talking to me all the time. They comment on everything, like 'You want that but it's too good for you, or you are so bad, or that man is going to kill you.'"
- "Sometimes I wonder: Is that a real memory, or not? Is that person trying to kill me? Will my thoughts hurt someone? My mother killed herself. I know why."
- "Please. Please, can you or one of your kind tell me what happened to me? Why are my thoughts like this? The last time I saw you, you were blue. Now you're red. I know you're an alien. Please tell me what is wrong with me!"
- "I don't remember much about my hospitalization. I do remember being afraid, terrified. I also remember a few people trying to help me, saying that I would be OK. Their reassurance could last me for days. It didn't happen very often."
- "Before the new medication, I spent all of my adult life in the hospital. Now that I'm being discharged I have some new problems I had never considered before, like 'How do I have fun?' And 'How do I prepare food?' These are not such bad problems to have."

Nursing practice is concerned with the client's response to illness, so the client's signs and symptoms are of interest to nurses. Box 8-2 ■ gives a description of the experience of schizophrenia by the real experts (people who have it).

The symptoms associated with schizophrenia may be placed into three major categories: positive, disorganized, and negative symptoms.

POSITIVE SYMPTOMS

The positive (or psychotic) symptoms seem to be an excess or distortion of normal functions (American Psychiatric Association, 2000). Positive (also called psychotic) symptoms include hallucinations, delusions, and disorganized thinking.

- **Hallucinations** are sensory perceptions that seem very real but occur without external stimulus. The client may or may not realize that these are not real sensory experiences. Auditory hallucinations are the most common type in schizophrenia, often experienced by the client as voices. Approximately 75% of people with

TABLE 8-1

Types of Delusions

TYPE OF DELUSION	CONTENT	EXAMPLES
Grandiose	The affected person has beliefs of inflated powers, knowledge, identity, or relationship to a deity or famous person.	"I am Spiderman."
Delusion of reference	Events, objects, or other people in the immediate environment have a particular and unusual personal significance.	"The newsman is talking to me through the TV."
Persecutory	The central belief is that the affected person is being conspired against, harassed, cheated, or persecuted.	"The food here is poisoned."
Somatic	The content of the delusion relates to the structure or function of the client's body.	"There is a machine inside my body."
Bizarre	Clearly improbable ideas that are not derived from real life experiences.	"My neighbor planted a fish inside my brain that tells me when to drink water."
Thought broadcasting	One's thoughts are being transmitted out loud so other people can hear them.	"I don't want to go to the store. Maybe I'll hurt somebody's feelings if I think they are fat."
Thought insertion	One's thoughts are not one's own, but are inserted into one's mind.	"You think I'm bad, but it's not me. The devil puts those ideas there."

schizophrenia hear voices at some time during their illness (Torrey, 2001). Visual hallucinations are the next most common. Hallucinations can also be tactile (touch), gustatory (taste), olfactory (smell), or somatic (involving body sensations, such as electricity).

■ **Delusions** are fixed false beliefs. These beliefs persist despite evidence that they are not true. A delusional belief is one not ordinarily accepted by the members of the person's culture or religion. Table 8-1 ■ provides a list of types of delusions, which are categorized by their content.

DISORGANIZED SYMPTOMS

Disorganized symptoms include disorganized thinking and disorganized behavior.

■ **Disorganized thinking** is a major feature of schizophrenia. Speech is an observable demonstration of a person's thinking. The client's speech (rate, organization, loudness, content) is a good way to assess thinking. Disorganized speech suggests disorganized thinking. Schizophrenia can cause an inability to sort and interpret incoming sensory information. As a result, people with schizophrenia cannot respond appropriately. Clients may have incoherent speech (with topics changing every few words). At its worst,

this becomes "word salad" in which words are thrown together without relationship to each other, such as "Dogs, bicycle, fight, door, happening, machine, quickly." Loose associations (also called *derailment*) can occur; this is a pattern of speaking in which a person's ideas move from one track to another frequently (American Psychiatric Association, 2000). An example of loose associations is: "You know I live in the zoo, I like animals, I plan to wear my new shoes when I go on the walk, are you coming?"

■ **Disorganized behavior** lacks goal orientation. The lack of goal orientation makes activities of daily living (personal hygiene or preparing meals) difficult. The client may have unusual or purposeless behavior such as walking in circles or pacing. Affected people sometimes dress in odd ways, perhaps wearing several hats on a hot day or wearing necklaces over the ears. Schizophrenia causes an altered sense of the self, affecting movements and behavior. Disorganized behavior may include unpredictable agitation (pacing, shouting, profanity), or inappropriate personal behavior, such as public masturbation (American Psychiatric Association, 2000). It may also include **catatonic behavior** (a marked decrease in response to the environment). Clients with catatonia may have a rigid posture, resisting efforts to be moved. They may have excessive purposeless movement or take on bizarre positions.

NEGATIVE SYMPTOMS

Negative symptoms of schizophrenia represent another major source of disability for clients. In contrast to the positive symptoms, the negative symptoms involve a deficit or decrease of normal functions. Negative symptoms include the following:

- *Flat affect.* **Affect** is the nonverbal expression of emotion. The person experiencing schizophrenia may have decreased (*blunt*) or absence of nonverbal emotional expression. The absence of emotional expression is called *flat* affect. This person does not show any facial expressions or other body language indicating feelings.
- *Alogia.* **Alogia** is decreased amount and richness of speech. This is also called poverty of speech. It is thought that this reduction in speech reflects a reduction in thinking. A person with alogia has brief verbal responses, with little emotional expression. The speech may also be *concrete*, meaning that it is confined to practical objects and events, lacking abstract ideas.
- *Avolition.* **Avolition** is a lack of motivation. Clients with avolition have difficulty initiating and persisting in goal-directed activities. This symptom can make it difficult for affected people to work or care for themselves.
- *Anhedonia.* **Anhedonia** means lack of the ability to feel pleasure.

Critical Self-Check. Review the symptoms of schizophrenia: positive, negative, and disorganized. Which of these symptoms would be the most difficult for you to live with if you had schizophrenia?

Course of the Disease

The onset of schizophrenia is usually in young adulthood, although it can affect people of any age. Most cases develop between the ages of 16 and 30 (Torrey, 2001). In addition to the thought and neurological symptoms, schizophrenia affects the person's abilities to relate to self and others, and to function in society. The positive symptoms tend to plateau within 5 to 10 years of diagnosis, and the negative symptoms tend to worsen over time (Beebe, 2003). Most people with schizophrenia do not marry and are more likely than their parents to be unemployed (American Psychiatric Association, 2000). However, many other people with schizophrenia are living fulfilling lives in the

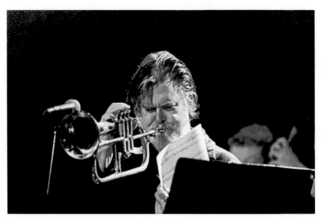

Figure 8-1. ■ Tom Harrell, American jazz trumpeter (who has schizophrenia) playing the trumpet on stage. *Source:* The Image Works.

community, especially when they are in the remission phase, or in recovery from the disease. Figure 8-1 ■ shows Tom Harrell, an American jazz musician (who has schizophrenia) during a performance.

Like many chronic illnesses, schizophrenia is characterized by *exacerbations* (recurrences) in which the client has psychotic and other symptoms, and then periods when the symptoms subside. Many clients experience a *prodromal phase* in which early symptoms occur, before they have a full psychotic episode. Symptoms can include peculiar behavior, unusual speech or affect, and bizarre ideas, such as thinking that one can communicate with inanimate objects (Beebe, 2003). Some people know a psychotic episode is coming on when they are unable to sleep for several nights. If individuals recognize the symptoms that make up their prodromal (or warning) phase, it may be possible for treatment with medication to prevent or lessen the psychotic episode that follows. For many individuals, the prodromal phase starts with negative symptoms. Often family members can look back and remember that the client spent a lot of time in bed, or became more distant or isolated before a psychotic episode.

The treatment and management of schizophrenia have been divided into three phases to coincide with major aspects of the course of the disease (National Collaborating Centre for Mental Health, 2002):

- Initiation of treatment at the first episode
- The acute phase
- Promoting recovery

In the acute phase of the disorder, the affected person may experience positive symptoms (hallucinations, delusions, disorganized speech or behavior) and negative symptoms (alogia, flattened affect, social isolation, loss of motivation, and anhedonia). The affected person is usually not able to keep a job, go to school, do housework, or even do activities of daily living (ADLs) while in an acute episode.

Medication appears to improve the long-term prognosis for many people with schizophrenia. After 10 years of treatment, 25% of those with schizophrenia have recovered completely (the symptoms of schizophrenia go away and never return), 25% have improved considerably, and 25% have improved moderately. Fifteen percent have not improved, and 10% are dead (Torrey, 2001).

People with schizophrenia die at an earlier age than other people do. Females have a 5.6 times greater risk of early death than the general population. Males have a 5.1 times greater risk of early death. Suicide is the largest contributor to this excess mortality rate. People with untreated schizophrenia who are experiencing depression and psychosis are the ones most likely to complete suicide. Other increased risks associated with schizophrenia are accidents, diseases (diabetes, heart disease, infections, and breast cancer), and homelessness. Homelessness probably contributes to the incidence of accidents and diseases (Torrey, 2001).

The brain disorder in schizophrenia renders many affected people unable to understand that they are mentally ill. It is a cruel irony that people with schizophrenia avoid effective treatments, because they lack the insight to use them. Some healthcare providers blame the failure of people with schizophrenia to take their disease seriously on denial. Denial is not the problem. In fact, lack of insight is part of the disorder of schizophrenia (Amador, 2001).

Early diagnosis and treatment of schizophrenia is important for prevention of frequent relapses and rehospitalizations. Early intervention may prevent the worst long-term outcomes (homelessness and death) (Torrey, 2001).

Dual diagnosis means that both mental illness and substance abuse coexist. Substance abuse is particularly common among people with schizophrenia. In combination, these problems lead to even more homelessness, disease, violence, incarceration, and death. People with schizophrenia may be using drugs and alcohol to treat the intolerable symptoms of the disease. The chapter on substance abuse covers this problem in more depth.

Recovery

In 2005, the Substance Abuse and Mental Health Services Administration (SAMHSA) created a plan to transform the mental healthcare delivery system. The plan includes a focus on consumers (people with mental illnesses) and their families who would be served by a coordinated care delivery system. The treatments or interventions would be evidence based (based on research that shows they are effective). The entire program is based on the idea of recovery from mental illness (SAMHSA, 2005).

Recovery is a process in which people with serious mental illnesses such as schizophrenia, major depressive disorder, or bipolar disorder reengage with life. They use new adaptive coping skills, achieve a new sense of self as a person first (not a disease), and feel a new sense of purpose in life (O'Connor & Delaney, 2007).

An important message of the recovery movement is that mental illnesses are treatable and people with mental illnesses can lead meaningful lives in the environment of their choice. Mental health professionals work with consumers, giving them more autonomy than in previous treatment models and help them to develop the skills and support they need to reach their goals. The ultimate goal is to function with as little professional help as possible (Anthony, Cohen, Farkas, & Cagne, 2002).

Recovery from a major mental disorder is not like recovering from an acute illness such as the flu, in which all the symptoms and the cause of the disorder go away. It is not a cure. The recovery from mental illness involves recovering a new sense of self and purpose within and beyond the limits of the disorder. The person in recovery accepts and overcomes the challenges of the disorder. It is through the process of recovery that people with mental and other disabilities become active and courageous participants in their own treatment (Deegan, 1988).

The best rehabilitation programs nurture, or ideally expect, recovery. These programs provide services in the context of supporting participants' efforts, avoidances, failures, learning, and new attempts. Participants must be able to pick up where they left off and try again, in a fail-proof environment where everyone is welcomed, valued, and wanted. A successful rehabilitation program must recognize that each person's recovery journey is unique. Although all people who recover from disabilities experience despair, transitioning to hope and achieving a willingness to take responsible actions is an individual achievement. Options and flexibility are important (Deegan, 1988). Figure 8-2 ■ shows a model of recovery.

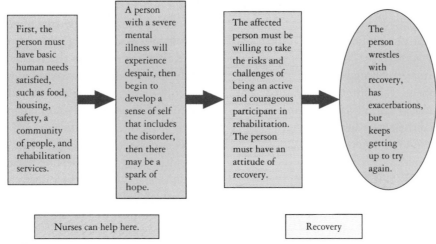

First, the person must have basic human needs satisfied, such as food, housing, safety, a community of people, and rehabilitation services.

A person with a severe mental illness will experience despair, then begin to develop a sense of self that includes the disorder, then there may be a spark of hope.

The affected person must be willing to take the risks and challenges of being an active and courageous participant in rehabilitation. The person must have an attitude of recovery.

The person wrestles with recovery, has exacerbations, but keeps getting up to try again.

Nurses can help here.

Recovery

Figure 8-2. ■ Recovery from severe mental illness.

Collaborative Care

CONTINUUM OF CARE

Even people in the recovery process can have exacerbations and require hospitalization during acute episodes of schizophrenia. People also have treatment needs that extend beyond the hospital. The treatment program that helps clients most is a continuum of care. This continuum provides services for people who have different needs and for individuals as their needs change:

- Hospitalization for management of acute episodes
- Case management, involving a case manager who is aware of the client's history and coordinates the client's services in the community
- Resources in the community for basic needs such as housing, food, medical care, transportation, and clothing
- A range of housing and care options for people with different functional levels, such as subacute care, day hospitalization, supervised/assisted living, group homes, foster care homes, and independent living situations
- Outpatient treatment in the client's community (including mental health clinics, community commitment, and medication supervision as indicated)
- Programs for employment, active community involvement, volunteer opportunities, or other ways for people to be with others, especially the opportunity to be with other people with mental disorders for the purpose of peer support and role modeling of recovery (Jacobson & Greenley, 2001)
- Support for families, including respite care, education, support groups, and referral services; local affiliates of

the National Alliance for the Mentally Ill are an excellent resource for families

People with schizophrenia have better outcomes if they begin treatment early and receive appropriate services throughout their lives. It is well known what services are required to meet the needs of this vulnerable population, yet the resources do not exist in many communities. There are many reasons for this lack of help for people with schizophrenia. One is that our society values independence so highly that we reject the idea of treating people against their will. In addition, schizophrenia has such a stigma that people do not value spending tax money on those who suffer from it. The stigma also prevents affected people from seeking help. Another reason is that because of the disease itself, the people who have it are not able to speak for themselves.

MILIEU THERAPY

For psychiatric inpatients, the environment, or **milieu,** can be used as part of therapy. The environment should be pleasant, simple, and safe. Each client in the milieu is responsible for his or her own environment and behavior.

A consistent nursing staff helps to promote development of trust. Nurses also serve as role models for normal behavior. The staff demonstrates how to interact with other people, how to dress, and how to ask people to change their behavior. Clients have the opportunity to practice and receive feedback on their behavior in the milieu. A common goal is learning how to react appropriately to stress and frustration. Every interaction with a client is an opportunity for the staff to be therapeutic.

Peer pressure can encourage behavior change. Peer encouragement and positive role modeling can give clients hope and practical ideas about how to promote their own recovery.

In milieu therapy inappropriate behavior by clients is dealt with as it happens. Punishment is avoided. The entire process of living in the milieu is an opportunity for clients to practice their new healthy behaviors and coping skills.

PSYCHOSOCIAL REHABILITATION

Rehabilitation is what happens after an acute phase of psychosis. For rehabilitation to have the best chance for success, the client must have a mindset of recovery. The change in terminology toward talking about recovery represents a change in the way people think about major mental illnesses. The illness model used to dominate the literature and treatment language. We now know that people with schizophrenia need to develop a sense of self that includes their disorder but includes the knowledge that they are more than the disorder. When they are able to incorporate the demands of the disorder into their roles as participating members of their communities, there is hope for recovery. They will still have schizophrenia and may still have acute episodes, but they will be community members, not psychiatric patients. Nurses have known for years that people are people first, not diseases: the client in room 103 is a tall soft-spoken 28-year-old Latina from Hillsboro who has schizophrenia, not a schizophrenic.

Traditional American values of individualism, competition, personal achievement, and self-sufficiency may not be the best goals for people with schizophrenia. Programs that allow clients (who often prefer to be called *consumers*) to work cooperatively may be best. Shared work and shared responsibilities for work goals can compensate for the individual during periods of relapse (Deegan, 1988).

Many consumers report that the most powerful form of rehabilitation for them has been helping others. Some consumers become mental health providers or advocates; some talk with individuals or groups of peers; some publicly tell the story of their experiences and recovery. These brave people are fighting the stigma against the mentally ill as well as inspiring others by demonstrating the reality of recovery (Jacobson & Greenley, 2001). Encouraging the client's hope for recovery is also an important nursing intervention.

PSYCHOPHARMACOLOGY

Medication is not the only treatment, but it is a cornerstone in the treatment of schizophrenia. Antipsychotic medications help relieve the hallucinations, delusions, and disordered thinking associated with the disorder.

Antipsychotic medications (also called **neuroleptics**) are used to treat disorders like schizophrenia that are characterized by psychosis. They are also used to treat the thought disorders sometimes associated with dementia, mania, or major depression with psychotic features. Table 8-2 ■ provides information about the three groups of antipsychotic medications and their implications for nurses.

Because schizophrenia affects people differently, any individual client may need to try several different antipsychotics before finding the one that works well. This trial process can be demoralizing. Each antipsychotic medication may take 3 to 6 weeks to have the desired effect. The nurse should explain this to clients, telling them that the healthcare provider will work with the client until the right one is found, and that no one will give up hope.

Medication compliance is a major problem in the psychiatric setting. Approximately 80% of those who stop taking their medication after an acute episode will have a relapse of psychosis within a year. Even people who continue to take their medications experience relapse at the rate of approximately 30% in a year (Torrey, 2001). Medication clearly improves the quality and quantity of life for people with severe mental illnesses such as schizophrenia. Unfortunately, the people who need medications the most often do not realize this. Also, medications cause side effects that further decrease compliance in clients who tend to have poor insight.

The goals of treatment with antipsychotic agents are to do the following:

- Relieve symptoms of psychosis
- Improve negative symptoms
- Prevent future episodes of psychosis
- Improve clients' function and quality of life

Psychosis is complicated and affects all aspects of a person's life. The healthcare team must assess and evaluate a variety of aspects of client behavior, thought, feelings, and functional ability to determine the effectiveness of the medications.

Typical (First-Generation) Antipsychotics

The typical antipsychotics tend to be effective in treating psychosis or the positive symptoms of schizophrenia. The typical antipsychotics are especially effective in the

TABLE 8-2

Antipsychotic Agents

AGENTS/DRUGS	ACTION AND USE	NURSING RESPONSIBILITIES	CLIENT TEACHING
Typical or First-Generation Antipsychotics ■ Chlorpromazine (Thorazine) ■ Fluphenazine (Prolixin) ■ Thioridazine (Mellaril) ■ Trifluoperazine (Stelazine) ■ Haloperidol (Haldol) ■ Droperidol (Inapsine) ■ Loxapine (Loxitane) ■ Thiothixene (Navane) ■ Molindone (Moban)	The typical antipsychotics are dopamine-2 (D_2) antagonists that block D_2 receptors and ↓ DA activity. Used to ↓ positive symptoms, to treat psychosis. Can be used to ↓ nausea (esp. droperidol). Haloperidol (IM) is used to ↓ psychosis with agitation in emergent situations. This group is being prescribed much less often than the atypicals because the typical agents (especially haloperidol) cause more abnormal movement SEs and are not effective against negative Sx.	Monitor for side effects (SEs): anticholinergic symptoms, weight gain, EPS, TD, hypotension, tachycardia, seizures, galactorrhea, impaired memory, NMS. EPS very likely with IM form: give anticholinergic drug. Treat SEs. **Drug interactions:** additive effect of CNS depressants (including alcohol), may ↓ effects of anticoagulants, may ↑ effect of antihypertensives (↑ risk of hypotension). **Lower doses needed in the elderly.**	Teach clients to describe subjective symptoms and to evaluate whether they are improving from their point of view. Efficacy takes several weeks. Teach about SEs, when to notify nurse or physician. Teach about EPS and to report to nurse so p.r.n. meds can be given. Avoid alcohol. If one medication does not work, there are many others: Keep hope alive. Many people have to try several drugs to find the one that works for them.
Atypical or Second-Generation Antipsychotics ■ Clozapine (Clozaril) ■ Risperidone (Risperdal) ■ Olanzapine (Zyprexa) ■ Quetiapine (Seroquel) ■ Ziprasidone (Geodon)	Second-generation antipsychotics are serotonin-dopamine antagonists. They treat psychosis as well as some negative symptoms. Used for schizophrenia, acute mania, bipolar maintenance, behavior disturbances in dementia, and disorders associated with impulse control. Clozapine is uniquely effective for psychosis that is resistant to other drugs. Not a first choice agent due to SE of agranulocytosis (a ↓ in WBCs).	Monitor for SEs: Clozapine can cause potentially fatal agranulocytosis, so WBC should be monitored weekly for first 6 months, then every 2 weeks throughout therapy. Other SEs for this group include weight gain (esp. olanzapine), sedation, orthostatic hypotension, hyperglycemia (can cause DM type 2), hypersalivation, risk of seizures, EPS (esp. risperidone), prolonged cardiac conduction (esp. ziprasidone), NMS (uncommon). **Drug interactions:** may ↑ effects of antihypertensives, may antagonize anti-Parkinson drugs, additive CNS depression with other depressants (alcohol), ↑ anticholinergic effects with other anticholinergics. **Lower doses needed in the elderly.**	Teach clients to describe subjective symptoms and to report if they are improving or not. Efficacy for positive symptoms may be within 1 week, but may take several weeks to take full effect. Teach about SEs and when to report to staff. May need exercise and nutrition teaching. Clients on clozapine must comply with WBC blood draws. Avoid alcohol. Client may require blood glucose testing. Many people have to try several meds before they find the one that works best for them: Keep hope alive.

(continued)

TABLE 8-2			
Antipsychotic Agents (continued)			
AGENTS/DRUGS	**ACTION AND USE**	**NURSING RESPONSIBILITIES**	**CLIENT TEACHING**
Third-Generation Antipsychotics ■ Aripiprazole (Abilify)	Dopamine stabilizer: ↓s DA when it is high, maintains DA when at normal level, also stabilizes mood. Used in schizophrenia and bipolar mania, same disorders as atypical agents.	Monitor for SEs: causes fewer EPS than second-generation atypicals, can cause akathisia, weight gain and sedation are also less frequent, NMS (rare), orthostatic hypotension, nausea, constipation. Same **drug interactions** as above. **Lower doses needed in the elderly.**	Teach client to describe psychosis symptoms and to report if they are subjectively improving. Efficacy for positive symptoms may be within 1 week, but may take several weeks to take full effect. If this medication is not effective, keep hope alive; many people must try several meds before the best one for them is found.

Note: SE = side effect, ↑ = increase, ↓ = decrease, DA = dopamine, EPS = extrapyramidal symptoms, TD = tardive dyskinesia, IM = intramuscular, CNS = central nervous system, NMS = neuroleptic malignant syndrome, DM = diabetes mellitus, Sx = symptoms, WBC = white blood cell.

treatment of acute psychosis with agitation. Negative symptoms are not very responsive to the typical antipsychotic medications.

It may take from 2 days to 2 weeks for clients to experience the sedating effects of the typical antipsychotic drugs. Full effect (efficacy) may take 4 weeks or longer. The atypical agents may take several months to achieve their full benefit. Clients and families must be informed that the wait for treatment response is expected to be long. Without this knowledge, they might give up hope and stop taking the medication too soon (Stuart & Laraia, 2005).

SIDE EFFECTS. Side effects are common with antipsychotic agents. Side effects are often the reason that clients stop taking their medications when they are at home. So, management of side effects is a critical part of the care of clients taking these medications.

Extrapyramidal Side Effects. Antagonism of D_2 receptors causes a reduction in psychosis and also causes extrapyramidal side effects (also called EPSEs or EPS for **extrapyramidal symptoms**). Box 8-3 ■ lists extrapyramidal side effects. EPSEs result from the effects of antipsychotic drugs on the extrapyramidal tracts of the central nervous system, which control involuntary movement (Kneisl, Wilson, & Trigoboff, 2004).

The client with untreated psychosis has an elevation of dopaminergic activity. The person's homeostatic (balancing) mechanism responds by increasing cholinergic

BOX 8-3	
Extrapyramidal Side Effects	

■ **Dystonia** (muscle rigidity)
■ **Pseudoparkinsonism** or **dyskinesia** (stiffness, tremors, shuffling gait)
■ **Akathisia** (restlessness, inability to be still)
■ **Tardive dyskinesia** (late-onset movement disorder)

activity. The neurotransmitters dopamine and acetylcholine must be balanced to maintain normal muscle function. When this client is given an antipsychotic medication, the dopaminergic activity is quickly decreased, but the cholinergic activity is still high (it can take a couple of weeks for cholinergic balance to return at the new low level of dopamine caused by the medication). As a result, dopaminergic and cholinergic activity are again imbalanced, causing EPS. A second medication, an anticholinergic drug, can restore this balance and relieve EPS. Figure 8-3 ■ diagrams the cause and treatment of EPS.

EPS are significant neurological symptoms that include the following:

■ **Dystonia**. Muscular rigidity, abnormal muscle contraction. If tongue or larynx is involved, choking can result. Acute dystonia can be painful and terrifying. It can be mild, such as jaw muscle tightening, or as

A. Balance occurs in schizophrenic client's steady state of high dopamine.

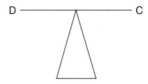

B. Antipsychotic med, decreases dopamine activity, putting dopamine, DA, and acetylcholine, ACh, out of balance, Client has EPS.

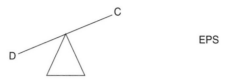

EPS

C. Anticholinergic med, is given to bring cholinergic activity down, restoring balance and treating EPS.

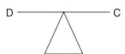

Figure 8-3. ■ Dopaminergic and cholinergic balance in extrapyramidal symptoms (EPS).

severe as *oculogyric crisis* (eyes uncontrollably rolled back), *torticollis* (neck twists head to side and back), or *opisthotonos* (generalized muscle spasms that result in arching of the back and neck). Dystonia occurs in approximately 20% of clients taking typical antipsychotics.

- **Pseudoparkinsonism** or **dyskinesia** (abnormal movement). Stiff, stooped posture; shuffling gait; tremor; slow movements; *cogwheel rigidity* (jerky, ratchet-like movements of the joints); *mask-like facies* (loss of facial expression). These movement symptoms are caused by the imbalance between dopamine and acetylcholine, not by real Parkinson's disease. Pseudoparkinsonism, or dyskinesia, affects 20% of clients taking typical antipsychotics.
- **Akathisia**. Restlessness, intense need to move. The client may report a sense of "jumping out of my skin"

or an inability to sit still. Akathisia may cause clients to pace the floor (walk back and forth continuously), to fidget with fingers, or to move arms and legs while sitting. Akathisia can make it impossible for a client to rest or sleep for days. It is the most common of the EPS, affecting 25% of clients, and it responds poorly to treatment (Keltner, Schwecke, & Bostrom, 2007).

EPS are very uncomfortable for clients. When a client experiences EPS, the provider may reduce the dose of the antipsychotic, prescribe a different antipsychotic medication, or try an anticholinergic or other medication to treat the symptoms. Anticholinergic medications are usually given orally, but some may be given parenterally in emergent situations. It is the responsibility of the nurse to ask whether the client is uncomfortable and to advocate for the client to obtain relief. Table 8-3 ■ lists the drugs used to treat EPS.

TABLE 8-3		
Anticholinergic Drugs Used to Treat Extrapyramidal Symptoms		
GENERIC (TRADE) NAME	**DRUG CLASSIFICATION**	**AVAILABLE IN INJECTABLE FORM?**
Benztropine (Cogentin)	Anticholinergic	Yes
Biperiden (Akineton)	Anticholinergic	Yes
Diphenhydramine (Benadryl)	Antihistamine (has strong anticholinergic side effects)	Yes
Procyclidine (Kemadrin)	Anticholinergic	No
Trihexyphenidyl (Artane)	Anticholinergic	No

- **Tardive dyskinesia** (late onset of abnormal movement) is an extrapyramidal side effect that develops after extended antipsychotic drug therapy. The symptoms of tardive dyskinesia (TD) include involuntary movements such as lip smacking, facial grimacing, tongue protrusion, tongue writhing, blinking, or other involuntary movements of the limbs and trunk. The most common TD symptoms involve abnormal involuntary movements of the face and tongue. The symptoms disappear during sleep. Sometimes clients can voluntarily suppress the abnormal movements briefly, but they recur when the client concentrates on something else.

TD may be due to development of hypersensitivity to dopamine. It is not caused by the same dopamine-acetylcholine imbalance as the other EPS. It does not respond to anticholinergic medications (Keltner et al., 2007).

Ironically, the same antipsychotic medications that cause TD can mask its early symptoms. It is important for clients on antipsychotic therapy to be assessed for abnormal involuntary movement with a scale such as the Abnormal Involuntary Movement Scale (AIMS) to identify it early. Table 8-4 ■ is a scale used by nurses to monitor for abnormal involuntary movement. There is no effective treatment for TD, but it can be prevented by the use of the lowest effective dose of antipsychotic medication. Changing to another antipsychotic may be able to arrest the progression of TD. It is often irreversible.

Critical Self-Check. A client is experiencing discomfort from muscle tightening in her jaws due to EPS. She asks: "Why should I keep taking this medicine? It makes me feel worse than I did when I wasn't taking any meds." How should the nurse respond? Is it ethical for the nurse to give a medication that is known to cause side effects?

Neuroleptic Malignant Syndrome. Neuroleptic malignant syndrome (NMS) is a potentially fatal side effect of antipsychotic drugs. The major symptoms are high fever, muscle rigidity, *autonomic instability* (unstable blood pressure, diaphoresis, pale skin), delirium, inability to speak, tremors, and elevated levels of enzymes that indicate muscle damage (creatine phosphokinase, or CPK). Temperatures may rise as high as 108 °F (42.2 °C).

Fewer than 1% of people who take antipsychotic drugs develop NMS, but for these it can be fatal. Early diagnosis and treatment are the keys to client survival.

Clients are at higher risk for developing NMS if they have dehydration, poor nutrition, or concurrent medical illness. Treatment involves discontinuing antipsychotic drugs and providing supportive treatment for dehydration and other symptoms (Videbeck, 2004).

Neuroleptic malignant syndrome is an idiosyncratic reaction to antipsychotic (neuroleptic) drugs. It usually, but not always occurs early in therapy. It is not a toxic or allergic effect. High potency typical antipsychotics are most frequently involved.

clinical ALERT

Neuroleptic malignant syndrome is a potentially fatal side effect of antipsychotic drugs. It usually occurs early in therapy. Nurses should monitor for high fever, muscle pain, and unstable vital signs, and report these to the physician immediately.

Endocrine Side Effects. Dopamine inhibits the hormone prolactin, which promotes breast enlargement and milk production. Typical antipsychotics elevate levels of prolactin because they inhibit dopamine. Chronic prolactin elevation can cause decreased *libido* (sexual drive), *gynecomastia* (breast

TABLE 8-4

Abnormal Involuntary Movement Scale (AIMS)

Dyskinesia Symptoms

THIS FORM HOLDS FOUR ASSESSMENTS TO SHOW CHANGES OVER TIME.	DATE	DATE	DATE	DATE
1. Muscles of facial expression				
2. Lips and area around mouth				
3. Jaw				
4. Tongue				
5. Upper body (arms, hands, fingers)				
6. Lower body (legs, knees, ankles, toes)				
7. Neck, shoulders, torso, hips				
Overall judgment Severity of abnormal movements				

Extrapyramidal and Other Symptoms

1. Rigidity				
2. Tremor				
3. Bradykinesia				
4. Akathisia				

Dental Problems

1. Current problems with teeth or dentures No = 0, Yes = 1				
2. Does client usually wear dentures? No = 0, Yes = 1				

Examination Procedure

Either before or after examination, observe the client at rest. Abnormal movements can sometimes be suppressed if the client concentrates on this. The chair used in the examination should be firm and without arms.

1. Ask the client if there is anything in his/her mouth (gum, candy) and if so, to remove it.
2. Ask the client about the current condition of his/her teeth. Ask if he/she wears dentures and if so do they bother the client now. Tongue and mouth movements associated with dental problems may be mistaken for abnormal involuntary movements.
3. Ask client whether he/she notices any movements in mouth, face, hands, or feet. If yes, ask to what extent to they currently bother the client or interfere with activities.
4. Have the client sit in a chair with legs slightly apart, hands on knees, feet flat on floor. Look at the entire body for movements while in this position.
5. Ask the client to sit with hands unsupported (between legs or hanging over knees). Observe hands and other body areas.
6. Ask the client to open his/her mouth. Observe tongue at rest in the mouth. Do this twice.
7. Ask the client to protrude tongue. Observe for abnormalities of tongue movement. Do this twice.
8. Ask the client to tap his/her thumb with each finger one at a time as rapidly as possible for 10 to 15 seconds, separately with one hand then the other. Observe face and legs. Concentration on finger movements may allow abnormal movements to become evident elsewhere.
9. Flex and extend client's arms one at a time. Note any rigidity.
10. Ask client to stand up. Observe in profile all body areas again, including hips.
11. Ask client to extend both arms outstretched in front with palms down. Observe trunk, legs, mouth.
12. Have the client walk a few paces, turn, and walk back to chair. Observe hands and gait. Do this twice.

Score each item on the following scale. Rate the highest severity observed. } None = 0, Minimal = 1, Mild = 2, Moderate = 3, Severe = 4

enlargement), and *galactorrhea* (leakage of milk) in women or men. It can also cause menstrual dysfunction in women.

The incidence of type 2 diabetes is increased in people who have schizophrenia, even in those who are not obese. This increase may be in part due to adverse effects on the endocrine system caused by antipsychotic medications. Nurses should be alert for the development of signs and symptoms of hyperglycemia in clients taking atypical antipsychotics.

Anticholinergic Side Effects.   Anticholinergic side effects often result from the use of antipsychotics. Box 8-4 ■ lists anticholinergic symptoms. Clients taking anticholinergic medications for EPS have an increased risk for these side effects.

Weight Gain.   Any of the antipsychotics can cause weight gain, especially clozapine, olanzapine, and risperidone. Weight gain with antipsychotics is associated with increased appetite, binge eating, carbohydrate craving, decreased satiety, and change in food preferences in some clients (Allison & Casey, 2001). Increased insulin may also contribute to weight gain in people taking antipsychotic drugs (Brown, Cooper, Crimson, & Enderle, 2002). Weight gain brings with it elevated risks for cardiovascular and other diseases. The best nursing approach is prevention, through teaching about exercise and nutrition.

Orthostatic Hypotension.   The hypotension caused by antipsychotics is an antiadrenergic effect. Normally the blood vessels can respond to changes in body position by constricting, ensuring adequate blood flow to the brain. When sympathetic alpha-1 receptors are blocked, the vessels are prevented from responding automatically to body position changes.

BOX 8-4	

Anticholinergic Effects

Dry mouth
Orthostatic hypotension
Constipation
Urinary hesitancy or retention
Pupil dilation (*mydriasis*)
Blurred near vision
Dry eyes
Photophobia
Increased heart rate

BOX 8-5	NURSING CARE CHECKLIST

Orthostatic Blood Pressure Measurement

☑ After the client has been lying down for at least 5 minutes, take the client's blood pressure and pulse.
The 5 minutes allows for the blood pressure to equilibrate in the supine position.

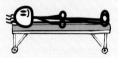

☑ Instruct the client to stand up. Wait for approximately 1/2–1 minute, and retake the blood pressure and pulse.
The 1-minute wait allows the orthostasis (drop in BP caused by position change) to develop. A longer wait may allow time for the client's vasculature to compensate for the position change. You are trying to determine whether the client's blood pressure drops significantly on arising, putting her/him at risk for injury.
A drop of 15–20 mmHg in systolic BP with increased pulse indicates orthostatic hypotension.

☑ Wait 2 more minutes and take the blood pressure and pulse again.
The additional time will allow for evaluation of whether the client can compensate with time for the change in position. If client can compensate, BP will return to near baseline.

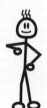

This orthostatic (position-related) hypotension happens when the individual stands up or changes position quickly. It is also called postural hypotension. Orthostatic hypotension is more likely to occur in older adults. It can create a safety hazard for the client who becomes dizzy or falls when the blood pressure drops. Box 8-5 ■ provides a reminder on how to measure for orthostatic hypotension.

Cardiac Side Effects.   Antipsychotics may cause increased heart rate as an anticholinergic side effect. They (especially ziprasidone) may also cause prolonged conduction time through the heart's electrical system. On EKG you would see a prolonged QT interval.

Seizures.   Antipsychotics tend to decrease the seizure threshold. This means that it would take a smaller stimulus to cause a seizure in a client taking these medications. Epilepsy or a history of seizures is not a contraindication for the use of antipsychotic drugs, but the physician should be notified of any such history.

Photosensitivity. Some clients taking antipsychotics experience *photosensitivity*, which is an increased sensitivity to the effects of the sun. Photosensitive clients experience severe sunburn with minimal sun exposure. Dark-skinned as well as light-skinned clients can experience photosensitivity. They should be counseled to avoid prolonged exposure to sunlight or to wear sunscreen on their skin whenever they are outdoors.

Atypical Antipsychotics

The atypical agents influence a variety of dopamine receptor sites, serotonin receptors, muscarinic receptors, alpha-receptors, and histamine receptors.

Atypical agents differ from typical antipsychotic agents in several important ways. The atypical agents (Rankin, 2000):

1. Are more effective in treating the negative symptoms of schizophrenia
2. Cause fewer extrapyramidal side effects
3. Are effective against the symptoms of schizophrenia for some people who do not respond to typical agents

SIDE EFFECTS. EPS are the side effects most commonly cited by clients as their reason for noncompliance with antipsychotic medications at home. As a group, the atypical agents cause fewer EPS, less prolactin increase, and less tardive dyskinesia. Because of their efficacy and more favorable side-effect profile, the atypical antipsychotics are currently prescribed more frequently for clients with psychosis.

Diabetes. Atypical antipsychotics increase the client's risk for developing type 2 diabetes. Clients receiving atypical antipsychotics are 9% more likely to have type 2 diabetes than people taking typical agents. Schizophrenia itself increases clients' risk of having impaired glucose tolerance. The medications may increase insulin resistance in body cells causing diabetes. Clients taking these drugs should be monitored regularly for development of hyperglycemia. Other risk factors, such as Native American, African American, or Latino ethnicity, obesity, female gender, and family history of type 2 diabetes, increase the client's risk (Brown et al., 2002; Ollendorf, Joyce, & Rucker, 2004).

Agranulocytosis. Even though their side-effect profile is favorable, the atypical agents still have side effects. The most notable is that clozapine can cause agranulocytosis, a life-threatening decrease in white blood cell production.

This effect happens to 1% of clients who take clozapine. Because of this serious possibility, clozapine is used only for clients who are resistant to treatment with other antipsychotics. Treatment resistance is established by failure to respond to at least two different antipsychotic agents. Clozapine is effective in treating 25–50% of clients whose symptoms do not respond to typical agents (Brown et al., 2002).

clinical ALERT

All clients receiving clozapine should have WBC measured once per week during the first 6 months of therapy, and every other week after that, to assess whether their white blood cell count is stable. If a client's WBC drops (indicating bone-marrow suppression), clozapine should be permanently discontinued.

Third-Generation Antipsychotics

The first third-generation antipsychotic is a dopamine system stabilizer called *aripiprazole* (Abilify, Abilitat). Unlike the other antipsychotic agents, aripiprazole has a stabilizing and modulating effect on brain dopamine. This drug is intended to reduce dopamine transmission when it is too high and to preserve it when it is too low, thus maintaining the dopaminergic-cholinergic balance. The drug causes a very low incidence of abnormal involuntary movements (EPS) but can cause akathisia (Stahl, 2001).

Depot Injection and Other Drug Forms

Several antipsychotic agents are currently available in long-acting *decanoate* (depot injection) form. The **depot injection** is an oil-based medication form of the drug injected intramuscularly for the purpose of slow release of the drug over several weeks. Haloperidol (Haldol) and fluphenazine (Prolixin) are among the typical agents available in depot form. They are supplied in a sesame oil solution. Haloperidol is repeated every 4 weeks, and fluphenazine every 1 to 4 weeks.

Risperidone is an atypical antipsychotic agent available in long-acting injectable form. It is supplied in a powder of microspheres, which is suspended in a saline solution and administered IM every 2 weeks. Olanzapine is also available in IM form. Its duration of action is 4 weeks with a peak 2 weeks after injection.

The advantages of the long-acting form of antipsychotic drugs relate to compliance with drug therapy. A client may be able to comply with a clinic visit once every few weeks more easily and consistently than taking oral medications daily.

Critical Self-Check. What do you think the disadvantages of taking antipsychotic drugs in a long-acting IM form might be?

Several antipsychotic agents are available in liquid oral concentrate forms. The liquid form can be used to prevent situations in which clients move pills to their cheeks instead of swallowing them and spit them out later. It is also helpful when the client has difficulty swallowing, or prefers liquid to the pill form. The liquid concentrates must be mixed with a small amount of juice or other liquid to improve the medication taste.

Critical Self-Check. Is it ever acceptable for the nurse to put a client's medication in juice, and then tell the client "drink your juice"? Why?

Abuse Potential

The antipsychotic medications do not cause euphoria, so there is virtually no abuse potential from these drugs. They also do not cause addiction or dependency. This lack of abuse potential is an important teaching point, because many consumers believe that any drug that affects the mind is addictive.

clinical ALERT

Nurses often hesitate to give p.r.n. medications, perhaps from fear of responsibility for making the decision to give them. If your client has EPS, do not hesitate to give these anticholinergics when they are ordered p.r.n. EPS are very uncomfortable for clients and are a major reason for noncompliance with antipsychotic medications.

NURSING CARE

ASSESSING

In mental health nursing the client's potential for violence is assessed first because it is a safety issue. Mentally ill people in general are no more violent than the general public, but there are groups of mentally ill people with increased risk for violence toward others (Torrey, 1997). These risk factors for violence include the following:

- Previous violent acts at home or in treatment
- History of substance abuse, especially if currently under the influence of substances

- Paranoid delusions
- Command hallucinations (commanding the client to hurt someone)
- History of being a victim of violence (violence is a learned behavior)

Certain behaviors may suggest that a client is becoming increasingly agitated and more likely to act out violently. These behaviors are clenching fists, talking loudly or yelling, threatening, increasing motor activity (was sitting, then walking, then pacing back and forth quickly), hitting walls or furniture, wincing, or looking afraid.

Mental Status Assessment

When asked, "What is the client's mental status?" the nurse will often reply: "Alert and oriented" or "Oriented times three." The major clinical findings in schizophrenia are not addressed by the "alert and oriented" assessment. A client could say, "I am Linda Eby. I am in the hospital. It is Tuesday at 8:00 P.M." This sounds pretty good, but does it show whether the client is experiencing hallucinations or delusions, or if her thinking is disorganized? When the assessment is charted, does the reader know if the client had flat affect or avolition? Look at the people in Figure 8-4 ■. You cannot hear what they are saying, but what can you tell about their feelings by observing their affect?

Since nurses do not read minds, systematic observation of the client's speech and behavior works best to assess thought content. Box 8-6 ■ is a sample mental status assessment. This assessment tool provides information about the various aspects of mental status that are pertinent in the psychiatric setting. See also the vocabulary of mental status assessment in Box 8-7 ■ (every specialty has its own language).

Cognitive Assessment

An assessment of the client's *cognitive ability*, which includes memory, judgment, and the ability to think abstractly, is included in mental status. These factors are especially important when planning client teaching and doing discharge planning. If a client replies that he would "call the mother ship" if he left his stove turned on, his judgment is not adequate to keep him safe if he lived alone.

To assess short-term memory, ask the client to remember three words (such as pen, watch, and flower) when you begin the mental status assessment. Ask again 5 to 10 minutes later what the three words were. If the client remembers accurately, short-term memory is said to be intact. For long-term memory, ask where the client went

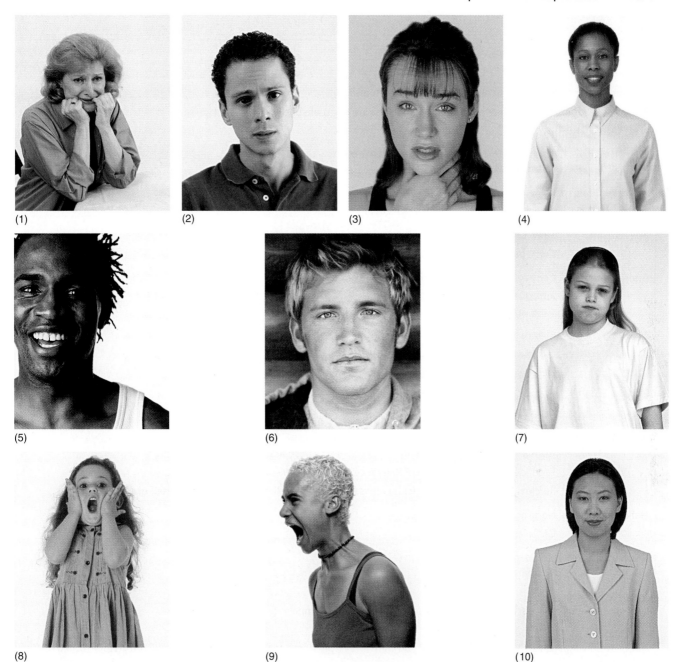

(1)   (2)   (3)   (4)

(5)   (6)   (7)

(8)   (9)   (10)

Figure 8-4. ■ What can you tell about these people's feelings by observing their affect? *Sources:* (1) Phototake NYC; (2) Phototake NYC; (3) Phototake NYC; (4) Dorling Kindersley Media Library; (5) Getty Images—Stockbyte; (6) Getty Images—Stockbyte (7) Dorling Kindersley Media Library; (8) Dorling Kindersley Media Library; (9) Getty Images Inc.—Image Bank; (10) Dorling Kindersley Media Library.

to school or about something that happened years ago (people do not usually make up an answer if they forget).

The ability to think abstractly is affected by many brain disorders, such as schizophrenia and dementia. One way to assess abstract thinking ability is to ask the client to interpret a proverb. Proverbs can be interpreted *concretely*, using only the literal meaning of the words, or *abstractly*, using ideas implied by the situation. For example, consider the

proverb "A stitch in time saves nine." A concrete interpretation is "One stitch taken in time saves nine stitches later." An abstract interpretation is "A problem treated early prevents a bigger problem later." A client with psychosis may even give a disorganized interpretation, such as "A stitch is an itch and we all go to Beaverton." This simple assessment can shed light on the client's thought processes. Consider the three interpretations in the previous example.

BOX 8-6	

Mental Status Assessment

Client's Name: _____ Date: _____ Time: _____

Reason for Admission (in client's own words, indicates insight): _____

Circle assessments that apply. When assessment findings are unusual, specify with a description.

Appearance (Grooming/hygiene):

Appropriate for situation	Disheveled (dirty, messy)	Unusual (specify)_____

Motor Activity:

Lethargic	Relaxed	Restless	Pacing
Threatening	Other (specify)_____		

Speech Rate:

Slow	Normal	Pressured (fast and difficult to interrupt)
Content of speech is appropriate to situation		Unusual (specify) _____

Interpersonal:

Cooperative	Oppositional/Resistant	Defensive
Intrusive (too close to others)	Other (specify)_____	

Mood: Client's rating of mood on 1–10 scale _____

Mood appears to be:	Normal	Euphoric	Irritable
	Depressed	Angry	Anxious

Affect:

Broad (can express both positive and negative emotion)	Blunted	Flat
	Labile (changeable)	

Thought Processes (assess through client's speech):

Normal	Blocking	Loose Associations	Grandiosity
Flight of Ideas	Ideas of Reference	Paranoia	Delusions
Suicidal Ideas	**Homicidal Ideas (ask directly if client feels like hurting self or others)**		

Hallucinations:

None noted	Auditory	Visual
Other (specify) _____		

Cognition: Short-Term Memory
(ask what client had for breakfast):   Intact   Impaired

Long-Term Memory
(ask where client went to school):   Intact   Impaired

Judgment
(problem solving, such as, "What would you do if you were away from home and remembered that you left the stove turned on?"):

Intact   Impaired   Unwilling/unable to answer

Abstract Thinking
(interpretation of proverbs, such as "What does it mean when they say, 'The early bird gets the worm'?"):

Abstract   Concrete   Unwilling/unable to answer

Signature _____

BOX 8-7

Vocabulary for Mental Status Assessment

Blocking: Abrupt interruption in train of thinking before a thought is finished, difficulty finding words.

Broad Affect: The expected finding of the ability to express a full range of emotions.

Blunted Affect: Severe reduction in the range of emotion displayed.

Catatonic: Severely slowed motor activity, decreased response to environment.

Circumstantial: Talking indirectly toward an idea with many unnecessary details or irrelevant additions.

Clanging: Association of words similar in sound but not in meaning; may include rhyming.

Delusion: A false belief that is inconsistent with reality. It is inconsistent with what the person's culture or religion accepts as real. Does not respond to reasoning or evidence that it is false.

Echolalia: Repeating words just said by another person.

Euphoric Mood: Elevated mood, very cheerful, often grandiose.

Flat Affect: Absence of any emotional expression; face is blank and voice is monotone.

Flight of Ideas: Rapid, continuous verbalization abruptly shifting from one idea to another.

Grandiosity: An inflated appraisal of one's abilities, power, or knowledge. May be of delusional proportions when severe.

Hallucination: A sensory experience that seems real but is not related to external stimuli. Most common is auditory, then visual. Can involve any of the senses.

Ideas of Reference: Interpretation that external events have a direct reference to oneself.

Labile Affect: Rapidly changing emotional expressions, without relation to external events.

Loose Associations: Flow of speech in which ideas shift from one to another without logical connections.

Neologisms: New words created by the client.

Restricted Affect: Reduced expression of range of emotion. Less severe than blunted affect, but still decreased emotional expression.

BOX 8-8   CULTURAL PULSE POINTS

Cultural Relativism

From the Client's Point of View

Mental health nursing across cultures can be challenging. Problems are created when the healthcare team misinterprets a client's behavior that is normal in his or her native culture. The definitions of psychosis include talking to voices that are not really present and bizarre behavior. In some traditional Latino cultures, it is normal for people to depend on spirits for guidance. People hear and speak to these spirits. To the European American nurse, communication with spirits may seem like hallucinations. Some African and Caribbean cultures recognize witches and sorcerers. Traditional Southeast Asians may use "coining," which involves healing by rubbing coins on the skin of a sick person. Navajos may attribute illness to "ghost sickness." Some American Indians attach amulets, such as those made from feathers, to an ill family member's clothing. These behaviors may seem bizarre or at least unnecessary to nurses who are not familiar with the cultures involved. A useful approach to cultural sensitivity in cases like these is to find a cultural facilitator, or person who can translate the client's language as well as the cultural meaning of the client's behavior and customs. The nurse should always take special care to try to interpret the client's behavior relative to the client's cultural background (which is cultural relativism), rather than by the cultural expectations of the nurse. Ask, "What meaning does this practice have for the client?" or "What need does this meet?" Mutual respect and willingness to compromise are critical to transcultural nursing.

How would the nurse use this assessment information to plan teaching these clients about taking their morning medications when they go home?

Cultural Issues

Interpreting the meaning of client behaviors can be difficult if the client is from a different culture from the nurse. The Cultural Pulse Points Box 8-8 ■ describes the concept of *cultural relativism*. Understanding this will help you see the client's behavior from the client's point of view. If the "Golden Rule" is to treat others as you would want to be treated, then the "Rule of Cultural Relativism" is to treat clients as *they* would want to be treated.

Physical Assessment in the Psychiatric Setting

Assessment is still the cornerstone of nursing, but why should the nurse avoid a routine full physical assessment of the psychiatric client every shift? Good question. When clients are hallucinating they may not be sure what is real and what is not. Physical touching may be perceived as part of a threatening hallucination. Delusional thinking may make even the well-intentioned nurse seem menacing. Physical assessment may be very stressful for the client. Some clients mistake physical touch for sexual advances. Therefore, only priority physical assessments should be done in the acute psychiatric situation. A physician or nurse practitioner will perform an initial physical assessment as part of the psychiatric client's admission process. Nurses will confine their physical assessment activities to pertinent illnesses or drug responses by clients, rather than screening assessments such as listening to every client's lungs every shift.

The brain is connected to the body and many physical problems, such as blood pressure and neurological changes, can accompany mental illness and its treatment. Psychiatric nurses must have good assessment skills because they are not free to take off every client's clothes to look and ask about every detail. They must know the difference between what is necessary to know and what is just nice to know. A trusting nurse-client relationship will make it easier for the nurse to gain client cooperation for necessary assessments.

Nurses must understand the desired effects and potential side effects of all medications and treatments received by their clients and assess for these. In addition, mental health clients may not be able to clearly articulate what is wrong with them. Careful listening is another important nursing skill. When a client with psychosis says, "The snake is squeezing my chest!" it is possible that this client is experiencing a heart attack.

Obtaining Additional Input from the Family

The client's family is a critical aspect of mental health care. It is important to obtain written permission from clients to communicate with anyone about them, including their family members. Assess the client's family in terms of who they are, where they live, how involved they are in the client's life, what their learning needs are, and what their questions and concerns about the client are. Families can make a big difference as allies in treatment for mental health clients, yet healthcare providers often overlook them, out of a mistaken sense of protecting the client's confidentiality. They can be important members of the treatment team.

DIAGNOSING, PLANNING, AND IMPLEMENTING

Data about the client's mental status, observation of the client's behavior and interactions with others, physical assessment findings, and information from family all contribute data for establishing nursing diagnoses.

In the psychiatric setting an interdisciplinary treatment team (nurse, psychiatrist, social worker, mental health therapist, occupational therapist, etc., and of course the client) provides treatment planning. In this context, client care plans and goals are written according to the medical and psychosocial models rather than the nursing process model. However, nurses must be able to document how they use the nursing process.

In the acute phase of psychosis, treatment should focus on the client's basic needs. Safety, nutrition, and rest are the priorities. Acute symptom management is also important.

Priority nursing diagnoses that often apply to clients with schizophrenia include the following:

- Risk for Violence, self-directed or directed at others
- Disturbed Thought Processes
- Sensory Perceptual Alterations (specify auditory or visual)
- Ineffective Coping
- Self-Care Deficit (specify bathing/hygiene, dressing, feeding, or toileting)
- Impaired Social Interaction

Desired outcomes for a client with schizophrenia include the following (Mills, 2000). The client will:

- Cause no harm to self or others
- Demonstrate reality-based thinking
- Use healthy adaptive coping skills
- Take medications regularly
- Continue to be active (employment, hobbies, exercise)
- Have a routine daily and weekly schedule
- Include enjoyable activities in schedule
- Perform activities of daily living independently
- Communicate regularly with family and important friends

Risk for Violence (Directed at Self or Others)

- Avoid touching an actively hallucinating client. *Touch may be perceived as part of a threatening hallucination and the client may hit in self-defense.*
- Intervene early as soon as you have identified agitation. Reassure the client that she or he is safe in the hospital. *Agitation can escalate quickly. Early intervention can prevent the situation from getting worse. Fear may motivate agitation. Clients often benefit from reassurance that they are safe.*
- Avoid confronting clients aggressively about their behavior. When inappropriate behavior arises, tell the

client simply and calmly that the behavior is not acceptable and redirect the client to another activity. *The client may not realize that her/his behavior is inappropriate. Aggressive behavior by the nurse may make the client feel defensive. The nurse's behavior and attitude are contagious: lend your self-control to the client instead of yelling and making the client more afraid.*

- Start with less restrictive interventions when the client exhibits inappropriate behavior: try to talk first, then redirect, offer meds, isolate/medicate, restrain last. *The client has the ethical and legal right to the least restrictive alternative treatment that is effective.*

- Maintain a low-stimulation environment. *Clients with schizophrenia may have difficulty processing multiple stimuli, and extra stimuli may lead to sensory overload and agitation.*

- Talk with the client about signs and symptoms of anxiety and agitation and triggers that start these feelings. Discuss options for appropriate behavior and anxiety management techniques. *If the client can recognize anxiety and agitation early, the client can notify staff who can help identify coping mechanisms to prevent violent acting out. Clients with schizophrenia often have short attention and inadequate coping skills and may have impulsive behavior. Cognitive and behavioral approaches to planning for future episodes are an effective way to help the client try appropriate new behavior.*

- Observe people experiencing paranoia or command hallucinations closely. *A person who has a nonviolent personality may act out violently when confronted with an apparently life-threatening hallucination or when terrorized by a paranoid delusion that threatens the person's life. Many people will never be violent unless they are in a life-threatening situation. Imagine how hard it is for a person to live with the constant threat of harm. When people with schizophrenia are violent, usually the violent act is a matter of self-defense from their point of view.*

Box 8-9 ■ lists suggestions for interacting with clients who are actively hallucinating.

Disturbed Thought Processes

- Provide antipsychotic medications as ordered and monitor effects. *It is the responsibility of nurses to assess the client's response to medications for the purpose of evaluating their effectiveness.*

- Look for the client's strengths and abilities when providing nursing care. *When a person has a severe mental illness such as schizophrenia, it is easy to see the pathology. It is important to look for the person's strengths and to acknowl-*

| BOX 8-9 | NURSING CARE CHECKLIST |

Interacting with a Person Who Is Hallucinating

☑ Only one person should interact with the client at a time. *The client is having difficulty interpreting stimuli, so it will be easier for the client to respond to one person.*

☑ Keep environmental noise to a minimum. Do not speak loudly. *The client is having difficulty filtering sensory stimuli and is easily overstimulated. A low-stimulation environment will make it easier for the client to differentiate real stimuli from the voices.*

☑ First specifically ask the client about the hallucinations (usually voices) and what they are saying or telling the client to do. *It is helpful to know if clients are experiencing voices commanding them to hurt themselves or others.*

☑ Focus on reality. Do not continually ask clients to describe the hallucinations. Do not react to clients' report of hallucinations as if they are real. *Often hallucinations are transitory experiences for clients. Describing the hallucination can form it more clearly in the client's mind and reinforce it. The nurse's role is to help clients recognize reality, not to further confuse them about their hallucinations or delusions. When the nurse keeps the conversation in reality, reality is reinforced and the hallucinations may be minimized.*

☑ Do not argue with the client's experience. Share your own perceptions. Reassure the client that she or he is safe. *The client is truly hearing the voices. The goal is to present reality, not to convince the client that she or he is wrong. Respectful disagreement can help the client understand what is real, such as "I know you hear voices, but I don't hear them." Reassurance may help the client see that she or he is not in danger and does not need to defend her- or himself.*

☑ Avoid touching a person who is actively hallucinating. *During a hallucination, any touch may be perceived by the client as part of the hallucination. If the hallucination is threatening, the client may strike out in self-defense.*

---

edge the normal parts of the person. Even the psychotic client has coping or survival skills that the nurse can draw on for the client's benefit.

- Reinforce reality. Talk about what is really happening. *Even conversations about the simple realities of daily life (the weather, doing laundry, meals, etc.) bring the client's attention away from disordered thoughts and into the here and now. The nurse's role is to help the client recognize what is real.*

- Encourage or assist the client to express feelings of fear or anxiety. Provide validation for the client's feelings. *The sense of losing contact with reality can be frightening.*

TABLE 8-5

Nursing Interventions for Psychotic Symptoms in Schizophrenia

CLIENT PROBLEM	DESIRED OUTCOMES	NURSING INTERVENTIONS	RATIONALE
Hallucinations	Client will have fewer than three hallucinations on my shift, and will state that they are less threatening. Client will participate in the real environment by talking with staff and attending one group activity each day. Client will verbalize a plan to decrease hallucinations.	1. Decrease environmental stimuli (noise). 2. Assist client to identify triggers for hallucinations. 3. Avoid reinforcing the reality of hallucinations. Call them "the voices." Tell client you do not hear them. 4. Avoid touching the client during a hallucination. 5. Distract the client with a simple task or conversation. 6. Teach client strategies for self-management of hallucinations.	1. Client has an inability to process multiple stimuli and can be overwhelmed. Sensory stimuli can trigger or increase hallucinations. 2. If the triggers are known, client can plan to avoid them. 3. Honesty by the nurse will reinforce that the hallucinations are not real. 4. Touch may be perceived by the client as a part of a threatening hallucination. Client may hit in self-defense. 5. Distraction can be an effective way to divert the client's attention to other thoughts away from the hallucination. 6. See text for distraction, activity, interaction, and social strategies for dealing with strange thoughts.
Delusions	Client will respond to reality-based interactions with others. Client will demonstrate ability to function without responding to delusions. Client will demonstrate an anxiety management technique.	1. Avoid arguing with the delusion. 2. Avoid reinforcing the delusion or suggesting its reality. 3. Engage the client in reality-based conversations and activities. 4. Help client to learn to manage anxiety (relaxation or breathing techniques).	1. Argument encourages the client to focus on the delusion to defend it. 2. The client has difficulty interpreting reality. Honesty by the nurse promotes trust and promotes the client's ability to test reality. 3. Distraction from thinking about the delusional ideas reinforces reality for the client. 4. Delusional thinking may be worsened by anxiety. Anxiety management may help client control delusions.

Expressing feelings to the nurse who accepts them without judgment and validates how difficult the situation must be can be affirming and helpful to clients.

■ Clients with schizophrenia may manifest disturbed thought processes in hallucinations or delusional thinking. Table 8-5 ■ describes nursing interventions and rationales for these client symptoms. *Clients with schizophrenia will be seen by nurses in every practice setting. It is important to be familiar with these interventions even if you don't plan to work in a psychiatric setting.*

Ineffective Coping

■ Establish a trusting relationship in which the client is safe to express true feelings, especially negative ones. Do not react to the client's negative feelings. *The client may feel that only positive feelings are appropriate and not know an appropriate way to express negative feelings. A nonthreatening relationship may provide the client with the opportunity to express unresolved feelings. A strong reaction to the client's feelings may indicate rejection (Townsend, 2006).*

- Offer medications in a confident way, expecting the client to take them. The same person should be assigned to the client each day if possible. *Antipsychotic medications will provide relief from the thought disorders that make the client's problems harder to manage. Confidence promotes trust. Consistency of staff promotes trust.*
- Role model how to interact and disagree with others. Teach the client stress management techniques such as going to her or his room and doing relaxation exercise. *Role modeling and behavioral approaches are effective ways to teach the client new coping skills.*

Self-Care Deficit (Specify Deficient Area)

- Encourage the client to do self-care but intervene if unable. *Personal hygiene is a safety issue and may not be omitted. Also, failure is demoralizing.*
- Demonstrate to the client how care should be done, helping the client the first time. Remind if the client forgets. *People with schizophrenia may not have the skill or motivation to proceed without direction. Concrete thinking may make it more difficult for the client to follow verbal directions.*
- Give the client positive reinforcement for successful self-care. *When the client is able to perform activities and is positively rewarded, it will promote self-esteem and continuing of the behavior. Ideally the client will do ADLs independently without prompts.*

Impaired Social Interaction

- Approach the client with an accepting attitude. Be honest and sincere. *Acceptance, honesty, and sincerity promote trust.*
- Interact with the client individually and model appropriate social behavior (body language, topics). *People with schizophrenia often lack social skills and benefit from role modeling as a way to learn them.*
- Give positive reinforcement for the client's voluntary interactions with others. *Positive reinforcement is an effective behavioral approach to behavior change.*
- Encourage the client to attend group activities in the hospital. Accompany the client at first if necessary. *The client may respond positively to encouragement from a trusted nurse. Trust is an important issue for the client with schizophrenia.*

EVALUATING

When evaluating the effectiveness of nursing care for clients with schizophrenia, the nurse looks to the desired outcomes. The nurse will determine whether the client:

- Demonstrates reality-based thinking
- Performs ADLs independently
- Demonstrates an understanding of medication management
- Interacts effectively with others

DISCHARGE CONSIDERATIONS

As the client recovers from psychosis and moves into the rehabilitation and recovery phase, the intervention focus changes to teaching and psychosocial rehabilitation issues. Medication teaching, group therapies, self-care skills, and social skills become more important. Clients can learn strategies to decrease the likelihood of relapse of schizophrenia. Box 8-10 ■ describes these strategies. Learning these strategies can give clients more control over their lives and disease processes. It may help the client to think about recovering.

Meeting the client's learning needs is an important aspect of nursing in every setting. In the psychiatric setting, an assessment of the client's readiness to learn is especially important. After it is determined that the client is ready and able to learn (adequate attention span, adequate insight), important topics include practical information about how to take medications at home, reasons for medications, side effects to report to the psychiatrist, relapse prevention (see Box 8-10), and symptom management at home.

Some people with schizophrenia will still have psychotic (delusional or hallucinatory) thinking when they are discharged. Research has been done in the area of helping people deal with strange thoughts. Strategies include *distraction*, including listening to music, reading aloud, counting backwards from 100, watching television, and describing an object in detail. *Interacting* is another strategy and includes telling the voices to stop, talking to the voices while pretending to use a cell phone, and agreeing to listen to the voices at certain times. The *activity* strategy includes walking, doing housework, taking a relaxing bath, playing the guitar, singing, and going to the gym. The *social* strategy involves talking to a trusted person, phoning a helpline, avoiding people, going to a drop-in center, and going to a favorite place (Mills, 2000).

Social skills are poor in clients with schizophrenia. Relating to others is difficult for them. Impaired social interaction is a common nursing diagnosis. In the acute stage, the positive symptoms force the client to focus on internal stimuli. In the long-term rehabilitative

BOX 8-10

Teaching Clients Relapse Prevention Strategies

Discuss the following suggestions with clients to help them reduce the chance of relapse of psychosis:

- Learn from your experience. In the past how did you feel in the weeks before you needed to be hospitalized? What feelings or symptoms did you experience? These are the **predictors of relapse** for you. Tell your family or friends about them, and watch for these symptoms. When they happen, get help from your psychiatrist who can change your treatment to help prevent or reduce the severity of the relapse.
- How do you feel about your **medication**? (Look for some positive aspect of client's attitude and repeat it.) What are your goals for the long term? Whatever you want to accomplish (getting a job, going to Disneyland) will not happen if you do not take your medication. If medication is part of your treatment, take it. It is what keeps you out of the hospital. Tell your prescriber about side effects; most can be treated.
- Do what you can to decrease the **stress** in your life. Keep it quiet around yourself. Go to a room alone or with one person if you want to. When someone argues with you, go to a quiet place. Know what is most stressful for you. If you know something is really stressful for you, avoid it.

- Know your **resources** and have a plan. Make a list of people who can give help when you need it. For example: Adam can take me to the pharmacy to refill my prescription. Betty can talk when I am lonely or scared. Carlos can take care of my fish if I am too tired. Dad can call the doctor or the hospital if I need to go, etc. Write down all their phone numbers.
- Think of some **things that make you feel better**. Write them on a list. Take it out and do them when you start to feel bad. Maybe you feel better when you take a walk, do relaxation techniques, have a snack, paint, draw, take a nap, look at pictures, listen to music, talk to a trusted person, or pet a dog. The list has to be things you would really do.
- **Avoid risky situations.** Stay away from people who want you to use drugs or alcohol with them. It is too hard to say no. Stay away from negative people who criticize you or make you feel bad about yourself. Avoid situations that increase the voices or your stress.
- **Keep healthy.** Eat right. Sleep regularly. Stay active with hobbies, work, and exercise.
- **Keep hope alive.** Remember how life is always changing. Do you agree that some days you feel bad and some days you feel better?

---

phase, there may be negative symptoms to deal with. It is difficult for clients to overcome the lack of motivation to socialize with other people. In the hospital, the nurse can schedule brief one-to-one interactions with the client or can encourage the client to attend group activities. In the community, the nurse can refer the client to community socialization programs at mental health clinics or day treatment programs or encourage the client to try recreational activities (such as bowling).

People with schizophrenia often need to learn how to behave in social situations. They also need a network of social contacts. Nurses are involved in psychosocial rehabilitation whether the client is in the hospital or in the community.

NURSING PROCESS CARE PLAN
Client with Neuroleptic Malignant Syndrome

You are a staff nurse on a medical-surgical unit where Roberto Valdez, a 56-year-old client, has been admitted with possible kidney stones (urolithiasis) and dehydration.

You notice on his chart that he also has been diagnosed with schizophrenia and has been taking fluphenazine for 3 weeks.

Assessment. Mr. Valdez expresses anxiety about this hospitalization and his treatment. He is having severe pain all over his body and just wants medication for the pain. He loses his train of thought easily and sometimes does not respond to your questions. You assess that Mr. Valdez has an unstable BP from 100/50 to 180/104 and an irregular pulse of 120. His oral temperature is 103°F. He is very diaphoretic. He is stiff and pale. Based on your knowledge of fluphenazine and other antipsychotic medications, you realize that Mr. Valdez might be experiencing neuroleptic malignant syndrome brought on by the medical crisis of renal colic while trying to pass a kidney stone and the dehydration. You immediately notify the RN charge nurse who contacts the physician.

Diagnosis. Several nursing diagnoses were identified for Mr. Valdez:

- Risk for Injury R/T adverse reaction to antipsychotic medication
- Pain R/T medication reaction and kidney stone
- Anxiety R/T not understanding his condition and treatment and possible reaction to antipsychotic medication

Expected Outcomes

- Client's physical condition will stabilize as evidenced by vital signs within normal limits within 24 hours.
- Client will state pain at a level of 3 or lower (on a 1–10 scale) within 1 hour of administration of pain medication.
- Client will state that he feels less anxious about his physical condition and treatment within 24 hours.

Planning and Implementation

- Monitor vital signs every 15 minutes.
- Monitor intake and output.
- Monitor mental status every 15 minutes.
- Prepare to transfer client to ICU.
- Explain all procedures to client simply and calmly.
- Discontinue fluphenazine as ordered by physician.
- Administer medication to reduce fever.

Evaluation. The client was transferred to the ICU. He was started on IV therapy and his vital signs stabilized. Within 24 hours, his BP returned to 130/86 and his pulse was 90 and regular. Temperature was 99° orally. Blood tests indicated no muscle or kidney damage. Mr. Valdez regained his alert mental status. He has not had hallucinations or delusions. The physician has asked for a psychiatric consultation to determine which antipsychotic medication should replace the fluphenazine. Pain was controlled with morphine, and he finally passed the kidney stone. He stated a reduction of his anxiety and expressed his thanks to the staff.

Critical Thinking in the Nursing Process

1. What could have been the result if you had attributed the client's signs and symptoms to possible kidney stones and had not considered other options?

2. What other antipsychotic medications could precipitate NMS? Which category of antipsychotic medications is least likely to result in this syndrome?

3. What symptoms will you expect to occur as the fluphenazine is eliminated from his system?

Note: Discussion of Critical Thinking questions appears in Appendix I.

Advocating for Clients

The treatments and knowledge needed to treat schizophrenia already exist. Financial commitment by the government and insurance companies and community priorities must change to bring the resources to the people who need them. The role of nursing in this process is in client advocacy.

Nurses are experts on the subject of how people are affected by diseases and disorders. Nurses can influence their legislators to prioritize funding for mental illness treatment. Nurses can act collectively through their legislators, unions, employers, and professional organizations to influence insurance companies to cover mental illness equally with physical illness, which is called *mental health parity*. They can advocate in their communities for improved housing and other social services for mentally ill people. They can raise the consciousness of the people in their communities by writing to local newspaper editors about the issue of mental illness treatment. Nurses can help stop the stigma by discouraging jokes or embarrassing comments about mentally ill people. We can work to make the invisible people with mental illness visible so our society will see who truly needs help.

Note: The references and resources for this and all chapters have been compiled at the back of the book.

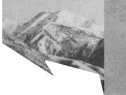

 ## KEY TERMS

Use the audio glossary feature of the Companion Website to hear the correct pronunciation of the following key terms.

affect

akathisia

alogia

anhedonia

avolition

catatonic behavior

delusions

depot injection

disorganized behavior

disorganized symptoms

disorganized thinking

dyskinesia

dystonia

executive function

extrapyramidal symptoms

hallucinations

milieu

negative symptoms

neuroleptics

positive symptoms

pseudoparkinsonism

tardive dyskinesia

KEY Points

- Schizophrenia affects approximately 1% of all people in the United States.
- Schizophrenia is a complex disorder caused by functional and structural abnormalities of the brain.
- It is among the most devastating of all illnesses to the quality and length of the lives of affected people, yet it is underrepresented in funding for research and client services.
- The disorder is characterized by positive, disorganized, and negative symptoms.
- People with schizophrenia have disordered thinking, decreased motivation, difficulty relating to other people and to themselves, and an increased risk of suicide.
- Schizophrenia usually starts in young adulthood and has periods of acute psychosis alternating with periods of reduced symptoms.
- Most people with schizophrenia require a range of services throughout their lives.
- Families can be important members of the treatment team.
- Antipsychotic medications improve the symptoms of the majority of people with schizophrenia.
- It is often necessary for an individual to try more than one antipsychotic medication to find the one that is the most effective. Nurses should inform clients about this frustrating possibility.
- Antipsychotic medications have side effects. Some (NMS and TD) are life-threatening or long-lasting; others (EPS) cause clients discomfort and may encourage noncompliance with medication therapy.
- There is hope for people with schizophrenia. Most people respond well to treatment.

 ## EXPLORE MediaLink

Additional interactive resources for this chapter can be found on the Companion Website at www.prenhall.com/eby. Click on Chapter 8 and "Begin" to select the activities for this chapter.

- Audio glossary
- NCLEX-PN® review
- Case study
- Study outline
- Critical thinking questions
- Matching questions
- Weblinks
- Video Case: Larry (Schizophrenia)

Caring for a Client Who Is Experiencing Psychosis

NCLEX-PN® Focus Area: Psychosocial Integrity

Case Study: Bob Goldman is a 40-year-old European American Jewish man who is diagnosed with schizophrenia. He has not been taking his ordered antipsychotic medication at home. He was admitted to the psychiatric unit today with the diagnosis of psychosis due to acute exacerbation of schizophrenia. It is time to give him his oral antipsychotic medication.

Nursing Diagnosis: Disturbed thought processes

COLLECT DATA

Subjective	Objective
_____	_____
_____	_____
_____	_____
_____	_____
_____	_____
_____	_____
_____	_____

Would you report this data? Yes/No

If yes, to: _____

Nursing Care

_____
_____
_____
_____
_____
_____
_____
_____
_____

How would you document this? _____
_____
_____
_____

Compare your documentation to the sample provided in Appendix I.

Data Collected
(use those that apply)

- History of benign prostatic hypertrophy
- History of suicide attempt at age 18
- BP 130/82
- Client states, "I don't need the medication. I am fine. The doctor is the one who is crazy."
- Weight loss of 15 pounds since last hospitalization 9 months ago
- Client states, "I like cereal for breakfast."
- Client is dirty and has strong body odor.
- Client takes the blanket off his bed, rolls it into a log shape, and swings it around.
- Client states, "I'll use this log to fight off the attackers!"

Nursing Interventions
(use those that apply; list in priority order)

- Tell the client, "You are safe here in the hospital."
- Take VS every 2 hours.
- Maintain a low-stimulation environment.
- Tell the client, "Yes, you do need the medication, and if you don't take it willingly, we can force you to take it."
- Teach the client about the chemical structure of his medication.
- Tell the client, "This medication will help to straighten out your thoughts. I think you should take it."
- Remove all bed linens from the client's room for the duration of his hospitalization.
- Communicate simply and calmly with the client.
- Say, "I will save you from the attackers."
- Say, "There are no attackers here."
- Ask, "Why don't you bathe?"
- Encourage the client to take a shower.
- Give the client a big hug to reassure him.

When you are taking any exam, put yourself into the best possible frame of mind. Get enough sleep the night before. Eat breakfast. Get to the test early enough that you will not have to hurry. Make sure that you are prepared and tell yourself that you have done everything you can. Your life does not depend on any test score. Really.

1 The belief expressed by a mental health client that an alien is creating sores on his body with a laser is classified as a(n):

1. Hallucination.
2. Neologism.
3. Idea of reference.
4. Delusion.

2 If a client were experiencing negative symptoms of schizophrenia, the nurse would expect to see:

1. Flat affect and little speech.
2. Rigid posture.
3. Excessive purposeless movements.
4. Inappropriate laughter.

3 Traditional, or typical, antipsychotic medications may help relieve which of the following symptoms of schizophrenia?

1. Anhedonia
2. Flat affect and alogia
3. Hallucinations, delusions, and disordered thoughts
4. Avolition

4 When a client newly diagnosed with schizophrenia asks the nurse about the Zyprexa she is now taking, the nurse's best response would be:

1. "This is an antipsychotic drug that will take 3 to 4 weeks to take effect."
2. "This is a new drug to help relieve your anxiety."
3. "This is an antipsychotic drug that will take effect immediately to eliminate your 'voices'."
4. "This drug is to help you sleep."

5 A newly admitted client with schizophrenia tells you that her dead grandmother sits in a chair in her room and tells her when it is safe to leave her room. The nurse's best response would be:

1. "If your grandmother is dead, she cannot be in your room."
2. "Your grandmother must have been very special to you."
3. "You don't feel safe here?"
4. "We are here to help you. You don't need your grandmother for protection."

6 In a psychiatric inpatient unit where milieu therapy is being used, one would expect the unit to have:

1. A television playing continuously on the news channel for reality orientation.
2. Structured daily activities.
3. Client-directed rules and regulations.
4. Little structure to avoid stress for the clients.

7 A nurse who is working on an inpatient psychiatric unit knows to observe which of the following clients most closely for potentially violent behavior?

1. A client experiencing catatonic symptoms
2. A client who has been pacing all day, talking loudly to an unseen voice
3. A client who refuses to participate in the morning arts and crafts activity
4. A client who has been following the nurse around all day

8 A young client with schizophrenia in an inpatient psychiatric unit shakes his fist at the nurse, threatening physical harm. The nurse's best response would be to:

1. Put an arm around him to show acceptance and support.
2. Grab his fist and say, "That is not acceptable behavior."
3. Talk to the client quietly and offer him medications to help him calm down.
4. Call for security to lock him in an isolation room.

9 When assisting the client who is taking an antipsychotic medication, a good nursing intervention to remember is to:

1. Encourage a high-fat diet.
2. Encourage daily time in the sun.
3. Remind the client to change positions slowly.
4. Take the medication with an antacid.

10 In a psychiatric unit specializing in psychosocial rehabilitation, which of the following would be expected to be part of a client's treatment plan? (Select all that apply.)

1. Teach the client how to play the piano
2. Teach the client how to access public transportation
3. Work with the client on job interview skills
4. Assist the client to prepare a meal
5. Supervise an arts and crafts group

Answers for Review Questions, as well as discussion of Care Plan and Critical Thinking Care Map questions, appear in Appendix I.

Chapter 9

Mood Disorders

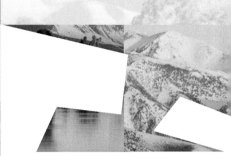

BRIEF Outline

MAJOR DEPRESSIVE DISORDER
Depression
Suicide

BIPOLAR DISORDER
Definition of Bipolar Disorder

LEARNING Outcomes

After completing this chapter, you will be able to:
1. Provide basic client or family teaching about the cause, clinical effects, and treatment of depression.
2. Assess suicide risk.
3. Assess a client using the Geriatric Depression Scale.
4. Provide basic client or family teaching about the cause, clinical effects, and treatment of bipolar disorder.
5. Safely administer antidepressant and mood stabilizing medications.
6. Apply the nursing process to the care of a client with a mood disorder (depression or bipolar disorder).

Everyone has felt happy and sad. We can all relate to a range of emotions that people normally experience in the course of a lifetime. When elation and tragedy are beyond the normal range of intensity, are persistent, are not a response to life experiences, and interfere with daily functioning, a mood disorder might exist.

Mood is a pervasive and sustained emotion that influences how a person perceives the world. *Affect* (nonverbal expression of feeling) indicates a client's current emotional state. It is more changeable than mood. There are several types of mood:

- **Elevated mood** is an exaggerated sense of well-being.
- **Euthymic mood** is a mood in the normal range.

- **Dysphoric mood** is a sad or unpleasant feeling or state.
- **Irritable mood** is a state of being easily annoyed, upset, or provoked to anger (American Psychiatric Association, 2000).

There are several disorders of mood (such as Major Depressive Disorder, Dysthymic Disorder, Bipolar I Disorder, Bipolar II Disorder, Mood Disorder Due to a General Medical Condition, and Substance-Induced Mood Disorder, among others). In this book we will use Major Depressive Episode/Disorder and Bipolar I Disorder as our prototypes for the nursing management of mood disorders. Box 9-1 ■ provides the diagnostic criteria for a major depressive episode according to the *DSM-IV-TR*.

MAJOR DEPRESSIVE DISORDER

Depression

Because everyone has experienced sadness and a low mood at some time, it seems that it would be easy for people to relate to how it feels to be depressed. The difficulty is that depression takes sadness and lack of energy to a lower level that is not in the usual experience of unaffected people.

BOX 9-1

DSM-IV-TR Diagnostic Criteria for Major Depressive Episode

A. Five or more of the following symptoms have been present during the same 2-week period and represent a change from the previous functioning; at least one of the symptoms must be (1) depressed mood or (2) loss of interest or pleasure.

1. **Depressed** mood most of the day, nearly every day, as indicated by either subjective report (for example "I feel sad or empty") or observation made by others (such as appears tearful). *Note:* In children or adolescents, mood can be **irritable**.
2. **Very diminished interest or pleasure** in all, or almost all, activities most of the day nearly every day (either by client report or report of others).
3. **Significant weight loss** while not dieting **or weight gain** (change of more than 5% of body weight in a month), or an increase or decrease of appetite nearly every day. *Note:* Children may fail to make expected weight gains.
4. **Insomnia** or **hypersomnia** (sleeping too much) nearly every day.
5. Activity changes: **psychomotor agitation** (increased physical activity associated with mental

processes) or **psychomotor retardation** nearly every day (observed by others, not just feeling restless or slow).
6. **Fatigue or loss of energy** nearly every day.
7. Feelings of **worthlessness or inappropriate or excessive guilt** nearly every day.
8. **Diminished ability to think or concentrate**, or indecisiveness, nearly every day.
9. **Recurrent thoughts of death** (not just fear of dying), recurrent suicidal ideation, a plan for committing suicide, or a suicide attempt.

B. The symptoms cause significant distress or impairment in social, occupational, or other important areas of functioning.

C. Symptoms associated with general medical conditions, side effects of substances, or bereavement are excluded.

Note: Do not include symptoms that are clearly due to a general medical condition.

Source: Reprinted with permission from the *Diagnostic and Statistical Manual of Mental Disorders, Text Revision*, copyright 2000. American Psychiatric Association.

Consider the statement of Bob, a man whose wife, Lee, has Major Depressive Disorder: "I knew Lee had depression when we got married, but I didn't realize what a battle it would be. When she is depressed, she can't get out of bed. I don't understand why she can't just cheer up. She doesn't have anything to be depressed about." Bob can still get up for work even when he is tired or does not really want to. He can still go to the store for medicine or food even when he does not feel well. He thinks that adults should be motivated to do necessary things that are important even though they are difficult for them. Bob may wonder whether his wife is not trying hard enough or if she really does not love him enough to do things with him even though she is experiencing a depressive episode.

Consider also the case of Pearl, a 70-year-old woman who lives in a long-term care facility. Pearl had a stroke a year ago and has hemiplegia on her right side. She does not feed herself and has little appetite. She cooperates with having her activities of daily living done for her, but she does not try to help. When she talks, it is only one or two words at a time. Her face always seems to look sad. The nurse thinks Pearl is depressed. In this chapter we hope to prepare nurses to help people like Pearl, Bob, and Lee live with this debilitating brain disorder.

Major Depressive Disorder is a disease that consists of one or more Major Depressive Episodes like the one described in Box 9-1. Depressive episodes can range from mild to severe, with a range of functional impairment as well. Figure 9-1 ■ depicts a young woman who is too depressed to get out of bed.

CAUSES

Major Depressive Disorder has a genetic component and a psychosocial component. Each contributes, but neither explains the disorder alone. Because multiple factors cause and affect the disorder, effective treatments usually include psychosocial (teaching and counseling) and physiological (medication or psychopharmacological) approaches.

Major Depressive Disorder is 1.5 to 3 times more common among first-degree biological relatives of affected people than among the general population (American Psychiatric Association, 2000). A genetic predisposition may interact with environmental factors to create the disorder. People can inherit the tendency to respond to life stressors with the development of depression. A gene variant has been found in a transporter for the neurotransmitter serotonin that, when combined with stress, increases the risk of depression (Caspi et al., 2003).

A hypothesis called **kindling** suggests that a stressful event may alter neurotransmitter function, causing a person to have a first episode of a mood disorder. The early episodes of depression or mania may be precipitated by psychosocial stressors in individuals who have the gene that makes them susceptible. The individual's brain becomes increasingly sensitive over time until mood episodes can occur without stimuli. *Kindling* explains the increased frequency of mood episodes over time. The fact that the neurotransmitters that are in low supply in depression inhibit kindling further reinforces this hypothesis (Stuart & Laraia, 2005).

Recent advances in brain imaging have been used to assess brain function of people with depression. Positron emission tomography (PET) shows abnormal function in the prefrontal cortex of the cerebrum and in the limbic system during depressive episodes. Figure 9-2 ■ shows a PET scan before and after medication for depression was administered.

There is also a lot of evidence that an abnormality in brain neurotransmitter physiology causes depression. Brain neurotransmitters such as serotonin, norepinephrine, dopamine, acetylcholine, and gamma-aminobutyric acid (GABA) are likely involved. We learned that in schizophrenia brain neurotransmitters are overactive. In depression, the opposite is true; the neurotransmitters have reduced function. The fact that antidepressant medications are so effective is evidence that neurotransmitter function affects mood.

The endocrine system is also involved. The hypothalamus, pituitary, and adrenal glands, together called the *HPA axis*, control the physiologic responses to stress. These glands may be hyperactive in people with depression. The HPA axis also affects the 24-hour day–night cycle of body rhythms (circadian rhythms). In both depression and mania, the normal circadian rhythms are

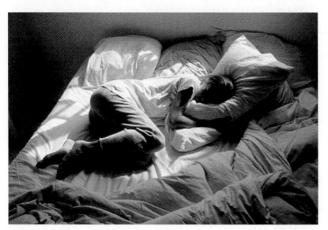

Figure 9-1. ■ Woman in bed, too depressed to get up. *Source:* PhotoEdit Inc.

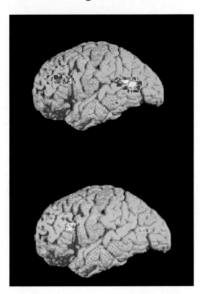

Figure 9-2. ■ PET scan of brain with depression before and after antidepressant treatment. Areas of low activity are red/yellow. Untreated depressed brain (top) shows low activity in prefrontal cortex and parietotemporal lobe. The lower brain, after treatment, shows normal function. *Source:* Photo Researchers, Inc.

BOX 9-2

Risk Factors for Depression

- Previous depressive episode
- Female gender
- Family history of depression
- Stressful life events
- Substance abuse or dependency
- Postpartum period
- History of suicide attempt
- Chronic general medical condition

disrupted. Circadian rhythms affect many physiological functions, including sleep and wakefulness, hormone secretion, mental alertness, and body temperature.

Women are twice as likely as men to develop depression. Children show no gender difference in risk, but at puberty women become more likely to be affected. A significant proportion of affected women report a worsening of depressive symptoms in the few days before menstruation. The lifetime risk of having a Major Depressive Episode is 10–25% for women and 5–12% for men. At any given time, 3–5% of people in the United States are experiencing a major depressive episode. Most of these are not diagnosed or treated. The disorder affects people of all ethnicities and socioeconomic groups equally (American Psychiatric Association, 2000).

Depression is thought to increase the risk of coronary artery disease, stroke, and diabetes. It is also linked to higher mortality rates following a heart attack or stroke and to slower rehabilitation after hip surgery (Spires, 2006).

Depressive symptoms may be caused by certain medications. Some antibiotics, antifungal, anti-inflammatory, antineoplastic, cardiovascular, and gastrointestinal drugs have been shown to cause depressive symptoms in some people. When a client has a new onset of depression, it should be determined if the client started any new medications.

COURSE OF THE DISEASE

The disorder may begin at any age. The average age of onset is in the mid-20s. A major life stressor precedes the first Major Depressive Episode for many people (American Psychiatric Association, 2000). However, it is not the stressor itself that causes depression. The person who becomes depressed is susceptible to developing depression after a stressful event. Box 9-2 ■ lists risk factors for depression and the development of a depressive episode.

Some people experience only a single episode. Most people who have one episode of depression continue to have episodes throughout their lives. Yet others experience almost a steady state of depressed mood. An untreated episode of depression can last for years.

Some clients experience psychotic symptoms, such as hallucinations or delusional thinking, associated with severe depression. This psychotic depression is more disabling and often requires more intensive treatment than a depressive episode without psychotic features.

OTHER TYPES OF DEPRESSION
Postpartum Depression

Depression after childbirth can range from the "postpartum blues" to psychotic depression. It is very common for women to experience tearfulness, anxiety, impaired concentration, and lack of energy immediately after delivery. This normal case of "the blues" usually starts within 3 to 4 days after delivery and lasts no longer than 2 weeks. It usually resolves without medical treatment. The client may benefit from reassurance by the nurse that the condition is common and will resolve with time, rest, and family support. The client and her family should be encouraged to notify the care provider if the depressive symptoms do not resolve after 2 weeks.

Postpartum psychosis usually develops within 3 weeks of delivery. It is characterized by depressed mood, lack of concentration, guilt, lack of interest in the baby, rejection of the baby, or unreasonable fear that something bad will happen to the baby. The client may have an abnormal attitude toward bodily functions. The risk of suicide and infanticide should be assessed. Affected women usually improve within 2 to 3 months of treatment. Treatment depends on the individual client's symptoms. Women with a history of psychiatric disorders are more likely to develop postpartum psychosis.

Seasonal Affective Disorder

Seasonal affective disorder (SAD) is depression that is associated with shortened exposure to daylight. It usually happens in the winter when the days become shorter, and resolves in the spring and summer. The symptoms are sleepiness, fatigue, lethargy, irritability, and increased appetite. It is thought to be a result of abnormal melatonin metabolism. The treatment is light therapy, depicted in Figure 9-3 ■. Antidepressant medications and cognitive behavioral therapy are also effective treatments. In light therapy the client is exposed to bright light for a prescribed number of hours each day. It is more effective if administered in the morning. Light therapy has been effective for clients with mild to moderate seasonal, nonpsychotic depression (Lurie, Gawinski, Pierce, & Rousseau, 2006).

CLINICAL FEATURES

Major Depressive Disorder is a disabling disease that affects occupational and personal functioning. An affected person will have a depressed or low mood every day and the symptoms listed in Box 9-1. A list of symptoms can never fully describe the human consequences of a disease. See the Reality Check on Depression (Box 9-3 ■) to see how people

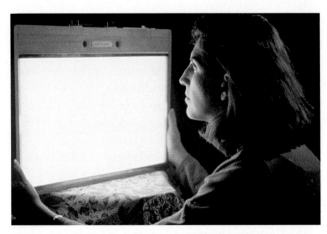

Figure 9-3. ■ Woman with seasonal affective disorder (SAD) is being treated with light therapy. *Source:* PhotoEdit Inc.

BOX 9-3

Reality Check on Depression

What people with depression say:

■ "The color, flavor, and spark of life are extinguished."
■ "Everywhere is another reason for me to feel sadness and regret. I am so sensitive. Every little thing makes me feel sad. I dwell on feeling bad and what I should have done."
■ "I feel like I'm in a deep dark hole and can't even try to get out."
■ "Everything worth living for goes out of focus."
■ "I've been too tired to chew."
■ "People can be overstimulating, especially when they are cheerful."
■ "People want me to do things that I should really want to do. It makes me feel guilty."
■ "My soul left and was replaced with lead."
■ "My kids want me to get up and play. It's not that I don't want to. I wish I could! I can't move. They must hate me."
■ "I am a failure in every sense of the word."
■ "My job was so important to me, so important, but I got to the point where I couldn't concentrate at work, then I was unable to go to work at all."
■ "Nothing matters, everything hurts, and you are always alone no matter who is around you."
■ "When I'm depressed I think about the time I heard a bird screeching outside. I ignored it, and later saw a cat eating a bird. The bird was crying to me for help and I failed it. This was ten years ago, and I think of it frequently."
■ "When I didn't answer your questions, it was because I didn't have the energy to talk."
■ "If I don't feel like living, why would anyone else want me to?"

---

with depression describe their feelings. Figure 9-4 ■ shows the symptoms of a major depressive episode.

Depression causes misery and disability (loss of function) for the people who have the disorder. It also causes difficulty in the relationships they have with other people. Depression causes people to lose the ability to enjoy the things in life that used to make them happy. It affects their ability to relate to other people. Depressed people miss work, lose their jobs, or have reduced effectiveness and productivity at work. Affected people often cannot continue their family and work responsibilities. They may not be able to do their activities of daily living. Most of the people who commit suicide are depressed at the time.

Depression has a high cost in human suffering as well as a financial cost to businesses that lose productivity. When a person has depression along with a general medical condition (such as diabetes or a stroke), the medical condition is likely to be worse than it would be if the depression were not present. Depression is associated

Mood depressed; Memory problems
Anxious; Apathetic; Appetite changes
"**J**ust no fun"
Occupational impairment
Restlessness; Ruminative

Doubts self; Difficulty making decisions
Empty feeling
Pessimistic; Persistent sadness; Psychomotor retardation
Report vague pains
Energy gone
Suicidal thoughts and impulses
Sleep disturbances
Irritability; Inability to concentrate
Oppressive guilt
"**N**othing can help" (Hopelessness)

Figure 9-4. ■ Characteristics of a major depressive episode. *Source: Contemporary Psychiatric Mental Health Nursing* by Kneisl/Wilson/Trigoboff, © Reprinted by permission of Pearson Education, Inc., Upper Saddle River, NJ.

with increased disability and even reduced life expectancy in hospitalized clients with serious medical conditions (Roach et al., 1998).

Depression in the Elderly

In older adults, depression may have different signs and symptoms from those that caregivers expect. Geriatric clients are more likely to report vague physical complaints (expressing mental disorders in the form of physical complaints is called **somatization**), such as headaches and abdominal complaints, rather than describing themselves as depressed. They are not even likely to tell the physician that they are feeling sad. The diagnosis of depression is further complicated by cognitive impairment. If clients are unable to answer questions about their feelings, the Geriatric Depression Scale is useless (Spires, 2006).

It is easy to see how so many older people go undiagnosed and untreated. Often their symptoms are seen as a normal response to aging. Only one in three primary care physicians routinely screens older clients for depression. The diagnosis and treatment of depression can be lifesaving. Nursing home residents with depression have a 1.5 to 3 times greater death rate than their nondepressed counterparts (Spires, 2006).

clinical ALERT

Depression is not a normal part of aging. Depression in the elderly is often overlooked. Older clients should be assessed for depression. Those with cognitive impairment may display anxiety, irritability, and social withdrawal instead of the usual depression symptoms.

STIGMA

Because of the stigma associated with mental illness, people are reluctant to seek help when they have the symptoms of depression (National Alliance for Mental Illness, 2006). People with depression are less likely to accept treatment, to comply with treatment recommendations, and to continue treatment than are people with general medical conditions without depression.

Evidence of the stigma against people with mental illness includes the following:

■ People are often required to report their mental illnesses when they apply for driver's licenses, jobs, security clearances, and other routine purposes, whereas those with other medical diseases are not (some of this has decreased since passage of the Americans with Disabilities Act).
■ Insurance companies reimburse for mental illness treatment at a reduced rate compared with general medical illnesses. There is often a limit on the amount of coverage for mental illness treatment that does not apply to general medical conditions.
■ Physicians may choose not to enter the diagnosis of depression into medical records because they want to protect their clients from the stigma.
■ At least 80% of all depression treatment takes place outside the mental health setting.

People with depression may fear being stigmatized or discriminated against in hiring, promotion, and other societal opportunities. Until mental illness is seen on an equal plane with general medical disorders attitudinally, economically, socially, and politically, it will be underreported, underdiagnosed, and undertreated.

The public is becoming more informed about mental illness as healthcare providers and mental health advocates provide them with information. Even when they understand that mental illness is treatable and appreciate advances in treatment, only 41% of people in one study said that they would take medication for depression. The stigma against psychotropic drugs remains especially high (Rihmer, 2007). The challenge for nurses to help reduce this stigma remains high also.

Suicide

In 1996 the World Health Organization urged member nations to create suicide prevention strategies. The U.S. Surgeon General published a call to action in 1999, which included the risks for suicide (Box 9-4 ■), protective factors for suicide (Box 9-5 ■), and the following statistics.

An average of 85 Americans die from suicide each day. The suicide rate in the United States has remained relatively stable since the 1970s. However, the rates for certain groups have increased significantly. The suicide

---

BOX 9-4

Risk Factors for Suicide

- Previous suicide attempt
- Mental disorders, especially mood disorders such as depression and bipolar disorder
- Co-occurring mental and alcohol or substance abuse disorders
- Family history of suicide
- Hopelessness
- Impulsive and/or aggressive tendencies
- Barriers to accessing mental health treatment
- Relationship, social, work, or financial losses
- General medical illness
- Easy access to lethal suicide methods, especially guns
- Unwillingness to seek help because of the stigma attached to mental and substance abuse disorders, and/or suicidal thoughts
- Influence of significant people—family members, celebrities, peers who have died by suicide—through either direct personal contact or inappropriate media representations
- Cultural or religious beliefs—for example, the belief that suicide is a noble resolution of a personal dilemma
- Local epidemics of suicide that have a contagious influence
- Isolation, a feeling of being cut off from other people

Source: U.S. Public Health Service. (1999). *The Surgeon General's call to action to prevent suicide.* Washington, DC: Author.

BOX 9-5

Protective Factors for Suicide

- Effective and appropriate clinical care for mental, physical, and substance abuse disorders
- Easy access to a variety of clinical interventions and support
- Restricted access to highly lethal methods of suicide
- Family and community support
- Support from ongoing medical and mental healthcare relationships
- Learned skills in problem solving, conflict resolution, and nonviolent handling of disputes
- Cultural and religious beliefs that discourage suicide and support self-preservation instincts

Source: U.S. Public Health Service. (1999). *The Surgeon General's call to action to prevent suicide.* Washington, DC: Author.

---

rate among adolescents and young adults has increased dramatically. Firearms-related suicides account for almost 100% of this increase in adolescent suicide. In the general population, firearms constitute the most common means of suicide in the United States (59%). Having a firearm in the home increases the risk of completed suicide. More Americans die each year from suicide than from homicide (National Institute for Mental Health, 2006).

Suicide rates are highest among older adults. Older white males are the group with the highest risk (Figure 9-5 ■). The suicide rate among older white men with depression is six times higher than that of the general population (Spires, 2006). There is no recent change in the rates for this

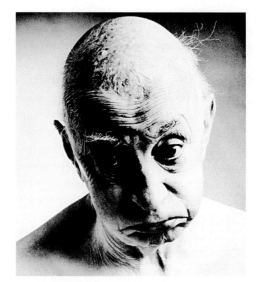

Figure 9-5. ■ Older white males have the highest suicide rate.
Source: Photolibrary.com.

BOX 9-6

Geriatric Depression Scale (Short Form)

1. Are you basically satisfied with your life?	Yes/**No**
2. Have you dropped many of your activities and interests?	**Yes**/No
3. Do you feel that your life is empty?	**Yes**/No
4. Do you often get bored?	**Yes**/No
5. Are you in good spirits most of the time?	Yes/**No**
6. Are you afraid that something bad is going to happen to you?	**Yes**/No
7. Do you feel happy most of the time?	Yes/**No**
8. Do you often feel helpless?	**Yes**/No
9. Do you prefer to stay at home, rather than going out and doing new things?	**Yes**/No
10. Do you feel you have more problems with memory than most?	**Yes**/No
11. Do you think it is wonderful to be alive?	Yes/**No**
12. Do you feel pretty worthless the way you are now?	**Yes**/No
13. Do you feel full of energy?	Yes/**No**
14. Do you feel that your situation is hopeless?	**Yes**/No
15. Do you feel that most people are better off than you are?	**Yes**/No

SCORING: Count **bold** responses. A score of 5 or more indicates need for referral to evaluate for depression. Score of 10 is almost always depressed.

Source: Sheikh, J. I., & Yesavage, J. A. (1986). Geriatric depression scale: Recent evidence and development of a shorter form. *Clinical Gerontologist, 5,* 165–172.

---

population. Most elderly suicide victims are seen by their primary care provider within a few weeks of their suicide and are experiencing a first episode of mild to moderate depression. This demonstrates a lost opportunity for identifying suicide risk and preventing suicide (National Institute of Mental Health, 2006). Physicians and nurses must assess the elderly for depression and suicide risk. See Box 9-6 ■ for the Geriatric Depression Scale, a screening assessment tool for depression. The nurse should report to the physician clients who score as depressed on the Geriatric Depression Scale and refer them for further assessment.

A dangerous myth about suicide is that discussing it with someone who is not contemplating suicide may suggest the idea. In fact, most people with depression, whether they are contemplating suicide or not, benefit from talking about their feelings. For people who are contemplating suicide, discussion of their feelings may be the only opportunity for prevention. Depression makes it hard for people to identify and explain their own feelings. Talking about and clarifying these feelings can help a depressed person gain perspective, interrupt negative thinking, or work on problem solving. Active listening is a powerful tool for nurses to use. Clients often express gratitude for the opportunity to express their feelings about suicide (National Institute for Mental Health, 2006).

Only when the nurse is aware of a client's suicidal thinking, or **suicidal ideation,** can the nurse intervene to help the client. The nurse can assess the dangerousness of the client's suicidal thoughts. Fleeting thoughts such as "I feel so bad, I wish I were dead" are not as dangerous as "I have a gun at home, and as soon as I am discharged I plan to shoot myself."

Imagine yourself asking a client: "Do you ever think about hurting yourself or other people?" This is a hard question. It is socially inappropriate. It is just not polite to talk about suicide or to suggest that a person may be thinking about it. So, what should a nurse do?

Remember why you are here. This is not a social relationship. It is a professional one. The nurse is the professional. The nurse's goal is to assess the client's safety and to intervene to protect the client or others as necessary. It is difficult to ask people if they feel like hurting themselves or others, but if nurses do not ask, how will they provide appropriate care for the client?

Every client in the mental health setting should be asked specifically about suicidal and homicidal ideation as a part of a mental status assessment.

In the general medical setting every elderly client with a chronic illness and every client who has the risk factors for suicide listed in Box 9-4 should be asked: "Do

BOX 9-7	NURSING CARE CHECKLIST

Talking with a Client Who Feels Hopeless

☑ Use open-ended questions, or broad opening statements when asking the client to express feelings.

NURSE: "Tell me about how you are feeling."

CLIENT: "I feel bad."

☑ Clarify the client's message.

Nurse: "Can you give me some examples of how you feel bad?"

CLIENT: "I am a failure, I lost my job, I hate myself, and I am so tired of it all."

NURSE: "Do you mean that you are tired of living?"

CLIENT: "Yes."

☑ Make the implied message explicit. This is very important to do, even if it feels awkward.

NURSE: "Charlie, do you mean that you are thinking about killing yourself?"

CLIENT: "Well, yes. I think about it a lot."

☑ Clarify and gather data for assessment.

NURSE: "Do you have a plan?"

CLIENT: "I have a gun at home."

☑ Validate the importance of the client's feelings, give information about next steps, and assess the client's current safety.

NURSE: "Charlie, this is important. I will be talking with Dr. Rodgers and the other team members about your thoughts. We will work on a plan to help you. Are you thinking about hurting yourself here in the hospital?"

CLIENT: "No."

☑ Obtain a **no self-harm contract** (an agreement with the client to disclose suicidal feelings before taking action to hurt himself or herself).

NURSE: "We want you to be safe. Will you promise me that if you do think you want to hurt yourself while you are here, you will not hurt yourself, but tell me or anyone on the staff, so we can help you?"

CLIENT: "OK, I promise. I wish I wanted to live."

☑ Validate the client's importance, reassure the client that treatment can help, offer hope.

NURSE: "You are in the hospital so we can help you through times like this. There are effective treatments for depression, and we will not give up until you feel better. OK?"

CLIENT: "OK."

---

you feel like hurting yourself?" Add ". . . or other people" if the client has delusional or psychotic thinking.

In the process of therapeutic communication, or even in casual conversation, the nurse may learn that the client is feeling hopeless. Hope that depression will improve is what keeps many people from self-harm. Box 9-7 ■ provides a process recording of a nurse talking with a person who is feeling hopeless.

Critical Self-Check. What is the appropriate response by the nurse when the client says: "I feel like killing myself, but don't tell anybody. You are the only one I trust"?

COLLABORATIVE CARE

A good reason for hope is that effective treatment for depression is available. Once it is accurately identified, depression can almost always be treated successfully with medications, psychotherapy, or a combination of the two. Clients are individuals and respond to treatment differently, but as with schizophrenia, when a client does not respond to one therapy, there are others

to try. The goals of medical treatment for depression are (Stahl, 2005):

■ To achieve complete remission of depression symptoms
■ To prevent recurrence

There are five medical treatments for depression:

1. Medication
2. Psychotherapy
3. Combination of medication and psychotherapy
4. Electroconvulsive therapy (ECT)
5. Light therapy

Clients experience the best treatment outcomes when their depression is treated with a combination of medications and cognitive-behavioral therapy (CBT). Some clients with mild to moderate depression achieve success with psychotherapy alone. Figure 9-6 ■ shows a client in therapy.

Psychotropic Agents

Medications have been shown to be effective for all types of depression. However, there is no single medication that works for everyone. There is also no single medication that is better or more effective than the others.

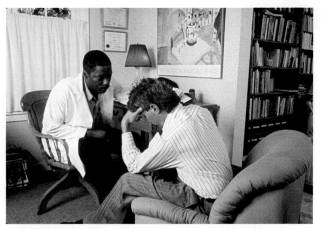

Figure 9-6. ■ The best treatment outcomes occur when clients combine medication and psychotherapy. *Source:* PhotoEdit Inc.

Although antidepressant medications have proved to be very effective, they do have limitations. People with depressive symptoms often wait until their symptoms are almost intolerable before they seek help. Then the antidepressants take 2 to 6 weeks to have their full effect. If the first medication is not effective for a client, the wait for effectiveness of a second or even third drug can seem endless. Some clients experience side effects that they are not willing to tolerate. Some people experience no improvement with antidepressant medications. Table 9-1 ■ provides a summary of medications that treat depression. Box 9-8 ■ lists the special considerations of antidepressant medications for the older adult.

The provider often chooses which antidepressant medication to prescribe based on the side effect profile or on which drug has been used effectively by a family member

TABLE 9-1

Antidepressant Agents

CLASSIFICATION/DRUG	ACTION AND USE	NURSING RESPONSIBILITIES	CLIENT TEACHING
Selective serotonin reuptake inhibitors (SSRIs) Citalopram (Celexa) Escitalopram (Lexapro) Fluoxetine (Prozac) Fluvoxamine (Luvox) Paroxetine (Paxil) Sertraline (Zoloft)	SSRIs ↑ 5-HT by blocking 5-HT reuptake in the presynaptic neuron. ↑s neurotransmission of 5-HT. Primarily used for depression, but also used for obsessive-compulsive disorder, panic disorder, social anxiety disorder, posttraumatic stress disorder (PTSD), generalized anxiety disorder, bulimia nervosa, and premenstrual dysphoric disorder.	Assess for SEs: sedation or agitation, headache, dizziness, tremors, sexual dysfunction (↓ libido, anorgasmia, erectile dysfunction, delayed ejaculation), GI effects (↓ appetite, nausea, diarrhea, constipation), dry mouth, bruising. These tend to be the first choice for treatment of depression in elderly, who require lower doses.	Some clients may experience relief of anxiety or insomnia early after starting therapy, but it usually takes 2–4 weeks for antidepressant effects. Most side effects go away with time.

Serotonin and norepinephrine reuptake inhibitors (SNRIs)
Duloxetine (Cymbalta)
Venlafaxine (Effexor)
	SNRIs ↑ 5-HT, NE, and DA. They block 5-HT and NE reuptake pumps, ↑ing their neurotransmission. They ↑ DA neurotransmission in frontal cortex, especially at higher doses.
	    Primarily used to treat depression. Also used for stress urinary incontinence, chronic and neuropathic pain, anxiety disorders.
		Assess for SEs: ↑ BP (dose dependent), insomnia, sedation, headache, nausea, decreased appetite, sweating, sexual dysfunction (↓ libido, impotence, abnormal orgasm), seizures (rare).	Therapeutic action takes 2–4 weeks. Most side effects go away with time.
			    Client should have regular BP monitoring.

Norepinephrine and dopamine reuptake inhibitor (NDRI)
Bupropion (Wellbutrin)
	↑s NE and DA, by blocking NE and DA reuptake, and increasing their neurotransmission.
	    Primarily used for depression and nicotine addiction, also used for bipolar depression, ADHD, and sexual dysfunction caused by other meds.
		Assess client for SEs: dry mouth, constipation, nausea, anorexia, sweating, tremor, insomnia, agitation, and headache. Rarely causes seizures (dose-related risk). Evaluate drug effectiveness.	Takes 2–4 weeks to achieve desired effects.
			    Teach client about constipation prevention. Most side effects go away with time.

TABLE 9-1			
Antidepressant Agents (continued)			
CLASSIFICATION/DRUG	**ACTION AND USE**	**NURSING RESPONSIBILITIES**	**CLIENT TEACHING**
Tetracyclic antidepressant, also called *noradrenergic-specific serotonergic antidepressant* **(NaSSA)** Mirtazapine (Remeron)	↑s 5-HT and NE by blocking presynaptic receptors, ↑ing neurotransmission of 5-HT and NE. Used for depression, also for panic disorder, anxiety, PTSD.	Assess for SEs: hypotension, dry mouth, constipation, ↑ appetite, weight gain, sedation, dizziness, abnormal dreams, confusion, flu-like symptoms, urinary retention, seizures (rare). SEs are dose dependent. Available in a form that dissolves on the tongue. Lower doses for elderly.	May begin to relieve insomnia and anxiety soon after starting therapy, but onset of antidepressant action usually takes 2–4 weeks. Teach client to rise slowly to reduce orthostatic hypotension. Teach constipation prevention.
Combined serotonin antagonists and reuptake inhibitors (SARIs) Trazodone (Desyrel) Nefazodone (Serzone)	↑s 5-HT by blocking reuptake in presynaptic neuron and by blocking serotonin 2A receptors. Used usually for insomnia and anxiety, can treat depression. Blocking of serotonin 2 also makes them effective against migraine headaches.	Assess for SEs: sedation, fatigue, dizziness, headache, lack of coordination, tremor, nausea, vomiting, edema, blurred vision, dry mouth, hypotension, syncope. Trazodone can cause *priapism* (painful prolonged penile erection). Nefazodone can rarely cause liver damage. Less likely to cause sexual SEs than the SSRIs. There is no development of tolerance to these drugs, so they can be used indefinitely for insomnia.	Teach client to rise slowly to reduce orthostatic hypotension. Teach constipation prevention.
Selective norepinephrine reuptake inhibitor (NRI) Reboxetine (Edronax)	↑s NE by blocking its reuptake. Can also ↑ DA in the frontal cortex. Used for depression, panic disorder, and ADHD.	Assess for SEs: anticholinergic effects, insomnia, anxiety, sexual dysfunction (impotence), hypotension (dose dependent).	Teach client to rise slowly to avoid orthostatic hypotension.
Tricyclic antidepressants (TCAs) Amitriptyline (Elavil) Amoxapine (Ascendin) Clomipramine (Anafranil) Desipramine (Norpramin) Doxepin (Sinequan) Imipramine (Tofranil) Maprotiline (Ludiomil) Nortriptyline (Pamelor) Protriptyline (Vivactil) Trimipramine (Surmontil)	TCAs ↑s NE and 5-HT activity by blocking the reuptake of norepinephrine and serotonin and also ↑s DA activity in frontal cortex. Used primarily for depression, often when the client's depression does not respond to drugs with fewer side effects. Also used for neuropathic and chronic pain, fibromyalgia, headache, low back and neck pain, anxiety, and insomnia.	Assess for SEs: as a group the TCAs tend to cause sedation, orthostatic hypotension, weight gain, and anticholinergic side effects. Can be cardiotoxic (especially Amitriptyline), especially in overdose. Avoid these meds in clients with suicidal thinking. Tell physician if client is pregnant, may change meds. Use with caution in elderly.	Onset of antidepressant action usually takes 2–4 weeks. Anxiety and insomnia may respond earlier than other depression symptoms. Teach client to rise slowly to reduce orthostatic hypotension risk. Teach constipation prevention.
Monoamine oxidase inhibitors (MAOIs) Isocarboxazid (Marplan) Phenelzine (Nardil)	↑s 5-HT, NE, and DA (which are monoamines) by stopping monoamine oxidase (an enzyme) from breaking them	Assess for critical side effect: hypertensive crisis, caused by interaction of MAOIs with tyramine-containing foods and	Client education about the many food and drug interactions that can cause hypertensive crisis with MAOIs is critical

(continued)

TABLE 9-1			
Antidepressant Agents (continued)			
CLASSIFICATION/DRUG	ACTION AND USE	NURSING RESPONSIBILITIES	CLIENT TEACHING
Tranylcypromine (Parnate) **Selective MAO-A Inhibitor** Moclobemide (Manerix) **Selective MAO-B Inhibitor** Selegiline (Emsam)	down so they stay longer in the synapse. Used for treatment-resistant depression, treatment-resistant panic disorder, and treatment-resistant social anxiety disorder. The newest MAOI, selegiline, is available in a transdermal form.	certain drugs (see text). Also assess for anticholinergic SEs, orthostatic hypotension, sedation, weight gain, sexual dysfunction, sleep disturbances, weakness, tremors. Moclobemide has a lower risk of hypertensive crisis, and selegiline does not require dietary restrictions at a low dose. They both cause anticholinergic SEs.	(see text). Clients unable to comply with these restrictions should not take MAOIs. Also teach client to rise slowly to avoid orthostatic hypotension.

Note: SEs = side effects, ↑ = increase, ↓ = decrease, 5-HT = serotonin, DA = dopamine, NE = norepinephrine.

BOX 9-8	

Antidepressants and the Older Adult

Older adults with depression tend to respond well to antidepressant drugs, but there are some special considerations for this group:

■ Due to less efficient metabolism, the elderly usually require **lower doses** of medications.

■ Elders are at increased risk for **orthostatic hypotension,** which increases their risk for falls and injury.

■ More severe anticholinergic effects, such as agitation, mental confusion, and paralytic ileus, may occur in older adults.

■ If older adults are **dehydrated,** they are at increased risk for medication side effects.

or the client in the past. In some situations, a drug may be chosen because its particular side effects might be useful. For example, an antidepressant with sedating effects can benefit a client who has trouble sleeping if it is taken at bedtime. Figure 9-7 ■ shows a diagram of neurotransmitters in depression and the action of antidepressant drugs.

With one exception antidepressants are only given orally. For the most part they act on two major brain neurotransmitters, serotonin (5-HT) and norepinephrine (NE), which regulate mood. A few new antidepressants have been developed to act on dopamine (DA) also.

TRICYCLIC AND RELATED AGENTS. The tricyclic antidepressants (TCAs) were the first-choice treatment for depression from the 1950s until the 1990s, when newer drugs with similar efficacy but fewer side effects were introduced. TCAs block the reuptake of serotonin and

norepinephrine, increasing the amount of these monoamine neurotransmitters in brain synapses.

A period of 2 to 4 weeks is required before TCAs and other antidepressants cause a significant relief of depression symptoms. This long lag time before the drug is effective is explained by the time required to cause a change in the receptors on postsynaptic neurons (Keltner, Schwecke, & Bostrom, 2007). The long wait for efficacy of antidepressants is also important because of the risk for suicide. Some people with depression have been unable to carry out their suicide plans until their antidepressant medications started to work. They probably felt increased energy before they experienced relief from the depression. This is not common, but nurses should assess for suicidal thinking in clients who are newly prescribed antidepressant drugs. It is this process that has given members of the public the mistaken idea that antidepressant medications can cause people to kill themselves.

clinical ALERT

It is important for nurses to know that clients with narrow-angle glaucoma may experience increased eye pressure due to mydriasis (excessive pupil dilation, an anticholinergic effect). The nurse should notify the physician of any mental health client's history of glaucoma.

The anticholinergic side effects tend to be the ones most often cited by consumers (clients) as the reason they quit taking TCA medications. Weight gain and sexual dysfunction are also reasons cited by clients for their noncompliance.

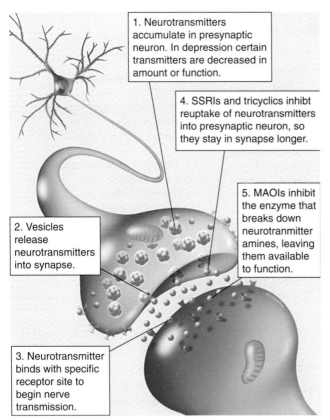

1. Neurotransmitters accumulate in presynaptic neuron. In depression certain transmitters are decreased in amount or function.

4. SSRIs and tricyclics inhibt reuptake of neurotransmitters into presynaptic neuron, so they stay in synapse longer.

5. MAOIs inhibit the enzyme that breaks down neurotranmitter amines, leaving them available to function.

2. Vesicles release neurotransmitters into synapse.

3. Neurotransmitter binds with specific receptor site to begin nerve transmission.

Figure 9-7. ■ Antidepressant agents increase the availability or function of neurotransmitters. *Source:* Phototake NYC.

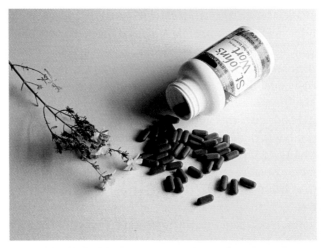

Figure 9-8. ■ St. John's wort, a natural remedy with antidepressant action. *Source:* Photo Researchers, Inc.

all antidepressants they do not cause euphoria or physical dependency.

Drug Interactions. The SSRIs are highly protein bound. As a result, they can increase the circulating levels of other protein-bound drugs that must compete for binding sites. TCA toxicity can result when SSRIs are given in combination with TCAs. When SSRIs are given with lithium, lithium levels increase (causing potential lithium toxicity). When SSRIs are combined with antipsychotics, EPS are increased. The SSRIs interact dangerously with MAOIs. The combination can cause serotonin syndrome.

Serotonin Syndrome. Serotonin syndrome can result from combining SSRIs with MAOIs, St. John's wort (an herbal antidepressant depicted in Figure 9-8 ■), or tryptophan (an amino acid in food that is a serotonin precursor). Serotonin syndrome appears to be related to excess serotonin activity. The signs and symptoms of serotonin syndrome include changes in mental status, agitation or restlessness, muscle spasms, hyperreflexia, diaphoresis, shivering, tremor, diarrhea, abdominal cramps, nausea, lack of coordination, and headache (Keltner et al., 2007).

clinical ALERT

The tricyclics can be fatal in overdose. Because suicide is a risk of depression, the healthcare team must consider the possibility of use of antidepressants as a method of suicide.

Overdose and Toxic Effects. Acutely suicidal clients should be hospitalized, and precautions should be taken for clients who are at risk. Currently, if a client has significant suicidal thinking, a history of suicide attempts, or impulse control problems, another class of antidepressant is usually prescribed.

SELECTIVE SEROTONIN REUPTAKE INHIBITORS (SSRIs). The SSRIs are usually the first-choice drugs for the treatment of depression because they have fewer side effects than the other types of antidepressants, with equal efficacy. The SSRIs act by inhibiting the reuptake of serotonin into the presynaptic neuron, thus increasing the amount of serotonin in brain synapses.

The SSRIs have a low potential for harm with overdose. They also have low potential for abuse, because like

clinical ALERT

Potentially fatal serotonin syndrome can result from combining SSRIs or TCAs with MAOI antidepressants. One drug must be cleared from the body before starting the other. A 2-week "washout" period should occur between the use of these two groups of drugs. If the nurse suspects serotonin syndrome, the SSRI should be held, and the physician notified immediately.

MONOAMINE OXIDASE INHIBITORS (MAOIs). The monoamine oxidase inhibitors (MAOIs) are effective antidepressant agents, but they are seldom prescribed because of their serious adverse effects. The MAOIs can cause potentially fatal drug interactions and hypertensive crisis. The MAOIs are usually prescribed for people who have not responded to other antidepressants and who can carefully comply with diet and drug restrictions.

The MAOIs act by inhibiting the breakdown of the monoamine neurotransmitters. They block the enzyme (monoamine oxidase) that breaks down neurotransmitters in brain synapses, causing increases in available serotonin, norepinephrine, and dopamine.

The MAOIs must be used with extreme caution because they can cause:

- Hypertensive crisis when combined with foods containing the amino acid tyramine
- Potentially fatal drug interactions with SSRIs, other MAOIs, TCAs, meperidine (Demerol), CNS depressants including general anesthetic agents, sympathomimetics (stimulants or decongestants such as over-the-counter cold, allergy, and weight loss remedies), methylphenidate (Ritalin), bronchodilators, and some antihypertensives
- Death in overdose

clinical ALERT

Symptoms of hypertensive crisis are a throbbing headache, sense of speeding or pounding heart, and stiff neck. If you suspect hypertensive crisis, don't administer the MAOI drug, take vital signs, and notify the physician. The treatment for hypertensive crisis is a single oral or sublingual dose of a calcium channel blocker.

Clients taking MAOIs must avoid foods high in tyramine. A list of high-tyramine foods is provided in Box 9-9 ■. Keep in mind that not all antidepressants cause these food and drug interactions. The nurse must recognize which type of antidepressant the client is taking. Client education is critical for people taking MAOI drugs.

A relatively new MAOI, moclobemide (Manerix), is a reversible selective inhibitor of MAO-A. It is shorter acting and it generally lacks the serious hypertensive side effects of the older, irreversible nonselective MAOIs, although combining it with an older MAOI can still cause hypertensive crisis. It does not require a low-tyramine diet. It should not be given with the older MAOIs or with narcotics (Stahl, 2005).

BOX 9-9

Foods to Avoid When Taking MAOIs

The following foods are high in tyramine and should be avoided by people taking MAOIs:

- Aged cheeses (all cheese is considered aged except cottage, cream, ricotta, and processed cheese slices)
- Foods containing aged cheeses, such as pizza or blue cheese dressing
- Preserved meats, such as pepperoni, sausage, salami, lunch meats, canned ham, pickled herring, dried fish
- Liver and other organ meats
- Broad fava beans, sauerkraut, and banana peel
- Draft beer (even alcohol-free), red wine
- Soy sauce, yeast, or protein extract (concentrated) products
- Although caffeine does not contain tyramine, large amounts of caffeine can cause a sympathomimetic effect; coffee, cola, and tea should be used only in moderation

---

The newest MAOI is selegiline (Emsam), which is a selective monoamine oxidase B (MAO-B) inhibitor. At recommended doses it selectively blocks MAO-B from breaking down dopamine. At higher doses it blocks both MAO-A and MAO-B from breaking down serotonin, norepinephrine, dopamine, and tyramine, which causes the risk of hypertensive crisis inherent in the other MAOIs. The transdermal patch form of selegiline was recently approved by the FDA. This is the first antidepressant available transdermally, or in anything other than an oral form. It is stated that the patch form does not cause a risk for hypertensive crisis at a low dose, and therefore does not require dietary restrictions (Stahl, 2005; Mayo Clinic, 2007).

Psychotherapy

Psychotherapy is usually used in addition to medication therapy for major depression. Some of the psychosocial problems associated with depression (ability to relate to others, motivation, problem-solving ability) can be resolved by medications. Psychotherapy may be used in addition to medications to help the client learn to live with a chronic depressive disorder, to manage the specific symptoms that plague the specific client, to promote effective coping skills, to change habitual negative thinking patterns, or for psychosocial rehabilitation. Some clients experiencing a mild to moderate depressive episode without psychotic symptoms may benefit from psychotherapy alone.

COGNITIVE THERAPY. Cognitive therapy is the most effective psychotherapeutic approach for depression. For depression, the objective of cognitive therapy is to reduce symptoms by identifying and correcting the client's distorted, negatively biased thinking (Beck & Rush, 2004). According to cognitive theory, depressed people have automatic negative thoughts even in the midst of positive life events. They have negative expectations of their environment, negative perceptions and expectations of self, and negative expectations for the future. Cognitive therapy approaches include identifying the client's erroneous negative thinking, and developing new thinking patterns. It is often combined with behavior therapy.

BEHAVIOR THERAPY.   Behavior therapy is often used along with cognitive therapy. The behavioral approach to therapy is based on learning theory. See Chapter 3 for a review of cognitive-behavioral and learning theories. The therapist and client work together to determine which behaviors to change. The client practices new ways to behave that are positive, replacing the old dysfunctional behavior. The principle in behavior therapy is that clients' thinking and feelings will follow their behavior. When people learn to act in a positive, self-confident way, they will feel positive and self-confident. Reinforcement of the client's successes will promote the persistence of positive effective behavior for coping.

INTERPERSONAL PSYCHOTHERAPY.   The interpersonal psychotherapy approach involves identifying and resolving the client's interpersonal difficulties. Interpersonal problems are viewed as causal or aggravating factors of depression. According to the interpersonal theorists, the difficulties that lead to depression may be social isolation, prolonged grief, or early development of dysfunctional social behavior. The treatment focus is interpersonal relationships and social functioning.

Exercise

Moderate physical exercise has been shown to relieve mild to moderate depressive symptoms. Exercise should be an adjunct to every other depression therapy if the client is able. The effects of exercise on depression may be due to the release of endorphins. The difficulty with exercise as a treatment for depression is that depressed people do not feel like exercising. Lack of energy and motivation are part of the disease. Exercise is best used as a preventive strategy. However, it is appropriate to teach clients that it is better to start exercising before they feel like it, rather than waiting until they feel like exercising. If clients can be motivated to exercise regularly, they are likely to feel much better.

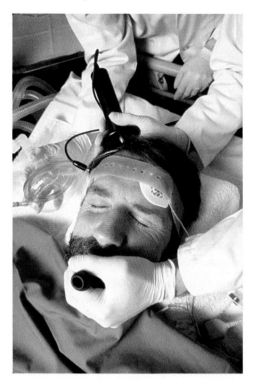

Figure 9-9. ■ A client prepared for electroconvulsive therapy (ECT). *Source:* Photo Researchers, Inc.

Electroconvulsive Therapy

Electroconvulsive therapy (ECT) is the application of electrical current to the brain, which induces a generalized seizure. The procedure is conducted while the client is under general anesthesia with muscle relaxation. The exact mechanism of action is not known, but ECT does increase circulating levels of brain neurotransmitters, which may be the way it relieves depression. Figure 9-9 ■ shows a client prepared for ECT.

ECT is not recommended for use as a first treatment for uncomplicated nonpsychotic major depression because less invasive treatments are available. It is used for clients who have intense, prolonged symptoms with marked disability, especially if the client has not responded to adequate trials with medications, or if psychotic features are present. ECT has been successful in inducing remission in people with severe psychomotor retardation. It may also be used for clients who cannot take medications or those at imminent risk of suicide or having dangerous delusions. Clients tend to respond more quickly to ECT than they do to medication therapy. Because of the history of misuse of ECT, there is a negative stigma associated with its use (Mendelowitz, Dawkins, & Lieberman, 2000).

The most common side effects of ECT are transient memory loss and mental confusion. The confusion usually resolves within 1 hour. The short-term memory loss may increase as the client has the series of treatments (usually three times per week for 2 to 6 weeks, depending on client response). Rare mortality associated with the procedure was due to myocardial infarction, stroke, or cardiac rhythm abnormalities. It should not be done on clients with increased intracranial pressure. Clients with cardiovascular disease should be treated and carefully assessed for the appropriateness of ECT. Approximately 50% of clients experience remission of depression after a series of ECT treatments (Rother, 2003).

Postprocedure nursing care for ECT includes the following (Rother, 2003):

- Take vital signs after the procedure
- Take frequent orthostatic blood pressures
- Provide frequent orientation and reassurance
- Document client's mental and physical status

Transcranial Magnetic Stimulation

Although it has not yet received approval for clinical use by the U.S. Food and Drug Administration (FDA), repetitive transcranial magnetic stimulation (TMS) is showing promise as a new therapy for treatment-resistant

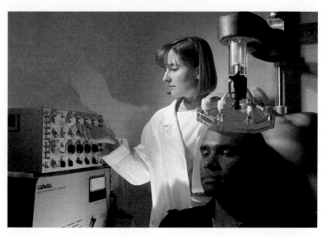

Figure 9-10. ■ Transcranial magnetic stimulation. *Source:* Photo Researchers, Inc.

depression. A series of magnetic impulses are applied to the left dorsolateral prefrontal cortex of the brain. Figure 9-10 ■ shows a client during the procedure. In one study, 30% of clients who received TMS had a positive response (improvement in depressive symptoms) and 20% experienced a remission of their depression. The study concluded that TMS can produce statistically significant antidepressant effects in clients with medication-resistant major depression (Avery et al., 2006).

BIPOLAR DISORDER

Definition of Bipolar Disorder

Bipolar disorder is our other prototype mood disorder. People with bipolar disorder, also called *manic-depressive disorder*, have experienced at least one manic episode (Box 9-10 ■ lists the diagnostic criteria) or one mixed mood episode (with rapid cycling of depression and mania in the same day). Often these individuals have also experienced one or more Major Depressive Episodes. **Bipolar** refers to the experience of both poles of mood: mania and depression.

CLINICAL FEATURES

The mood a client feels while in a manic episode may be described as elated, euphoric, high, or unusually good. The mood is characterized by constant and indiscriminate enthusiasm. Frequently the person alternates between elation and irritability. An affected person may play basketball enthusiastically for 24 hours, becoming angry when someone tries to take the ball. He or she may go on an extended shopping spree, buying gifts for everyone

on credit, or gamble away an entire paycheck (see Figure 9-11 ■). The flurry of activity seems productive to the client, but can be really disorganized and unproductive.

Grandiose delusions are common. The client may believe that he is a famous musician or a successful novelist, without having any skill at music or writing. The client may feel qualified to give advice on any subject, such as how to conduct brain surgery or send a rocket to Mars. The client may believe that s/he is a superhero.

People in mania almost always have a decreased need for sleep. They may awaken several hours earlier than usual, feeling alert and energetic. When mania is severe, the affected person may go for days with no sleep and not feel tired (American Psychiatric Association, 2000).

Manic speech is rapid and **pressured speech,** which means that it is so fast and determined that it is hard to interrupt. The person's expressions may be dramatic or may be related to sounds more than words, such as in clang association. The following is an example of *clang association*:

BOX 9-10

DSM-IV-TR Criteria for Manic Episode

A. A distinct period of abnormally and persistently elevated, expansive, or irritable mood, lasting at least 1 week (or any duration if hospitalization is necessary).

B. During the period of mood disturbance, three (or more) of the following symptoms have persisted (four if the mood is only irritable) and have been present to a significant degree:

1. inflated self-esteem or **grandiosity**
2. **decreased need for sleep** (e.g., rested after only 3 hours of sleep)
3. **more talkative** than usual or pressure to keep talking
4. **flight of ideas** or subjective experience that thoughts are racing
5. **distractibility** (i.e., attention too easily drawn to unimportant or irrelevant external stimuli)
6. increase in **goal-directed activity** (either socially, at work or school, or sexually) or psychomotor agitation

7. **excessive involvement in pleasurable activities** that have a high **potential for painful consequences** (e.g., engaging in unrestrained buying sprees, sexual indiscretions, or foolish business investments)

C. The mood disturbance is sufficiently severe to cause marked impairment in occupational functioning or in usual social activities or relationships with others, or to necessitate hospitalization to prevent harm to self or others, or there are psychotic features.

D. The symptoms are not due to the direct physiological effects of a substance (e.g., a drug of abuse, a medication, or other treatment) or a general medical condition (e.g., hyperthyroidism).

Source: Reprinted with permission from the *Diagnostic and Statistical Manual of Mental Disorders, Text Revision,* copyright 2000. American Psychiatric Association.

Figure 9-11. ■ During a manic episode, a client has grandiose thoughts, poor judgment, and poor impulse control. These may result in risking a whole paycheck on lottery tickets. *Source:* AP Wide World Photos.

"I went to the store, tell me more, open the door, I like to eat cake, may I have a rake?" If irritability is present, the person may make long speeches about angry subjects, such as why anyone would ever want to do nursing care plans. Rapid speech reflects rapid thinking. The person's thinking may be going so fast that the thoughts are disorganized and incoherent. Box 9-11 ■ describes bipolar disorder in the words of people who experience it.

The affected person is likely to be easily distractible. **Distractibility** is evidenced by an inability to screen out excess sensory stimuli. The person may not be able to distinguish which thoughts are pertinent to the situation

BOX 9-11

Reality Check on Bipolar Disorder

These are statements by people with bipolar disorder:

■ "Yes, I am feeling better. I am a CEO. Did you know that I put grocery departments in Sears? You and your family can join all the clients here for free groceries. I will also have free medications for everybody who needs them. Just go to any Sears and mention my name. They'll give you some new clothes for work."

■ "I think faster and faster. Sometimes the thoughts fly so fast I can't keep up with them and I am lost in the confusion."

■ "I am not crazy, and I do not require the meds that are so important to you. The side effects are unbearable; the trembling in my hands makes me unable to play the piano; I feel like my intelligence is dampened. Would you put up with that?"

■ "You know, I really am a smart person. Intellectually it is logical to take my meds, but they make me feel stupid and slow-thinking. I have had three divorces and lost my house because of gambling. I don't care to remember how many jobs I've lost. My family doesn't speak to me any more. I wonder if I should take the meds, but I don't want them. I think I should be able to control myself without them."

■ "Believe me; I have tried every drug I can find. Nothing feels so good as the natural high I get. I am smarter, stronger, quicker, happier, more alive, everything. When I get depressed, I think nothing can feel as bad as that. It is not like being alive. My life is a roller coaster, only more so."

and which are not. Manic clients may be distracted from a conversation by someone's clothing, colors, sounds, or even furnishings in the room (American Psychiatric Association, 2000).

Excess goal-directed activity may involve planning and doing multiple activities, such as having sexual encounters with multiple partners, producing great volumes of work that later turn out to be confusing, or getting involved in multiple financial dealings. Affected people may hold several conversations at the same time, in person and on the phone. They may start many different projects without being able to finish them (American Psychiatric Association, 2000).

Unwarranted optimism, grandiosity, and poor judgment characterize behavior in mania. Clients may spend an entire paycheck on lottery tickets, gamble, drive recklessly, and engage in unsafe sexual behavior ignoring possible painful consequences. Affected people may spend money they do not have, participate in illegal activities that have serious penalties, or hurt themselves or others in the moment without foreseeing future consequences (American Psychiatric Association, 2000).

What may look like an exciting experience at the beginning can be devastating to affected people and their families (see Box 9-11). Manic episodes impair affected individuals' ability to function and may threaten their lives. Excess energy expenditure without adequate rest can lead to exhaustion. Often during a manic episode, people will be too busy to eat, thus decreasing their energy supply even more. Figure 9-12 ■ shows the characteristics of a manic episode.

Critical Self-Check. What can a nurse say in response to a client with mania who says: "I have never felt so great! Why do you think I should take drugs to make this feeling go away?"

People in a manic episode frequently lack insight about their illness and its effects on themselves and others. They often resist treatment. Sometimes involuntary hospitalization is necessary to protect clients from their own behavior. Involuntary hospitalization is indicated when a person is dangerous to self or others.

CAUSE OF THE DISORDER

Like Major Depressive Disorder, Bipolar I Disorder has a tendency to recur in families. There is evidence of a genetic etiology, but not of a single gene inheritance. First-degree biological relatives of a person with bipolar disorder have a 4–24% chance of having the disease, the same recurrence rate as depression. Any given manic episode is likely to follow a stressor. Disordered sleep (such as experienced when traveling across time zones or working the night shift) may be a trigger (American Psychiatric Association, 2000).

The brain neurotransmitters norepinephrine and dopamine are implicated in the cause of manic episodes. The same monoamine neurotransmitters whose decreased activity is implicated in depression are increased in mania. Hormones also interact with neurotransmitters in mood disorders. Hypothyroidism is correlated with depression and with rapid cycling of mood between depression and mania.

Mania is considered to be a biological condition. Psychosocial factors are more important in the timing of

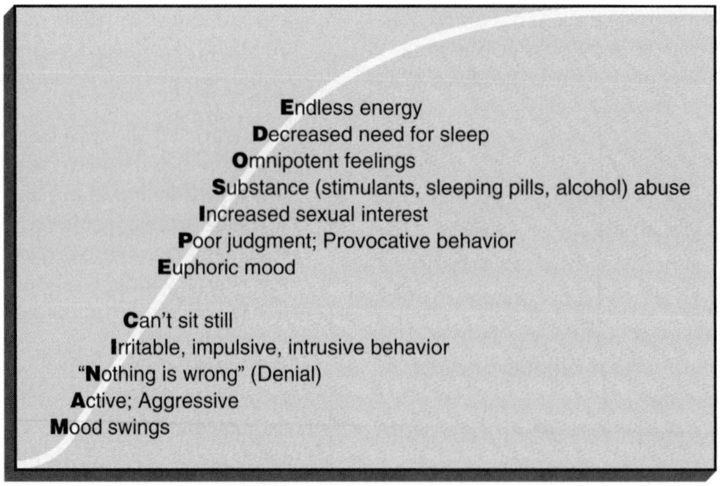

Endless energy
Decreased need for sleep
Omnipotent feelings
Substance (stimulants, sleeping pills, alcohol) abuse
Increased sexual interest
Poor judgment; Provocative behavior
Euphoric mood

Can't sit still
Irritable, impulsive, intrusive behavior
"**N**othing is wrong" (Denial)
Active; Aggressive
Mood swings

Figure 9-12. ■ Characteristics of a manic episode. *Source: Contemporary Psychiatric Mental Health Nursing* by Kneisl/Wilson/Trigoboff, © Reprinted by permission of Pearson Education, Inc., Upper Saddle River, NJ.

manic episodes than in their cause. Stressful events may precede manic episodes.

The person with bipolar disorder will probably be taking a mood-stabilizing drug, which prevents and treats the manic aspect of the disorder. In addition to the mood stabilizer, an antidepressant is often prescribed, often in lower doses than for people who have depression alone. The dose is kept low because antidepressant medications can trigger a manic episode in a person with bipolar disorder.

COURSE OF THE DISORDER

The average age of onset of a first manic episode is in the early 20s. It affects women and men equally. More than 90% of all individuals who have one manic episode will go on to have more. The exact pattern of recurrence is individual, but without treatment the average rate of manic episodes is four in 10 years. A few individuals have more rapid cycling (four or more episodes per year). Most clients have more depressive episodes than manic episodes over time.

Some children show a history of behavior problems before their first actual manic episode. Like depressive episodes, manic episodes tend to occur following psychosocial stressors. The episodes usually begin suddenly and last from a few weeks to several months. Manic episodes are briefer and end more abruptly than depressive episodes. Fifty to 70% of the time, a major depressive episode will come immediately before or after a manic episode. When a manic episode is accompanied by psychosis (hallucinations and delusions) it is more serious and more likely to lead to aggression or suicide (American Psychiatric Association, 2000).

CONCURRENT DISORDERS

Disorders of substance abuse occur commonly with bipolar disorder. People with substance use disorders that have bipolar disorder tend to experience more rapid cycling between mania and depression and have more *dysphoric* (unpleasant, unhappy) feelings in the manic phase (Sonne & Brady, 1999).

COLLABORATIVE CARE

In the acute phase of a manic episode the treatment priorities are ensuring client safety and treating the mood disorder. Medication continues to be the mainstay of treatment for bipolar disorder.

As the focus of mental health treatment moves from disease management to promotion of recovery, the attitude toward treatment of bipolar disorder is changing. Formerly, management of the acute phases of depression or mania was the priority, or for some clients their only treatment. Currently, clinicians are using a more comprehensive approach that includes more client education, pays more attention to psychotherapy while clients are in remission, and expects clients to take a more active role in their treatment and recovery.

Psychotropic Agents

The desired treatment outcomes for clients with bipolar disorder are to:

- Eliminate the symptoms of the mood episode (either depression or mania)
- Stabilize the mood to prevent cycling between depression and mania and cause complete remission of symptoms
- Improve the client's self-care ability, function, and quality of life

The classes of drugs used to treat manic episodes are mood stabilizers (antimanic agents), anticonvulsants (which act as mood stabilizers), benzodiazepines (to decrease anxiety and agitation while the other drugs are starting to work), and antipsychotics (if the client has psychotic symptoms). This chapter focuses on the mood-stabilizing or antimanic agents. Table 9-2 ■ provides the specifics about these agents (Stahl, 2005).

LITHIUM.   Lithium, a naturally occurring element, is the classic mood-stabilizing drug. It is a first-line treatment for acute mania due to bipolar disorder and for long-term prevention of recurrent episodes. Target symptoms of mania include irritability, euphoria, pressured speech, flight of ideas, motor hyperactivity, aggressive behavior, grandiosity, delusions, impulsiveness, and hallucinations. The target symptoms of depression include sadness, anhedonia, guilt, worthlessness, slowed thinking and movement, helplessness, hopelessness, suicidal thinking, and sleep disturbances. The symptoms of bipolar depression are the same as those of major depressive disorder. Sometimes a client with depression is given an antidepressant and is thrust into a manic episode because the healthcare provider did not realize that the client had bipolar disorder. A thorough client history is important in mental health.

Before a client starts on lithium therapy, a full history and physical exam should be done. Lithium is excreted by the kidneys and can have toxic effects on renal function. It inhibits several steps in thyroid hormone synthesis and metabolism, so thyroid function should be assessed. Lithium has a narrow therapeutic index, and toxicity is close to therapeutic blood levels. Blood lithium levels should be drawn 12 hours after the last lithium dose, for the "trough" or lowest level of lithium in the blood.

Lithium is a salt. Because of this, the sodium and fluid balance of the body affect lithium levels. If the kidneys

TABLE 9-2

Mood Stabilizers/Antimanic Agents

CLASSIFICATION/DRUG	ACTION/USE	NURSING RESPONSIBILITIES	CLIENT TEACHING
Mood Stabilizers Lithium (Eskalith, Lithobid)	Action is unknown and complex. Lithium alters sodium transport across cell membranes in nerve and muscle cells and alters metabolism of neurotransmitters including epinephrine, NE, and 5-HT. It is a first-line drug for treating manic episodes and as maintenance (preventive) treatment for people with bipolar disorder to stabilize mood (decreasing episodes of both mania and depression). It tends to work better for preventing manic than depressive episodes. Most people with bipolar disorder need more than one medication to maintain remission.	Before starting treatment, client should have baseline kidney and thyroid function tests and an EKG if client is over 50. Kidney and thyroid function should be monitored throughout treatment. Monitor for potentially fatal SEs: renal impairment, cardiac dysrhythmias, nephrogenic diabetes insipidus, and lithium toxicity. Toxicity Sx include coarse tremors, ataxia, diarrhea, vomiting, sedation, slurred speech, hypotension, irregular pulse. DC immediately for signs of toxicity. Check therapeutic blood levels as "trough" levels about 12 hrs. after the last dose. Other SEs: weight gain, sedation, fine hand tremor, nausea, acne, rash, alopecia (hair loss), memory problems, subjective feeling of mental dullness, leukocytosis. SEs tend to ↑ with ↑ blood levels. Lower doses for elderly.	It takes 1–3 weeks for lithium to have a therapeutic effect. Benzodiazepines may be used to treat manic symptoms until lithium efficacy is achieved. Rapid discontinuation of lithium ↑s the risk of a relapse. Taper off over 3 months. For stomach upset, take with food. For fine hand tremor, avoid caffeine. Drugs that can ↑ lithium levels and ↑ risk of toxicity: NSAIDs, ACE-Inhibitors, some diuretics, calcium channel blockers, phenytoin, carbamazepine, and metronidazole. Notify all your physicians that you are taking lithium to avoid these drug interactions. Dehydration ↑s risk of toxicity. Lithium should generally be discontinued before planned pregnancies (risk category D).
Anticonvulsant (for multiple seizure types), mood stabilizer, migraine prophylaxis, voltage-sensitive sodium channel modulator Valproate has several brands, but the only one used for mania is Divalproex sodium (Depakote ER)	Blocks voltage-sensitive sodium channels in CNS, increases brain concentrations of gamma-aminobutyric acid (GABA). It is especially effective for rapidly cycling bipolar disorder, for mania caused by a general medical condition, and for mixed episodes, a condition of frequently alternating manic and depressive symptoms.	Clients should have liver function tests before starting valproate because rarely it can be liver toxic. Monitor liver function and platelet count during therapy. Contraindicated in clients who already have advanced liver disease. Assess for SEs: sedation, tremor, dizziness, ataxia, headache, abdominal pain, nausea, constipation, weight gain (frequent), alopecia (rare), pancreatitis (rare), thrombocytopenia (with high doses). Lower doses for elderly.	For acute mania, efficacy occurs in a few days, but mood stabilization takes several weeks to months. Take at bedtime to reduce sedation during the day. Should not be stopped abruptly. Rapid discontinuation can trigger relapse. Taper slowly. Pregnancy risk category D: positive evidence of risk to human fetus.
Anticonvulsant, voltage-sensitive sodium channel antagonist carbamazepine (Tegretol) (Equetro=extended release version)	Blocks voltage-sensitive sodium channels, inhibits the release of glutamate. Used to treat seizures, trigeminal neuralgia pain, as a second-line augmenting agent for bipolar disorder, and as an adjunctive treatment for psychosis in schizophrenia. Used as a second- or third-line treatment for mania.	Before therapy begins, and during therapy, clients should have blood count, liver, kidney, and thyroid function tests. Assess for SEs: sedation (common), dizziness, headache, nausea, vomiting, diarrhea, blurred vision, rash. Rarely causes bone marrow suppression: agranulocytosis (↓ in WBCs) or aplastic anemia. Rare severe skin reactions (Stevens-Johnson syndrome).	Takes a few weeks for efficacy in acute mania. Can decrease blood levels (and effectiveness) of hormone contraceptives. Teach client to report unusual bruising or bleeding (signs of clotting disorder). Pregnancy risk category D: positive evidence of risk to human fetus.

TABLE 9.2

Mood Stabilizers/Antimanic Agent (continued)

CLASSIFICATION/DRUG	ACTION/USE	NURSING RESPONSIBILITIES	CLIENT TEACHING
	Equetro is used for the treatment of acute mania and mixed episodes.		
Anticonvulsant, mood stabilizer, voltage-sensitive sodium channel antagonist Lamotrigine (Lamictal)	Blocks voltage-sensitive sodium channels (stabilizing cell membranes), and inhibits the release of glutamate. Used to treat seizures and bipolar disorder. Appears to be more effective at treating the depressive symptoms than the manic ones. Truly stabilizes mood: prevents both manic and depressive episodes. Used in combination with lithium and atypical antipsychotics in acute mania. One of the best tolerated mood stabilizers.	Valproate ↑s lamotrigine levels. When they are used together, lamotrigine dose should be ↓d by half. Assess for SEs: blurred vision, sedation, dizziness, ataxia, headache, fatigue, tremor, insomnia, nausea, vomiting, abdominal pain, constipation, can cause benign or serious rash. The risk of this serious skin reaction (Stevens-Johnson syndrome) is greater if the client is also taking divalproex or if lamotrigine is being started with rapidly increasing doses. Rarely causes dyscrasias (blood formation abnormalities).	Takes several weeks to improve bipolar disorder. Teach client to report development of rash. Pregnancy risk category C.

Note: SEs = side effects, Sx = symptoms, ↑ = increase, ↓ = decrease, 5-HT = serotonin, NE = norepinephrine.

are conserving sodium (like they do when the client is dehydrated) lithium is also conserved, and the client may develop toxic lithium levels.

Treatment Compliance. Compliance with lithium therapy is an important issue. Clients sometimes find the side effects of the drug to be intolerable. There is a relatively high dropout rate for people on lithium therapy. Tolerability of treatment is especially important in bipolar disorder. People with bipolar disorder tend to be high functioning between episodes. They are often reluctant to take a medication that makes them feel sedated because they expect to live full occupational and social lives.

Trials of several drug combinations may be required before the most effective and agreeable treatment plan for an individual is found. It is no longer necessary for the treatment team to encourage a client to endure intolerable discomfort in exchange for prevention of mania (Bowden, 2003).

Client Education. Part of client education about lithium therapy is how to maintain consistent lithium and sodium levels. This is achieved with consistent hydration levels. For example, if a person taking lithium played basketball for hours, losing sodium through perspiration, he would be at risk for lithium toxicity unless he replaced the lost sodium, maybe with a sports drink or a salty snack. He would also need to replace the water lost during exercise by drinking at intervals during the basketball game (remember: dehydration can cause lithium toxicity). The management of lithium therapy is difficult and can be a challenge for clients.

For the client to have the best possible outcomes, the nurse must ensure that the client understands and participates in the treatment plan. Lifestyle changes are necessary to maintain lithium/fluid and electrolyte balance and to prevent toxicity. People taking lithium require ongoing psychotherapeutic support.

ANTICONVULSANT MOOD STABILIZERS. Some anticonvulsants have proved to be clinically effective both in treating the symptoms of mania and in preventing recurrence of episodes. The anticonvulsant valproate (Depakote) is endorsed as a first-line drug for mood stabilizing in bipolar disorder. It is used alone or in combination with lithium, or atypical antipsychotic agents, to meet individual client needs (Stoner & Dubisar, 2006).

clinical ALERT

Valproate has been known to cause fetal anomalies and should not be taken by clients during pregnancy or by those who are planning to become pregnant.

Carbamazepine (Tegretol) is another anticonvulsant proven effective for the treatment of bipolar disorder. Carbamazepine is used for clients who do not respond to lithium or valproate. Carbamazepine can cause bone-marrow suppression with decrease in red and white blood cell formation. Clients need regular blood cell counts while taking this drug. CBC, platelet, and liver function tests should be done every 2 weeks for the first 2 months of treatment and then every 3 months thereafter (Stoner & Dubisar, 2006). Use of carbamazepine for bipolar disorder may be declining due to the emergence of anticonvulsants with better documentation of efficacy and improved tolerability in bipolar disorder (Stahl, 2005).

Lamotrigine (Lamictal) is also used as a mood stabilizer in conjunction with other standard drug therapy such as divalproex, carbamazepine, lithium, or an atypical antipsychotic. It acts by stabilizing nerve cell membranes and inhibiting neurotransmitter release. It is generally well tolerated by clients, but has approximately 1% risk of rash development, which may be a benign self-limiting rash or Stevens-Johnson syndrome, a potentially fatal skin reaction involving the skin and mucous membranes. Skin loss can lead to infections, fevers, dehydration, and even death.

Although the previously mentioned medications are used for treating the mania component of bipolar disorder and for maintenance therapy, there is another medication approved specifically for the depression associated with the disorder. Symbyax is a combination of olanzapine, an atypical antipsychotic drug, and fluoxetine, an antidepressant. It acts on the neurotransmitters of dopamine, norepinephrine, and serotonin, although its exact mechanism of action is unknown. Common side effects are drowsiness, diarrhea, weight gain, and dry mouth (Stoner & Dubisar, 2006).

Psychotherapy

Although bipolar disorder has a largely physiologic etiology, psychosocial therapy is still valuable. Living with bipolar disorder is challenging. At some point in a manic episode, clients may feel so wonderful that taking medications to stop it seems absurd. They may lack the insight to connect untreated mania with its many negative outcomes. Compliance with medication therapy is challenging and often a problem for these clients. But the mania will be a relatively brief time, and the rest of the time the client is living with the consequences.

Psychotherapy, in any of the same styles described under depression, can be a valuable tool to help clients with bipolar disorder. It can assist clients to learn about their disorder, learn to manage and live with it, discuss and organize their feelings about having a chronic mental illness, discuss the dilemma of treatment, and work on development of insight into the real consequences of untreated bipolar disorder.

Group Therapy

When the acute phase of mania or depression has passed, client outcomes shift to coping with the disorder over the long term. Group therapy can be very valuable toward the goal of living with a chronic mental illness (or any chronic illness). The therapy or support group is composed of people who all experience the same chronic mental illness. There may or may not be a mental health professional group facilitator.

The group discusses topics relevant to managing and coping with the disorder. For example, one session may be about dealing with medication side effects. Another may be on what to do if a client is unable to work. A third may be on how to respond to family members. People who have actually lived through these challenges may share with the group what they have learned from their experiences. The newly diagnosed member receives valuable advice from real experts on how to cope. The more experienced members receive the benefit of being able to help others, and the validation that comes from being knowledgeable. Local affiliates of the National Alliance for the Mentally Ill have support groups for clients and their families.

NURSING CARE

ASSESSING

Mood is reflected in the client's behavior and speech. When a client has a mood disorder, it is good to do a mental status assessment (described in Chapter 8) on admission to provide baseline information. Then briefer assessments can be made of pertinent parts of mental status, and then compared to the original assessment to document client progress. It is also the responsibility of the nurse to assess the client's response to drug therapy for any mood disorder.

Most cases of depression are not diagnosed or treated. Nurses in every area of specialty work with depressed people. It makes sense for nurses to routinely do screening assessments for depression. The Geriatric Depression Scale (see Box 9-6) was mentioned earlier in this chapter and is used for the elderly. The Beck Depression Inventory, short form (Table 9-3 ■) can be used to identify adults who are

TABLE 9-3

Beck Depression Inventory, Short Form

Instructions: This is a questionnaire. On the questionnaire are groups of statements. Please read the entire group of statements in each category. Then pick out one statement in that group that best describes the way you feel today, that is, right now! *Circle the number beside the statement you have chosen. If several statements in the group seem to apply equally well, circle each one.* Be sure to read all the statements in each group before making your choice.

A. (Sadness)
   3 I am so sad or unhappy that I can't stand it.
   2 I am blue or sad all the time and I can't snap out of it.
   1 I feel sad or blue.
   0 I do not feel sad.

B. (Pessimism)
   3 I feel that the future is hopeless and that things cannot improve.
   2 I feel I have nothing to look forward to.
   1 I feel discouraged about the future.
   0 I am not particularly pessimistic or discouraged about the future.

C. (Sense of failure)
   3 I feel I am a complete failure as a person (parent, husband, wife).
   2 As I look back on my life, all I can see is a lot of failures.
   1 I feel I have failed more than the average person.
   0 I do not feel like a failure.

D. (Dissatisfaction)
   3 I am dissatisfied with everything.
   2 I do not get satisfaction out of anything anymore.
   1 I do not enjoy things the way I used to.
   0 I am not particularly dissatisfied.

E. (Guilt)
   3 I feel as though I am very bad or worthless.
   2 I feel quite guilty.
   1 I feel bad or unworthy a good part of the time.
   0 I don't feel disappointed in myself.

F. (Self-dislike)
   3 I hate myself.
   2 I am disgusted with myself.
   1 I am disappointed in myself.
   0 I don't feel disappointed in myself.

G. (Self-harm)
   3 I would kill myself if I had the chance.
   2 I have definite plans about committing suicide.
   1 I feel I would be better off dead.
   0 I don't have any thought of harming myself.

H. (Social withdrawal)
   3 I have lost all of my interest in other people and don't care about them at all.
   2 I have lost most of my interest in other people and have little feeling for them.
   1 I am less interested in other people than I used to be.
   0 I have not lost interest in other people.

I. (Indecisiveness)
   3 I can't make any decisions at all anymore.
   2 I have great difficulty in making decisions.
   1 I try to put off making decisions.
   0 I make decisions about as well as ever.

J. (Self-image change)
   3 I feel that I am ugly or repulsive-looking.
   2 I feel that there are permanent changes in my appearance and they make me look unattractive.
   1 I am worried that I am looking old or unattractive.
   0 I do not feel that I look any worse than I used to.

K. (Work difficulty)
   3 I can't do any work at all.
   2 I have to push myself very hard to do anything.
   1 It takes extra effort to get started at doing something.
   0 I can work about as well as before.

L. (Fatigability)
   3 I get too tired to do anything.
   2 I get tired from doing anything.
   1 I get tired more easily than I used to.
   0 I don't get any more tired than usual.

M. (Anorexia)
   3 I have no appetite at all anymore.
   2 My appetite is much worse now.
   1 My appetite is not as good as it used to be.
   0 My appetite is no worse than usual.

Scoring: 0–4 = None or mild depression.   5–7 = Mild depression.
            8–15 = Moderate depression.   16 + = Severe depression.

Source: Beck, A. T., Ward, C. H., Mendelson, M., et al. (1961). An inventory for measuring depression. *Archives of General Psychiatry, 4,* 561–571. Copyright 1961. American Medical Association.

BOX 9-13 CULTURAL PULSE POINTS

Is Depression the Same Everywhere?

The answer to the above question is *yes* and *no*. People from all over the world suffer from depression. According to the World Health Organization (2007), there is a worldwide epidemic of it. People from various cultures tend to respond to antidepressant medications. However, the signs and symptoms of depression vary from one culture and even subculture to another. Nurses must be aware of this in order to make accurate assessments and interpretations of client symptoms. African Americans, Asian Americans, and Latinos tend to experience more physical symptoms, such as headache, abdominal pain, and body aches than European American clients do (European Americans may have physical symptoms also). European Americans are more likely to describe psychological symptoms, such as sadness and guilt feelings. When clients from these cultures have symptoms that are not explained by medical tests, depression should be considered.

likely to be depressed. The client's cultural background is another important aspect of assessment. The Cultural Pulse Points Box 9-13 ■ discusses the relationship between culture and symptoms of depression.

In a depressed client, suicidal thinking must be assessed. The nurse can assess suicidal ideation as follows:

1. Start with an assessment of whether the person has suicidal ideation (thinking): "Are you thinking about hurting yourself?" Or "Do you think about killing yourself?"
2. If clients have suicidal ideation, determine if they have organized their thoughts about it enough to have a plan: "Do you have a plan?"
3. Assess lethality of the plan: "What is your plan?" or "How would you do it?" (more serious if planned means is firearm or hanging).
4. Assess if the client has access to the planned means of suicide: "Do you have access to a gun? drugs?" (the means in the client's plan).
5. **Inform the treatment team.** Failure to report suicidal ideation constitutes breach of the nurse's legal duty to protect the client.

Mental Status

Client Self-Assessment

One way to monitor a client's mood over time is to use a mood scale. Ask the client, "Please rate your mood on a scale of 1–10, where 1 is the lowest and 10 is the best possible mood." Although the numbers themselves do not have real measurement value, the client's perception of how s/he feels may be quantified in this way. The nurse can compare the numbers to see if the client is feeling better or worse. The mood assessment is done at least once per shift and documented in the nurses' notes.

Appearance and Affect

Other aspects of mental status that are pertinent to a person with a mood disorder are appearance, affect (nonverbal expression of mood), behavior, motor activity, and thought processes. The appearance of a person with depression may be disheveled, if s/he does not have the energy to bathe and change clothes. Mania may be expressed with flashy, bright clothing and outrageous makeup and jewelry.

Normal affect is called *broad*, meaning that the client can express a broad range of emotions from happiness to sadness. A person with depression cannot usually express the full range of emotions. Depression limits emotions (affect) to sadness. This finding is expressed as "blunted or restricted affect" (blunted affect is more limited than restricted affect). Emotions in mania may be restricted to excitement, elation, rage, or irritability.

Psychomotor Activity

Psychomotor activity would be slow in depression and agitated in mania. The depressed client may have psychomotor retardation and may lie in bed all day, or sit moving very little. The manic person may be so active that s/he is in danger of exhaustion.

Documenting Findings

The nurse's assessment should be documented as specifically as possible. It is more clear when the nurse documents the findings that led to a conclusion rather than stating the conclusion only. Charting "agitated" is not as clear as "Client has been pacing up and down the halls all night, except when he washed the windows and floors in the lounge with a paper towel, and ran-in-place near the nurses' station for 30 minutes. He has blisters on the soles of his feet and states that he is fine, not tired, and is ready to run a marathon."

Thought Processes

Clients' thought processes also demonstrate how they are affected by mood disorders and how they are responding to treatment. Everyone has occasional thought blocking, in which it is difficult to think of a word that you intended to say. However, thought blocking is very common and more severe in . . . uh . . . wait a minute . . . uh . . . umm . . . depression.

Flight of ideas, in which thoughts are moving so fast that the client's speech jumps from one subject to another frequently, is common in mania. Grandiosity is also common in mania. "I am the world's most famous author, and I will be glad to write my next book about you, if you will give me a candy bar" is a grandiose statement that would more likely be used by a person in mania than one in depression.

Thought processes might include psychotic features in either severe depression or severe mania. The content in depressive delusions or hallucinations would likely be frightening, persecutory, or very negative ("My boss hates me and wants to kill me."). In mania, delusions or hallucinations would be expansive and fantastic, such as "I will fly on over to my department store to pick up a new TV. No need for a plane."

The nurse also assesses and documents any side effects from psychotropic medications. Review the section on Psychotropic Agents for side effects of drugs used for mood disorders.

DIAGNOSING, PLANNING, AND IMPLEMENTING

Common nursing diagnoses for clients with either depressive disorder or bipolar disorder include:

- Risk for Violence (self-directed with major depressive disorder, self- or other-directed with bipolar disorder)
- Impaired Social Interaction
- Imbalanced Nutrition

Hopelessness, Powerlessness, Chronic Low Self-Esteem, and Self-Care Deficit are common among people with depression. Disturbed Thought Processes is a common nursing diagnosis for clients with bipolar disorder.

The desired outcomes for clients with psychiatric disorders are found in four categories: thinking (cognition), feeling (mood), physiology, and behavior (acting or coping). Figure 9-13 ■ shows a diagram of desired outcomes for clients with mood disorders. These outcomes are used as appropriate for the individual client.

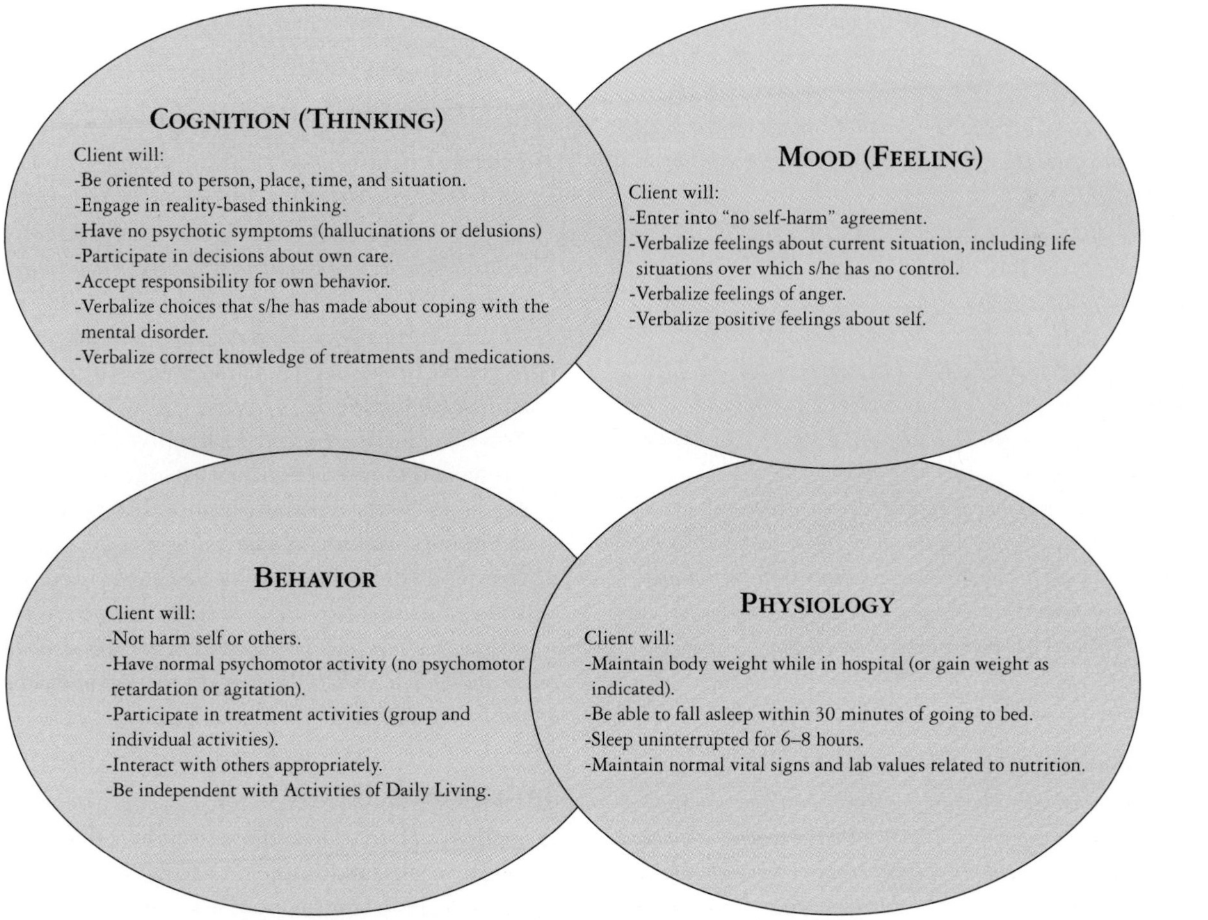

COGNITION (THINKING)

Client will:
- Be oriented to person, place, time, and situation.
- Engage in reality-based thinking.
- Have no psychotic symptoms (hallucinations or delusions)
- Participate in decisions about own care.
- Accept responsibility for own behavior.
- Verbalize choices that s/he has made about coping with the mental disorder.
- Verbalize correct knowledge of treatments and medications.

MOOD (FEELING)

Client will:
- Enter into "no self-harm" agreement.
- Verbalize feelings about current situation, including life situations over which s/he has no control.
- Verbalize feelings of anger.
- Verbalize positive feelings about self.

BEHAVIOR

Client will:
- Not harm self or others.
- Have normal psychomotor activity (no psychomotor retardation or agitation).
- Participate in treatment activities (group and individual activities).
- Interact with others appropriately.
- Be independent with Activities of Daily Living.

PHYSIOLOGY

Client will:
- Maintain body weight while in hospital (or gain weight as indicated).
- Be able to fall asleep within 30 minutes of going to bed.
- Sleep uninterrupted for 6–8 hours.
- Maintain normal vital signs and lab values related to nutrition.

Figure 9-13. ■ Desired outcomes for clients with mood disorders.

Nursing care must be personalized for each individual client. The suggested interventions in this chapter are based on common concerns for clients with mood disorders. If a client has different concerns, creativity will be needed. Creativity is one of the cornerstones of nursing.

Risk for Violence (Self-Directed)

- Assess mental status, including suicidal ideation. *Mental status assessment includes information about client's mood and whether client has psychosis (increases suicide risk due to abnormal reality testing).*
- If client does have suicidal ideation, assess for plan and whether client has the means to complete the plan. *The nurse can assess the dangerousness of the client's suicidal plan (more dangerous if client has a specific lethal plan and the means to complete it).*
- Share information about suicidal thinking with the treatment team. *Team must be involved to ensure client safety.*
- Remove potentially dangerous items from client's area (knives, lighters, razors, belts, glass, etc.). *Removing dangerous items promotes safety by decreasing client's opportunity for impulsive use for self-harm. People experiencing mania have impaired judgment, so the nurse must anticipate the risks and must control the environment to promote safety.*
- Assess client safety frequently during the night. *Client may feel unsupervised at night.*
- Remain with a client who is having feelings about harming self. *The nurse's presence shows regard for the client's safety and worth. The nurse can prevent harmful behavior. A client at high risk for suicidal behavior requires close observation, ideally in a psychiatric facility.*
- Create a "no self-harm" contract with the client. *Although an agreement by the client not to harm self is not really binding, it suggests that the client is in control and responsible for her/his behavior. The contract emphasizes the worth of the client and the concern by the staff for his/her safety.*

Risk for Violence (Directed at Others)

- Provide low-stimulation environment for a manic client. *People experiencing mania have a reduced ability to filter and process stimuli. The more sensory stimuli, the more difficult it is for the client to determine what is real, and to maintain control over behavior.*

- Make expectations for client behavior clear to client as soon as possible. Staff must be consistent in expectations of client. *Having clear, structured expectations can make it easier for client to comply with behavior expectations. Consistency among staff is important to avoid confusion and client manipulation of staff to change expectations.*
- Observe client closely and respond quickly to increasing agitation. Start with least restrictive approach: redirection, p.r.n. medication, isolation, finally restraint. *Early intervention may prevent violent behavior and injury to client and others.*
- Minimize group activities for client in mania. *Client in mania becomes easily overstimulated and may have difficulty responding appropriately with multiple people. One-to-one interactions are less stimulating and easier for client to manage.*
- Provide appropriate opportunities for physical activity. Walking is the ideal activity. Client may prefer another activity, such as Ping-Pong or basketball. *Client may feel compelled to be physically active and would thus find confinement very stressful. Walking is active without being exhausting if prolonged.*

Impaired Social Interaction

- Establish a trusting relationship with the client. *The nurse-client relationship is the foundation for nursing care and for understanding the client's needs. When the client trusts the nurse, s/he has an opportunity to have a sense of emotional security. A client who feels secure will be more likely to interact positively with others. The nurse provides a role model for how to communicate and behave in an individual relationship.*
- Provide structured activities to allow the client with depression to interact with others. Encourage client to participate (arts and crafts groups, listening to music in a group, walking or exercising in a group, discussing medications, reminiscing groups, etc.). *The depressed client is more likely to be able to interact with others if the situation is structured because the demands on the individual are less. Positive interactions with others reinforce socializing.*

Imbalanced Nutrition

- If client is lethargic and overweight, offer lighter foods, snacks, and liquids. Discuss the value of regular exercise in improving one's spirits. Encourage the client to set a plan of regular, light exercise. *Client may be unable to focus on weight loss until depression is resolved and may be too depressed to think of exercising. It is better to have a regular time for exercise than to try to get up and exercise when the depression is at its worst. Light, brief efforts are more possible to achieve and thus can improve self-esteem.*

- The client may feel too depressed to eat. *Offer fluids frequently and small amounts of nutritious foods as the client tolerates.*

- If client is highly active, pacing, or too busy to eat, provide nutritious "finger foods" (sandwiches, fruit, etc.) that client can eat while walking. Offer food and fluids frequently. *Client has high energy needs while in a manic phase and may not be able to meet nutritional needs. Client may be able to eat foods that can be held in her/his hands when s/he is unable to sit down for a meal. Client is also at risk for dehydration from excessive activity, especially in hot weather.*

Hopelessness

- Allow client to talk about feelings and life events. Use therapeutic communication techniques to help client see that s/he has survived difficulties in the past and that s/he has strengths. *The knowledge that one has overcome obstacles before suggests that it is possible to do so again. When client recognizes own strengths, it provides a foundation for hope that the current trouble can be overcome.*

- Teach the client about the disorder and medications and that the treatment team will not give up hope until the client feels better. *Knowledge that the client is likely to have a positive response to treatment is hopeful. It may be beneficial to point out that depression has episodes and that this one will eventually resolve. Many clients worry that the staff will abandon them if they do not respond to treatment.*

Disturbed Thought Processes

- Provide antipsychotic medications as ordered and monitor effects. *It is the responsibility of nurses to assess the client's response to medications for the purpose of evaluating their effectiveness and detecting side effects.*

- Look for the client's strengths and abilities when providing nursing care. *When a person has a severe symptom like psychosis, it is easy to see the pathology. It is important to look for the person's strengths and to acknowledge the normal parts of the person. Even the psychotic client has coping or survival skills that the nurse can draw on for the client's benefit.*

- Reinforce reality. Talk about what is really happening. *Even conversations about the simple realities of daily life (the weather, doing laundry, meals, etc.) bring the client's attention away from disordered thoughts and into the here and now. The nurse's role is to help the client recognize what is real. Disordered thoughts can be improved by reality-based conversations. Talking about delusions with the client reinforces the abnormal thinking.*

- Encourage or assist the client to express feelings of fear or anxiety. Provide validation for the client's feelings. *The sense of losing contact with reality can be frightening. Expressing feelings to the nurse who accepts them without judgment and validates how difficult the situation must be can be affirming and helpful to clients.*

- Pay attention to the content of the client's speech (and therefore thoughts). *If a client is yelling about being attacked, he or she might mistake the nurse for an attacker. Be careful when approaching agitated clients. Remain calm, and your attitude will be contagious to the client and the staff around you. Keep enough distance between yourself and the client to be safe from swinging arms. Even peaceful people may strike out when they think they are defending themselves.*

EVALUATING

In the evaluation phase, the nurse looks back at the desired outcomes, and asks "Were the outcomes met?" If the outcomes are not met, the nurse must report that the nursing care plan was unsuccessful. Perhaps the outcomes were not realistic in the first place. Maybe the interventions were appropriate, but did not work toward the identified goal. The LPN/LVN would give feedback to the charge nurse so that the care plan could be revised.

DISCHARGE CONSIDERATIONS

Clients with mood disorders face many challenges related to their disorder and its treatment. Education is an important role for the nurse. The nurse should reinforce client teaching about medications, side effects, and the interaction between medication and diet or activities. Most clients will need ongoing psychotherapeutic support. Information about support groups, as well as emergency numbers, should be provided. The National Alliance for the Mentally Ill has support groups in many localities.

Nurses can also help to create a healthier environment for clients with mood disorders by being active in their communities. Box 9-14 ■ describes opportunities for nurses to advocate for clients with mental disorders.

BOX 9-14

Community Care: Advocating for Clients with Mental Disorders

Roles Outside the Workplace

Nurses have responsibilities outside the walls of the workplace. As healthcare professionals, we have the responsibility to help our society learn to be healthier. One way nurses can make a difference is to encourage people to be diagnosed and treated for depression. Another is to work through national and local regulations to decrease the availability of firearms to adolescents. Also, by stopping the habit of telling or laughing at jokes about mentally ill people, we can be role models for others, including our children, about the fact that mental illness is not a joke any more than diabetes is.

Teaching Organizations

Finally, nurses can cooperate with an organization created by the National Alliance for the Mentally Ill called StigmaBusters. StigmaBusters works to reduce the stigma against mental illness and mentally ill people in our society. They target advertising, the media, and public policy. Through education of the public, legislators, advertisers, and others, they work to change attitudes and laws. Visit their website and learn about their latest projects at www.nami.org.

NURSING PROCESS CARE PLAN
Client with Depression

Remember Pearl from the beginning of this chapter? Pearl G. is a 70-year-old African American widowed woman who is a resident in a long-term care facility. She had a stroke a year ago and has hemiplegia on her right side. She is right-handed. She does not feed herself and has little appetite. Ms. G. is alert and oriented to person and place. She cooperates with having her activities of daily living done for her, but she does not try to help. When she talks, it is only one or two words at a time. Her face always seems to look sad. The nurse has worked with Ms. G. for the 11 months since she has been in this facility. The nurse thinks Ms. G. is depressed. The nurse assessed her with the Geriatric Depression Scale. Ms. G. scored 12. In the conversation they had about the depression scale, Ms. G. said that she missed her family.

Assessment. The nurse collected all the assessment findings in the case study above. In addition, the chart stated that Ms. G. had an adult daughter and a married son with one teenage granddaughter living nearby.

Diagnosis. Three priority nursing diagnoses were identified for this client:

- Powerlessness R/T disability and impaired communication
- Self-Care Deficit, bathing/hygiene, dressing/grooming, feeding, and toileting R/T hemiplegia and lack of motivation
- Impaired Social Interaction R/T lack of motivation and lack of opportunity to socialize with family and peers

Expected Outcomes. The expected outcomes for the plan of care are:

- Client will identify two areas in which she feels some control.
- Client will assist with all her ADLs, feeding herself independently within 2 weeks.
- Client will interact with the staff, her peers, and her family.

Planning and Implementation. Before beginning to work on independent nursing actions, the charge nurse consulted with Ms. G.'s physician about the possibility of treating her depression. The physician agreed that Ms. G. is depressed. She prescribed fluoxetine 20 mg to be given to Ms. G. PO each morning. The LPN (Kevin) looked up fluoxetine and found it to be a selective serotonin-reuptake inhibitor type of antidepressant drug. The following interventions were planned and implemented:

- *Offer simple choices first.* Ms. G. is given a choice of clothes to wear each day. She is asked if she wants to take her shower before or after breakfast, and where she wants to eat lunch (there are three dining rooms in this facility). Ms. G. has some cognitive deficit after the stroke. She is asked which radio station she wants to listen to.

- *Encourage self-care.* The aides who supervised meals were asked to help her use her left hand to feed herself. Self-feeding was tried months before, and it worked until Ms. G. became unwilling to do it.

- *Encourage social contact.* Kevin, the nurse, called each of Ms. G.'s children and encouraged them to visit. He also arranged to visit with Ms. G. for a few minutes each day that he worked. (We know that Kevin would have liked to have time to talk longer with her, but this is a real story.) He had Ms. G. put on the list of residents who attend the news group (where the activity aide reads parts of the newspaper each morning).

Evaluation. Two weeks after the plan was started, Kevin evaluated its effectiveness. With encouragement, Ms. G. had started to make choices about her clothes, radio stations, social activities, and visitors. Ms. G. assisted in washing herself during her shower. She tried feebly, but was not much help with dressing. She was able to feed herself about 50% of her meals, and was able to call for help to get to the bathroom about 75% of the time.

Within 10 days after starting her new medication, she was smiling, more interested in her surroundings, had more appetite, and was more active. She was more talkative and enjoyed visits from her family.

Critical Thinking in the Nursing Process

1. Was Outcome 1 met, and why was it important for Ms. G.?
2. How successful was Outcome 2 of Ms. G.'s plan? How might it be adapted after evaluation?
3. Discuss how the range of social interactions that were set up for Ms. G. increased the likelihood that Outcome 3 would be met.

Note: Discussion of Critical Thinking Questions appears in Appendix I.

Note: The references and resources for this and all chapters have been compiled at the back of the book.

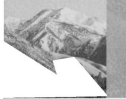

 KEY TERMS

Use the audio glossary feature of the Companion Website to hear the correct pronunciation of the following key terms.

distractibility

dysphoric mood

electroconvulsive therapy (ECT)

elevated mood

euthymic mood

flight of ideas

irritable mood

kindling

mood

pressured speech

psychomotor agitation

psychomotor retardation

seasonal affective disorder (SAD)

somatization

suicidal ideation

KEY Points

- Mood disorders are caused by an interaction of genetic predisposition, brain function abnormalities, and environmental stressors (biological and psychosocial factors).

- Depression is the most common mental disorder in the world.

- Nurses in every specialty area work with people who have mood disorders, especially depression.

- Most people who commit suicide were depressed.

- Suicide is more common than homicide in the United States.

- There is a recent increase in suicide among adolescents. This increase is due to firearm-related suicide.

- Mood disorders are treatable and most people respond positively to medications.

- There is a stigma against people with mood disorders, as well as other mental disorders.

- Desired outcomes for people with mood disorders are in the areas of cognition (thinking), mood, behavior, and physiology.

- People with depression may experience anhedonia, lack of energy, lack of motivation, difficulty relating to other people, and psychomotor retardation, as well as sadness.

- There are serious possible side effects associated with the MAOI antidepressants, including hypertensive crisis when clients combine foods containing tyramine with taking these drugs.

- Serotonin syndrome can occur when MAOIs are combined with SSRIs or St. John's wort. Symptoms include agitation, muscle spasms, tremor, nausea, abdominal cramps, and headache.

- People with bipolar disorder in the manic phase have several challenges including lack of insight, poor judgment, and impulsive behavior.

- Lithium and valproate are both first-line drugs for bipolar disorder.

 EXPLORE MediaLink

Additional interactive resources for this chapter can be found on the Companion Website at www.prenhall.com/eby. Click on Chapter 9 and "Begin" to select the activities for this chapter.

- Audio glossary
- NCLEX-PN® review
- Case study
- Study outline
- Critical thinking questions
- Matching questions
- Weblinks
- Video Case: Everett (Major Depressive Disorder)

Caring for a Client Who Has Bipolar Disorder

NCLEX-PN® Focus Area: Physiologic Integrity

Case Study: John Nguyen is a 36-year-old Vietnamese American male client with a diagnosis of Bipolar Disorder. He is hospitalized for a surgical repair of an ankle injury he experienced while he was playing basketball. Mr. Nguyen is a certified public accountant. He is having a manic episode that is less severe than his untreated episodes were, but he has been sleepless for three nights. He stayed home from work yesterday to play basketball all day. He did not eat or drink all day when he was playing basketball. He takes lithium carbonate extended release (Eskalith CR) 450 mg twice a day at home, and this is also ordered in the hospital. The morning dose is due now.

Nursing Diagnosis: Risk for injury R/T lithium toxicity

COLLECT DATA

Subjective	Objective
_____	_____
_____	_____
_____	_____
_____	_____
_____	_____
_____	_____
_____	_____

Would you report this data? Yes/No

If yes, to: _____

Nursing Care

_____
_____
_____
_____
_____
_____
_____
_____
_____
_____

How would you document this? _____
_____
_____
_____

Data Collected
(use those that apply)

- Weight 185 lbs.
- BP 130/80
- Pulse 108, irregular
- Client states, "My hands won't stop shaking."
- Slept 6 hours last night
- Skin is warm and dry.
- Client's mother had bipolar disorder.
- Client states, "Would you please read the menu to me? I can't see very well."
- When the physical therapist was teaching him to use crutches, the client was too weak to bear his own body weight on his unaffected leg.
- Client is allergic to tree pollen.
- Refused dinner last evening and breakfast today
- Client's wife states, "He has been under a lot of pressure at work lately."

Nursing Interventions
(use those that apply; list in priority order)

- Look in the client's chart to find his baseline vital signs.
- Call the physician to request an order for a sleeping pill to help the client sleep to regain his strength.
- Teach client to drink 3 gallons of water daily.
- Hold the lithium dose that is due now.
- Call the physician to report the presence of symptoms of lithium toxicity.
- Teach the client and his wife that his strenuous exercise (playing basketball all day) is a good way to improve his cardiovascular fitness.

Compare your documentation to the sample provided in Appendix I.

When a question is asked about psychosocial concerns, first clarify what the client is telling you, and then ask for more information. If the client says, "I feel like dying," you might say, "You feel like you want to die?" then, "Tell me more about what you're feeling."

1 A newly married woman tells the nurse that she attempted suicide in high school due to an unhappy relationship. She says she is afraid to become pregnant for fear that having a new baby might bring on those same feelings. The nurse knows that the client:

1. Is no more likely than any other young woman to experience postpartum depression.
2. Was probably just making a suicidal gesture in high school for attention and has no risk of future depressive episodes.
3. Is at greater risk for another depressive episode considering her past experience and the added stress of a new baby.
4. Is worrying needlessly and should be encouraged to consider pregnancy.

2 When a client comes in for her 6-week postpartum checkup the office nurse notices that the client looks "drained." The client tells the nurse that the baby just won't leave her alone and that she has no time for herself. She makes no attempt to pick up the baby even though he is crying. She states, "I can't handle this much longer." The nurse's best response would be:

1. "I can assure you it will get better. All new mothers feel as you do."
2. "Being a new mother is stressful. Tell me about the changes that have occurred in your life since the baby came."
3. "Pick up your baby. When you hold him close, that should help both of you to feel better."
4. "You're probably experiencing a little bit of postpartum depression. It is normal and will pass with time."

3 A client complains to the nurse that every winter she experiences feelings of extreme fatigue and irritability. She has been diagnosed with seasonal affective disorder. The most effective treatment for this type of depression is:

1. Light or photo therapy.
2. Melatonin supplement.
3. Psychoanalysis.
4. Electroconvulsive treatment.

4 When the psychiatrist describes the client's symptoms as including anhedonia, it would mean that the client was:

1. Hallucinating.
2. Incapable of forming personal relationships.
3. Overeating.
4. Incapable of feeling pleasure.

5 People suffering from depression are often undiagnosed. The most likely reason for this is that:

1. Physicians do not recognize the condition.
2. General practitioners feel underqualified to treat a mental disorder.
3. Clients underreport their feelings, for fear of the stigma of being "mentally ill."
4. Physicians do not value the depth of the psychological feelings a client reports.

6 When the client asks the nurse how soon the new antidepression medication will work, the nurse's best response would be:

1. "You should feel over the depression immediately."
2. "It will take 2 to 6 weeks for the medication to reach its full effect."
3. "The medication usually takes 1 week to reach its potential."
4. "It may be 6 months before you feel the full effects of the medication."

7 A severely depressed client tells the nurse that he will be receiving an electroconvulsive therapy treatment in the morning. He says he is nervous about the therapy, because he has heard "horror stories" about it. The nurse's best response would be:

1. "You may experience some temporary memory loss and mild confusion, but ECT has been highly successful in relieving severe depression such as yours."
2. "ECT is an experimental procedure for severe depression, but the physician thinks it will be helpful in your situation."
3. "ECT has been used for years as the first-line treatment for severe depression. It works quickly and well for all depressed clients."
4. "Permanent memory loss is definitely a side effect for most people receiving ECT, but it is better than being depressed."

8 Clients experiencing a manic episode will most likely be noncompliant with treatment, because:

1. They do not realize they need treatment.
2. They are too busy.
3. They want to be liked by others.
4. They enjoy the "high."

9 A client with bipolar disorder is pacing constantly today while other clients are having a birthday party. There is music, noise, and food. The client walks over to the table and starts grabbing handfuls of cake to eat as he paces up and down the halls. The nurse's best response to this behavior would be to:

1. Let him continue to pace and eat.
2. Medicate him with a p.r.n. antianxiety drug.
3. Restrain him in his room.
4. Invite him to go outside and take a walk with the nurse.

10 Which of the following nursing interventions would be appropriate for a client admitted with a major depressive disorder and suicidal ideation? (Select all that apply.)

1. Ask the client if he is currently having any thoughts of harming himself.
2. Assure the client that any information he shares with you will be just between the two of you.
3. Remove potentially dangerous items from the client's area.
4. Provide the client with privacy while he is adjusting to his new environment.
5. Create a "no self-harm" contract with the client.

Answers for Review Questions, as well as discussion of Care Plan and Critical Thinking Care Map questions, appear in Appendix I.

Personality Disorders

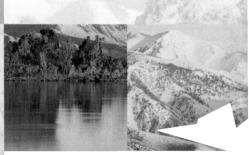

LEARNING Outcomes

After completing this chapter, you will be able to:

1. Describe the behaviors associated with personality disorders.
2. Adapt the nurse-client relationship to the special concerns of the client who has a personality disorder.
3. Apply the nursing process to clients with personality disorders.

As you recall from Chapter 3, *personality* is the relatively stable way that a person thinks, feels, and behaves. Personality includes the psychosocial (not physical) traits and characteristics that make a person an individual.

Personality begins to develop during childhood in part based on genetic foundations, and also in response to the challenges and experiences of living (De Clercq & De Fruyt, 2007). Based on these individual differences of genetics and life events, people think, feel, and behave in a variety of ways. One of the strengths of the human race is our diversity. Those thoughts, feelings, and behaviors stem from personality. Although the overall pattern of personality is unique to each individual, there are enough similarities observed in people that some generalizations can be made.

Personality Disorders

Although the normal range of human behavior, feelings, and thought is broad, it is possible for personality to be outside the normal range. A personality disorder is an enduring pattern of inner experience and behavior that has the following characteristics (American Psychiatric Association, 2000):

- It deviates markedly from the expectations of the individual's culture.
- It is pervasive and inflexible.
- It begins in adolescence or young adulthood.
- It is stable over time.
- It leads to distress for the individual or impairment of functioning.

A person's personality significantly affects how this person responds to life events, including illnesses. The response a client has to a mental disorder will be affected by that client's personality as well. A client's culture also affects the client's behavior and personality. Box 10-1 ■ shows the importance of considering a client's cultural background when interpreting behavior.

DIAGNOSTIC CRITERIA

Personality disorders are not considered to be the same as mental disorders or diseases. Personality disorders are coded as Axis II in the axis system of the *Diagnostic and Statistical Manual of Mental Disorders* (American Psychiatric Association, 2000). Axis I covers the major mental disorders such as Schizophrenia, Major Depressive Disorder, and Bipolar Disorder.

Diagnosing personality disorders requires an evaluation of the person's long-term patterns of functioning.

BOX 10-1	CULTURAL PULSE POINTS

Personality and Culture

Any judgment about a client's personality must take into account that person's ethnic, cultural, and social background. People who are immigrants from other cultures are especially at risk of being diagnosed with disorders of mental function and personality when they are acting or thinking in a way that is accepted in their culture of origin but not in their new home. For example, a Cuban immigrant stated to the nurse that her dead father talked to her and told her to be careful when talking to strangers. In the Cuban culture, "talking" with deceased people may mean the same as "This is what my father would have wanted me to do" in the European American culture. The nurse can become more culturally sensitive to this client by talking with other Cuban people or learning more about the client's culture.

Personality patterns must be persistent to be significant. For a personality disorder to be present, the individual's symptoms cannot be caused by a general medical disorder or by substance abuse. The personality characteristics used for diagnosis must have persisted since the individual was an adolescent or young adult. Finally, they must be consistent over different situations (American Psychiatric Association, 2000).

Whether there are early signs of personality disorders in children is a current research question. Studies have found that both personality traits and environmental experiences in childhood appear to contribute to the development of personality disorders in adulthood. There is not a direct correlation, but children who have conduct disorder are statistically more likely to develop Antisocial Personality Disorder as adults. Children with self-mutilating behavior and impulse control problems are more likely to develop Borderline Personality Disorder. Obsessive-Compulsive Personality Disorder appears to have a more clearly genetic basis. Adults with Obsessive-Compulsive Personality Disorder often had a history of symptoms beginning in childhood (De Clercq & De Fruyt, 2007).

The American Psychiatric Association (2000) describes 11 types of personality disorders. These disorders are grouped into three clusters by their similarities. The clusters are based on similar observed behaviors. These include the following:

1. Odd and eccentric
2. Dramatic and emotional
3. Anxiety- and fear-based personality disorders

Table 10-1 ■ provides an outline of the categories.

TABLE 10-1

Personality Disorders by Cluster

CLUSTER	PERSONALITY DISORDER
A: Odd-eccentric	Paranoid Personality Disorder Schizoid Personality Disorder Schizotypal Personality Disorder
B: Dramatic-emotional	Antisocial Personality Disorder Borderline Personality Disorder Histrionic Personality Disorder Narcissistic Personality Disorder
C: Anxious-fearful	Avoidant Personality Disorder Dependent Personality Disorder Obsessive-Compulsive Personality Disorder

Source: Diagnostic and Statistical Manual of Mental Disorders (4th ed., Text Revision), copyright © 2000. American Psychiatric Association.

Personality disorders that do not meet the diagnostic criteria for any of the above may be diagnosed as Personality Disorder Not Otherwise Specified (the 11th disorder). In some clients, there will be features of more than one disorder of personality. Such a client may have a diagnosis of "mixed" personality disorder.

COMMON CLINICAL FEATURES

Impaired sense of self is a central problem in disorders of personality. Self-identity is a part of normal personality development. It begins in infancy as the child begins to separate from the mother or caregiver. Identity includes the ability to differentiate the self from others, an integration of social and occupational roles, chosen values and behaviors, gender roles, beliefs about sexuality and intimacy, goals, and political and religious beliefs. The sense of identity is often not adequately formed in people with personality disorders. Sense of self, or identity, is necessary for goal-directed behavior and for satisfying interpersonal relationships (Limandri & Boyd, 2005).

Thinking patterns are distorted in personality disorders. The individual's ability to decode stimuli and to interpret environmental events is impaired. Maladaptive thinking patterns cause individuals to misinterpret the actions of others. The misinterpretations result in maladaptive responses by the affected person.

Emotions, in their intensity and quality, appear to be affected by disorders of personality. People affected by personality disorders have blunted or distorted emotional experience. They tend to have more negative emotional experiences. Their ability to function in daily life and even to learn new things is affected.

Behavior is a part of personality. First, personality disorders cause *impulsive behavior*. These disorders appear to make it more difficult for people to foresee the consequences of their actions or to control their impulses despite probable negative consequences.

Second, these disorders cause *inflexibility* of behavior. Affected people tend to be rigid. They are unable to change their usual behavior when circumstances suggest that a change is indicated. Usually, people learn to change their behavior when they try new actions and receive positive reinforcement from the new approach. The inflexibility in personality disorders makes it difficult for people to learn new ways to behave or cope.

This inflexibility traps the client in a **vicious cycle of behavior** that are self-defeating. They become rigid and inflexible in role functions and personal interactions. The inflexibility provokes predicaments and problems. The more inflexible they are, the more problems they have. The more problems they have, the more inflexible they become. This vicious circle reduces learning opportunities and alienates other people (Millon & Davis, 1999). Figure 10-1 ■ illustrates this vicious cycle.

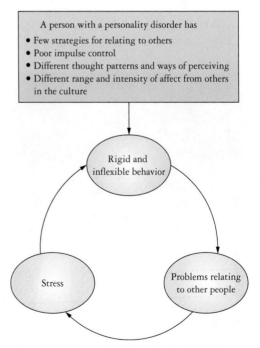

A person with a personality disorder has

- Few strategies for relating to others
- Poor impulse control
- Different thought patterns and ways of perceiving
- Different range and intensity of affect from others in the culture

Rigid and inflexible behavior

Problems relating to other people

Stress

Figure 10-1. ■ Vicious cycle of personality disorders.

Challenges for Nurses

Often nurses find it frustrating to work with clients with disorders of personality. These clients can be manipulative, socially inappropriate, and difficult. When nurses see the rigid, inflexible behavior patterns, they often believe that these clients could change and act appropriately if they tried. However, personality represents a *persistent* pattern of thought, emotion, and behavior. It is not within the ability of these clients to change their personalities completely. Such clients need all the patience and skill nurses have to offer. Remember that the goal of the nurse is to provide professional care, not to be the friend of the client. To work successfully with clients who have personality disorders, nurses must adapt the nurse-client relationship to the special concerns of the client. These adaptations are discussed further in the Nursing Care section of this chapter.

Cluster A Personality Disorders: Odd-Eccentric

PARANOID PERSONALITY DISORDER

Paranoid Personality Disorder is a pattern of distrust and suspiciousness that other people are acting maliciously toward the affected individual. People with this disorder automatically assume that others will hurt or deceive them, even if there is no factual evidence that this is true. On the basis of imagined evidence, they may think that people are plotting against them or may attack them without reason (Figure 10-2 ■ shows a man with a suspicious

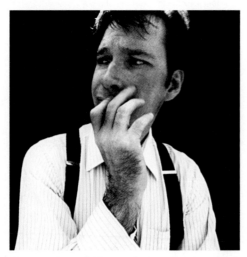

Figure 10-2. ■ Paranoid Personality Disorder is associated with automatic suspiciousness about the motives of others. *Source:* CORBIS- NY.

affect). They may fight back when their victim never attacked in the first place. People with Paranoid Personality Disorder often imagine hidden threatening or demeaning messages in innocent remarks or actions. They find it difficult to forgive and hold grudges. They perceive that others are attacking their character or reputation even when it does not appear so to others (American Psychiatric Association, 2000).

Difficulty with interpersonal relationships is a hallmark of this disorder. Affected people tend to be so suspicious of the malicious intentions of others that they cannot form mutually satisfying relationships. They may form relationships in which they are in power or control. They avoid confiding in others due to their pervasive suspiciousness. Paranoid Personality Disorder causes people to interpret the actions of others as deception and betrayal. They especially distrust the faithfulness or trustworthiness of a partner or friend (Millon & Davis, 1999).

This disorder causes a hostile and defensive nature. When the client's hostility arouses a hostile response in others, the suspicion that others are against the affected person is confirmed (American Psychiatric Association, 2000).

Because this disorder occurs in approximately 0.5–2.5% of the general population, and in 10–30% of inpatients in the psychiatric setting (American Psychiatric Association, 2000), nurses encounter clients with Paranoid Personality Disorder in a variety of settings.

Collaborative Care

Personality disorders are difficult to treat, because personality is resistant to change. Cognitive-behavioral therapy is the most effective psychotherapy for people with personality disorders, but it takes time, commitment, and insight on the part of the client. Many people with personality disorders lack the insight to realize that they have a problem. There are no medications that affect personality directly. Sometimes medications are effective in treating the symptoms of personality disorders. Antidepressants may be useful for avoidant and borderline personalities. People with the cluster A disorders may find antipsychotic medications helpful if they experience psychosis (Nathan & Gorman, 2002).

Because a person's personality is such an integral part of the individual's identity, nurses cannot just identify a problem, plan an intervention, and make personality changes. Nurses must identify short-term outcomes that are realistic for people with disorders of personality. For a person affected with Paranoid Personality Disorder, these outcomes will be related to small changes in thinking patterns and behavior, such as realistic interpretation of events, taking medications, eating meals, and cooperating with treatment. The long-term treatment goal for the client with Paranoid Personality Disorder is increased flexibility and trust. This client will challenge the nurse who is accustomed to forming trusting relationships with clients easily. A matter-of-fact, business-like approach is indicated with a person with paranoia.

Although people with paranoia often appear to be aggressive, their inner feelings are often fear and insecurity. These feelings generally respond to reassurance about the person's safety. These clients are very aware of power relationships. They may respond better to information directly from the physician rather than from the nurse.

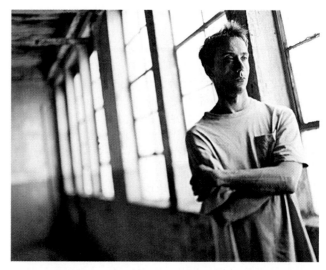

Figure 10-3. ■ People with Schizoid Personality Disorder avoid relationships and contact with others. *Source:* Corbis/Bettmann.

CASE EXAMPLE

Consider the case of Peter, who was admitted to the general hospital for abdominal surgery. He was alert and oriented. The surgeon met only briefly with him on the night before surgery. As a result, he believed that the surgeon cared so little for his welfare that she might kill him during surgery. He said that the nurses were afraid that he might file a lawsuit, so they might try to give him someone else's medications to punish him. *The nurse finds it difficult to relate to Peter because he is so suspicious. What can Peter's nurse do to make it possible for the staff to provide care for Peter while decreasing his level of stress?*

SCHIZOID PERSONALITY DISORDER

The most important features of Schizoid Personality Disorder are a pervasive pattern of detachment from social relationships and a restricted range of emotional expression (*affect*). People with this disorder of personality avoid relationships (Figure 10-3 ■). They appear to receive little satisfaction from being part of a family or group. They prefer to be alone and even choose hobbies that can be done in isolation from other people. They have little interest in sexual or other intimate relationships. They lack friends and they appear indifferent to the opinions of others. People with Schizoid Personality Disorder show a reduced and flattened range of emotions. They rarely experience strong emotions such as anger or joy. They may confide only in their parents or sisters and brothers (American Psychiatric Association, 2000).

Schizoid Personality Disorder may cause impairment in occupational as well as social functioning unless the affected individual can find a suitable job working alone. Affected people find pleasure in few if any activities.

Collaborative Care

People with Schizoid Personality Disorder experience little positive emotion and want to isolate themselves from other people. The goals of nursing cannot realistically include the client becoming socially active. Realistically, these clients need enough interpersonal contact to keep them oriented to reality, but not so much that they experience undue stress. Treatment outcomes would focus on finding individual activities that provide satisfaction for the client.

CASE EXAMPLE

Consider the case of Sid, who has Schizoid Personality Disorder. He works as a night inventory auditor. He was riding to work on the bus when the bus was involved in a crash. Several people on the bus were badly injured. Sid suffered a laceration on his arm. In the emergency department, he seemed passive, not very expressive, and did not return the nurses' smiles or expressions of concern. His brother came to the emergency department to be with him and Sid seemed distant, even with him. *What could the nurse do to find out if Sid is so badly shocked that he is unable to respond, or if this behavior is part of his personality?*

SCHIZOTYPAL PERSONALITY DISORDER

People with Schizotypal Personality Disorder have a consistent pattern of interpersonal deficits. They have discomfort in and reduced capacity for close relationships. They also have cognitive (thinking) or perceptual distortions, and eccentric behavior. The cognitive deficit may be **ideas of reference,** in which clients misinterpret everyday events as having a personal meaning for them. For example, the client may believe that her thoughts about the plants being dry caused it to rain, or that the arrival of the bus at exactly this moment is because she thought about it coming. Ideas of reference are not as severe as the delusions of reference (discussed in the context of schizophrenia in Chapter 8). Delusions are more fixed, despite evidence that they are false (American Psychiatric Association, 2000).

People with Schizotypal Personality Disorder may be superstitious or preoccupied with paranormal activity that is outside the realm of belief of their culture, such as clairvoyance, telepathy, or mind reading. Their thinking and speech are likely to be odd. They may have suspicious or paranoid thoughts. Affect is likely to be restricted or inappropriate. *Inappropriate* affect occurs when the client has an emotional response that is not culturally appropriate for the situation, such as laughing when someone's pet dies. The behavior and appearance of affected people are also likely to be eccentric or peculiar. The client depicted in Figure 10-4 ■ is demonstrating eccentric appearance and behavior. These clients will probably not have friends. They have excessive social anxiety that does not resolve as people become more familiar. Their social anxiety is more likely to be due to paranoid fears than to negative ideas about themselves (American Psychiatric Association, 2000).

Collaborative Care

Like others with odd or eccentric personality disorders, people with Schizotypal Personality Disorder usually do not seek treatment for it. If they did seek treatment, it would probably be for the associated symptoms such as anxiety or depression rather than for the personality disorder itself.

When people with Schizotypal Personality Disorder are under stress, they may have delusional thinking or perceptual alterations. Nurses should reinforce reality for these clients. It is not helpful to argue with a client about delusional thoughts, which clients believe are true despite evidence otherwise. It is helpful to have brief concrete conversations (talk about the client's current experiences rather than abstract ideas). Maintain a matter-of-fact, businesslike approach to all the clients with the odd and eccentric personalities. It helps them respect care providers. They may believe that joking or informality are mocking or untrustworthy behaviors by the nurse.

These clients' odd behavior may isolate them from others. Social skills training is a valuable therapy. It can help them behave in more socially appropriate ways, thus making it easier for them to interact in the community.

CASE EXAMPLE

Consider the case of Sylvia, who is a resident of a long-term care facility after having a CVA (stroke). Sylvia never socializes with the other residents. Other residents seem to be suspicious of her and avoid her. She has always acted and looked eccentric. She wears necklaces over her ears and wears her many earrings as pins on her sweaters. She frequently accuses others of stealing her things and believes that she can tell who is stealing by the colors in their eyes. She states: "The lies in the eyes cannot be disguised." *What can the nurse do to help this client have more positive social interactions and be more comfortable in the facility?*

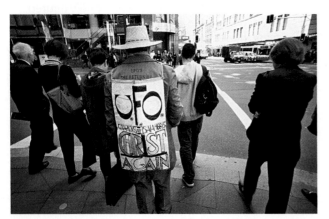

Figure 10-4. ■ People with Schizotypal Personality Disorder may appear to be eccentric in their dress and behavior. *Source:* Photolibrary.com.

Cluster B Personality Disorders: Dramatic-Emotional

ANTISOCIAL PERSONALITY DISORDER

The essential characteristic of *Antisocial Personality Disorder* is a pervasive pattern of disregarding and violating the rights of others. To receive this diagnosis, clients must be at least 18 years old. They must have had *Conduct Disorder* in childhood by the age of 15. Conduct Disorder includes cruelty to people or animals, deceitfulness or theft, destruction of property, and serious violations of rules (American Psychiatric Association, 2000). See Chapter 13 for more information about Conduct Disorder.

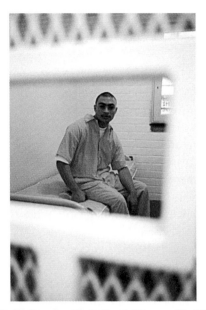

Figure 10-5. ■ People with Antisocial Personality Disorder tend to believe that rules and laws do not apply to them.
Source: PhotoEdit Inc.

People with Antisocial Personality Disorder tend to disregard societal expectations by breaking the law (Figure 10-5 ■). They repeatedly commit acts that are illegal, whether they are arrested or not. For example, they may destroy the property of others, harass others, steal, or engage in illegal occupations (drug dealing, dog fighting, selling stolen property). People with this disorder are frequently deceitful. They manipulate others for their personal gain or pleasure (for money, sex, and power). They disregard the rights, feelings, and safety of others. They lie repeatedly and may use false names or other methods to deceive others (American Psychiatric Association, 2000).

Impulsiveness is a major feature of Antisocial Personality Disorder. People with this disorder make decisions suddenly, without planning ahead. They do not consider how others will be affected, or even how they will be affected themselves. This leads to frequent change of jobs, residences, and relationships. People with this disorder tend to be aggressive and irritable. They may fight repeatedly or assault others frequently, including partners and children. Affected people may be friendly and likeable until they are frustrated. This disorder results in disregard for the safety of self or others. Fast, reckless driving, substance use, or irresponsible sexual behavior may illustrate this aspect of the disorder (American Psychiatric Association, 2000).

Irresponsibility is another aspect of this personality disorder. Affected people are irresponsible in all aspects of their lives: family, employment, interpersonal relationships, and finances. They may ignore personal and financial promises and responsibilities. They live in the moment and are not concerned with the past or the future. Rules are made for other people, not for them.

People with Antisocial Personality Disorder show little remorse for the negative consequences of their behavior. They may believe that they should do anything necessary to ensure that others will not control them. These clients often blame their victims for weakness or foolishness, without any guilt or sorrow over their suffering or loss (American Psychiatric Association, 2000).

Antisocial Personality Disorder affects men more often than women. Approximately 1% of females are affected, whereas 3% of males have the disorder. The difference in gender rates may be due to the fact that the symptoms are different in men and women. Nurses will encounter clients with this disorder much more often in substance abuse treatment or in forensic (legal) settings, such as prison (American Psychiatric Association, 2000).

Collaborative Care

The first-priority short-term goal is no harm to others. The person with Antisocial Personality Disorder may be manipulative and physically violent, so these issues should be managed first. Other issues include anger management, coping skills, increasing self-awareness (insight), and learning to see an event from another person's point of view. The best personal approach to a client with this disorder is the most direct one. Nurses should tell the truth, clearly and concisely. The nurse should share perceptions about the emotional consequences of the client's behavior for others.

Facility rules should be communicated to the client and followed consistently by all staff. Antisocial clients are expert at getting staff to sympathize and break the rules "just this once." The staff must work together to help this client see that the rules apply to him or her as well as everyone else.

Group interventions can be especially helpful for people with this disorder. The group provides an opportunity for feedback to the client about other people's perceptions. Empathy is the biggest challenge for the client affected by Antisocial Personality Disorder.

CASE EXAMPLE

Consider the case of Andrew. He is a client on an orthopedic surgical unit. He sustained multiple fractures in a motor vehicle crash in which he was driving while intoxicated. A pedestrian was killed in the crash. He stated that the victim should not have been in the crosswalk when he was. Andrew stated to his nurse: "You are the best nurse in this hospital. Those other nurses never give me enough pain medicine. Can't you just give me a little extra this time? I really need it." All the nurses on the unit are struggling with this client. Some of the nurses are angry at each other for not caring enough for him. Others are angry with the client for manipulating the staff. *How can this client's nurse manage the care of this challenging client who has upset the entire unit?*

BORDERLINE PERSONALITY DISORDER

A psychoanalyst named Stern first used the term *Borderline Personality Disorder* in 1938. He was describing clients who seem to be on the border between *neurosis* (an outdated term for anxiety) and psychosis.

Marsha Linehan is a leading contemporary theorist on Borderline Personality Disorder. She and her colleagues believe that the disorder is caused by an interaction between biological and social learning influences (nature and nurture). Their research focuses on the behavior patterns in the disorder, which include the following (Linehan, 1993):

- *Emotional vulnerability.* A pattern of difficulty managing negative emotions; high sensitivity to negative emotional stimuli; and slower than normal return to baseline emotional level than the average person.
- *Self-invalidation.* Failure to recognize own emotions, thoughts, behaviors; setting unrealistically high expectations for self, making it impossible for self to be successful; intense shame and self-directed anger; and blaming others for unrealistic expectations because client has no insight.
- *Unrelenting crises.* Experiences frequent, stressful negative events, some caused by self, others not.
- *Inhibited grieving.* Client tries to overcontrol negative feelings, especially those associated with grieving such as guilt, sadness, shame, and anxiety.
- *Active passivity.* Affected person fails to work actively on solving own life problems; actively seeks out help from others for problem solving, resulting in helplessness and hopelessness.
- *Apparent competence.* Tends to appear to be more competent than s/he really is; may be unable to apply what is learned in one situation to other situations; may fail to display nonverbal cues of early emotional distress.

The biosocial theorists propose that Borderline Personality Disorder occurs when a vulnerable individual interacts with an invalidating environment. An invalidating environment is one in which the individual's feelings and emotions are negated. Their emotions are constantly dismissed, disrespected, trivialized, and punished by powerful others. The invalidating environment is often abusive. The ultimate invalidation is sexual abuse, which is a common experience of people with the disorder (Linehan, 1993; Zanarini, 2000).

The biological theorists suggest that people predisposed to the disorder have impaired regulation of the neural circuits that regulate emotion. Deficits in the ability to activate parts of the prefrontal cortex may cause inability to suppress negative emotion. The prefrontal cortex inhibits activity of the amygdala, which regulates negative emotion, including fear and arousal (Davidson, Jackson, & Kalin, 2000).

Clinical Features

Borderline Personality Disorder includes a pattern of impulsiveness and instability in interpersonal relationships, self-image, and emotions. These symptoms begin by early adulthood and are present in a variety of contexts in the affected person's life. Affected people have intense fear of abandonment. They make frantic efforts to avoid real or imagined abandonment by others. When the client perceives that separation, rejection, or loss of external structure are going to occur, the client can experience abrupt and profound changes in self-image, emotions, thinking, and behavior. Affected people are very sensitive to environmental circumstances. Being left by others may suggest to people with Borderline Personality Disorder that they are bad. They experience intense fears and inappropriate anger even when faced with expected separations (such as when a friend goes on vacation, someone is late for an appointment, or a favorite nurse has a day off work). They are intolerant of being alone. Clients may even injure themselves in an effort to prevent abandonment (American Psychiatric Association, 2000).

Affected people have a pattern of intense and unstable relationships. They may begin by idealizing a potential friend or partner, spending extensive amounts of time with them, and confiding their innermost thoughts early in the relationship. They might quickly and unexpectedly change to devaluing the person, saying that the formerly "perfect" friend or mate does not care or give enough. People with this disorder are able to cultivate relationships with others. However, they expect that the others will provide nurturance and be there to meet their considerable needs, on demand, at any moment (American Psychiatric Association, 2000).

Borderline Personality Disorder is also characterized by an unstable self-image or sense of self. Life goals, plans, values, sexual identity, and friends may change abruptly and impulsively. The self-image of affected people is based on the feeling that they are bad. They may also have the sense that they do not exist at all, or that they have no feelings. This is most likely to occur when they are feeling a lack of support. People with this disorder respond best to a predictable, structured environment (American Psychiatric Association, 2000).

Impulsivity is another hallmark of Borderline Personality Disorder. The diagnosis requires impulsivity in at least two areas that are potentially self-damaging (such as gambling, spending money irresponsibly, binge eating, unsafe sex, abusing substances, or self-injuring behavior) (American Psychiatric Association, 2000).

Self-harm is a common occurrence in this disorder. Completed suicide occurs in 8–10% of affected people. Self-injury without suicide intent (also called parasuicidal behavior), such as cutting, scratching, or burning self (Figure 10-6 ■), occurs much more frequently (Miller, 2006). Box 10-2 ■ lists clients' own reasons for cutting themselves.

The self-injuring behavior often starts when the client is concerned about abandonment or rejection, when the client is expected to assume more responsibility (such as just before graduation or a promotion at work). The self-harming behavior may occur during

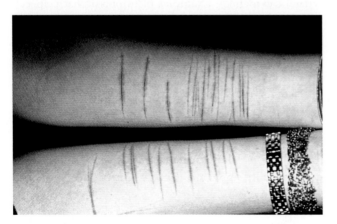

Figure 10-6. ■ Self-inflicted cuts by a young woman with Borderline Personality Disorder. *Source:* Photo Researchers, Inc.

BOX 10-2

Reality Check on Self-Injury

When asked why they cut themselves, clients with Borderline Personality Disorder have said:

- "Tension builds up and gets out of control until I feel the pain, then it is released."
- "When I have no feelings, cutting or burning myself makes me feel alive."
- "Other people can see how much they hurt me when I am bleeding."

---

dissociative or depersonalized experiences. *Depersonalization* (dissociation) is an alteration in the perception of the self in which the client feels like she is looking at herself from outside her body and does not feel pain from injury. Some clients state that the pain of the cutting or burning reaffirms that they are alive (American Psychiatric Association, 2000).

People with Borderline Personality Disorder also experience unstable emotions. Their mood is very reactive. This means that they have intense episodes of low mood, irritability, or anxiety that last only a few hours (or at most a few days) in reaction to various stressors. Their baseline low mood is often interrupted with episodes of anger, panic, or despair. They rarely have periods of well-being or satisfaction. These clients often express intense or inappropriate anger or have difficulty controlling their anger. They may have sarcastic or bitter outbursts. Inappropriate angry outbursts are often followed by shame and guilt and contribute to the affected person's feeling of being bad or evil. During periods of extreme stress, they may experience transient episodes of paranoia or depersonalization (American Psychiatric Association, 2000).

Borderline Personality Disorder is much more common in women than in men, with women making up 75% of cases. It is estimated that 2% of the general population is affected and 20% of psychiatric inpatients. Borderline Personality Disorder is five times more common among first-degree relatives of affected people than it is in the general population. There is also an increase in Substance-Related Disorders, Antisocial Personality Disorder, and Mood Disorders among family members (American Psychiatric Association, 2000).

The course of Borderline Personality Disorder often involves intense use of health and mental health resources. The most common pattern includes chronic instability with an increased rate of suicide attempts in early adulthood, followed by a gradual decrease in severity of the disorder with age (American Psychiatric Association, 2000).

Collaborative Care

Although there is no medication for Borderline Personality Disorder directly, it is commonly associated with depression. When it is, appropriate medications should be given to treat the depression.

The first treatment priority in psychosocial treatment is no self-harm. Other treatment issues are dysfunctional mood and impulsive behavior. Treatment of this disorder is long-term. It involves a treatment team of professionals (nurses, psychiatrist, social worker, psychologist, therapists) and the client working together.

Dialectical behavior therapy is a cognitive and behavioral therapy used specifically for Borderline Personality Disorder. Dialectical behavior therapy (DBT) has been shown to decrease suicidal behavior, hospitalization, and treatment dropout while improving interpersonal functioning and anger management. DBT theory begins with a validating treatment environment. Treatment focuses on client education and prioritizing treatment goals. Treatment techniques include behavior analysis, skills training and coaching, and management of responses to behavior (Swenson, Sanderson, Dulit, & Linehan, 2001).

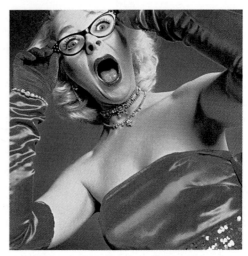

Figure 10-7. ■ Clients with Histrionic Personality Disorder may dress dramatically, and experience exaggerated emotions. *Source:* Photolibrary.com.

CASE EXAMPLE

Consider the case of Barbara. She is a 22-year-old European American woman who was admitted to the psychiatric unit of a general hospital after she went into a rage at a coffee shop. The police were called and found her to be screaming incoherently. She has many scars on her left arm. In the hospital she was initially screaming and pounding the walls with her fists. At this time, she is quiet and states that she is worthless. She hates herself for making such a scene at the coffee shop because her friend was late and she was given the wrong order.

Barbara said to the nurse: "I feel like cutting myself. When the pressure builds up this bad, only the cutting can make those feelings go away." *What can the nurse say to help Barbara? What can the nurse do to reduce the risk that Barbara will cut herself while she is in the hospital or at home?*

HISTRIONIC PERSONALITY DISORDER

The most important features of *Histrionic Personality Disorder* are excessive emotionality and attention-seeking behavior. People with Histrionic Personality Disorder need to be the center of attention. When they are not, they are uncomfortable or unhappy. They will often create a scene to bring attention to themselves (American Psychiatric Association, 2000).

The appearance of affected individuals is often inappropriately sexually provocative. Affected people often behave seductively in social, work, and other settings. Their seductive behavior is beyond what is socially appropriate for the setting. Their emotional expression may be shallow and changeable. Affected people use physical appearance to draw attention to themselves (Figure 10-7 ■). They spend inordinate time, energy, and money on clothes, jewelry, and grooming. Unflattering comments easily upset people with this disorder (American Psychiatric Association, 2000).

The speech of these clients is lacking in detail and excessively impressionistic (gives a general impression without evidence). Examples of impressionistic speech are "That nurse is the most insensitive person in the world," and "My dog is the greatest of his breed" with no reason for these conclusions. Affected people have strong opinions and express them dramatically, yet there is rarely any foundation for the opinion. Their emotions are exaggerated theatrically. They may embarrass friends and acquaintances by being too intimate, sobbing uncontrollably over minor sentiments, or having temper tantrums. The emotions, though dramatic, are turned on and off quickly and may seem insincere (American Psychiatric Association, 2000).

People with Histrionic Personality Disorder are very suggestible and easily influenced by others. They may be overly trusting, especially of authority figures. They often consider relationships to be more intimate than they really are. They have difficulty achieving close relationships. They may act dependent, while trying to control their partners with emotional manipulation. Affected people often alienate friends with their demands for attention. They may crave novelty and excitement. They have little tolerance for frustration or delayed gratification (American Psychiatric Association, 2000).

Gender role stereotypes can affect the way people express this disorder. For example, a man with Histrionic Personality Disorder may spend lots of time bodybuilding, buy a sports car that he cannot afford, and exaggerate his sexual exploits. An affected woman may dress in seductive clothes, demand that her friends admire her new outfits, and exaggerate what a "dear friend" some important person is.

Collaborative Care

People with this disorder do not often seek mental health care for it. When they do, it is often because they have experienced rejection, disapproval, or a period without satisfying relationships. These clients often have developed a negative self-concept. They may feel that they are incapable of successfully managing life on their own. They seek out others to complete their lives and to take care of them. The treatment goal is for clients to begin to focus on themselves for problem solving rather than expecting others to fulfill all their needs (Limandri & Boyd, 2005).

CASE EXAMPLE

Consider the case of Hester. She is a 30-year-old European American woman who is being seen in the sexually transmitted disease clinic for a case of *Chlamydia* infection. She is crying loudly and states to the nurse: "This is the worst thing that has ever happened. I don't know what to do! I think I should call my dear friend the Surgeon General!" The nurse knows that the clinic sees clients with *Chlamydia* infections daily and that it is treatable with antibiotics. *How can this nurse best help Hester cope with this stressful situation?*

NARCISSISTIC PERSONALITY DISORDER

Narcissistic Personality Disorder is characterized by a pervasive pattern of grandiosity, need for admiration, and lack of empathy for others. Affected people have an inflated sense of self-importance. They routinely overestimate their abilities and inflate their accomplishments. They expect that others will have the same high opinion of

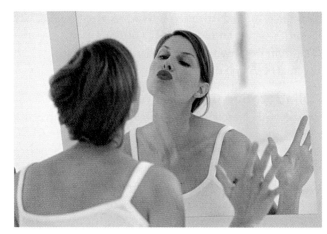

Figure 10-8. ■ A woman with Narcissistic Personality Disorder appreciates her reflection in the mirror. *Source:* Getty Images Inc.-Stone Allstock.

them. They may be surprised if they do not receive the fame and fortune they think they deserve. While these clients inflate their own abilities, they tend to underestimate the abilities of others (American Psychiatric Association, 2000).

People with Narcissistic Personality Disorder often have fantasies of unlimited success, power, beauty, or ideal love and compare themselves with famous people (Figure 10-8 ■). Affected people see themselves as superior to others and expect to be so recognized. They prefer to associate with other "special" people like themselves and may ask to see the head surgeon, head nurse, or head hairdresser. Only the best is good enough. People with this disorder require excessive admiration and have a sense of entitlement. They feel entitled to especially favorable treatment and automatic compliance with their wishes (American Psychiatric Association, 2000).

Affected people tend to exploit others and have little empathy for others' feelings. They assume that others are concerned about their feelings and needs. They present an emotional coldness and lack of reciprocal interest. Narcissistic Personality Disorder causes people to have arrogant, conceited behavior and attitudes. These people are often envious of others or believe that others are envious of them. They are quick to criticize, yet hate to be criticized. Their interpersonal relationships are usually impaired because of their insensitivity to others' feelings, their need for constant admiration, and the problems with entitlement. Their functioning as employees may be impaired when they are unable to take risks due to fear of the humiliation of failure. Many people with this disorder also have depression, eating disorders, and substance-related disorders. Narcissistic Personality Disorder occurs in less than 1% of the general population, more commonly in men than in women (American Psychiatric Association, 2000).

Collaborative Care

People with Narcissistic Personality Disorder are only seen in the inpatient setting when they are admitted for another disorder. It is often difficult for nurses to relate to these clients because of their poor social skills and arrogance. To work with clients with personality disorders, nurses must understand themselves first. Nurses must have the insight to know what type of behavior is stressful to them so they can manage their own stress without giving it back to the client. Direct communication with clear expectations for client behavior and clear and consistent limits is important for these clients. Treatment goals for this personality disorder include developing coping skills that involve independent problem solving without exploitation of others.

CASE EXAMPLE

Consider the case of Nate. Nate is a 58-year-old European American male who was admitted to the postsurgical unit after a partial gastrectomy. He is demanding of the staff. He refuses to allow the nursing assistant to take his blood pressure, demanding that the surgeon or the charge nurse do it. When his assigned nurse comes in to assess his surgical wound he says, "Bring the Chief of Surgery in here! I want the best to take care of me, not the likes of you." *What can the nurse say to this client? How can the nurse communicate the reasonable boundaries for this person's behavior?*

Cluster C Personality Disorders: Anxious-Fearful

AVOIDANT PERSONALITY DISORDER

People with *Avoidant Personality Disorder* have a pervasive pattern of social shyness, feelings of inadequacy, and hypersensitivity to negative evaluation. Because they fear disapproval or rejection, they avoid work or school activities that involve significant contact with other people. They may decline offers of job promotion to avoid potential criticism of coworkers. They avoid making new friends unless they are sure to be accepted without criticism. They assume other people to be critical and disapproving. Affected people would like to have social relationships, but

they hesitate to join in social activities. They are preoccupied with thoughts of being criticized or rejected. They view themselves as socially inept, unappealing, or inferior. Their self-esteem is very low. They limit themselves in intimate relationships due to the fear of shame or ridicule. They are unusually reluctant to engage in new activities because of the chance of embarrassment. They may have a fearful and tense manner (American Psychiatric Association, 2000).

In contrast to other personality disorders in which affected people have no desire to socialize with others, people with Avoidant Personality Disorder want to have contact with other people but find themselves unable to take the risk of rejection. Other personality disorders may combine with this one. This disorder affects women and men equally. It occurs in an estimated 0.5–1% of the general population (American Psychiatric Association, 2000).

Collaborative Care

Treatment goals for clients with this disorder include improving self-esteem, developing a trusting relationship, developing adaptive coping skills, and improving social skills. Symptoms in some people with Avoidant Personality Disorder are reduced when they take antianxiety and antidepressant medications.

CASE EXAMPLE

Consider the case of Andrea. Andrea is a 28-year-old Latina with Avoidant Personality Disorder. She has never had a boyfriend, although she secretly fantasizes about being the girlfriend of a rock musician. She is hospitalized in the general hospital after being injured while riding her bicycle. The nurse expects that Andrea should be in severe pain because of the type of injuries she has, but Andrea has never asked for pain medication. In fact, she has never asked for anything. *How can the nurse assess and evaluate Andrea's level of pain? How can Andrea be made comfortable in the hospital?*

DEPENDENT PERSONALITY DISORDER

A need to be taken care of characterizes *Dependent Personality Disorder*. People with this disorder have submissive and clinging behavior; they fear separation and abandonment. They have difficulty making everyday decisions without excessive help and advice from others. They are passive and allow others to take responsibility for major areas of their lives. They have difficulty expressing disagreement due to fear of loss of support or approval. Doing things independently is difficult for these people because they have so little self-confidence. They believe that others can do things better than they can, so they take no initiative and allow others to start projects (American Psychiatric Association, 2000).

Affected people may fear abandonment so much that they will act as though they are incompetent and in need of help just to maintain the support of others. They submit to the will of others, even if the demands are unreasonable. They make great self-sacrifices and submit to abuse, even though other choices are available. When they are alone, affected individuals feel fearful and helpless because they feel unable to take care of themselves (American Psychiatric Association, 2000).

When a close relationship ends, a person who has Dependent Personality Disorder may urgently seek another relationship to replace the care that they so desperately need. They may quickly and indiscriminately attach to another person. Fear of the necessity for self-care and responsibility may become an obsession. Even when there are no grounds to justify these fears, they have excessive and unrealistic fears of abandonment. These individuals have a pessimistic outlook and tend to minimize their own abilities and strengths. Their self-esteem is determined by the reactions of others (American Psychiatric Association, 2000).

The disorder may affect an individual's occupational functioning if a job requires initiative or decision making. People with Dependent Personality Disorder try to avoid positions in which they will be required to make decisions. Their social behavior tends to be warm and giving. Social relationships are usually limited to the few people on whom the individual is dependent (American Psychiatric Association, 2000).

Like the other personality disorders, Dependent Personality Disorder is difficult to diagnose across cultures. *The degree of dependent behavior that is considered normal varies across ages and cultures.* So, the cultural expectations of the client must be considered when interpreting the client's behavior. An individual must have dependency behavior clearly in excess of what is expected by her/his culture to be diagnosed with this disorder (American Psychiatric Association, 2000).

Collaborative Care

This is one of the most common disorders to be seen in mental health clinics, although clients usually seek help for other complaints (American Psychiatric Association, 2000). Nurses will be likely to encounter clients with Dependent Personality Disorder in various practice settings. These clients will probably expect the nurse to make their decisions for them. The challenge for the nurse is to support the client to make her/his own decisions without giving advice on how to act.

Nurses often have the opportunity to reinforce the need for long-term psychotherapy or counseling. This is the most effective way for people to change their personalities or to learn adaptive ways to cope with the personalities they have. The nurse should determine whether a client has outpatient providers for psychotherapy when clients are admitted for inpatient care. When clients are in an inpatient setting (usually for some other problem than their personalities), nurses can encourage them to continue with their therapy after discharge. Nurses may also consult with physicians and social workers on the treatment team about referral of clients to therapists or therapy groups when they are discharged.

CASE EXAMPLE

Consider the case of David. David is an 18-year-old Nigerian American male client admitted to the hospital for peritonitis following an appendectomy for a ruptured appendix. He sees a therapist weekly to work on his Dependent Personality Disorder. The nurse asked David during the nursing admission history if he is going to school or working. He states that his mother wants him to attend Portland Community College to study computer technology. He has been an ideal client: he drinks, eats, and ambulates when he is told, even if he is not hungry or thirsty or has too much pain to want to ambulate. He is anxious when his mother leaves the hospital to buy some school clothes for him. David will have a wound drain with a simple dressing change that must be done daily when he goes home. When the nurse wants to teach him how to do the dressing change, he says, "My mother will do it. Please wait to teach her. She'll be back in 15 minutes." *How can the nurse promote David's independence?*

OBSESSIVE-COMPULSIVE PERSONALITY DISORDER

Obsessive-Compulsive Personality Disorder is characterized by a preoccupation with orderliness, perfectionism, and mental and personal control. Affected individuals are so orderly and controlling that they cannot be flexible, open, or efficient. People with this disorder try to maintain a sense of control through painstaking attention to rules, trivial details, lists, and schedules, until the main point of the project is lost. Extraordinary attention is paid to detail and to checking repeatedly for possible mistakes. Affected people are oblivious to the fact that other people find the delays caused by their behavior to be aggravating. They expect themselves to be perfect. When this is not possible, it causes significant stress and dysfunction. They may be so involved in making every detail of a job perfect that they can never finish it. They are excessively devoted to work to the exclusion of other activities such as family, friends, and fun. If they have hobbies, they treat the hobby like a job with meticulous detailed requirements. If they do play, it is always by the rules, and play becomes work or a lesson (American Psychiatric Association, 2000).

They are overly conscientious and inflexible about matters of morality. They adhere to very strict rules of performance and may force others to do so as well. People with this disorder defer to authority and insist on following rules without exception for any reason. They may criticize themselves without mercy for their own mistakes (American Psychiatric Association, 2000).

People with Obsessive-Compulsive Personality Disorder may be unable to throw away things that are worn out or worthless, even when they have no sentimental value (Figure 10-9 ■). They are reluctant to delegate tasks to others. They insist that everything be done their way, because only they can do things right. They stubbornly and unreasonably expect others to do things according to their detailed instructions and are surprised and irritated by others' creative alternatives. Affected people may be miserly. They may hoard their resources out of an attitude that spending must be limited to provide for future emergencies. They may live far below their means. They are known for being rigid, indecisive, and stubborn. They

plan ahead in meticulous detail and will not consider changes to their plans. It is difficult for people with this disorder to consider the perspectives of others. Their expression of emotion is tightly controlled and they are often uncomfortable around people who are emotionally expressive (American Psychiatric Association, 2000).

Hoarding items such as newspapers, magazines, canned foods may be associated with Obsessive-Compulsive Personality Disorder. Even collecting stray animals may fall into this category. Clients with this symptom acquire goods (as in compulsive shopping) and then are unable to discard any of their possessions. Their living spaces become compromised and unusable due to the accumulation of clutter. These clients are subjected to extraordinary anxiety when faced with discarding any of their items. Health issues such as fire hazards and sanitation may become concerns as well (Bohrer & Haynes, 2005).

Obsessive-Compulsive Personality Disorder occurs in approximately 1% of the general population and 3–10% of clients in mental illness clinics. It is diagnosed about twice as often in men (American Psychiatric Association, 2000).

Obsessive-Compulsive *Personality* Disorder is not the same as Obsessive-Compulsive Disorder (OCD). OCD is characterized by true *obsessions* (uncontrollable desire to continue thinking about an idea or feeling) and *compulsions* (repetitive stereotyped acts done to relieve anxiety that are a response to obsessive thoughts). Another difference is that people with OCD recognize the limitations placed on them by the disorder, whereas people with OCPD do not, as their behavior is so ingrained in their personality. See Chapter 11 for more information on OCD.

Collaborative Care

As with the other disorders of personality, long-term therapy is the only effective treatment for the pervasive pattern of Obsessive-Compulsive Personality Disorder. In the short term, clients with the disorder may seek medical help for anxiety or related symptoms. In these time-limited situations, antianxiety medications may be prescribed. The nurse will focus on how the client is affected by the disorder in such areas as coping, sleeping, nutrition, and interpersonal relationships.

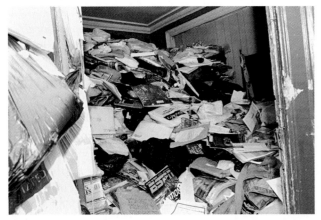

Figure 10-9. ■ A client with Obsessive-Compulsive Personality Disorder hoarded these magazines. When the stacks fell over, he was trapped beneath them. *Source:* The Image Works.

CASE EXAMPLE

Consider the case of Oscar, a 77-year-old Mexican American who has Obsessive-Compulsive Personality Disorder. Oscar is a resident of a subacute treatment facility where he is recovering from a total hip arthroplasty (replacement). Every time the nurse leaves extra dressing supplies in the room, they disappear. Oscar asks for extra medicine cups and saves dishes from his meal trays in his room. He becomes agitated when anything is moved. The housekeeper found a hoard of hospital supplies in his closet and piles of hospital linens under his bed. *What should the nurse do about this behavior?*

NURSING CARE

ASSESSING

The physician or psychiatrist will make the medical diagnosis of a personality disorder. The role of the nurse is to help clients deal with the effects of the disorder. Personality is developed over years of learning to cope with the challenges of life. So, a client's personality itself is very resistant to change. As part of the treatment team, nurses encourage clients to begin or to continue psychotherapy (with nurse practitioner, psychologist, psychiatrist, clinical social worker, or other therapist on an outpatient basis). Nurses also assess the client's short-term needs related to

the disorders of personality. These needs become apparent as the nurse assesses the client's functional ability, mental status, and interpersonal relationships.

The nurse often gains information about clients' personality from their significant others. Because personality is so integral to a person's self-identity, individuals usually do not see abnormalities in their own personality. However, the disorders of personality covered in this chapter are evident to those who are close to the client. A friend or family member may be of great help to the nurse in identifying how a client behaves or copes with problems at home.

DIAGNOSING, PLANNING, AND IMPLEMENTING

Table 10-2 ■ provides common nursing diagnoses for people with specific personality disorders, divided by cluster.

Critical Self-Check. Look at the nursing diagnoses presented for personality disorders. Do you see patterns of problems there? Are some problems common to most of the disorders?

TABLE 10-2

Common Nursing Diagnoses for People with Personality Disorders

CLUSTER A: ODD-ECCENTRIC DISORDERS	CLUSTER B: DRAMATIC-EMOTIONAL DISORDERS	CLUSTER C: ANXIOUS-FEARFUL DISORDERS
Paranoid Personality Disorder ■ Defensive Coping ■ Disturbed Thought Processes ■ Impaired Social Interaction	**Antisocial Personality Disorder** ■ Risk for Other-Directed Violence ■ Ineffective Coping ■ Noncompliance (specify) ■ Impaired Social Interaction	**Avoidant Personality Disorder** ■ Chronic Low Self-Esteem ■ Social Isolation ■ Ineffective Coping
Schizoid and Schizotypal Personality Disorders ■ Impaired Social Interaction ■ Chronic Low Self-Esteem ■ Disturbed Thought Processes	**Borderline Personality Disorder** ■ Risk for Self-Mutilation ■ Risk for Other-Directed Violence ■ Ineffective Coping ■ Noncompliance (specify) ■ Chronic Low Self-Esteem ■ Risk for Suicide ■ Social Isolation	**Dependent Personality Disorder** ■ Ineffective Coping ■ Chronic Low Self-Esteem ■ Impaired Social Interaction ■ Social Isolation ■ Powerlessness
	Histrionic Personality Disorder ■ Ineffective Coping ■ Chronic Low Self-Esteem ■ Impaired Social Interaction	**Obsessive-Compulsive Personality Disorder** ■ Anxiety ■ Impaired Social Interaction ■ Ineffective Coping
	Narcissistic Personality Disorder ■ Impaired Social Interaction ■ Ineffective Coping	

Following each section on a personality disorder, there was a case study in which you were asked to consider a client situation. There were questions about nursing interventions for problems relating to the clients' personality disorders. Each of the questions from the case studies is covered in this section. You will learn more from this section if you think about the questions before you read the answers and rationales. The suggested interventions here can be used in a variety of situations, not only with the specific personality disorders listed.

Paranoid Personality Disorder

Our first case is Peter, who has Paranoid Personality Disorder. He is going to have surgery, and he thinks the surgeon might kill him. He thinks the nurse might try to give him another client's medications. The question is about how the nurse can make it possible for the staff to provide care for this client while decreasing his level of stress.

- Remember that people with paranoid personality are very aware of who has the power. *The nurse may need to ask the surgeon to reassure this client that she will take good care of him.*
- Do not ignore the client's suspicion about medications, but do not overemphasize the fears of the client, either. If the client requests complicated confirmation that the medications are his, the nurse should respectfully and briefly reassure him that they are the correct medications, but not engage in any elaborate unnecessary plans. *His suspiciousness about the medications is common in people with his disorder. It may be enough to tell the client confidently that the nurse checked these medications personally and they are accurate. The nurse could bring the medications still wrapped in their individual dose wrappers to reassure the client that they are his medications. When the reason for a client's suspiciousness is paranoia, excessive and elaborate proof (bringing in the client's chart with every medication, calling the pharmacist, etc.) does not really help.*
- Approach this client with a matter-of-fact, professional attitude. *This client will not respond to a friendly approach by the nurse and may even see friendliness as weakness.*
- Reassure the client that he will be safe and that the staff is making every effort to provide accurate, quality care for him. *The nurse's confidence may be reassuring to the client. People with paranoia seem to be aggressive, but their feelings are often fear and insecurity.*

Schizoid Personality Disorder

Our client in this case is Sid, who has Schizoid Personality Disorder. He is in the emergency department after a bus accident and the nurse wonders why his affect is so flat. Is he in shock, or is he always like this?

- If possible, enlist the help of family in understanding the client. *Sid is unlikely to have enough insight into his own personality to explain to the nurse why he does not express emotions. His brother, who is in the emergency department with him, is probably the best source of information about his usual behavior. When the brother tells the nurse that Sid has always been like this, the nurse can be reassured that his affect is not due to the acute situation, but is due to his personality.*
- Ask if the client would like help with problems related to the personality disorder. *Sid is in the hospital for a cut on his arm, not for treatment of his personality. The nurse may ask if he would like help with any other problems; if so, he can be given a referral. If not, he can be discharged when his laceration is treated.*

Schizotypal Personality Disorder

Sylvia lives in a long-term care facility and has Schizotypal Personality Disorder. She has some eccentric behaviors that don't bother her, but the other residents avoid her. She thinks that people are stealing her things and that she can find thieves by looking in their eyes. The question is "What can the nurse do to make this client socialize more and be more comfortable in the facility?"

- Provide low-stress opportunities for Sylvia to be with other people, such as eating at a table with others at mealtime. *This client does not really want to socialize with other people, but the nurse knows that some contact with other people is important for mental health. It would be unrealistic for the nurse to expect Sylvia to do lots of socializing with other residents; this is not in her nature.*
- Provide some social skills training, such as asking her if she would like to wear her necklaces around her neck instead of over her ears. *If she dresses and behaves in ways that the other residents accept, she may be more accepted. The nurse should not take the idea of conformity too far, however. (People have a right to self-expression.) This concept is best used when a client's appearance is frightening or disagreeable to others and the client wants to interact with people more.*
- Find out if people really are stealing from the client. (Just because she is always suspicious does not mean that her suspicions are always unfounded.) If this is a

Corrective Statements for Distorted Thoughts

Thought Distortion: "This is the worst thing that has ever happened."
Corrective Statement: "True, this is a bad thing, but it is not the worst thing that ever happened." (*Giving perspective allows client to see the real placement of this stressful event as it relates to life priorities.*)
Thought Distortion: "I could NEVER do anything like you are suggesting."
Corrective Statement: "You have already done things like this before, such as . . ." (*Giving examples makes the implied generalization specific.*)
Thought Distortion: "If only I hadn't made him mad, he wouldn't have beat me up."
Corrective Statement: "He is an adult and responsible for his own behavior. You are responsible for your own behavior, not his." (*Stating the mature reality of the situation helps the client see it from another point of view.*)
Thought Distortion: "My boyfriend left me. This will kill me. I can't go on."
Corrective Statement: "You have survived disappointments before. You are strong enough to handle this. Let's talk about how you feel." (*Allowing client to discuss and examine feelings increases insight and promotes the ability to learn from past experiences and to apply current learning to future situations.*)
Thought Distortion: "Nobody understands me."
Corrective Statement: "Let's talk about how you feel, so I can understand." (*Suggesting a problem-solving approach promotes adaptive coping.*)

distortion of thinking, reassure her that no theft has occurred. *An example of a helpful comment by the nurse might be: "See, Sylvia, here is your diamond tiara, nobody took it." An example of a not-so-helpful comment by the nurse would be: "Sylvia, you are so suspicious. Nobody is stealing your things."*

■ Try some corrective statements. Box 10-3 ■ gives examples of how to adjust unfounded observations toward more realistic thinking.

Antisocial Personality Disorder

Andrew has Antisocial Personality Disorder. He was in a motor vehicle crash in which he killed a pedestrian. He has multiple fractures and has an order for p.r.n. pain medication. The nurses are upset and angry at each other. Some sympathize with him and think he needs nurturing; others think he is manipulating the staff. What is the nurse to do?

This situation (where client has staff upset and angry at each other) is more common than you may realize.

Box 10-4 ■ provides some ideas on how to respond when the client tries to pit the staff against each other.

■ Understand your own attitudes and behave professionally. *Sometimes it can be frustrating to work with people with personality disorders. When nurses realize that the client's behavior is related to a personality disorder, and not an intentional effort to aggravate the staff, it is easier for the nurse to be objective.*

■ In charting, provide specific, objective observations and avoid judgmental comments. This note is clear: "The client stated: 'I am the king of the world and you are all fired. You are a bunch of lazy dogs.'" This note is not clear: "The client rudely insulted the staff." *The chart of this client may be used in court because he broke the law before he was admitted to the hospital. Sometimes nurses' assessments and comments in charts are used to help the court decide whether a client is legally competent to stand trial. Charting can also be used to document the quality of a client's care.*

Borderline Personality Disorder

Barbara is a 22-year-old woman with Borderline Personality Disorder. She had an overreaction to a small frustration. The police brought her to the psychiatric hospital. She has scars on her left arm from self-injury. She tells the nurse that she feels like cutting herself to release the pressure she feels. What can the nurse do to decrease the risk that she will cut herself now and when she goes home?

■ Ask the client how she got the scars. *She will probably say that they are the result of cutting herself. They are on her left arm, and she is probably right-handed. This suggests that she regularly uses self-mutilation as a coping mechanism.*

■ Help the client identify early internal cues of distress (such as pounding heart, sense of uneasiness, nervousness) (Linehan, 1993). *Identifying the symptoms of distress early can allow the client time to respond in an adaptive way.*

■ Write the cues of distress listed by the client on a card and give it to the client (or the client can write the list on a card herself). *The client can refer to the card later in a time of distress.*

■ Teach the client skills for tolerating a stressful event. The mnemonic "Wise mind ACCEPTS" can help the client remember the steps:
  Activities to distract from stress
  Contributing to others such as volunteering or visiting a sick neighbor
  Comparing yourself to people less fortunate than you
  Emotions that are opposite what you are experiencing
  Pushing away from the situation for a while
  Thoughts other than you are currently thinking
  Sensations that are intense, such as holding ice in your hand

BOX 10-4	NURSING CARE CHECKLIST

Preventing Personality Disordered Clients from Upsetting the Unit

☑ Make the unit rules clear. *People with some personality disorders (such as Antisocial, Borderline, Histrionic, and Narcissistic) may not have adaptive social and coping skills. They may be practiced in manipulating people in charge to give them exceptions to the rules. They may not believe that the rules are for them.*

Example: Unit policy is that televisions are turned off at 10 P.M. A client wants to watch TV until 3 A.M. "just this once."

☑ Stick to the rules consistently. This means everybody. *When staff responds to the manipulative client inconsistently, there is opportunity for the client to pit the staff against each other.*

Example: A client asked a nurse if he could have his pain medication a little bit early. The nurse gave it 30 minutes before it was scheduled. He asked the next nurse to do the same thing. She refused. The client told the first nurse that she is his favorite and that he only wants her to care for him, not the mean nurse who won't help him with his pain. Now the client wants the nurse to give him "just a little extra medicine, just this once, I really need it." Some of the nurses sympathize with the client's apparent pain, others think he is manipulative, and the entire unit is upset.

☑ When a client is causing staff to be upset, have a conference. *In the above situation, some nurses think one thing, others think another, and still others are unaware that there is a controversy. The client is treated differently every shift. The client is focusing on manipulating the staff and the staff is focusing on controlling the client's behavior. When everyone works together and receives the same information (including the client), the client is best served.*

Example: A systematic approach to the situation would include an assessment of the client's problem (pain) with an appropriate prescription by the physician; an around-the-clock dosing schedule instead of p.r.n. doses so the client does not need to ask for the med—it will automatically be given; adherence to the schedule by all nurses in the same way; and feedback from the client about how pain is managed.

☑ Include the client in problem solving. *When a client's behavior is problematic, the client has an opportunity to learn how to change to more adaptive behavior only if the client is included in discussions of problem-solving strategies. Clients with personality disorders can benefit from discussion on how their behavior affects others because they often do not understand others' perspectives.*

Example: A client asks every staff member to give him coffee. He is drinking 20 cups of coffee a day. His nurse realizes this and tells the rest of the staff to limit the coffee. The client continues to ask; sometimes he receives coffee, other times he doesn't. He asks for coffee 50 times a day. When the client is included in the discussion and is told that he will be given three cups of regular coffee and three cups of decaffeinated coffee each day, and that he can choose when he drinks them, he limits his requests to the designated times.

☑ Remember who is the client and who is the professional. *It is easy to react emotionally when clients act inappropriately or make personal comments. When clients flatter or insult nurses, it is challenging not to respond personally, but it is critical for nurses to respond to clients professionally. The goal is not a friendship with the client, but professional client care. Maladaptive behavior by the client is a learning opportunity.*

Example: A client stated: "I don't want that fat one to be my nurse. I want my favorite nurse." A good response by the nurse is: "Your nurse is Jack. When you talk like that, it hurts people's feelings. How could you ask for what you want in a nicer way?"

■ Write the coping skills on the back of the symptom card so the client will have everything available when a distressing situation arises. *The client is to identify when the feelings suggesting distress are beginning. Then, the client uses the coping skills that go with Wise mind ACCEPTS.*

Linehan (1993) also proposed the Five Senses Exercise to help people who have used self-harm for coping to find more enduring and adaptive ways to comfort themselves. The Five Senses Exercise follows:

1. **Vision** (for example, go outside and look at the stars or flowers or autumn leaves)

2. **Hearing** (for example, listen to beautiful or invigorating music or the sounds of nature or the city)

3. **Smell** (for example, light a scented candle, boil a cinnamon stick in water)

4. **Taste** (for example, drink a soothing, warm nonalcoholic drink)

5. **Touch** (for example, take a hot bubble bath, pet your dog or cat, get a massage)

■ Tell all clients who have thoughts about self-mutilation, self-injury, or suicide to notify the staff if they feel like hurting themselves while they are in the hospital. An agreement to notify staff of thoughts of self-harm is called a "no self-harm contract." Some nurses write out a statement for the client to sign that says, "I promise that if I feel like hurting myself I will tell the staff before I do it." *The idea is that the client is stating that s/he is in control of her/his own behavior and will try not to hurt self. When the client does tell the nurse of these feelings, the nurse will begin with encouraging the client to talk about and examine the feelings that led to the self-harm thinking. Alternatives to self-harm are then discussed. After the talking if the client still feels like harming self, the nurse will consult the treatment team. Antianxiety medication or other interventions may be indicated.*

Histrionic Personality Disorder

Hester has Histrionic Personality Disorder. She feels like having a sexually transmitted disease is "the worst thing that has ever happened." The question is about how the nurse can help Hester cope with this stressful situation.

It is true that having an STD is not a good thing, but it is not really the worst thing that *ever* happened. This is a thought distortion, which is a common occurrence in this disorder. People tend to exaggerate the severity of their problems and the grandeur of their triumphs. They tend to take a kernel of truth and use it to paint a whole picture that is not founded in reality.

- See Box 10-3 for examples of how to present a problem in a more realistic light.

Narcissistic Personality Disorder

Our client here is Nate, who has Narcissistic Personality Disorder. He is hospitalized after surgery and he thinks that the world revolves around him. He is making many unreasonable demands for special treatment (a feature of his disorder). He demands that only the charge nurse or surgeon take his blood pressure and wants the chief of surgery to do his nursing care. How can the nurse respectfully set appropriate limits for this client?

Nate is experiencing a thought distortion. He thinks that he is the most important client and that the hospital should change to cater to him. It would be good for Nate to understand that although he is important, every client is important. The chief of surgery and the charge nurse have their own responsibilities, which do not include doing his nursing care. The chief of surgery would probably not know how to do his nursing care anyway.

- In a matter-of-fact and professional manner, the nurse must tell Nate that the nursing assistant is the one who takes blood pressure in this hospital. She is the most experienced person at this job and takes an accurate measurement. Ruth, the nurse, will be caring for

him and if he has any questions, Ruth will be glad to answer them. The surgeon will visit once each day for approximately 10 minutes. If he has any questions for the surgeon, they can be asked then. *This communication is clear, professional, caring, and contains the information the client needs. An overly friendly attitude with this client might suggest weakness to the client. The client needs a confident approach in order for him to trust that the nurse has the authority to decide what to do.*

- Repeat the message calmly if necessary. Do not take this client's criticism personally. *The nurse is setting reasonable limits. Catering to this client's every whim would be more than a full-time job. The role of the nurse is to provide professional care for this and all clients, not to be a friend to them.* His criticism is related to his disorder, not to the nurse's competence.

Avoidant Personality Disorder

Our client in this case is Andrea, who has Avoidant Personality Disorder. She was injured in a bicycling accident and is in pain. She never asks for pain medication or anything else. How can the nurse assess this client's pain and keep her comfortable?

- Establish a trusting relationship. When possible, a consistent nurse should be assigned to this client. *Andrea has such low self-esteem that she is unable to ask the nurse to help her. When she trusts the nurse she will be more likely to express her feelings and needs openly.*
- Offer this client medication frequently if it seems that she is in pain. *Pain management is a critical priority.*
- Help the client practice asking for what she needs, giving positive reinforcement when she asks for something. Correct the client when she says she does not deserve help. *This client could benefit from a discussion of her thought distortion (that she does not deserve help). Practicing new behavior (asking for help) can encourage the client to continue this behavior.*

Dependent Personality Disorder

David is the ideal client. Watch out for this. He has Dependent Personality Disorder and expects others to make all his decisions for him. He plans to let his mother decide what job he does and what he wears to school. He always does what the nurse asks without question. He needs to have a daily dressing change at home and wants his mother to do it. How can the nurse promote his independence?

- Begin by suggesting to the client, without his mother present, that it would be appropriate for him to do his own dressing change. He could even be allowed time to think about it. If he agrees, the nurse could teach him how using the three-step teaching process: The nurse demonstrates; nurse helps client do it; client does it alone. *This is a growth opportunity for the client.*

- If necessary, teach the mother to do the dressing change. *The priority is that the dressing will be changed. Although the nurse wants this client to change his dependent behavior, clients only change their behavior when THEY want to do so.*

Obsessive-Compulsive Personality Disorder

Our final client is Oscar, who has Obsessive-Compulsive Personality Disorder. He has a new total hip replacement, and yet he is up and about in his room checking on his piles of things. What should the nurse do about this behavior?

- Make certain that Oscar has all the information he needs to ambulate safely. *He will follow the rules if he understands them.*

- Provide medication to keep his pain under control. *It is often difficult to get clients out of bed after surgery to ambulate and move around to decrease their risks of deep vein thrombosis, pneumonia, and skin breakdown. Oscar is up and taking care of his potential risks of immobility, but he is likely to be in pain.*

- Tell Oscar that the housekeeper must mop the floor, and that an accumulation of linens under his bed is a fire or infection hazard. The dirty dishes may also be an infection hazard. *The nurse must try to compromise whenever possible, but safety takes priority. The client must be told gently but authoritatively that the potential dangers must be removed. Emphasize that the reason is safety. If the client is very stressed by the process, he might prefer to wait outside his room while the items are removed. The nurse might be able to find some compromise, such as allowing him to keep his extra medicine cups or packaged crackers.*

- Give the client choices about his care whenever possible. *Choices, such as those relating to daily activities (when to bathe, meal choices, when to ambulate, where to put items at the bedside, etc.) can help the client have a sense of control. A sense of control can decrease anxiety. If he feels better having a supply of dressing materials in his closet, the nurse could use these instead of hospital stock (they came from hospital stock originally).*

EVALUATING

The desired outcomes for clients with personality disorders relate to resolving the effects these disorders have on clients. Nurses will intervene based on the individual client's needs and determine whether the client experiences the following effects as a result of the interventions. The client will demonstrate the following:

- Effective, adaptive coping behavior
- No harm to self or others
- Adequate sleep to feel rested during the day
- Appropriate interactions with other people
- Making positive statements about self
- Taking initiative to solve problems
- Following unit rules
- Asking for help directly and appropriately
- Reality-based thinking

A client's personality is a stable way the client responds to the world. It is difficult to change. The most successful nursing interventions will be based on realistic, practical, and attainable goals.

NURSING PROCESS CARE PLAN
Client with Borderline Personality Disorder

Brenda Bacon is a 23-year-old Bulgarian American female client admitted to the short-stay unit for multiple lacerations she received when she ran through a glass door. She seems to be a very passionate person, who expresses her concerns loudly and with emotion. She told the admitting nurse that she ran through the door because her boyfriend was planning to leave her and she could not stand it. The client was seeing a psychiatrist and a therapist regularly for Borderline Personality Disorder but stopped treatment because "It wasn't helping."

Assessment. Ms. Bacon's lacerations on her head, shoulders, and right knee are sutured and the dressings are clean and dry. On admission the chart says that she was loud and emotional. Now she is quiet and expressing remorse for her impulsive behavior. She states that she is worthless and that her boyfriend is too good to deserve such a terrible person. She is right-handed and has multiple healed laceration scars on her left arm. When the nurse asked about them, Brenda stated, "Sometimes I have to cut myself to know that I'm alive. Sometimes I do it to stop the stress." When it was time for the nurse's shift to end, Brenda cried and begged the nurse not to leave her like everyone else has.

Diagnosis

- Risk for Self-Directed Violence
- Ineffective Coping
- Impaired Skin Integrity

Expected Outcomes. The client will:

- Not harm herself.
- Notify the nurse when she feels increasing stress or when she feels like cutting herself.
- Express her feelings to the nurse.
- List adaptive coping methods that she could use during stress.
- Keep lacerations clean and dry.
- Heal without signs or symptoms of infection.

Planning and Implementation

- Assign consistent staff to this client and have consistent expectations for behavior.
- Show client how to contact nurse.
- Teach client to call nurse when she is feeling stressed, so the nurse can talk with her about adaptive coping to avoid self-injury.
- Actively listen to the client's concerns.
- Help client list alternative healthy coping mechanisms that are realistic for her.

- Teach basic wound healing information (have good nutrition, keep lesions clean and dry).

Evaluation. Brenda was hospitalized for 2 days. During that time she had several angry outbursts at staff members when she perceived that her needs were not being met. She had long discussions with the nurse about her feelings and abuse history. She did not injure herself while she was in the hospital. Her boyfriend decided to stay with her, because she needs him so badly. Her lacerations healed well.

Critical Thinking in the Nursing Process

1. The nurse suggested that Brenda try listening to music when she feels stressed. Brenda found this to be helpful. Will this resolve her problem with ineffective coping?
2. The nurse believes that Brenda should return to therapy for the personality disorder. What can the nurse do to ensure that this will happen?
3. When Brenda said, "You won't give me more medication, I hate you! Give me another nurse," what response by the nurse is the best for Brenda?

Note: Discussion of Critical Thinking questions appears in Appendix I.

Note: The references and resources for this and all chapters have been compiled at the back of the book.

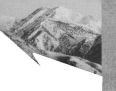
 KEY TERMS

Use the audio glossary feature of the Companion Website to hear the correct pronunciation of the following key terms.

ideas of reference

vicious cycle of behavior

KEY Points

- Personality disorders cause people to have abnormalities in perception or cognition, affect, interpersonal functioning, and impulse control.

- Nurses often see people with personality disorders when they are hospitalized for reasons other than their personality disorder.

- Personality develops over years starting in childhood and is very resistant to change.

- There is no medication to treat disorders of personality. Some people respond to long-term psychotherapy for changing the pervasive patterns of personality. Sometimes medications are used to treat symptoms.

- Most people with personality disorders do not know that they are affected.

- Nurses can help people with personality disorders achieve personal growth.

- It can be very challenging to care for people with personality disorders. Nurses who work with them must understand themselves and their professional responsibilities to be most effective.

- The most successful nursing interventions will be based on realistic, practical, attainable goals.

 EXPLORE Media Link

Additional interactive resources for this chapter can be found on the Companion Website at www.prenhall.com/eby. Click on Chapter 10 and "Begin" to select the activities for this chapter.

- Audio glossary
- NCLEX-PN® review
- Case study
- Study outline
- Critical thinking questions
- Matching questions
- Weblinks
- Video Case: Paul (Antisocial Personality Disorder)

Caring for a Client with Impaired Communication

NCLEX-PN® Focus Area: Psychosocial Integrity

Case Study: Ann Lu is a 36-year-old Asian American female client with Dependent Personality Disorder. Yesterday she had a partial bowel resection because of acute diverticulitis. She is very compliant with requests made by the staff. She has never asked the staff for anything. The physician wrote an order for Demerol 75 mg every 4 hours IM p.r.n. for incisional pain.

Nursing Diagnosis: Impaired verbal communication

COLLECT DATA

Subjective	Objective
_____	_____
_____	_____
_____	_____
_____	_____
_____	_____
_____	_____
_____	_____

Would you report this data? Yes/No

If yes, to: _____

Nursing Care

_____

_____

_____

_____

_____

_____

_____

_____

_____

How would you document this? _____

_____

_____

_____

Compare your documentation to the sample provided in Appendix I.

Data Collected
(use those that apply)

- Client is married.
- BP 158/90, P110, R24, T 99.0
- Client states, "Yes, whatever you say."
- When asked if she needs pain medication, she states, "No, I don't want to bother you."
- When asked if she needs anything, she states, "I don't know."
- Weighs 168 lbs.
- Awake on all 2-hour checks during the night
- Bowel sounds hypoactive
- Ate 100% of clear liquid breakfast tray
- Ambulates when asked
- Abdominal surgical incision is dry and intact, without exudate. Incision is well-approximated.
- Grimaces and sweats when ambulating or moving in bed
- Client asks nurse, "What do you think I should do?"

Nursing Interventions
(use those that apply; list in priority order)

- Teach the client now about dressing changes at home.
- Call the physician immediately about the VS.
- Notify the physician about the elevated temperature.
- Ask the client, "Are you in pain?"
- Tell the client, "Most people have a lot of pain after surgery. You have signs of pain. Does your incision hurt?"
- Tell the client, "It is no trouble to give you some pain medication. I will be glad to get some if you need it."
- Say to the client, "Sometimes people don't like to ask for help. While you are in the hospital, we want to help you, so please tell us what you need."
- Tell the client, "Because you don't seem to want any help, I will leave you alone."
- Help the client practice identifying her needs.
- Document that the client is passive, inappropriate, and dishonest.
- Encourage the client to take the ordered pain med.
- Include offering pain med regularly (every 4 hours) in the plan of care.
- Visit the client regularly (every 1 to 2 hours) to determine whether she needs help.
- Discuss outpatient referral for therapy with treatment team.

1 The client with a Paranoid Personality Disorder responds best to a nurse who uses which of the following approaches?

1. Friendly, outgoing
2. Self-confident, matter-of-fact
3. Shy, hesitant
4. Quiet, using brief encounters

2 A client with cancer who has a Schizoid Personality Disorder. says little to staff and has a flat affect. He has no visitors or phone calls. The nurse would conclude that:

1. This is the client's usual behavior.
2. The client is ashamed of his condition.
3. The client is depressed about his diagnosis.
4. The client is lonely.

3 A resident with Schizotypal Personality Disorder always refuses to eat in the dining room with other residents. She does not attend social functions, preferring to stay in her room. The best approach to this client would be to:

1. Insist she attend all social functions.
2. Encourage other residents to visit her daily.
3. Invite her to eat at least one meal a day in the dining room.
4. Leave her alone.

4 A young male is admitted to the detoxification unit after beating up his wife while intoxicated. He wants to go outside more often than the three times a day allowed for clients. He tells staff, "If you will let me go out an extra time today, I'll make sure your supervisor knows what a good nurse you are." He has been diagnosed with an Antisocial Personality Disorder. The staff should:

1. Allow him to go out four times a day.
2. Refuse to let him go outside to smoke at all unless his behavior changes.
3. Bend the rules for just one day as a reward for good behavior.
4. Stick to the rules consistently.

5 The treatment priority for a client suffering Borderline Personality Disorder is:

1. Teaching appropriate social skills.
2. Preventing self-injury.
3. Teaching problem-solving techniques.
4. Medicating for sleep disturbances.

6 A client on a psychiatric unit is disruptive in group sessions directing all attention to herself. She is constantly asking the group to help her solve her problems. She dramatically refers to everyone as her "dearest friends" and gushes over the assistance they will give her. This person probably has which personality disorder?

1. Borderline
2. Avoidant
3. Schizotypal
4. Histrionic

7 A client has been admitted to the medical-surgical unit after gallbladder surgery. He belittles the nurses and wants the surgeon called in the middle of the night to complain about his care. The nurse suspects that he has a Narcissistic Personality Disorder. The night charge nurse's best approach would be to:

1. Apologize that he is unhappy with his care, but it is not appropriate to call his surgeon. He is welcome to voice his complaints when the surgeon visits in the morning.
2. Tell him his surgeon will be called and then do not call. If he asks, tell him no one answered.
3. Tell him he is not the only client on the unit and there is no time to cater to his every demand.
4. Ask for suggestions on how to make him happier. Promise to pass his complaints along. Assure him his care will improve.

8 An orthopedic client with Avoidant Personality Disorder refuses to go to physical therapy. She says that she knows she will not be successful with her therapy and will disappoint her doctor. The best approach for the nurse is:

1. Tell her she does not have to go. Explain her feelings to the doctor. Suggest that she work on exercises at home.
2. Reassure her that the physical therapy is for her benefit, not the doctor's. Suggest the therapist come to the unit to work with the client in her room before encouraging her to go to the PT gym.
3. Tell her that the staff will be so proud of her accomplishments in therapy.
4. Call a PT assistant to assist her into the wheelchair. Tell her she must go to physical therapy, because it has been ordered and she will not get better without it.

9 Which of the following medications might be prescribed for someone with Obsessive-Compulsive Personality Disorder?

1. Anxiolytic
2. Antidepressant
3. Antipsychotic
4. Hypnotic

10 Which of the following nursing interventions would be most appropriate for a client with a Dependent Personality Disorder? (Select all that apply.)

1. Give the client an opportunity to participate in his/her care.
2. Encourage family members to participate in client decision making to alleviate anxiety.
3. Support the client in decision-making process without giving advice.
4. Protect the client from the opportunity for self-injury.
5. Encourage the client to become part of a support group for others experiencing Dependent Personality Disorder.

Answers for Review Questions, as well as discussion of Care Plan and Critical Thinking Care Map questions, appear in Appendix I.

Chapter 11

Anxiety Disorders

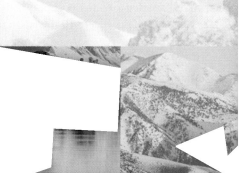

BRIEF Outline

Biological Basis of Anxiety	Anxiety Disorders
Coping with Anxiety	Collaborative Care

LEARNING Outcomes

After completing this chapter, you will be able to:

1. Analyze the special needs of clients who have anxiety disorders.
2. Conduct basic client teaching about anxiety disorders.
3. Safely administer antianxiety medications.
4. Apply the nursing process to the care of clients with anxiety disorders.

Anxiety is one of the most common feelings of humankind. Everyone has experienced anxiety. You might be feeling anxious now if you are worrying about the test on the anxiety disorders chapter. **Anxiety** is a feeling of uneasiness that activates the autonomic nervous system in response to a vague, nonspecific threat (Carpenito-Moyet, 2006). Anxiety differs from fear, because fear is a response to a known threat. If an alligator is chasing a person, that uneasy feeling is fear. If the person feels impending doom while sitting in a classroom (no alligators involved), that feeling is anxiety.

Biological Basis of Anxiety

The experience of anxiety appears to originate in the subcortical or primitive brain, specifically in the limbic system (Braun & Anderson, 2007). During anxiety there is an increase in blood flow to the limbic system and the cerebral cortex. Figure 11-1 ■ shows the structures of the limbic system. Table 11-1 ■ describes the functions of these structures and what happens when they function abnormally (dysfunction). The limbic system conducts stimuli to the autonomic nervous system. Sympathetic (part of autonomic system) stimulation causes the symptoms we recognize as anxiety. From the limbic system, neural messages are also conducted to the cerebral cortex. In the association areas of the cerebral cortex, the individual experiences thoughts about anxiety. Thus, feelings,

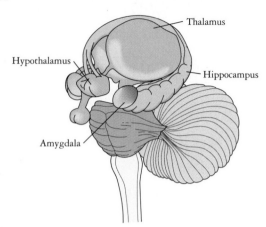

Figure 11-1. ■ The limbic system. The limbic system is surrounded by the cerebral cortex. It plays a role in motivation, emotion, and memory. It is composed of the thalamus, amygdala, hippocampus, and hypothalamus. *Source: Psychology 3/E* by Kassin, Saul, © 2001. Reprinted by permission of Pearson Education, Inc., Upper Saddle River, NJ.

physiological responses, and thoughts are all part of the anxiety experience.

Fear has survival value. When a person sees an alligator, fear motivates the person to move away. Anxiety is not so focused and often has no realistic source. Even when the individual experiencing anxiety knows the reason for it, the **dysphoric** (uncomfortable and dissatisfied) feeling is usually out of proportion to the real danger. Low levels of anxiety can arouse the individual's attention

TABLE 11-1	
Functions of the Limbic System	
LIMBIC STRUCTURE	**FUNCTION AND DYSFUNCTION**
Thalamus	Relays sensory input from spinal cord. Regulates emotional aspects of sensory experiences. Dysfunction is involved in OCD, mood disorders, and schizophrenia.
Amygdala	Coordinates actions of autonomic nervous system and endocrine system. Involved in control of emotions, nurturing behavior, fear conditioning. Controls memory of fear experiences. Dysfunction contributes to inappropriate fear and rage, anxiety, PTSD.
Hippocampus	Processes information between parts of the brain that receive sensory input and those that translate the input into action. Regulates immune system and memory storage. Dysfunction results in memory and learning impairments.
Hypothalamus	Composed of neurons that produce hormones. Integration center. Concentrates dopamine. Converts thinking and feelings into hormones that cause changes throughout the body through the autonomic nervous system. Dysfunction can cause excessive thirst and hunger. May be involved in eating disorders and schizophrenia. Implicated in side effects of psychotropic drugs.

Manifestations of Sympathetic Stimulation

- Increased heart rate
- Increased blood pressure
- Dilated pupils
- Cool skin
- Piloerection (hair "standing on end")
- Decreased GI motility

and alertness, and even make it easier to learn new things, but as anxiety becomes more severe, it causes impairment of function. Anxiety and fear have the same physiological responses related to sympathetic nervous system stimulation, as shown in Box 11-1 ■.

Like other emotions, thoughts, and behaviors, anxiety is a common and normal human experience under usual circumstances. It only becomes abnormal when its frequency or severity interferes with the development or function of the individual.

LEVELS OF ANXIETY

Hildegard Peplau described four degrees of anxiety (O'Toole & Welt, 1989). Table 11-2 ■ shows the four levels and the behaviors the nurse might observe in a client at each level.

Coping with Anxiety

People use **coping** behaviors to adapt to or manage stress or change. To control anxiety, people develop patterns of coping behavior. Coping behaviors can be adaptive or maladaptive.

CASE EXAMPLE

Consider these two students: Linh is a student who received a failing grade on a midterm exam. She went to the instructor, asked where her problems were, and studied those areas harder before the final exam. Her coping method is active problem solving, which is adaptive. Tran also received a failing grade on the midterm exam. He did not seek out help or advice. He continued his regular pattern of study hoping that he would pass the final exam. His coping method here is avoidance, which is a maladaptive approach.

RESILIENCE

Some people seem to be more resilient, or able to recover from stress (Rosenbaum & Covino, 2005). Others cannot cope or they become physically ill under similar circumstances. Some children who have lives of seemingly intolerable poverty or stress grow up unable to function in society, and others grow up to be resourceful and well-adjusted

Four Degrees of Anxiety

DEGREE OF ANXIETY	SUBJECTIVE EFFECTS	OBSERVABLE BEHAVIOR
Mild	Perceptual field widens slightly. Increased ability to see relationships among data.	Alert, more perceptive, able to recognize anxiety. Promotes motivation and growth.
Moderate	Perceptual field narrows slightly. Concentrates on the immediate focus, ignoring peripheral stimuli. Can change attention if directed.	Able to sustain attention on a focal point. Inattentive to stimuli outside this focus. May talk faster. Vital signs begin to increase (except temp.). Able to recognize and express anxiety.
Severe	Perceptual field is greatly reduced. Does not notice external events. Unable to redirect focus even with outside direction.	Attention is focused on a small part of a specific area. Assumptions made may be erroneous due to incomplete perception. May be unaware of anxiety. VS increasing. Coping/relief measures used.
Panic	Perception is reduced to a detail. Perception is distorted. May jump from one detail to another, as in flight of ideas. Experienced as a threat to survival. Affected person feels dread, terror.	Feelings of unreality, confusion, terror, self-absorption. May be expressed with violence toward self or others. Loss of control. May include pacing or running. Automatic coping/relief behaviors used. Can result in exhaustion if prolonged.

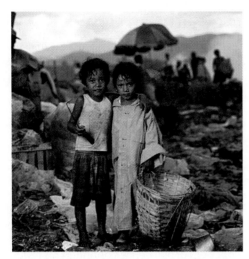

Figure 11-2. ■ These two children survive their hard life on the Payatas Smoking Mountain (a giant garbage dump in the Philippines) because of their resilience. *Source:* Peter Arnold, Inc.

adults. The difference is **resilience** (the ability to withstand and recover from stress). Figure 11-2 ■ shows children who are resilient enough to survive under the harshest of conditions.

A study on resilience was done on 750 servicemen who were held captive during the Vietnam War. They were prisoners of war (POWs) for 6 to 8 years. During that time they were tortured and/or kept in solitary confinement. The study tried to determine why some of these men did not develop depression or Posttraumatic Stress Disorder after the extreme stress of their ordeal. What protected them? The study by Rosenbaum and Covino (2005) found 10 critical characteristics of the resilient men:

1. **Optimism**. Those who are extremely optimistic tend to show greater resilience, which has implications for cognitive therapies (it may be helpful to enhance the client's positive view of the situation).
2. **Altruism**. Those who were resilient often found that helping others was one way to handle extreme stress. This can be used therapeutically as a tool for recovery.
3. **Moral values**. It helps for a person to have a set of beliefs that cannot be shattered. It may be beneficial to help clients to clarify their values.
4. **Faith and spirituality**. For some, prayer was a daily ritual, although other resilient POWs were not involved or interested in religion.
5. **Humor**. A sense of humor allows for relief of stress and another way of seeing the situation.
6. **Having a role model**. Many people with role models draw strength from this. For treatment, using a role

model, role modeling, or helping someone find a role model can be beneficial.
7. **Social supports**. Having contact with others who can be trusted, either family or friend, someone with whom one can share the most difficult thoughts and feelings is important in recovery.
8. **Facing fear**. The ability to leave one's comfort zone, both for the act of doing what must be done and the feeling of empowerment.
9. **Having a mission**. Having a sense that one's life has meaning. This helps clients recover because they feel that they can be productive and empowered.
10. **Training**. One can train or learn to become a resilient person. Resilience can be developed through experience in meeting and overcoming challenges. This helps clients and teaches us how to prepare young people for adulthood.

CONSCIOUS COPING METHODS

The automatic or unconscious ways that people cope with stress are called *defense mechanisms* (listed in Chapter 3 in Table 3-1). There are also conscious ways to cope with stress, each of which can be used adaptively or maladaptively. They include the following:

- Active problem solving
- Withdrawal behavior
- Compromise

Active Problem Solving

Active problem solving means actively removing obstacles through problem solving, while considering the rights of others. An example of *adaptive* problem-solving behavior is a nurse asking another nurse to help figure out why a client's condition is changing. *Maladaptive* problem solving includes anger and hostility. It might be expressed by negative or aggressive behavior toward others. An example of maladaptive behavior is a nurse shouting at a nursing assistant who made a mistake.

Withdrawal Behavior

Withdrawal behavior involves removing oneself either physically or emotionally from a stressful situation. Adaptive examples of withdrawal include a person who is feeling overstimulated or frustrated leaving the room to decrease the negative stimuli and to avoid an argument or acting out. A maladaptive example is staying away from other people to avoid the stress of personal contact and interaction.

Compromise

Compromise involves cooperative problem solving that includes giving up something that an individual wants or taking less than originally wanted in order to achieve a partial goal that is still acceptable. Compromise is usually adaptive. For example, a client in the state psychiatric hospital is ready to return to the community, and he is discussing a pass from the hospital with the treatment team (limited time away from the hospital to practice community reintegration skills). He wants to take a 1-week pass to stay with his girlfriend. The treatment team has decided that a 1-day pass with his parents is more appropriate for his treatment goals. He accepts the compromise plan. A maladaptive approach might be for the client to say he agrees then fail to keep his part of the agreement, and not come back to the hospital (in which case the police would probably have to bring him back).

Critical Self-Check. What behaviors do you use to manage your own anxiety? Which behaviors are adaptive and which are maladaptive?

Anxiety Disorders

The *Diagnostic and Statistical Manual of Mental Disorders* lists several anxiety-related disorders. They have many different manifestations. The feature they all have in common is anxiety (American Psychiatric Association, 2000).

- Generalized Anxiety Disorder
- Panic Disorder with or without Agoraphobia
- Agoraphobia without Panic Disorder
- Obsessive-Compulsive Disorder
- Acute Stress Disorder
- Posttraumatic Stress Disorder
- Anxiety Disorder due to a general medical condition
- Substance-Induced Anxiety Disorder

CAUSES

Studies of twins and families, and human genetic studies confirm that there is a genetic basis for anxiety disorders. As with other mental disorders, genetics is not the sole etiology (cause) of anxiety disorders. Life experiences also play an important part (nature and nurture again). Researchers are looking at how genetics and experience interact in anxiety disorders. They hope to find clues to prevention and treatment of these disabling disorders (National Institute of Mental Health [NIMH], 2006).

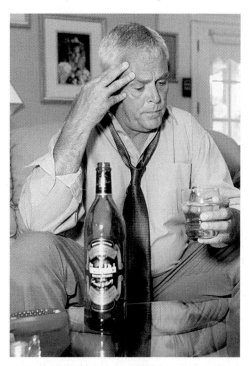

Figure 11-3. ■ Many people try to "medicate" or treat their own anxiety with alcohol. *Source:* PhotoEdit Inc.

Anxiety disorders are likely to have comorbidities (other disorders that occur with them). People with Major Depressive Disorder often also have anxiety disorders. Substance dependence is commonly associated with anxiety and other mental disorders as well. One hypothesis is that people self-treat their emotional pain with alcohol or street drugs. Figure 11-3 ■ shows a man who may be medicating his anxiety with alcohol. Chapter 12 covers substance use in more detail.

From a behavioral point of view, experience can teach people different ways to respond to stressful events. An individual's experiences in both childhood and adulthood determine the nature of situations that cause anxiety.

Cognitive function can moderate how often a person thinks about anxiety-producing stimuli. If a person focuses her or his thoughts on stressful events, this individual will be more prone to anxiety. Intelligence and the personality trait of introspection may put people at a higher risk for anxiety.

GENERALIZED ANXIETY DISORDER

Excessive anxiety and worry occurring on most days for at least 6 months characterize Generalized Anxiety Disorder (GAD). The anxiety is about a number of different events or activities, and the individual finds it difficult to control the feelings. The affected person also has at least three of the following (American Psychiatric Association, 2000):

- Restlessness
- Fatigue
- Difficulty concentrating
- Irritability
- Muscle tension
- Disturbed sleep

For children to receive the diagnosis of Generalized Anxiety Disorder, they would need only one of the above symptoms in addition to the persistent anxiety.

People with GAD report that they feel significant stress, have difficulty controlling the worry, or have related impairment in social or occupational functioning. In this disorder, the intensity, frequency, and duration of the anxiety are far out of proportion to the realistic likelihood or impact of the feared event. Thoughts of the feared event intrude on the individual's thinking, distracting her/him from other tasks. The focus of worry may shift from one concern to another. A few potential examples of concerns for these individuals are being late, personal performance, illness, family, job responsibilities, financial responsibilities, and household chores (American Psychiatric Association, 2000).

People with Generalized Anxiety Disorder usually realize that their anxiety is more intense than makes sense in the situation, but they still cannot control their worries. Their anxiety is accompanied by physical symptoms, especially fatigue, headaches, muscle tension, muscle pain, irritability, sweating, nausea, difficulty swallowing, trembling, and hot flashes. Relaxation seems impossible (NIMH, 2006).

Unlike people with other anxiety disorders, people with this disorder do not usually avoid anxiety-producing situations as a result of their disorder. When the disorder is mild, affected people can function, but at its worst, they have substantial functional impairment (Antai-Otong, 2005).

Generalized Anxiety Disorder is the most common anxiety disorder and affects about twice as many women as men in the general population. In treatment settings, the nurse can expect to see about equal numbers of women and men seeking treatment. In any given year, approximately 3% of the population will have this disorder. Over a lifetime, any individual has about a 5% chance of having it. This disorder is commonly associated with Major Depressive Disorder (American Psychiatric Association, 2000).

CASE EXAMPLE

A person with Generalized Anxiety Disorder said:"I'd have terrible sleeping problems. There were times I'd wake up wired in the middle of the night. I had trouble concentrating, even reading a newspaper or a novel. Sometimes I'd feel a little lightheaded. My heart would race or pound. And that would make me worry more. I was always imagining things were worse than they really were: when I got a stomachache, I'd think it was an ulcer. When my problems were at their worst, I'd miss work and feel just terrible about it. Then I worried that I'd lose my job. My life was miserable until I got treatment" (NIMH, 2006).

PANIC DISORDER

People with Panic Disorder have recurrent, unexpected panic attacks followed by at least 1 month of persistent concern about having another one. They may worry about the possible complications of the attacks or have a significant behavioral change associated with the attacks (American Psychiatric Association, 2000).

A **panic attack** is characterized by an episode of intense fear or discomfort. During this episode four or more of the following are present (American Psychiatric Association, 2000):

- Palpitations, pounding heart, or increased heart rate
- Sweating
- Trembling or shaking
- Sensations of shortness of breath or smothering
- Feeling of choking
- Chest pain or discomfort
- Nausea or abdominal distress
- Feeling dizzy, unsteady, lightheaded, or faint
- *Derealization* (feeling of unreality) or *depersonalization* (feeling detached from oneself)
- Fear of losing control or going crazy
- Fear of dying
- Paresthesias (numbness or tingling)
- Chills or hot flashes

People with Panic Disorder have panic attacks without warning. Sometimes the attacks are associated with a stressor and sometimes they are not. Figure 11-4 ■ depicts a professor experiencing a panic attack. He may be short of breath, have chest pain, and feel that he is going to die. There is no way to predict when an attack will occur, so people often spend much time worrying about when the next one will strike. Panic attacks can occur at any time, even during sleep. An attack usually peaks in severity within 10 minutes, but some symptoms

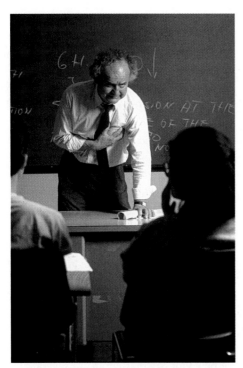

Figure 11-4. ■ A person having a panic attack may feel like he is dying. *Source:* Pearson Education/PH College.

last much longer. Untreated, the disorder can be very disabling. Affected people often fear returning to the site or situation of a previous attack. This, of course, can severely limit an individual's ability to function. For example, if a person experienced one anxiety attack at a grocery store and another attack on a bus, this individual may not be able to shop for groceries or go to work.

Not everyone who has a panic attack will go on to have Panic Disorder. Some people have one attack, with no recurrence.

clinical ALERT

People experiencing Panic Disorder often visit the hospital emergency department several times before they are accurately diagnosed. They may go for years before they find out that they have a real, treatable illness (NIMH, 2006). It is critical for emergency department nurses and physicians to be aware of Panic Disorder.

Imagine a person who comes to the hospital for help with a really terrifying panic episode, believing that she is dying. Physical assessment and EKG are done and show no abnormalities. The episode is resolving by the time the tests are done. The client is told that there is nothing wrong. She may even be told that she has misused the emergency department. This client is suffering not only the effects of the panic attack, but also the devastation of not being taken seriously. Many people with treatable mental illnesses avoid treatment because they fear not being believed by health professionals.

Panic Disorder is often associated with other serious disorders such as depression, substance abuse, or alcoholism. The incidence of suicide is increased in people affected by this disorder. The disorder affects three times as many women as men and affects 1–2% of the general population. The onset is usually between late adolescence and the mid-thirties, although it can begin at any age (American Psychiatric Association, 2000).

CASE EXAMPLE

People with Panic Disorder state the following:

■ "I had my first attack in my nursing clinical. I felt fine, and then all of a sudden I thought I was going to die. I didn't know what hit me. I was losing control. It was unreal. Not only have I never been so scared, I didn't know it was possible to be so scared."

■ "In between attacks there is this dread and anxiety that it is going to happen again. I'm afraid to go back to places where I've had an attack. Unless I get help, there soon won't be anyplace where I can go and feel safe from panic."

AGORAPHOBIA

Agoraphobia is characterized by anxiety about being in places or situations where escape may be difficult (or embarrassing), or when help might not be available in the case of a panic attack. Agoraphobic fears typically include situations that involve being alone away from home in a crowd or standing in line; on a bridge; or traveling in a plane, train, bus, or automobile. The person avoids fear-producing situations, endures them with much anxiety and distress, or requires the presence of a companion (American Psychiatric Association, 2000).

Agoraphobia is commonly associated with Panic Disorder. People who seek treatment for the disorder almost always also have Panic Disorder. Figure 11-5 ■ shows a woman who is afraid to leave her home. It is more likely to occur in females than in males. It can severely impair social and occupational functioning when the individual avoids multiple anxiety-producing situations (American Psychiatric Association, 2000).

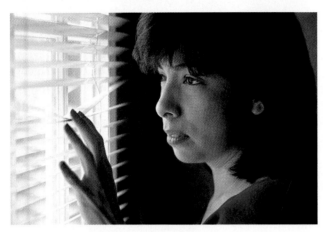

Figure 11-5. ■ People with agoraphobia do not feel safe outside their own homes. *Source:* The Image Works.

Not everyone who stays in the home all the time has Agoraphobia, however. In some cultures women are expected to remain at home, and their public activities are greatly limited. If a woman from such a culture stays at home, she is acting in accordance with culture expectations and does not have a diagnosis of Agoraphobia.

CASE EXAMPLE

A person with Agoraphobia said: "I have always been a 'worrier,' but recently it has been much worse. At first I was uneasy about being in crowds of people, like at the mall. Then I became paralyzed with fear when I got on the bus. I felt trapped, like I would die if I couldn't get off the bus. I lost my job because I couldn't get to work without the bus. I don't feel safe unless I am at home. I never go out alone anymore."

OBSESSIVE-COMPULSIVE DISORDER

Obsessions are recurrent and intrusive thoughts that cause marked distress. The affected person recognizes that these thoughts are from her or his own mind and tries to ignore or suppress them. **Compulsions** are repetitive behaviors or mental acts that the affected person feels driven to perform in response to obsessive thoughts. The objective of these behaviors is to reduce stress or to prevent some dreaded event. The compulsive behaviors are not realistically connected with the situations they are supposed to neutralize, or they are clearly excessive (American Psychiatric Association, 2000).

Obsessive-Compulsive Disorder (OCD) is characterized by compulsions or obsessions that the affected person recognizes are excessive or unreasonable. The obsessions or compulsions cause marked distress and take more than 1 hour each day, or significantly interfere with daily occupational, academic, or personal functioning (American Psychiatric Association, 2000).

Common obsessive thoughts involve dirt and germs, numbers or counting, symmetry and order, ideas that are against the individual's religious beliefs, or sexual thoughts that are disgusting to the affected individual. Some examples of compulsive rituals performed to control the obsessive thoughts are cleaning, handwashing, counting, touching or doing things in a certain order, or praying. Figure 11-6 ■ shows people in common OCD situations: compulsive handwashing, obsessive fear of germs with compulsive cleaning, and measuring the height of books on a shelf due to a compulsive need for symmetry. There is no pleasure for the affected individual in performing the compulsive rituals, only temporary relief from the anxiety caused by not doing them (NIMH, 2006).

Many people without OCD can identify with some compulsive behavior, such as checking several times that the stove is really off before leaving home. This behavior does not become OCD until it becomes distressing, consumes over an hour a day, or interferes with daily life.

OCD usually begins in adolescence or early adulthood. It can begin in childhood. It tends to affect males at an earlier age than females. Affected children often do not realize that the behavior is unreasonable. The majority of affected people experience OCD with a waxing and waning course. The disorder becomes more severe in the presence of stress. OCD occurs more often in first-degree relatives of people with OCD and Tourette's syndrome than in the general population. OCD occurs in many cultures around the world. It affects approximately 1–2% of people at some time in their lives (American Psychiatric Association, 2000).

When diagnosing personality or anxiety disorders, the client's culture must be considered. Some religious practices require repetition of certain prayers and behaviors over and over again, maybe several times each day. Behavior that originates in religious or other cultural expectations is not a part of OCD, even if the participants doing the behavior state that they do not really want to do it.

Some people with OCD also have depression or other anxiety disorders. Some have eating disorders as well as OCD. The disorder can affect people so severely that their development and ability to function in their daily lives are changed.

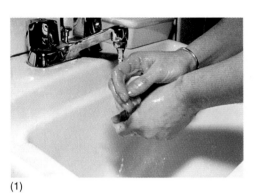
(1)

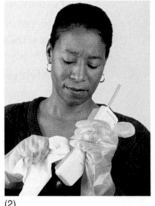
(2)

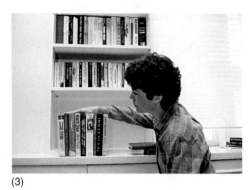
(3)

Figure 11-6. ■ These three photos show people who suffer from OCD in typical situations: (1) compulsive handwashing, (2) obsessive fear of germs with compulsive cleaning, and (3) a woman compulsively measuring the height of books to ensure their "correct" placement. *Sources:* (1) The Image Works; (2) PhotoEdit Inc.; (3) Pearson Education/PH College.

CASE EXAMPLE

A person with Obsessive-Compulsive Disorder said: "I couldn't do anything without rituals. They invaded every aspect of my life. Counting really bogged me down. I would wash my hair three times as opposed to once, because three was a good luck number and one wasn't. It took me longer to read because I'd count the lines in a paragraph. When I set my alarm at night, I had to set it to a number that wouldn't add up to a 'bad' number.

"Getting dressed in the morning was tough because I had a routine, and if I didn't follow the routine, I'd get anxious and would have to get dressed again. I always worried that if I didn't do something, my parents were going to die. I'd have these terrible thoughts of harming my parents. That was completely irrational, but the thoughts triggered more anxiety and more senseless behavior. Because of the time I spent on rituals, I was unable to do a lot of things that were important to me.

"I know the rituals didn't make sense, and I was deeply ashamed of them, but I couldn't seem to overcome them until I had therapy" (NIMH, 2006).

POSTTRAUMATIC STRESS DISORDER

Posttraumatic Stress Disorder (PTSD) was first recognized in war veterans. It is a debilitating condition that follows an extreme traumatic stressor. The traumatic stressor may be an event that threatens the individual's life, serious injury, or personal integrity. It may be witnessing an event, including death or serious injury of another. It may be learning about an event, such as the unexpected or violent death of or serious harm to a family member or significant other. The person's response to the event must involve intense fear, helplessness, or horror.

Children respond with agitated or disorganized behavior. The characteristic symptoms of PTSD, which are present for more than 1 month, include the following (American Psychiatric Association, 2000):

■ Persistent reexperiencing of the traumatic event
■ Avoidance of stimuli associated with the trauma
■ Numbing of general responsiveness (also called "psychic numbing" or "emotional anesthesia")
■ Increased arousal (difficulty sleeping, nightmares, exaggerated startle response, and hypervigilance or alertness for danger)

Traumatic events resulting in PTSD include, but are not limited to, violent personal assault (sexual assault, physical attack, robbery), military combat, being taken hostage, terrorist attack, torture, imprisonment as a prisoner of war or in a concentration camp, disasters, transportation crashes, or diagnosis of life-threatening illness. Figure 11-7 ■ shows survivors of the World Trade Center attacks. Many of them suffer from PTSD. Children may develop PTSD as a result of sexual abuse even if there is no actual or threatened injury. The disorder is more likely to occur and to be more long lasting when the stressor is of intentional human action, such as rape or torture (American Psychiatric Association, 2000). Box 11-2 ■ describes one cultural aspect of PTSD.

People with PTSD can reexperience the traumatic event in various ways. Commonly, the person has repeated intrusive memories or dreams of the event. Some people experience flashbacks in which they relive the event, believing that it is actually happening. A flashback may include sights, sounds, smells, or feelings from the traumatic event.

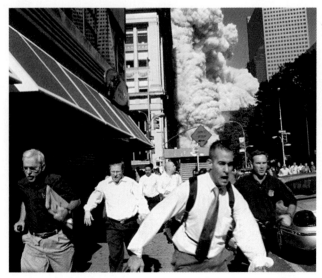

Figure 11-7. ■ Many people who survived the World Trade Center attack on 9-11-01 are experiencing PTSD. *Source:* AP Wide World Photos.

Affected people feel distressed by situations that remind them of the event and avoid these situations. For example, a person who was raped in an elevator may avoid all elevators. A person who was held in a prison camp with military guards may avoid anyone in uniform. Ordinary events can trigger memories and a flashback in susceptible individuals.

People with PTSD may have difficulty with interpersonal relationships. They may have difficulty trusting or being affectionate. Things they formerly enjoyed may not provide pleasure for them anymore. Irritability, aggression, even violence may be expressed when these would be out of character for the person before the incident.

BOX 11-2	CULTURAL PULSE POINTS

Monitoring for PTSD

As a nurse in the United States you will care for clients from all over the world. Refugees who emigrate from areas of war and unrest probably have increased rates of Posttraumatic Stress Disorder. Because of the nature of the disorder and the individual circumstances, affected people may be reluctant to discuss their experiences of torture and trauma. Refugees should be asked specifically about traumatic experiences and symptoms of PTSD. The nurse might ask, "Do you have nightmares about things that happened in your country?" or "Do you have recurring thoughts about bad things that happened to you?" Clients should be referred for treatment if it is indicated.

Depression sometimes occurs in people with PTSD. As with people affected by other anxiety disorders, people with PTSD may use alcohol and other substances to medicate their anxiety symptoms.

After extreme trauma, people often have some of the same symptoms as PTSD. The disorder is only diagnosed if symptoms persist for longer than a month. If a person is going to develop PTSD, it usually occurs within 3 months of the traumatic experience.

PTSD can occur at any age. Approximately half of affected people experience complete resolution of symptoms within 3 months. The most important factors affecting the likelihood of developing this disorder are severity of the traumatic event, duration of the trauma, and proximity of the individual's exposure. Approximately 8% of people in the United States will be affected at some time in their lives. Prevalence information from other countries is not currently available.

CASE EXAMPLE

A person with Posttraumatic Stress Disorder said: "I was raped when I was 25 years old. For a long time, I spoke about the rape as though it was something that happened to someone else. I was very aware that it had happened to me, but there was just no feeling.

"Then I started having flashbacks. They kind of came over me like a splash of water. I would be terrified. Suddenly I was reliving the rape. Every instant was startling. I wasn't aware of anything around me; I was in a bubble, just kind of floating. And it was scary; having a flashback can wring you out.

"The rape happened the week before Thanksgiving, and I can't believe the anxiety and fear I feel every year around the anniversary date. It's as though I've seen a werewolf. I can't relax, can't sleep, don't want to be with anyone. I wonder whether I'll ever be free of this terrible problem."

MILITARY SEXUAL TRAUMA

The U.S. Veterans Administration has identified a condition called *military sexual trauma* that refers both to sexual harassment and sexual assault that occur in military settings. Both men and women can be the victims of military sexual trauma and the perpetrator can be of the same or opposite gender. In 1995 the Department of Defense conducted a large study of sexual victimization among active duty populations and found that 78% of women and 38% of men had experienced sexual harassment during a 1-year period. Rates of completed or attempted sexual assault were 6% for women and 1% for men. Research in the Persian Gulf War found that the rates of sexual assault and harassment actually increased during wartime (Street & Stafford, 2004).

Victims of military sexual trauma are at increased risk for PTSD. Men have a 65% risk and women a 45.9% risk of developing PTSD after military sexual trauma (Figure 11-8 ■). Military sexual trauma causes a greater risk for PTSD than even military combat, which causes PTSD at a general rate of 38.8%. In addition military veterans with PTSD due to military sexual trauma have higher rates of Major Depressive Disorder, difficulty adjusting following discharge, poorer psychological and physical health, and increased incidence of substance abuse (Street & Stafford, 2004; Yaeger, Himmelfarb, Cammack, & Mintz, 2006).

The implication for healthcare providers is that veterans should be assessed for military sexual trauma carefully due to the stigma associated with sexual victimization and the reluctance of victims to report or even acknowledge that it happened. Military camaraderie and the fact that the perpetrators often work closely with the victims make accurate data collection difficult. Rather than asking about "rape" or "sexual harassment," nurses should ask questions such as "While you were in the military did you ever experience any unwanted sexual attention, such as verbal remarks, touching, or pressure for sexual favors?" and "Did anyone ever use force or the threat of force to have sex with you against your will?" The Veterans Administration mandates universal screening of veterans for a history of military sexual trauma (Street & Stafford, 2004).

CASE EXAMPLE

A woman who experienced military sexual trauma said the following. "One of my superior officers was always making sexual jokes or comments to the enlisted women. We just tried to ignore it, or smile so he wouldn't get angry. I had to deliver papers to his tent on a regular basis. I always hoped to do it when someone else was there. On the time that he raped me, I couldn't scream, I tried to push him away and tell him not to, but I couldn't even fight too hard because he was my commander. I never felt so helpless. I never felt safe again. Later I thought, 'We are both in the U.S. Army. Who is on my side now?' I never told anyone while I was deployed. I thought they would believe him, or I would get in trouble, or that nobody would believe that it happened at all. When I got out, the nurse at the VA asked me if I had anything like this happen. I was so thankful that someone acknowledged what happened. Now I'm in a women survivors' group. I still have trouble sleeping. I've thought about it every day since it happened. I feel guilty and always afraid. This was the worst thing that happened to me during the war."

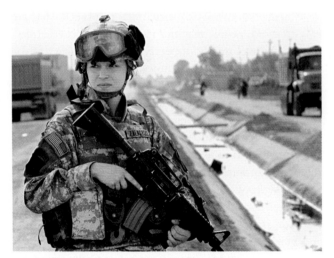

Figure 11-8. ■ Veterans who experience military sexual trauma are at higher risk to develop PTSD than those who experience combat. *Source:* Corbis/Reuters America LLC.

SOCIAL PHOBIA

Social Phobia (also called *Social Anxiety Disorder*) is characterized by a marked and persistent fear of social or performance situations in which embarrassment may occur. A **phobia** is a persistent and irrational fear. Exposure to the social or performance situation (such as public speaking or speaking to a supervisor) almost always results in an immediate anxiety reaction. Adults and adolescents with Social Phobia recognize that their fear is excessive. Affected children may not. People usually avoid the risky situations, but may endure them with dread. Social Phobia only exists if the fear, avoidance, or anxiety about encountering the social situation interferes significantly with daily routine or social, academic, or occupational life, or if the person is markedly distressed by the disorder. Anticipatory anxiety may begin weeks before an anticipated social event (American Psychiatric Association, 2000).

In people younger than age 18, the symptoms must have lasted for more than 6 months. Temporary social anxiety in childhood or adolescence is quite common and does not constitute Social Phobia. Neither does fear of speaking in situations in which fear may be justified, such as when the teacher calls on you and you have not done the homework.

Physical symptoms often go along with the anxiety in Social Phobia. These include blushing, excessive sweating, nausea, GI distress, tremors, and difficulty talking. Although they realize that their fears are irrational, people with this disorder are unable to control it. Even after they have done the dreaded deed, people with this disorder continue to feel anxious about how they were perceived and judged by others. Making or keeping friends may be difficult. People with Social Phobia may medicate themselves with alcohol or drugs to make it possible for them to endure social situations.

CASE EXAMPLE

"In any social situation, I felt fear. I would be anxious before I even left the house, and it would escalate as I got closer to a college class, a party, or whatever. I would feel sick at my stomach—it almost felt like I had the flu. My heart would pound, my palms would get sweaty, and I would get this feeling of being removed from everybody else.

"When I would walk into a room full of people, I'd turn red and it would feel like everybody's eyes were on me. I was embarrassed to stand off in a corner by myself, but I couldn't think of anything to say to anybody. It was humiliating. I felt so clumsy; I couldn't wait to get out.

"I couldn't go on dates, and for a while I couldn't even go to class. My sophomore year of college I had to go home for a semester. I felt like such a failure" (NIMH, 2006).

SPECIFIC PHOBIAS

A Specific Phobia is an excessive fear of a specific object or situation. It might be triggered by the presence or even the anticipation of the feared object. Affected people have an immediate anxiety reaction in response to the feared situation, which may take the form of a panic attack. Some examples of Specific Phobias are animals, flying, heights, or needles. Figure 11-9 ■ shows a man with claustrophobia. Table 11-3 ■ gives examples of Specific Phobias and their clinical names. Adults with phobias recognize that their fears are unreasonable. They usually avoid the phobic stimulus, but may endure it with intense anxiety or dread. A phobia seriously affects the person's daily routine, occupational or academic functioning, social life, or quality of life (American Psychiatric Association, 2000).

Children often have fears of things that seem irrational to adults. A child with a fear is not diagnosed with a

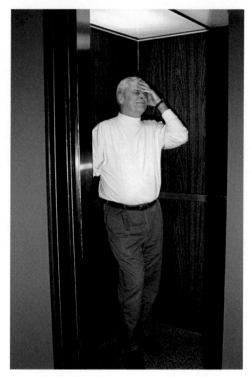

Figure 11-9. ■ An elevator can be a terrifying place for a person with claustrophobia. *Source:* PhotoEdit Inc.

Specific Phobia unless the fear is specific, extreme, causes great distress, and has affected school or daily functioning for at least 6 months. Children with phobias may not realize that their fears are irrational. Anxiety in children may be expressed by crying, clinging, the inability to move or "freezing with fear," or tantrums.

When phobias involve situations or objects that are easy to avoid, people may not feel the need to seek treatment. Phobias involving everyday experiences can be disabling. Fears of specific objects or situations are very common. Specific Phobia is not diagnosed unless the phobia significantly interferes with the individual's functioning or causes severe distress.

Specific Phobias often occur in people who also have other anxiety disorders, mood disorders, and substance-related disorders. People who have a blood-injection-injury–type phobia have a history of fainting from a vasovagal response in about 75% of cases. A vasovagal response is indicated by an initial rise in the heart rate and blood pressure, followed by a drop in heart rate and blood pressure that often causes fainting (American Psychiatric Association, 2000).

The first symptoms of Specific Phobias usually occur in childhood, but can be in adulthood. Factors that predispose

TABLE 11-3

Specific Phobias

CLINICAL NAME	FEARED OBJECT OR SITUATION
Acrophobia	Heights
Agoraphobia	Open spaces
Ailurophobia	Cats
Apiphobia	Bees
Astraphobia	Lightning
Aviophobia	Flying
Claustrophobia	Closed spaces
Cynophobia	Dogs
Entomophobia	Insects
Gephyrophobia	Bridge crossing
Hematophobia	Blood
Iatrophobia	Doctors
Hydrophobia	Water
Microphobia	Germs
Monophobia (or Autophobia)	Being alone
Mysophobia	Dirt
Nyctophobia	Darkness, night
Pyrophobia	Fire
Xenophobia	Strangers

people to develop Specific Phobias include the following (American Psychiatric Association, 2000):

- Traumatic events such as being trapped in a closet or attacked by an animal
- Unexpected panic attacks in the feared situation
- Observing others in the feared situation (seeing someone fall from a height)
- Seeing others demonstrate fear in the situation (mother is afraid of going to the dentist)
- Informational transmission (media coverage of bombing, natural disasters, plane crashes, or repeated parental warnings about dangers of some situation)

The subject of Specific Phobias differs from one culture to another. Women are more frequently affected by phobias than men are, at a rate of 2:1. The prevalence of phobias decreases in the elderly. Some phobias tend to run in families, especially the fears of blood and injury (American Psychiatric Association, 2000).

CASE EXAMPLE

A person with *aviophobia* (fear of flying) stated: "I'm scared to death of flying, and I never do it anymore. I used to start dreading a plane trip a month before I was due to leave. It was an awful feeling when the airplane door closed and I felt trapped. My heart would pound and I would sweat bullets. When the airplane would start to ascend, it just reinforced the feeling that I couldn't get out. When I think about flying, I picture myself losing control, freaking out, climbing the walls, but of course I never did that. I'm not afraid of crashing. It's just that feeling of being trapped. Whenever I've thought of changing jobs I think 'Would I be under pressure to fly?' These days I only go places where I can drive or take a train. My friends always point out that I couldn't get off a train traveling at high speeds either, so why don't trains bother me? I just tell them it isn't a rational fear" (NIMH, 2006).

Collaborative Care

Because the symptom of anxiety is associated with so many different physiological and psychosocial problems, an accurate diagnosis must be made before treatment begins. Some general medical disorders that frequently present with anxiety are listed in Box 11-3 ■.

Critical Self-Check. Why is it so important to have an accurate diagnosis of the reason for a client's anxiety before treatment begins?

There are effective treatments for anxiety disorders. Each disorder is treated specifically, but generally the

BOX 11-3

General Medical Conditions Associated with Anxiety

Hypoglycemia

Hyperthyroidism

Asthma

Pneumonia

Chronic Obstructive Pulmonary Disease

Pulmonary Embolism

Encephalitis

Cardiac Dysrhythmias

Vitamin B_{12} Deficiency

Pheochromocytoma (adrenal tumor)

Vestibular Dysfunction

Neoplasms

most effective treatments are cognitive-behavioral therapy and medications (Satcher, Delgado, & Masand, 2005).

COGNITIVE-BEHAVIORAL THERAPY

A major goal of cognitive-behavioral therapy (CBT) is to reduce anxiety by eliminating maladaptive beliefs or behaviors that help to maintain the anxiety disorder. CBT is effective for most anxiety disorders. It has two parts. In the **cognitive** part, clients are helped to change thinking patterns that stop them from overcoming their fears. Cognitive therapy includes helping clients discover the erroneous thoughts that initiate their anxiety. Cognitive therapy is based on the idea that thinking errors by the client produce mistaken negative beliefs that continue despite evidence to the contrary.

Cognitive restructuring is a therapeutic technique in which the client works to change patterns of negative thoughts that occur automatically. The client is helped to see the process of automatic negative anxiety-producing thoughts and negative self-talk. When the client sees the basis for the erroneous negative thinking, s/he can work on seeing the situation realistically, and can then be helped to replace the negative self-talk with more supportive and self-calming thinking.

People with anxiety disorders tend to put the worst possible interpretation on physical symptoms. For example, a woman with Panic Disorder may think that her panic attacks are heart attacks. She can be helped to see that they are panic attacks and are not life threatening. She can learn to replace the thought "I am dying!" with "I'm OK. This is a panic attack." She can discuss her experiences, looking for symptoms and events that come before the panic attacks to help identify triggers. Finally, she can be helped to find new ways to think about the triggers that start panic attacks. In a similar way, a person with Social Phobia can be helped to see that other people are not really judging him to be incompetent when he walks into class.

The goal of the *behavioral* part of CBT is to change the client's behavioral reaction to anxiety-provoking situations. One behavioral approach is to teach the client deep breathing or relaxation techniques. People can use these techniques to cope with anxiety by deliberately relaxing or deep breathing in situations they expect to provoke anxiety, thus interrupting the automatic anxiety responses.

Exposure is an important aspect of behavioral therapy for anxiety disorders. In this therapy, clients confront the thing they fear. There are several approaches to the use of exposure in behavioral therapy. One approach called *exposure and response prevention* is often used in

OCD. For example, if clients fear dirt and germs, the therapist may encourage them to dirty their hands and then to wait a certain amount of time before washing. The therapist helps the client to cope with the anxiety that results, and the client experiences a coping success. This technique helps the person test rational thoughts about the danger of dirt. By repeating this technique, the client will have a series of successful experiences of surviving dirt, and the anxiety will decrease over time (NIMH, 2006).

In another type of exposure exercise, a person with Social Phobia may be encouraged to spend a certain amount of time in a feared social situation while fighting the desire to run away. The client may be asked to recall a small social error and to relate how others responded. The therapist then discusses the reaction of others and helps the client see that the fear of judgment by others is not as brutal as the client feared. Repeated practice and discussion of feelings and coping techniques with the therapist can help reduce Social Phobia.

For a person with Posttraumatic Stress Disorder, exposure might consist of recalling the stressful event in detail, allowing the client to reexperience it in a safe environment. If this exposure is done with the support of a therapist, it may be possible to reduce the anxiety associated with the traumatic memories (NIMH, 2006).

Behavioral therapy alone has long been used effectively to treat Specific Phobias. The person is gradually exposed to the feared object or situation. Initially the exposure may only be to pictures of the feared object. Later, when the client feels ready, s/he confronts the actual feared situation in a safe setting. The therapist usually goes with the client to provide support and guidance (NIMH, 2006).

CBT usually take about 12 weeks and can be done individually or in groups. As with all psychotherapy, CBT must be directed at the client's specific concerns. What is an effective approach for one person may not be effective for another.

PSYCHOTROPIC AGENTS

It is preferred that a client can be helped to overcome anxiety or learn how to manage it for the long term without medications. As a general rule, people are better off if they can develop the tools to solve their own problems without using drugs to solve the problems. This is especially true for people who have transient or low-level anxiety or poor coping skills. The best approach to anxiety treatment for these clients is to promote adaptive coping skills.

However, when an anxiety disorder is present, clients may have abnormal neurotransmitter or neurohormonal function, and their anxiety may not respond to CBT or other psychotherapy. These clients have the best treatment response to a combination of CBT and medication therapy. Medications from several classifications treat anxiety effectively. Antidepressants are widely used for people with anxiety because it frequently co-occurs with depression (Satcher et al., 2005).

Most antianxiety medications are central nervous system (CNS) depressants. A few people abuse CNS depressant drugs by taking them in large doses for a euphoric effect. The CNS depressant effect is increased when these drugs are combined with alcohol. CNS depressants depress the respiratory system, and clients who abuse them or take them with alcohol are at risk for respiratory depression and death.

Despite the potential hazards of antianxiety drugs for a few clients, they are generally quite safe and there are many situations in which they are indicated. Some forms of anxiety, such as Specific Phobias, respond best to behavioral therapy alone, but most anxiety disorders require a combination of medication and psychotherapy for effective treatment. People with Panic Disorder may require the long-term prescription of antianxiety drugs because they would not be able to function without them.

Nurses should be aware that many people with mental disorders require medications in order to function. People with depression require antidepressants; those with psychosis require antipsychotics. Similarly, those with anxiety disorders often require antianxiety medications in order to achieve their developmental tasks (education, family responsibilities, or working) and to function. Whereas the antianxiety medications are contraindicated as a problem-solving approach for the otherwise normal client, they are required for the well-being of many people with severe anxiety disorders. Nurses must be supportive of these individuals who need medications, because there is a loud message in our culture that says "Just Say No to Drugs" in any situation. The message from mental health-care providers is: "Take medications if you need them to treat mental disorders."

Nurses should educate clients that if one treatment is not effective, it is worth trying other treatment modalities. A combination of psychotherapy and medications proves to be the most effective for the most people. If one medication is not effective, another one is likely to work. People often must try several drugs before they find the one that works best for them. Sometimes clients have to try very hard to have enough hope to seek out medical help, and when the first treatment does not work, it might be the nurse's job to keep hope alive with the assurance that "We will keep trying."

Antianxiety Agents

Benzodiazepines (BZs) are the most widely prescribed drugs in the world today. They are used for anxiety, insomnia, alcohol withdrawal, skeletal muscle relaxation, acute management of seizures, severe agitation, social phobia, generalized anxiety disorder, and panic disorder. Table 11-4 ■ provides information about these drugs.

> **Critical Self-Check.** Why do you think that the benzodiazepines are the most widely prescribed drugs in the world?

Sedative-Hypnotic Agents

The target symptoms for sedative-hypnotics are insomnia and sleep disorders. **Insomnia** includes difficulty falling asleep, difficulty staying asleep, or awakening too early and not being able to go back to sleep. The provider can choose the specific BZ based on matching its duration of action with the client's sleep problem (for example, a short-acting agent would be best for someone who has difficulty falling asleep). Table 11-5 ■ lists their duration of action.

Occasionally clients have a **paradoxical** (contradictory, opposite) response to the BZs (either the antianxiety agents or the sedatives). Instead of relaxation, they experience agitation or unstable emotions. The elderly, children, and people with brain damage are at increased risk. When a client has a paradoxical reaction, the BZ should be discontinued.

DRUG INTERACTIONS. Overdoses of benzodiazepines alone are not usually fatal. However, fatalities involving BZs combined with alcohol are relatively common. An additive CNS depressant effect occurs when BZs are taken with alcohol, TCAs, MAOIs, anticonvulsants, antihistamines, antipsychotics, or other CNS depressants.

BARBITURATES. The barbiturates, such as secobarbital and pentobarbital, are rarely used. The other sedative-hypnotic agents described above are more effective and safer. The barbiturates cause dependence and tolerance, they have a dangerous withdrawal syndrome, they are dangerous in overdose, and they can cause fatalities due to interactions with alcohol and other CNS depressants.

TABLE 11-4			
Antianxiety Agents			
CLASSIFICATION AND DRUG	ACTION AND USE	NURSING RESPONSIBILITIES	CLIENT TEACHING
Benzodiazepine antianxiety agents (BZs)			
Alprazolam (Xanax) Chlordiazepoxide (Librium) Clonazepam (Klonopin) Clorazepate (Tranxene) Diazepam (Valium) Lorazepam (Ativan) Oxazepam (Serax)	The BZs are thought to reduce anxiety by enhancing the inhibitory effects of the neuro-transmitter GABA. GABA makes the neuron less responsive to excitatory neurotransmitters such as norepinephrine, serotonin, and dopamine. The BZ binds to GABA at its postsynaptic receptor site, (probably in the amygdala-centered fear circuits) increasing the inhibitory effects of GABA, thus reducing anxiety. The target symptoms for the antianxiety drugs are nervousness, sweating, increased heart rate, sense of dread, fearfulness, phobias, com-pulsiveness, nausea, vomiting, diarrhea, dizziness, irritability, headache, and dry mouth. BZs are also used to treat alcohol with-drawal, seizures, for skeletal mus-cle relaxation, and for the emer-gency treatment of agitation. They are frequently combined with antidepressants to treat anxiety associated with depres-sion. If taken for a prolonged period (> 2 weeks), dose should be tapered to avoid withdrawal symptoms of CNS stimulation. Clients tend to become tolerant of the sedating effects over time, but not necessarily of the anti-anxiety effects (Stahl, 2005).	Evaluate effectiveness of drug for treating target symptoms. Assess for side effects: sedation, ataxia, dizziness, weakness, for-getfulness, and confusion. Older adults may have diffi-culty metabolizing the long-acting BZs, and may have increas-ing blood levels. The shorter acting agents are a better choice for older adults. They are also more likely to suffer cognitive or memory side effects from long-term BZ therapy than are younger adults. BZ doses should be tapered down when drug is discontinued. Overdose of BZs alone almost never causes death. There is an antidote flumazenil (Romazicon) that can reverse BZ actions if needed. The antianxiety BZs are classified Pregnancy Category D (positive evidence of risk to human fetus, potential benefits may still justify their use during pregnancy). Avoid especially early in pregnancy.	Teach clients to avoid alcohol when taking BZs. Antacids and food in the stomach make the BZs absorb more slowly into the blood. Side effects decrease with time. Clients should avoid dri-ving or being in situations where muscle coordination is a safety issue until they know how these drugs will affect them. Do not stop taking BZs abruptly. Doses should be tapered down to avoid with-drawal symptoms. Teach client about the con-traindication of taking these drugs during pregnancy, so clients should report to physi-cian in advance if they are plan-ning pregnancy.
Nonbenzodiazepine Antianxiety Agents			
Classification: **Azaspirone** Buspirone (BuSpar) Classification: **Beta-blockers** Propranolol (Inderal)	Buspirone probably acts as a serotonin agonist, increasing serotonin activity. It is not sedat-ing, does not cause euphoria, and has no *cross-tolerance* with seda-tives or alcohol. (An example of cross-tolerance is when clients are tolerant to large amounts of alcohol; they will also be tolerant to BZs, even if they have never taken them before.)	Evaluate for drug effectiveness at reducing anxiety. Assess for side effects that include dizzi-ness, headache, nausea, nervous-ness, and excitement. It is a remarkably safe drug. Because it has no abuse potential, it is not a controlled substance. Evaluate for effectiveness on target symptoms of anxiety. Assess for side effects: bradycardia,	Buspirone begins to have antianxiety effects within 7–10 days, but may take up to 6 weeks to achieve full effect. If this drug does not work, there are other drugs that can be tried. Teach client to rise slowly to prevent orthostatic hypoten-sion. Instruct client to take drug 30–60 minutes before the antici-pated anxiety-producing activity

TABLE 11-4			
Antianxiety Agents			
CLASSIFICATION AND DRUG	**ACTION AND USE**	**NURSING RESPONSIBILITIES**	**CLIENT TEACHING**
	Buspirone does not cause dependence or withdrawal. It has virtually no abuse potential. It is not effective against seizures, muscle spasm, or alcohol withdrawal, nor does it treat panic disorder effectively. If a client is going to change from a BZ to buspirone, the dose of BZ should be tapered to avoid withdrawal. Propranolol is a blocker of beta-adrenergic receptors (beta-blocker). Rather than acting directly on anxiety, it decreases some anxiety symptoms, such as increased heart rate. It is used in the treatment of social phobia. The target symptom is performance anxiety or other anxiety related to social situations, usually on a p.r.n. basis.	fatigue, weakness, dizziness, and hypotension. Hold for heart rate < 50. Onset is 30 min and peak at 60 min after oral dose.	(such as public speaking or musical performance).
Benzodiazepine Sedative-Hypnotic Agents			
Estazolam (ProSom) Flurazepam (Dalmane) Temazepam (Restoril) Triazolam (Halcion) Quazepam (Doral)	Pharmacologic action is the same as BZs used for anxiety. Target symptom is insomnia. The specific agent used will be chosen to match with clients' sleep disorder. Those who awaken too early and cannot go back to sleep will be given long-acting drugs, those who cannot fall asleep are given short-acting drugs).	Evaluate client's length and quality of sleep. Assess for side effects: sedation, fatigue, depression, dizziness, forgetfulness, confusion, and respiratory depression (when combined with alcohol or other CNS depressants). The BZ sedative-hypnotics are classified Pregnancy Category X (positive evidence of risk to human fetus, contraindicated during pregnancy, can cause neonatal flaccidity or withdrawal effects when taken in late pregnancy).	Clients should avoid drinking alcohol with these drugs. The additive CNS depression can cause fatal respiratory depression. Teach clients to tell physician in advance if they are planning pregnancy, so these drugs can be tapered off.
Nonbenzodiazepine Sedative-Hypnotic Agents			
Classification: Cyclopyrrolones Eszopiclone (Lunesta) Imidazopyridines	These drugs are not BZs but they also interact with the GABA receptors, enhancing GABA inhibitory functions, and causing sedation. The target symptom for these drugs is insomnia. They	Evaluate the client's length and quality of sleep. Clients should not awaken in the morning with a "hung over" feeling due to the short duration of action. Side effects: sedation, dizziness,	Teach client to take these medications only at bedtime. The client will become too sedated to function safely if taken during the day. Onset of action is rapid.

(continued)

TABLE 11-4

Antianxiety Agents (continued)

CLASSIFICATION AND DRUG	ACTION AND USE	NURSING RESPONSIBILITIES	CLIENT TEACHING
Zolpidem (Ambien) Pyrazolopyrimidine (Sonata)	should increase the amount of sleep and decrease the latency (wait) of falling asleep. They also should decrease the number of nighttime awakenings. They have a more rapid onset than BZs and a shorter duration of effect.	ataxia. Lower dose is indicated in the elderly, who are also at increased risk for falls. If taken for more than a few weeks, dose should be tapered to prevent withdrawal effects.	Avoid use of alcohol with these drugs due to additive CNS depression.
Classification: **Antihistamines** Diphenhydramine (Benadryl) Hydroxyzine (Atarax, Vistaril)	The antihistamines are sometimes used for their sedating side effect. They act by blocking histamine 1 receptors. These are available in both injectable and oral forms. The target symptoms are anxiety and insomnia. These agents would be preferred for clients with anxiety or insomnia related to pruritis.	Evaluate the drug's ability to achieve the target effects. Assess for side effects: sedation, dry mouth, constipation, palpitations, tremor. Lower dose is indicated in the elderly. They may be more sensitive to sedative and anticholinergic effects.	Teach clients, especially the elderly, constipation prevention measures (high fiber diet, fluids, and exercise).

TABLE 11-5

Duration of Action of Benzodiazepine Antianxiety and Sedative-Hypnotic Agents

DRUG	DURATION OF ACTION	AVAILABLE IN INJECTABLE (IM AND IV) FORM?
Antianxiety Agents		
Alprazolam (Xanax)	Intermediate acting	No
Chlordiazepoxide (Librium)	Long acting	Yes
Clonazepam (Klonopin)	Long acting	No
Clorazepate (Tranxene)	Long acting	No
Diazepam (Valium)	Long acting	Yes
Lorazepam (Ativan)	Intermediate acting	Yes
Oxazepam (Serax)	Intermediate acting	No
Sedative-Hypnotic Agents		
Estazolam (ProSom)	Intermediate acting	No
Flurazepam (Dalmane)	Long acting	No
Temazepam (Restoril)	Intermediate acting	No
Triazolam (Halcion)	Short acting	No
Quazepam (Doral)	Long acting	No

NURSING CARE

ASSESSING

During the nursing history, the nurse may identify that the client has a general medical condition that commonly has anxiety as a symptom (see Box 11-3). In these clients, treating the general medical disorder treats anxiety symptoms. For example, if a client has anxiety symptoms due to hypoxia from an asthma attack, the treatment is her inhaler for bronchodilation, not an antianxiety medication.

The physical symptoms of anxiety usually begin with increased heart rate, blood pressure, and respiratory rate. (See Table 11-2, which summarizes the subjective effects and observable behavior of a person experiencing anxiety.) The nurse assesses not only whether the client has anxiety but also the level of anxiety.

Important assessments by nurses always include how clients respond to their illnesses and how they respond to their treatments. Nurses must document their objective findings, such as the client's vital signs and observed behaviors, as well as subjective symptoms such as the clients' statements on how they are feeling. Documentation should also include what factors cause or worsen anxiety, if these are observed. The nurse will use these in the intervention phase of the nursing process. Nurses use assessment findings to help the client recognize factors that increase and decrease anxiety and to improve the client's insight.

Licensed nurses who are responsible for the care of clients who receive medications must know the desired effects and potential side effects of those medications. The nurse assesses the client's response to medications. Box 11-4 ■ provides an example of a narrative charting entry on a client with anxiety. It includes objective and subjective assessment information and how the client responded to treatment. Note that the nurse tried non-pharmacological interventions before medicating this client with her p.r.n. dose of diazepam.

If a client were experiencing an episode of anxiety, the nurse would ask about the client's perception of the threat represented by the situation. This is an important assessment. The nurse should also assess the client's use of alcohol or drugs as self-medication for anxiety at home. A history of insomnia or the regular use of medications for sleep may indicate chronic anxiety. Information about the client's usual coping methods can be helpful in planning care for the anxious client. Box 11-5 ■ lists some questions that might obtain information about the client's usual coping methods.

BOX 11-4

Narrative Charting Example on Client with Anxiety

The client is an 82-year-old woman who has been a resident of a long-term care facility for 1 year, since she had a CVA. She is unable to ambulate due to hemiplegia. She also has a diagnosis of Generalized Anxiety Disorder.

Nurse charting on narrative notes: *Vital signs increased (HR 105, R 24, BP 154/96). Client was restless, unable to focus on one activity, moving items around on her bedside table repeatedly. Client states: "I am so nervous! I don't know what to do!" Client refused a backrub or music to decrease anxiety. Gave client p.r.n. dose of Valium 2.5 mg 30 min ago with desired results. Client is working on a puzzle and states that she feels better and not so nervous now.—Ima Nurse, LPN*

The nurse's own anxiety level is another important assessment. When the nurse is anxious, it is much easier for the client to feel anxious. Anxiety is "contagious" in this way. The nurse needs enough insight to recognize his or her own anxiety and the situations that promote it. Then the nurse can use adaptive coping methods to reduce the anxiety and present a calm demeanor with the client. A calm nurse makes it easier for the client to remain calm.

It can be stressful for a client to discuss anxious feelings. Sometimes the client finds it less stressful to deny anxiety and may resist confronting these dysphoric feelings. The resistive client may not be consciously trying to make it difficult for the nurse, but may be using behaviors that have been learned as a way to avoid stress. Some resistive behaviors used by clients to avoid recognizing anxiety include the following (Stuart, 2005):

■ *Hostility.* The client uses offense to defend her/himself and relates to others aggressively. The nurse may take this behavior personally and respond with anger, which reinforces the client's avoidance of anxiety.

BOX 11-5

Assessing Clients' Coping Methods

"When you have a lot of stress, what do you do?"
"What do you usually do in situations like this?"
"What usually helps you when this happens?"
"Who can help you at a time like this?"
"Do you ever drink alcohol to help you through stressful times?"
"Where could you go for help?"
"What helps you get through a really bad day?"

- *Screening symptoms.* The client focuses on minor physical complaints to avoid acknowledging difficult feelings.
- *Emotional seduction.* The client tries to manipulate the situation by causing the nurse to feel sympathy or pity.
- *Superficiality.* The client keeps the conversation on a shallow, surface level, never going deeply into real feelings.
- *Intellectualization.* The client expresses ideas about clients in general or analyzes feelings on an intellectual level, without talking about her/his own real feelings.
- *Withdrawal.* The client speaks in a vague or unclear way.
- *Forgetting.* The client purposely forgets (or pretends to forget) an incident to avoid exploring it with the nurse.

These resistive behaviors may cause nurses to respond with frustration, anger, or anxiety. Nurses must be aware of this potential so they can respond in the most therapeutic way toward the client. The client's behavior does not have to determine the nurses' behavior. When nurses feel angry or frustrated with the client, they have an opportunity to develop personal insight into how they are affected by client behavior. This insight can free them from the frustration of reacting to certain clients negatively.

DIAGNOSING, PLANNING, AND IMPLEMENTING

Anxiety is a nursing diagnosis. Nurses can diagnose and treat the symptom of anxiety independently. When a person has disabling anxiety such as in an anxiety disorder, a physician makes the diagnosis and care is collaborative. Some common nursing diagnoses for clients experiencing anxiety are as follows:

- Anxiety
- Fear
- Ineffective Coping
- Impaired Social Interaction
- Social Isolation
- Powerlessness
- Posttrauma Syndrome

The desired outcomes for people with anxiety are generally on three levels. First, during the *acute phase* of anxiety, the desired outcomes are that clients will be free from self-inflicted harm and will experience decreased anxiety symptoms. Second, during the *stabilization phase* of therapy clients will begin to learn to verbalize their own feelings, understand their own stress response, and try new methods

for anxiety reduction. Finally, *in the community,* clients will develop adaptive methods for coping with stress, use support systems, and demonstrate adequate social and occupational function (Schultz & Videbeck, 2005).

Acute Phase

During the acute phase of anxiety, the client is at greatest risk.

- Assess for risk of self-harm. *People with some anxiety disorders (especially panic disorder and PTSD) are at risk for suicide.*
- Observe closely and provide a safe environment. *People at risk for suicide require close observation, support, and no access to means of self-harm.*
- Have a calm, nonthreatening attitude while caring for the client. *Anxiety is easily transmitted from one person to another. Clients feel more secure when the nurse is confident, calm, and nonthreatening.*
- Assure the client that s/he is safe. Do not leave an acutely anxious person alone. *People with high anxiety may fear for their lives. The presence of the nurse can convey protection and safety.*
- Maintain a low-stimulation environment (avoid loud noise, bright light). *Environmental stimuli can worsen anxiety because high anxiety reduces the client's ability to filter stimuli.*
- Keep communication simple and direct. *High levels of anxiety make it impossible for clients to focus on any more than brief concrete messages.*
- If the client has a p.r.n. order for an antianxiety medication and needs it, give it. *Nurses often hesitate to give p.r.n. medications. Withholding a needed antianxiety medication may communicate to the client that there is something wrong with taking this medication. Antianxiety drugs are safe and effective and should be given as needed.*

Stabilization Phase

After the acute phase, when anxiety symptoms are resolved, the stabilization phase begins.

- Encourage the client to express feelings. Engage in therapeutic use of self by nurse (using interpersonal and communication skills as therapeutic nursing interventions). Provide time for 1:1 interaction. *Therapeutic use of self by the nurse helps establish trust and a foundation for a therapeutic relationship. One-on-one interactions provide time for the client to express feelings in a nonthreatening place.*

BOX 11-6	

Teaching Progressive Relaxation Exercise

Explain to the client that progressive relaxation is an exercise involving first tightening then relaxing the major muscle groups from one end of the body to the other. This exercise can be done with the client sitting or lying down. Dim the lights. The exercise is best done with the client's eyes closed so s/he can concentrate on relaxation. The nurse reads the following:

■ Take a deep breath in and hold it. Hold it in until it collects all the tension in your body, and then slowly let it out. The tension is leaving with the air. Take another slow deep relaxing breath. Let out the tension as you let out the air.

■ Now tighten the muscles in your feet. Your toes are all tightened up. Now let them go. Wiggle the toes and let them relax. Now your calves and ankles. Point your feet up toward your head and hold them tight. Then point them to the floor and hold tight. Now wiggle your feet and relax them. They are free now. Tighten your thighs. Press them down and feel the tension. OK; shake your legs and loosen them up.

■ Contract your abdomen. Hold the muscles down flat. Hold it tight. Now release. Hold your arms close to your body. Closer, tighter. Then release. Shake your arms to loosen them up. Now your hands. Tighten them into fists. Make them tight. Now let them go. Wiggle your fingers. Let them dance as they relax. Last, your mouth. Clench your teeth. Press your tongue to the roof of your mouth. Now let your tongue rest. Open your mouth and take a deep breath.

■ Your whole body is relaxed now. Hold the breath in, then let it out, and with it goes that last bit of tension. You are relaxed.

■ Use therapeutic communication techniques. *Therapeutic communication techniques help clients analyze their own feelings and actions.*

■ Help the client to explore factors that lead to anxiety. *Understanding what comes before anxiety can begin the process of disarming these precipitating factors and learning to respond to them adaptively without anxiety.*

■ Explore options for responding adaptively to stressors, and practice them if possible. *New coping skills can be discussed and planned first, but will be best incorporated into the client's life if an opportunity can be made to practice them.*

■ Teach the client to recognize anxiety as it develops and to take control of stopping the anxiety from escalating (relaxation or breathing techniques, exercise, meditation). *If the client can recognize anxiety early while s/he can still focus on problem solving, s/he can employ various techniques to reduce anxiety responses. The techniques listed under interventions can all be effective. Client preference indicates which one to use.*

An effective intervention for the relief of anxiety is progressive relaxation. The directions for assisting the client through a progressive relaxation exercise are provided in Box 11-6 ■. Note that in the directions the nurse tells the client to first tighten and then relax each muscle group. The tightening serves to show the contrast between tension and relaxation and makes it easier for the client to determine how the muscle group feels when relaxed. The nurse guides the client through the exercise the first time. Then the client practices it alone. Finally, the client learns to use the relaxation technique when a stressful situation arises to stop the progression of anxiety.

It is not the goal of the nurse to relieve all anxiety. Some anxiety is a necessary protective mechanism that allows people to be alert for danger and to learn new things. Nurses try to help clients understand themselves so they can learn new coping skills and keep anxiety at a manageable level.

The nurse may be able to help clients recognize their own anxiety by describing client behavior and connecting it to anxious feelings. For example, the nurse could say: "I saw you pacing up and down the hall (or wringing your hands, or shaking, etc.). Were you feeling nervous or anxious then?"

EVALUATING

In the evaluation phase of the nursing process, the nurse looks back to the desired outcomes for the client. Were they fully met, partially met, or unmet? If they were not fully met, why not? Perhaps the goals were unrealistically high for the client. Perhaps the nursing interventions were not adequate or not frequent enough. When the entire plan for nursing care has been reviewed, it may be revised to ensure that the client care outcomes can be met.

NURSING PROCESS CARE PLAN
Client with Generalized Anxiety Disorder

Mrs. Miedo is a 70-year-old Latina with mild dementia who lives in a long-term care facility. She was transferred to the skilled unit when she returned from the hospital to recover from a fractured hip. She was diagnosed with Generalized Anxiety Disorder as a young woman. She has not had severe anxiety symptoms for several years, until after the hip surgery. The nurse in the skilled unit is Marc.

Assessment. Mrs. M.'s heart rate is 110, her respiratory rate is 26, and her BP is 158/98. She is oriented to person and place and is very alert, carefully watching anyone who enters her room. Her skin is pale and cool. She is having surgical pain. She is not sleeping well. When the nurse tries to teach Mrs. Miedo about her medications, she is not able to pay attention. She is restless. Her hands are always busy pulling and fiddling with the covers on her bed. She states: "I don't know what to do. I am so scared. Don't leave me." For Mrs. M.'s anxiety, the physician ordered diazepam 5 mg PO three times a day and an additional 2.5 mg p.r.n., also three times a day.

Diagnosis. The following nursing diagnoses were identified for Mrs. Miedo:

■ Pain R/T injury and surgery on hip
■ Anxiety R/T unfamiliar situation
■ Ineffective Coping R/T inadequate coping skills in new situation

Expected Outcomes. The following outcomes were identified to help plan for Mrs. Miedo's care:

■ Client's surgical pain will remain at less than 3 on a scale of 1 to 10 throughout her stay in the skilled unit.
■ Client will have reduced anxiety symptoms (VS will be within normal limits, she will state that she feels less afraid, and she will sleep at least 7 hours per night) within 2 days.
■ Client will be able to express her feelings to the nurse within 1 week.
■ Client will develop and use her own strategies to relax herself within 1 week.

Planning and Implementation

■ Marc (the nurse) introduced himself and asked if Mrs. M. had any questions about her care in the skilled unit. He told her that he would be her nurse and he would take care of her.
■ Marc gave Mrs. Miedo the pain medication that the physician ordered every 4 hours p.r.n. on a regular schedule instead of waiting for her to ask for it. He planned her ambulation schedule so she would ambulate when the pain medication was at its peak (about 1 hour after the oral dose).
■ Marc gave the regularly scheduled dose of diazepam and the p.r.n. dose 2 hours later on the first day he

cared for Mrs. M. because her anxiety level was consistently so high.

■ He tried to keep her environmental stimuli to a minimum. He turned the TV off and turned on her radio when she requested to listen to music. He closed the drapes to keep out the bright light in her room.
■ Marc kept a calm and confident manner with Mrs. M. He kept his questions short and his communication concrete and simple.
■ The nurse and the nursing assistant checked on Mrs. M. as often as they could. He assigned the same nursing assistant to work with her every day.
■ Marc helped her with a progressive relaxation exercise.

Evaluation. When Mrs. M. took the pain medication on a regular schedule, her pain came under control very quickly. She needed less medication as time went on.

She came to trust the staff in the skilled unit. She was able to call the nurse when she started to feel anxious. Sometimes she needed p.r.n. diazepam; other times she responded to reassurance. She slept 8 hours each night after her pain was under control and she started taking the antianxiety medication. After 4 days she no longer needed the additional p.r.n. doses of diazepam. Her behavior indicated that she was feeling more relaxed. She smiled more, and the restlessness resolved. Her vital signs were within normal limits. Her anxiety was under control with the combination of the regular dose of diazepam and the nonpharmacological nursing interventions. However, she was not able to do the relaxation technique independently.

Critical Thinking in the Nursing Process

1. Explain why the regular dosage of pain medication was better than p.r.n. dosage for Mrs. M. to control both her pain and her anxiety.
2. What is the purpose of keeping the same nursing assistant on assignment to Mrs. M. every day?
3. What factor(s) might prevent Mrs. M. from doing self-relaxation exercises independently? Was this outcome realistic for Mrs. M.?

Note: Discussion of Critical Thinking questions appears in Appendix I.

Note: The references and resources for this and all chapters have been compiled at the back of the book.

Chapter Review

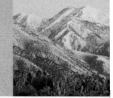

 KEY TERMS

Use the audio glossary feature of the Companion Website to hear the correct pronunciation of the following key terms.

anxiety

compulsions

coping

dysphoric

insomnia

obsessions

panic attack

paradoxical

phobia

KEY Points

- Anxiety is a universal human experience. It makes people alert to danger and more open to new learning. When it becomes so severe that it affects activities of daily living, occupational functioning, or quality of life, an anxiety disorder is present.

- Anxiety disorders are the most common psychiatric disorders in the United States, affecting 25% of the population each year.

- Many people with anxiety disorders do not seek help because they do not realize that they have a psychiatric problem or they fear the stigma of mental illness.

- There are effective medications and therapies for anxiety disorders.

- Client responses to anxiety include physiological, behavioral, and cognitive changes.

- A calm and confident nurse is most therapeutic with anxious clients.

- Some client behaviors result in frustration, anger, and anxiety in nurses. Nurses can prevent these reactions by developing insight about how they react to client behavior.

 EXPLORE MediaLink

Additional interactive resources for this chapter can be found on the Companion Website at www.prenhall.com/eby. Click on Chapter 11 and "Begin" to select the activities for this chapter.

- Audio glossary
- NCLEX-PN® review
- Case study
- Study outline
- Critical thinking questions
- Matching questions
- Weblinks
- Video Case: Dave (Obsessive-Compulsive Disorder)

Caring for a Client with Anxiety

NCLEX-PN® Focus Area: Psychosocial Integrity

Case Study: Kayla is a 22-year-old European American female client admitted to the surgical unit of a general hospital with abdominal pain. She had a cholecystectomy yesterday. She told the night nurse that she thinks she might die. She is scheduled for discharge tomorrow.

Nursing Diagnosis: Anxiety, severe

COLLECT DATA

Subjective	Objective
_____	_____
_____	_____
_____	_____
_____	_____
_____	_____
_____	_____

Would you report this data? Yes/No

If yes, to: _____

Nursing Care

_____
_____
_____
_____
_____
_____
_____
_____

How would you document this?_____
_____
_____
_____

Compare your documentation to the sample provided in Appendix I.

Data Collected
(use those that apply)

- VS: T 99° F, P 108, R 32, BP 130/86
- Client is married.
- Has 1 child, age 10 months
- Client asks, "Am I going to die from this?"
- Weight 152 lbs.
- Skin is cool, diaphoretic.
- States, "I think my incision is going to tear open."
- Client's hands are constantly moving, picking at the sheets.
- Nurse stated in report: client slept approximately 3 hours last night.
- Abdominal incision is well-approximated, without exudate.
- Dry oral membranes
- Eyes are glancing around the room, darting from one thing to another.
- Complains of feeling dizzy

Nursing Interventions
(use those that apply; list in priority order)

- Encourage the client to talk about her feelings.
- Accept the client as she is.
- Tell the client that she is fine, and that she should quit worrying so much.
- Acknowledge that client is anxious.
- Assign a nursing assistant to sit with the client 24 hours per day.
- Keep communication simple and concrete.
- Explain the pathophysiology of cholecystitis, the procedure of cholecystectomy, and analgesic therapy in detail.
- Provide comfort measures.
- Be calm and confident with the client.
- Discuss healthy ways to talk about and relieve anxiety.
- Assess coping skills the client has used successfully in the past.
- Assess client's resources for support.
- Use progressive relaxation to help client relax.
- Give the client her p.r.n. pain medication to treat the anxiety.
- Give the client a book to read to distract her from her problems.

1 A client expresses nervousness about the MRI he will have in the morning. He is fidgeting with his sheets. The nurse's first response to the client is to:

1. Bring him his p.r.n. alprazolam.
2. Validate that he is anxious, and ask him to state what he thinks is the source of his "nervousness."
3. Reassure him that MRIs are safe procedures and nothing to worry about.
4. Turn on his television to divert his attention to something else.

2 A client has been admitted with Generalized Anxiety Disorder to a psychiatric unit. The client tells the nurse she knows she is dying, and no one will tell her. She paces constantly and wrings her hands. Interventions for this client might include:

1. Putting the nurse's arm around the client and assuring her she is safe.
2. Calling her family to come in and walk with her.
3. Reassuring her that if she were dying she would have been placed in a different unit of the hospital.
4. Using a calm approach to the client, describe her anxious behavior as the nurse sees it. Encourage her to talk about what feelings she is having.

3 A client has just experienced her first panic attack. She asks the nurse if that means she will have attacks for the rest of her life. The nurse's best response would be to say:

1. "One panic attack is likely to be followed by a series of attacks."
2. "I would not worry about it if I were you. That will probably bring on another attack."
3. "Some people have one attack and that is all."
4. "You are young and healthy; this was just a one-time incident."

4 Agoraphobia is the fear of:

1. Flying.
2. Open spaces.
3. Heights.
4. Water.

5 When a nurse brings a new client on the medical-surgical unit his medications, he asks the nurse to pour them out on a sterile dressing. He counts the pills three times before taking any of them. Every time he takes a pill, he counts the remainder of the pills three times before taking the next one. This client is most likely suffering from which anxiety disorder?

1. Panic Disorder
2. Obsessive-Compulsive Disorder

3. Generalized Anxiety Disorder
4. Posttraumatic Stress Disorder

6 A nursing student is assigned a client in Room 306. When she starts to enter the room, she bursts into uncontrollable sobbing. When the nurse approaches her to find out what is wrong, she states that her mother died suddenly in that same room 2 months ago. This student is probably experiencing:

1. Posttraumatic Stress.
2. Panic attack.
3. Phobic attack.
4. Acute Stress Disorder.

7 A significant part of cognitive restructuring for the client suffering from an anxiety disorder is to assist the client to:

1. Avoid the situation or object that produces anxiety.
2. Discuss his negative thoughts about certain anxiety-producing situations and objects.
3. Replace negative self-talk with more supportive and positive self-talk.
4. Accept his negative thoughts about certain situations and objects as being part of his normal life responses.

8 Medications may be used along with behavioral interventions to treat anxiety disorders. The nurse should be aware that one of the biggest dangers with the use of medications for anxiety is:

1. Suicide.
2. Increased risk for depression.
3. Drug dependency and tolerance.
4. Increased blood sugars over time.

9 In helping the anxious client to adopt effective coping strategies, an effective approach by the nurse would be to:

1. Teach the client relaxation and/or deep-breathing techniques.
2. Leave the client alone to develop her own plan.
3. Provide reading material on coping strategies.
4. Tell the client what the nurse would do in similar circumstances.

10 Anxiety may manifest itself with a number of physiological responses. Select which of the following would contribute to an overall assessment of anxiety.

1. Constricted pupils
2. Cool skin
3. Increased heart rate
4. Lowered blood pressure
5. Piloerection ("goose bumps")

Answers for Review Questions, as well as discussion of Care Plan and Critical Thinking Care Map questions, appear in Appendix I.

Chapter 12

Substance Abuse and Dependency

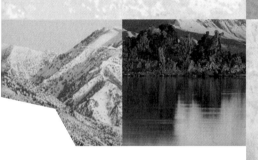

BRIEF Outline

Delayed Diagnosis

Substance Abuse and Dependency

Collaborative Care

Dual Diagnosis

Substance Dependency Among Nurses

LEARNING Outcomes

After completing this chapter, you will be able to:

1. Explain substance abuse, substance dependency, tolerance, and withdrawal.
2. Assess clients for substance abuse symptoms.
3. Apply the nursing process to clients with nursing problems related to substance abuse and dependency.
4. Respond appropriately when a colleague is impaired by substance abuse at work.

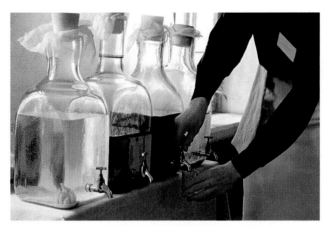

Figure 12-1. ■ Homemade alcohol being served in a restaurant in St. Petersburg, Russia. *Source:* AGE Fotostock America, Inc.

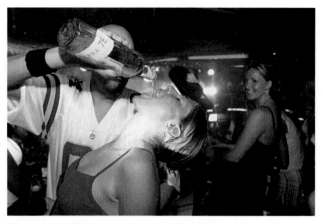

Figure 12-2. ■ Man pouring tequila down the throat of a young woman at a Spring Break celebration. *Source:* AP Wide World Photos.

It is natural for animals to seek an altered state of mind. Pigs eat fermented grain; elephants eat fermented fruit until they get drunk. People alter their state of mind by watching horror movies, riding carnival rides, climbing mountains, running marathons, meditating, relaxing, praying, and sometimes by taking substances. Figure 12-1 ■ depicts homemade alcohol being served in a Russian restaurant.

People use substances for a variety of reasons: to alter their perceptions; to elevate mood; to relieve pain, fear, anxiety, or boredom; to enhance socialization with their friends; or to aid in religious ceremonies. Although all substance use is not problematic, the abuse of substances can destroy people's lives. Substance use becomes a problem when:

- It interferes with the ability to function at work or at home.
- It puts anyone in danger.
- It continues despite negative consequences.

Substance abuse is one of the biggest health problems in North America in the 21st century. As many as 20% of adults in the United States meet the diagnostic criteria for an alcohol- or substance-related disorder (American Psychiatric Association, 2000). Up to 8.3% of the population age 12 and older are current (within the last month) illegal drug users. Among people age 12 to 17, 11.6% are current illegal drug users (Bailey, 2004). Fully half of all the alcohol consumed in the United States is done by underage drinkers and adults who drink excessively (Keltner, Schwecke, & Bostrom, 2007). Figure 12-2 ■ shows a young woman drinking excessively at a Spring Break celebration. Unfortunately, alcohol is a factor in many fatal events.

Figure 12-3 ■ shows how often alcohol is a factor in fatalities in the United States. Note that alcohol is involved in half of all motor vehicle deaths and half of all deaths due to domestic violence (Figures 12-4 ■ and 12-5 ■).

Delayed Diagnosis

Denial is the reason that the exact number of people with substance abuse and dependency is not known. Denial is a common coping mechanism for people with substance abuse disorders. Ironically, denial is also common in health professionals who work with these clients. Think about it: are 2 of every 10 clients in the facilities where you work or have clinical courses diagnosed with substance abuse or dependency? Healthcare providers do not assess or diagnose it, even though substance abuse and dependency are common and cause significant health effects. Another factor in the many undiagnosed cases is that people with substance-related disorders do not tend to consult healthcare providers. People usually wait until they experience the severe physical deterioration of late-stage substance dependency before they seek help.

Critical Self-Check. Why do you think healthcare providers fail to ask clients about substance use and abuse? Why do clients fail to seek treatment?

The stigma against substance abuse is very strong. Health professionals often hesitate to ask the questions that could determine who is affected by substance use. Sometimes health professionals are not aware of how they can help. This chapter helps nurses identify clients with substance-related disorders and suggests interventions to help them.

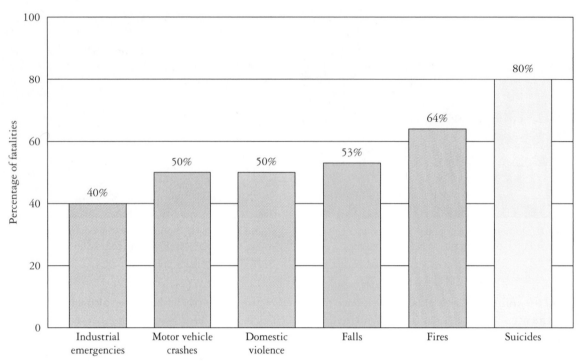

Figure 12-3. ■ Fatal events in which alcohol is a factor. *Source:* Reprinted with permission from *Mental Health Nursing, 5/E,* Fontaine and Fletcher, 2003, Prentice Hall.

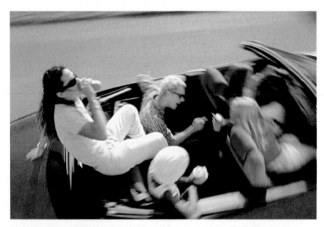

Figure 12-4. ■ Alcohol is involved in over half of all motor vehicle deaths. The risk is increased when the drivers are young. *Source:* Photo Researchers, Inc.

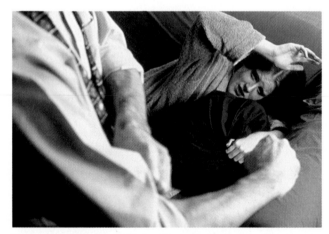

Figure 12-5. ■ Alcohol is involved in half of all deaths caused by domestic violence. *Source:* Photo Researchers, Inc.

Substance Abuse and Dependency

There are two different levels of substance use:

Substance abuse is a maladaptive pattern of substance use despite adverse outcomes (American Psychiatric Association, 2000). Box 12-1 ■ provides the *DSM-IV-TR* diagnostic criteria. People who abuse substances suffer the harmful consequences of repeated use. **Substance dependency** is more severe. It involves tolerance, withdrawal,

and compulsive use (see Box 12-1). The definitions from the *DSM-IV-TR* apply to all substances of abuse and dependence.

The most commonly abused substances are those that rapidly change a person's mental state, either by stimulating or by depressing the central nervous system (CNS). The *DSM-IV-TR* lists 11 substances of abuse:

- Alcohol
- Opioids
- Sedatives, hypnotics, and anxiolytics (antianxiety drugs)

BOX 12-1

DSM-IV-TR Diagnostic Criteria and Key Terms for Substance Abuse and Substance Dependency

Substance abuse:
A maladaptive pattern of substance use leading to significant impairment or distress manifested by one or more of the following:
1. Inability to fulfill major role obligations at work, school, and home (poor work performance, expulsions from school, neglect of children)
2. Recurrent substance use in physically hazardous situations (driving a car, operating a machine)
3. Recurrent legal or interpersonal problems
4. Continued use despite persistent social and interpersonal problems caused by use of the substance (arguments with spouse about intoxication, fights, problems at work)

Substance dependency:
A maladaptive pattern of substance use leading to significant impairment or distress, manifested by three or more of the following:
1. Tolerance to the substance
2. Withdrawal syndrome
3. Substance either taken in higher amounts or for longer periods than intended
4. Unsuccessful or persistent desire to cut down or control use
5. A great deal of time spent in obtaining, using, and recovering from effects of the substance
6. Reduction of important social, occupational, or recreational activities due to substance use

7. Continued substance use despite knowledge of a persistent physical or psychological problem that is likely caused by the substance

Key Terms in Substance Dependency
Tolerance:
Defined by either of the following:
   a. A need for increased amounts of the substance to achieve the same effect, or
   b. Diminished effect with continued use of the same amount of the substance

Withdrawal:
Due to discontinuing or reducing use of a substance that has been heavy and prolonged:
   a. A substance-specific withdrawal syndrome develops (see Table 12-2)
   b. The same or related substance is taken to relieve or avoid withdrawal symptoms
   c. Significant distress or impairment in social or occupational functioning occurs

Compulsive substance use:
Repetitive substance use behavior for the purpose of reducing distress. **Compulsive substance use** is often unwanted and time-consuming.

Source: Reprinted with permission from the *Diagnostic and Statistical Manual of Mental Disorders,* 4th ed., *Text Revision,* copyright 2000, American Psychiatric Association.

- Cocaine
- Amphetamines and similar drugs
- Hallucinogens
- Phencyclidine (PCP) and similar drugs
- Inhalants
- Cannabis (marijuana)
- Caffeine
- Nicotine

ALCOHOL

The most commonly abused substance in the world is beverage alcohol (ethanol or ethyl alcohol). Alcohol is quickly absorbed into the blood and acts as a central nervous system depressant. Initial symptoms of alcohol **intoxication** (a reversible set of physical, psychological, and behavioral symptoms caused by use of a substance) are relaxation, loss of inhibition, euphoria (an exaggerated feeling of well-being), and decreased mental concentration. With higher doses, symptoms progress to slurred speech, ataxia (staggering gait), labile (changeable) mood, aggressive behavior, incoherent speech, vomiting, coma, respiratory depression, and death. Blood alcohol concentrations and the symptoms they produce are shown in Table 12-1 ■.

Tolerance and Withdrawal

With continued use, the user develops **tolerance** (see Box 12-1). When an individual regularly drinks large amounts of alcohol, the CNS is repeatedly depressed. To maintain balance (homeostasis) for survival, the CNS increases its own stimulation to keep the person conscious and functioning. As this person's CNS is continually forced to produce excess chemical stimulation, the individual will require more alcohol to achieve intoxication. Eventually, over years of alcohol dependency, the individual must drink almost constantly to avoid the distressing symptoms of CNS stimulation.

When the alcohol-dependent individual (alcoholic) stops drinking, the homeostatic mechanism that balanced the depressant effects of the alcohol takes time to

TABLE 12-1	
Symptoms of Alcohol Intoxication by Blood Alcohol Concentration	
BLOOD ALCOHOL CONCENTRATION	**SYMPTOMS**
0.05–0.15 g/dl (0.08–0.10 is legal level of intoxication in most states)	Relaxation, euphoria, decreased inhibitions, impaired judgment, changeable mood, decreased mental concentration, decreased fine motor coordination
0.15–0.3 g/dl	Slurred speech, decreased motor function, ataxia, mood outbursts, aggressive behavior
0.3–0.4 g/dl	Incoherent speech, mental confusion, stupor, vomiting, labored breathing; blood alcohol concentrations above this level are life threatening
0.4–0.5 g/dl	Unconsciousness, coma, death
>0.5 g/dl	Respiratory depression, death

return to normal. The CNS is still stimulated, and the individual suffers **withdrawal** symptoms. Alcohol withdrawal syndrome includes elevated vital signs, anxiety, tremors, diaphoresis, slurred speech, GI disturbances (vomiting, cramping, diarrhea), ataxia, nystagmus, disorientation, and, at its most severe, hallucinations, seizures, and death. Figure 12-6 ■ illustrates how the CNS responds to chronic alcohol use with tolerance and

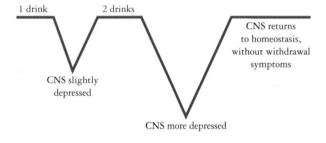

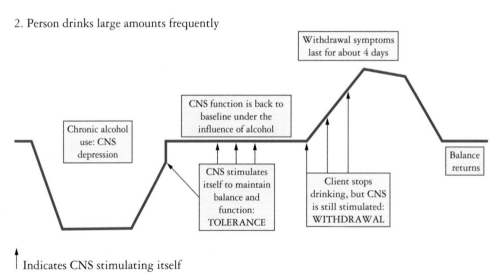

Figure 12-6. ■ CNS mechanism for development of alcohol withdrawal.

withdrawal. **Addiction** refers to psychological and physiological dependence and drug-seeking behavior.

Alcohol withdrawal delirium (*delirium tremens* or DTs) is diagnosed when withdrawal causes severe cognitive symptoms such as confusion, delusions, and terrifying hallucinations. This delirium happens to people with a long (5- to 15-year) history of alcoholism.

clinical ALERT

Alcohol withdrawal delirium is a medical emergency. When it is accompanied by seizures, it can be fatal.

Notice how the symptoms of alcohol withdrawal are generally the opposite of those of alcohol intoxication. The individual repeatedly takes the CNS depressant substance; the CNS stimulates itself to maintain homeostasis. When the substance is withdrawn, the CNS is still stimulated. The individual has CNS stimulation symptoms until the CNS eventually regains balance without alcohol, and the symptoms subside. Alcohol withdrawal syndrome usually lasts about 4 days. Table 12-2 ■ describes the effects, overdose symptoms, and withdrawal symptoms of alcohol and other CNS depressants.

The alcohol-dependent individual (*alcoholic*) may experience many episodes of withdrawal symptoms that he or she treats with alcohol. The statement, "I feel bad (nervous, tired, angry, lonely, etc.); I need a drink," may be evidence of withdrawal symptoms. Substance withdrawal symptoms are often behind a client's desire to leave the hospital against medical advice.

Critical Self-Check. A client says that he wants to check himself out of the hospital against medical advice. If the nurse believes that he wants to leave so he can drink alcohol, what should the nurse do?

Pattern of Use

Individuals vary in their pattern of alcohol use. Some people start drinking alcohol in childhood or adolescence, some in old age. Some drink daily, starting with "one or two drinks with dinner" and progressing to greater amounts and frequency. Some drink heavily on weekends or go on a drinking binge after a long "dry" period.

Alcohol dependency (alcoholism) is a progressive disease. It begins with alcohol abuse. The abuse of alcohol involves drinking alcohol even though it causes problems. A person may break the law by driving under the influence of alcohol, or lose a job due to multiple absences, or suffer an injury while intoxicated, or damage family relationships due to drinking behavior and its consequences (or even do all these things), and then continue to drink afterward. The alcohol abuser denies that alcohol is a problem.

As the disorder progresses to alcohol dependence, the person needs more and more alcohol to feel its influence. If the person stops drinking, withdrawal symptoms occur. The alcohol dependent individual may have blackouts of memory (forgetting what happens when drunk), anger, aggression, social isolation, loss of interest in pleasurable activities, and malnutrition. Alcoholics may lose their jobs, families, and self-respect. They still deny that alcohol is a problem for them. Eventually alcohol dependent people cannot control their drinking. They do not have a choice of whether to drink. They disintegrate physically and emotionally. Every body system suffers damage and life-threatening effects after years of alcohol dependency. Figure 12-7 ■ depicts these physical effects. Abstaining from alcohol causes the torture of life-threatening withdrawal. At this stage people often contemplate suicide.

The gastrointestinal system is often the first to show the effects of chronic alcoholism. Alcohol causes gastritis by inflaming the stomach lining. It damages the protective mucous lining of the stomach, allowing hydrochloric acid to erode the stomach wall. Bleeding can occur. Ulcers may form in the stomach (Figure 12-8 ■ shows a gastric ulcer). Symptoms include gastric distress, nausea, vomiting, black stools, and abdominal distension. Alcohol causes esophagitis (inflammation of the esophagus) by irritating the esophagus, and by causing frequent vomiting. The primary symptom is esophageal pain.

Pancreatitis, either acute or chronic, may also be caused by chronic alcohol use. Chronic pancreatitis leads to malnutrition, weight loss, and diabetes mellitus. Acute pancreatitis happens 1 or 2 days after a binge of drinking alcohol. The symptoms include severe, constant epigastric pain, nausea, vomiting, and abdominal distension.

Alcoholic hepatitis affects an already damaged liver. It usually happens after a prolonged binge of excessive alcohol consumption. The client has right upper quadrant abdominal pain, jaundice, an enlarged liver and spleen, vomiting, weakness, profound fatigue, and possibly *ascites* (accumulation of fluid in the abdomen due to impaired venous return through the liver). Palmar erythema (Figure 12-9 ■) is caused by an accumulation of chemicals that cannot be metabolized by the damaged liver.

TABLE 12-2

Comparison of Commonly Abused CNS Depressants and Stimulants

DRUG	EFFECTS OF USE	OVERDOSE SYMPTOMS	WITHDRAWAL SYMPTOMS AND THEIR ONSET (AFTER LAST DOSE)
CNS Depressants			
Alcohol, Beer, Wine, Liquor	Euphoria, loss of inhibition, ataxia, lack of coordination, reduced cognition, impaired judgment, nausea, tolerance with prolonged use	Respiratory depression, mental confusion, unconsciousness, death	6–8 hours CNS irritability, anxiety, increased vital signs (T, P, R, BP), tremors, ataxia, diaphoresis, slurred speech, GI disturbance, disorientation, hallucinations, seizures, death
Opioids Naturally occurring derivatives of opium (morphine) Semisynthetics (methadone, meperidine, oxycodone, codeine, heroin)	Analgesia, cough suppression, euphoria, loss of inhibition, lack of coordination, apathy, impaired judgment, nausea, constipation, constricted pupils, tolerance with prolonged use	Sedation, respiratory depression, mental confusion, unconsciousness, death	12–72 hours Watering eyes, CNS irritability, increased vital signs, tremors, diaphoresis (similar to alcohol withdrawal but less likely to cause death)
Sedatives, Hypnotics, Antianxiety Agents (Benzodiazepines), Barbiturates	Sedation, muscle relaxation, apathy, reduced cognition; antianxiety agents cause less sedation in low doses, tolerance with prolonged use	Muscle weakness, respiratory depression, mental confusion, unconsciousness, death; antianxiety drug overdoses are usually only deadly when combined with other CNS depressants	Onset depends on type of sedative (short- or long-acting). CNS irritability, increased vital signs, tremors, slurred speech, diaphoresis, seizures; barbiturate withdrawal can be fatal
CNS Stimulants			
Cocaine	Local vasoconstriction (therapeutic use), sudden rush of euphoria, elation, energy, talkativeness, impaired judgment, anorexia, weight loss, elevated VS, grandiosity, anger, aggression	Chest pain, slurred speech, mental confusion, vomiting, hallucinations, myocardial infarction, severe elevation of BP and P, shock, death	Acute depression, craving drug, fatigue, irritability, suicidal thoughts, loss of pleasure (anhedonia), not life threatening
Amphetamines and Methamphetamines	Amphetamines cause euphoria, elation, talkativeness, anorexia, weight loss, elevated VS, grandiosity; methamphetamines are closely related but more habit forming, longer acting, and more toxic to the CNS; methamphetamine use may cause memory loss, compulsively repetitive behavior, such as grinding the teeth or picking the skin (the skin lesions are called "speed bumps"), prolonged use causes severe dental problems	Overdose may cause mental confusion and aggression, cardiac dysrhythmias (potentially fatal), hallucinations, delusions; may cause death by cardiovascular collapse	Withdrawal symptoms similar to cocaine; withdrawal severity depends on amount of drug use

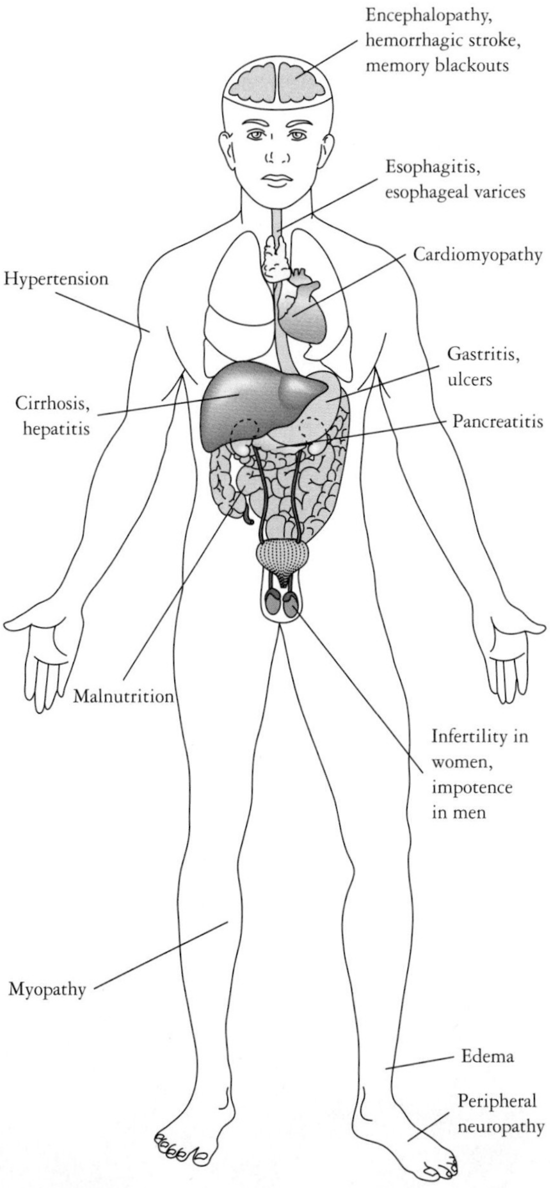
Encephalopathy,
hemorrhagic stroke,
memory blackouts
Esophagitis,
esophageal varices
Cardiomyopathy
Hypertension
Gastritis,
ulcers
Cirrhosis,
hepatitis
Pancreatitis
Malnutrition
Infertility in
women,
impotence
in men
Myopathy
Edema
Peripheral
neuropathy

Figure 12-7. ■ Physiological effects of alcohol dependence.

Cirrhosis of the liver is the end stage of chronic alcoholic liver disease. In cirrhosis, destroyed liver cells are replaced by scar tissue, making this disease irreversible. Cirrhosis causes portal hypertension, ascites, *esophageal varices* (varicose veins in the esophagus that can rupture and hemorrhage), and hepatic encephalopathy. Figure 12-10 ■ depicts a specimen of liver cirrhosis caused by alcoholism.

Hepatic encephalopathy is caused by accumulation of ammonia (due to the damaged liver's inability to metabolize protein). It results in impaired mental function and progresses to death. As clients' ammonia levels rise, they

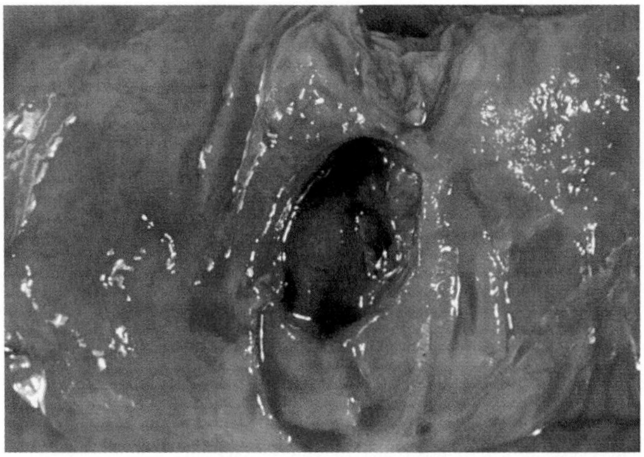

Figure 12-8. ■ Alcohol damages the protective mucous barrier of the stomach lining, and can cause or irritate gastric ulcers, as in this specimen. *Source:* Photo Researchers, Inc.

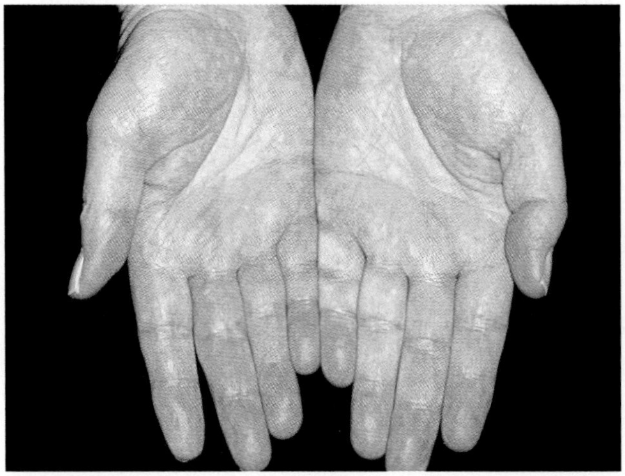

Figure 12-9. ■ Palmar erythema (in a 59-year-old male) is caused by the accumulation of by-products that the liver is unable to metabolize in chronic alcohol dependency. *Source:* Photo Researchers, Inc.

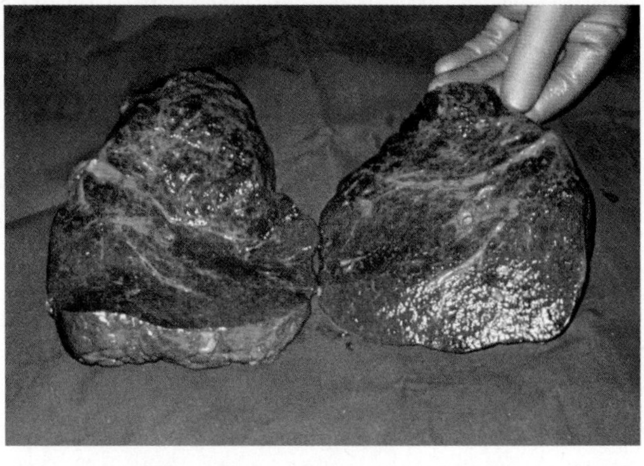

Figure 12-10. ■ Specimen of liver with cirrhosis due to chronic alcohol dependence. *Source:* Photo Researchers, Inc.

experience restlessness and agitation and also a loss of ability to understand what appropriate behavior is. When the liver is too damaged to remove ammonia from the blood, Cephulac (lactulose) is given. It lowers ammonia by increasing its excretion via the bowel (and usually causes diarrhea). As ammonia levels drop, the client's cognitive function improves.

The cardiovascular system is also affected by chronic alcohol use. Cardiomyopathy (weakening and enlargement of the heart), heart failure, and cardiac dysrhythmias may occur. The risk of hemorrhagic stroke is increased. Hypertension (especially diastolic elevation), tachycardia, and edema can also occur.

Chronic use of alcohol produces neurological changes as well. **Blackouts** are an early sign of alcoholism. The affected individual remains conscious and appears to be functioning normally, but is completely unable to remember anything that occurred while intoxicated.

After many years of alcohol abuse, a person may develop Wernicke's syndrome and Korsakoff's syndrome, which affect the entire neurological system. These syndromes usually occur together and are often called Wernicke-Korsakoff's syndrome.

clinical ALERT

Early treatment of vitamin B_1 deficiency can prevent alcoholic encephalopathy (Wernicke's syndrome) or stop its progression. The nurse should expect to give vitamin B_1 (thiamine) to all clients with alcohol dependency.

Wernicke's syndrome (alcoholic encephalopathy) is the result of severe vitamin B_1 deficiency caused by poor nutrition. It is characterized by ataxia, paralysis of eye muscles, nystagmus (rapid involuntary movement of the eyeballs), and mental confusion. If it is treated early, this brain dysfunction may respond well to large doses of parenteral thiamine. If not treated early, Wernicke's syndrome progresses to an irreversible, fatal condition.

Korsakoff's syndrome is a group of symptoms caused by a deficiency in the B vitamins, including thiamine, riboflavin, and folic acid. Clients exhibit amnesia, disorientation to time and place, severe peripheral neuropathy, and **confabulation** (a response to memory loss where the client makes up information to fill in gaps in memory). Symptoms of the neuropathy include tingling; muscle weakness; sore, burning muscles; abnormal sensation;

and pain with movement. The extremities are affected, especially the legs. Because of their extreme pain, care must be taken when moving these clients.

The reproductive system is also affected by chronic alcohol use. Men may become impotent. Women may stop menstruating and become infertile. Further, the unborn child of a pregnant woman who abuses alcohol may be seriously affected. Fetal alcohol syndrome (FAS) gives rise to low birth weight, microcephaly (small brain and small head circumference), facial abnormalities, and developmental disorders (learning disabilities, distractibility, poor coordination). Figure 12-11 ■ shows two girls with some of the facial features of FAS: flat nasal bridge, thin upper lip, and narrow eye openings. They also have developmental disabilities.

Alcohol abuse can affect the musculoskeletal system through the development of osteoporosis. Also, acute or chronic myopathy may occur, characterized by muscle cramps of sudden onset and later development of pain, tenderness, and edema of the skeletal muscles, especially of the legs. In chronic myopathy there is wasting and weakness of the skeletal muscles.

OTHER CNS DEPRESSANTS

Other CNS depressants are similar to alcohol in their effects on the CNS, intoxication symptoms, tolerance effects, and withdrawal symptoms (see Table 12-2).

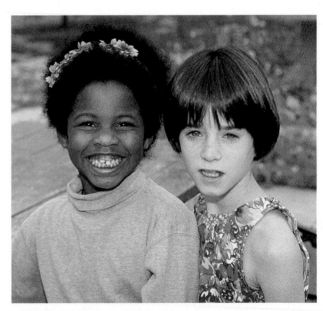

Figure 12-11. ■ Two girls with fetal alcohol syndrome show some of the facial features of the disorder (flat nasal bridge, thin upper lip, narrow eye openings). They are also developmentally delayed. *Source:* PhotoEdit Inc.

Opiates

Opiates are naturally occurring substances derived from opium (such as morphine), semisynthetics (such as heroin), and drugs that resemble them (such as methadone, meperidine, oxycodone, or codeine). These drugs have alleviated immeasurable human pain, but when abused they have caused immense suffering as well.

EFFECTS OF OPIATES.   Opiate (narcotic) drugs are prescribed to relieve pain or diarrhea or to reduce cough. Opiates can cause physical dependence (tolerance and withdrawal). Intoxication symptoms are similar to those of alcohol. Common effects include drowsiness, analgesia, euphoria, mood changes, nausea, constipation, and constriction of the pupils. In high doses, opiates cause hypotension by reducing vascular resistance.

Nurses especially need to know about the respiratory depressant effects of opioids. These drugs, which can be used to suppress cough, depress the respiratory center in the medulla of the brain. Respiratory depression is not likely to happen in therapeutic doses. However, **high doses may cause life-threatening respiratory depression.** Chronic respiratory depression predisposes the client to pneumonia and other respiratory infections.

Clients who take opiates for severe persistent pain, such as cancer pain, may become tolerant to usual therapeutic doses of narcotics. They will require increasing doses to achieve pain relief. This tolerance is expected and the increasing dose is appropriate. These clients are at less risk for respiratory depression than the "narcotic naive" client, who is new to taking narcotic medications. Nurses may be hesitant to give opiate/narcotic drugs to clients who need them, out of a fear of causing clients to become addicted. This fear is not founded in fact. People who take opiates for pain are not likely to develop dependency as a result (Morrison, 2000).

Opioids also affect sexual functioning. People who use opioids regularly in high doses have decreased libido (sexual drive) and may have lack of orgasm. Men can have ejaculation abnormalities and impotence. Women often have menstrual irregularities and infertility.

Opiate overdose is a medical emergency. The client may have pinpoint pupils, depressed (slow, shallow) respiration, seizures, and coma. Death can result from respiratory arrest. The treatment for opiate overdose is a narcotic antagonist drug, such as naloxone hydrochloride (Narcan). This drug competes for opiate receptors and blocks the action of narcotics.

PATTERNS OF SUBSTANCE USE.   Unlike alcohol, opiates either are available only by prescription or are illegal under all circumstances (such as heroin). So, opiate dependence is often associated with a history of crimes committed to obtain drugs or money to buy them. Healthcare professionals with opiate dependency may steal medications from clients or their employers, write prescriptions for themselves, or manipulate physicians to write prescriptions for them.

Although opioid dependence may begin at any age, problems are most commonly observed in the late teens or early twenties (American Psychiactric Association, 2000). Dependence develops over a period of years, with periods of **abstinence** (complete lack of drug use). **Relapse** (return to drug use after abstinence) is very common. Men are more commonly affected than women. People with opiate dependency have increased risk of developing hepatitis B or C, HIV infection, or other blood-borne diseases from needle use. Mortality in opiate dependent people may be 2% per year. Death often results from overdose, accidents, or injuries (American Psychiactric Association, 2000).

SEDATIVE, HYPNOTIC, OR ANXIOLYTIC-RELATED DISORDERS

Prescription sleeping medications and most of the antianxiety drugs are included in this group. Like alcohol and the opiates, these substances depress the CNS.

Overdose

It is important for nurses to know that CNS depressant drugs have additive effects when taken together. So, when people use alcohol and a sedative drug at the same time, the CNS depressant effect is beyond what either substance would cause alone. Although the amount of sedative may be a usual dose and the amount of alcohol may be what the person usually drinks, the two together could cause fatal respiratory depression. It is not uncommon for people to die as a result of this additive effect.

> ### clinical ALERT
>
> Many of the psychotropic medications cause CNS depression and are dangerous when taken with alcohol due to additive CNS depression. Nurses should teach clients with prescriptions for psychotropic drugs to avoid alcohol completely.

The substance-dependent individual commonly has a drug of choice, but uses a variety of other substances, including alcohol. This combination of abused substances is called *polysubstance abuse*.

CNS STIMULANTS: AMPHETAMINES, METHAMPHETAMINES, AND COCAINE

The only clinical usefulness of the amphetamines is for treatment of attention deficit hyperactivity disorder. Cocaine is used as a potent topical vasoconstrictor for surgery involving the mucous membranes of the nasopharynx.

Cocaine is a popular drug of abuse because it causes immediate euphoria. Table 12-2 describes its effects. The cycle of cocaine use, which also applies to the other stimulant drugs, is depicted in Figure 12-12 ■.

There is currently an international epidemic of methamphetamine abuse. In 2005, 10.4 million Americans had tried methamphetamines at least once. The methamphetamine involved in this epidemic is largely manufactured in small illegal laboratories where its production endangers the people in the labs, their neighbors, and the environment. It is more potent, long lasting, and harmful to the CNS than the related amphetamines (McGuinness, 2006). With prolonged use, it causes damage to the terminals of brain neurons in the serotonin and dopamine systems, causing problems with memory, cognition, and mood. Transmission of blood-borne pathogens (such as HIV and

hepatitis) is associated with the use of any drug that is used intravenously. Methamphetamines can be used orally, intranasally, intravenously, or by smoking. Young adults aged 18 to 25 are the most likely to have used methamphetamine in the last year. Giving clients the knowledge they need to have the power to resist using methamphetamine is the nurse's best weapon to fight the epidemic (National Institute on Drug Abuse, 2007). Figure 12-13 ■ shows a poster used in an anti-drug abuse campaign in the United Kingdom. It shows the physical deterioration of a woman after only 4 years of methamphetamine abuse.

Withdrawal

Just as the brain elevates its stimulation to balance regular use of depressants, it also depresses its function to balance regular use of a stimulant. When the stimulant-dependent individual abstains from stimulant drugs, the withdrawal syndrome includes CNS depression. The individual feels lethargic and depressed. Withdrawal from stimulants is uncomfortable but not life threatening and may last several days.

HALLUCINOGENS

Hallucinogens distort the user's perception of reality. The most common hallucinogens are LSD (lysergic acid diethylamide), mescaline, and PCP (phencyclidine). The CNS

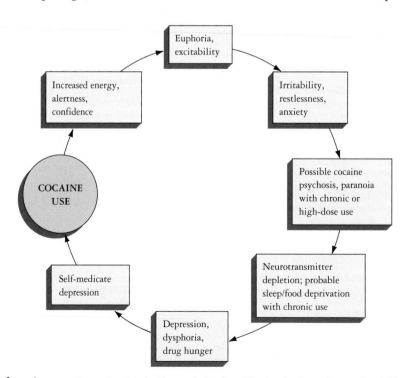

Figure 12-12. ■ Cycle of cocaine use. *Source:* Reprinted with permission from Mim Landry, Danya International, Silver Spring, Maryland.

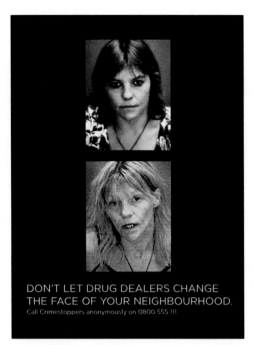

Figure 12-13. ■ Poster used in an anti-drug campaign in the UK. It depicts a woman before and after 4 years of methamphetamine abuse. *Source:* The Image Works.

effects are unpredictable and may be influenced by the expectations of the user. Hallucinations can lead to violent behavior. Some individuals have frightening psychotic experiences. When people with mental illnesses take hallucinogens, the outcome is less predictable. The combination of schizophrenia and hallucinogenic drugs can cause hallucinations that are prolonged and frightening.

There is no withdrawal syndrome associated with hallucinogens. However, flashbacks can occur for months after the last dose is used. During flashbacks, the individual has similar symptoms to those associated with use of the drug. Table 12-3 ■ describes effects of use, overdose symptoms, and withdrawal symptoms (if any) of hallucinogens and other categories of frequently abused substances.

Synthetic or "designer" drugs have become increasingly popular. MDMA, or Ecstasy, for example, is derived from amphetamine and methamphetamine, so it acts as both a stimulant and a hallucinogen.

INHALANTS

Two kinds of inhalants are commonly abused: hydrocarbons and nitrites. The hydrocarbons (solvents, glue, and aerosols) produce euphoria, loss of inhibitions, altered sensations, and hallucinations. Figure 12-14 ■ shows some of the common household products that can be used as a source of hydrocarbon inhalants. The hydrocarbons

can cause cardiac depression, renal injury, respiratory depression, and death from cardiac dysrhythmias, aspiration of vomitus, or accidents while intoxicated. Because these inhalants are readily available in stores (in the form of spray paint, certain glues, and even gasoline) they are the drug of choice for many young people who have difficulty buying alcohol (see Table 12-3).

The second source of inhalant abuse is the nitrites group. Amyl nitrite, butyl nitrite, and nitrous oxide are included. The nitrites are used to prolong penile erection and to enhance intercourse. They may cause euphoria and perceptual alterations. Some individuals experience panic, nausea, confusion, headache, and hypotension from their use.

CANNABIS

Delta-9-tetrahydrocannabinol (THC) is thought to be the chemical responsible for the psychoactive effects of marijuana and hashish. Cannabis effects include euphoria, a sense of serenity, and perceptual changes in vision, hearing, taste, touch, or smell (see Table 12-3).

Cannabis is the most widely used illegal substance in the United States. It has been therapeutically used to treat anorexia, nausea, and vomiting associated with AIDS and cancer.

CAFFEINE AND NICOTINE

It may be surprising to find caffeine and nicotine listed as substances of abuse. Still, these substances fit the model of dependence defined in the *DSM-IV-TR*. Both substances cause tolerance and withdrawal.

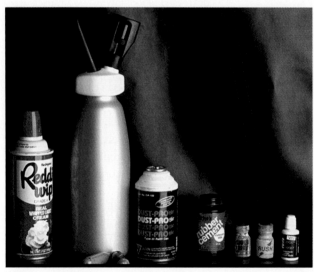

Figure 12-14. ■ Common household products can be used for inhalant abuse. *Source:* PhotoEdit Inc.

TABLE 12-3

Hallucinogens, Inhalants, Cannabis, Caffeine, and Nicotine

SUBSTANCE	EFFECTS OF USE	OVERDOSE SYMPTOMS	WITHDRAWAL SYMPTOMS
Hallucinogens			
LSD, DMT, Mescaline, MDMA (Ecstasy)	Hallucinations and distorted perceptions, distortions of time and space, illusions, emotional lability, tremor, nausea and vomiting	Panic (may be drug reaction, not OD), seizures (rare)	No withdrawal, may experience flashbacks for several months after last dose
Phencyclidine (PCP)	Bizarre perceptions, disorientation, hallucinations, agitation, grandiosity, withdrawn or agitated or both, paranoid, dilated pupils, dry red skin	Seizures, coma, death	No withdrawal
Inhalants and Cannabis			
Inhalants Hydrocarbons: Glue, gasoline, aerosol spray, solvents	Hydrocarbons: Euphoria, impaired judgment, nystagmus, ataxia, slurred speech, perceptual changes, sense of invulnerability	Hydrocarbons: Stupor, coma, cardiac depression and dysrhythmias, respiratory arrest, renal complications	Similar to alcohol
Nitrites: Amyl nitrite, nitrous oxide	Nitrites: postpone ejaculation or enhance intercourse	Nitrites: Panic, hypotension. Both: Brain damage	
Cannabis Marijuana Hashish	Mild euphoria, pleasure, confidence, grandiosity, relaxation, red eyes, dry mouth, increased appetite	None	No physical withdrawal; may have craving
Caffeine and Nicotine			
Caffeine	Increased alertness, increased pulse, anxiety, insomnia	Jitters (tremors)	Headache, fatigue, irritability
Nicotine	Pleasure, alertness, increased BP, P, decreased blood flow to heart muscle	None	Anxiety, depressed mood, anger, craving, increased appetite

Caffeine, the most commonly used stimulant drug, is primarily a performance enhancer. It prolongs the time the user can continue to work (which makes it popular among nurses), improves mental alertness, and elevates mood. However, it also increases anxiety and can cause insomnia, irritability, diuresis, tremors, and tachycardia (see Table 12-3).

The amount and frequency of caffeine use determine its effects and whether tolerance and withdrawal develop. Withdrawal symptoms include headache, fatigue, irritability, and nervousness. Figure 12-15 ■ shows common sources of caffeine and their doses. The average adult coffee drinker consumes 360–450 mg of caffeine per day.

Intake of more than 600 mg of caffeine per day is considered excessive (Kneisl, Wilson, & Trigoboff, 2004).

Nicotine dependence is the most common substance dependence in the United States (Centers for Disease Control, 2007). Symptoms of use include increased performance, decreased appetite, reduced anxiety, and increased alertness initially, followed by relaxation. Smoking is especially common among people who use alcohol and other substances.

The consequences of smoking are also due to other substances present in tobacco. Cancer of the lungs, oral cavity, esophagus, pancreas, and prostate is increased significantly among tobacco users. The risk of cardiovascular disease (stroke, myocardial infarction, and peripheral arterial disease) is increased by tobacco use as well. Accidents related to fire are also a concern (smoking in bed or while drinking alcohol can be deadly). Withdrawal symptoms include irritability, restlessness, drowsiness, anxiety, craving, and a transient increase in appetite.

Hospitalized clients often experience caffeine or nicotine withdrawal. Nurses may find that the headache clients have after surgery responds better to a cup of coffee than to medication. Some clients may consider checking themselves out of the hospital against medical advice so they can smoke cigarettes. These situations require the nurse's problem-solving skills.

Collaborative Care

In the acute phase of alcohol withdrawal, medical treatment focuses on physiological safety. Priorities are symptom management, seizure prevention, stabilizing vital signs, and minimizing the effects of CNS stimulation. In the rehabilitation phase, management is supportive. Nurses, physicians, therapists, social workers, and others cooperate on the healthcare team.

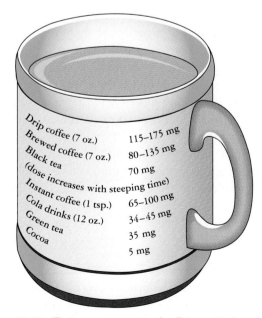

Figure 12-15. ■ Common sources of caffeine, with doses.

Drip coffee (7 oz.)	115–175 mg
Brewed coffee (7 oz.)	80–135 mg
Black tea (dose increases with steeping time)	70 mg
Instant coffee (1 tsp.)	65–100 mg
Cola drinks (12 oz.)	34–45 mg
Green tea	35 mg
Cocoa	5 mg

A person who is dependent on heroin or alcohol will be tolerant to other CNS depressants as well. This phenomenon of tolerance to several drugs in the same classification is called **cross-tolerance.** The anesthesiologist may find that the client needs more than the usual anesthetic to put him to sleep. Physicians and nurses may discover that the client needs a higher than usual analgesic dose to relieve pain.

There are several theories about the causes and best treatment for chemical dependency. Basically, substance dependency is viewed as a chronic, progressive medical illness that is characterized by remissions and relapses and is eventually fatal if untreated. Its etiology is a combination of genetic and cultural influences (nature and nurture). Box 12-2 ■ supplies some cultural information about alcoholism.

People with substance dependency have learned to use substances to cope with their problems. They must have new skills to replace the role substances play in their lives. **A promise of abstinence alone is not a long-term solution**. The ultimate goals of substance dependency treatment are:

1. To abstain from substance use.
2. To develop effective coping mechanisms to replace substances as a way to solve problems.

ACUTE PHASE OF TREATMENT

Substance dependency treatment has two major phases: acute and rehabilitation. In the acute phase, the person may be in a hospital, a detoxification center, a drug treatment facility, or another inpatient or outpatient setting. The client often enters treatment while intoxicated. **Detoxification,** or removal of the substance from the body, begins the acute phase. The withdrawal syndrome also occurs acutely. Medical and nursing supports are often needed during withdrawal.

Medications are used in the acute phase of treatment to provide safe withdrawal from CNS depressant drugs and alcohol. Alcohol withdrawal is usually managed with a benzodiazepine antianxiety agent. This agent is given in a decreasing dose over several days to treat the CNS withdrawal symptoms. Clients who abuse alcohol are given vitamin B_1 (thiamine) to prevent alcoholic encephalopathy (Wernicke-Korsakoff's syndrome).

There is a dangerous assumption that allowing clients to suffer agonizing withdrawal will "teach them a lesson" about why they should stop drinking alcohol or using drugs. In fact, withdrawal causes a person to crave and be preoccupied with the substance. There is no ethical justification for allowing clients to suffer needlessly. Alcohol and barbiturate withdrawals can be life threatening.

BOX 12-2	CULTURAL PULSE POINTS

Cultural Aspects of Alcoholism

Asian Americans: As a group they are less likely to seek treatment for alcoholism than the general population. Men tend to drink more alcohol than females.

Filipino Americans: Fifty percent of Filipina American women totally abstain from alcohol use. Of men, 80% drink alcohol. Heavy drinking is almost exclusively a male activity.

Japanese Americans: Lower rate of alcohol consumption than the general population. Low reported rates of alcoholism may be due to factors such as the following: affected people are shielded by their family; they only seek treatment in late stages of disease; they seek treatment from sources other than health providers.

Alaskan Natives (Aleut, Eskimo, Indian): Binge drinking has been associated with the stress of acculturation. Alcoholism is common, especially among men. Suicide is also common. Alcoholics Anonymous and other programs set up by White people have been relatively unsuccessful in this group. Culturally relevant programs are more effective.

European Americans: Alcoholism is a major health problem. Denial is common coping mechanism. This group relies more than other groups on the healthcare system for treatment. Four percent of women drink heavily.

Irish Americans: In Ireland adolescents drink less alcohol than their American counterparts, but both Irish and Irish American adults have high incidence of alcoholism and social problems associated with drinking. Affected people cite need for reassurance and escape from intolerable burdens as the reasons they drink alcohol.

Jewish Americans: There is a common belief by this group that alcoholics are unkempt homeless men. Regular drinking and problem behavior are not acknowledged as alcoholism. Behaviors that characterize the alcoholic—denial, isolation, and guilt—are intense in Jewish alcoholics because of the myth of Jewish sobriety.

Mexican Americans: Male role may be associated with the ability to drink large amounts of alcohol. This group has an increased death rate due to illnesses related to chronic alcohol use compared with alcoholics from other groups. Mexican Americans have lower drug abuse rates than the general population.

Russian Americans: Alcoholism rate is increasing in Russia, especially among adolescents and women. Incidence decreases as people emigrate from Russia to America.

African Americans: Alcoholism is a major problem. Contributes to reduced life expectancy. Rate is related to unemployment. Escape from problems is cited as a common reason for drinking. In studies that controlled for age and socioeconomic status, more African Americans abstain and generally consume less alcohol than European Americans. A higher percentage of women in this culture drink more heavily than the general population. This group is least likely to seek treatment for problem drinking.

This article was published in *Transcultural Nursing: Assessment and Intervention, 4/E*, J. N. Giger and R. E. Davidhizar, "Transcultural Assessment Model," © 2004, Mosby.

RECOVERY PHASE

Recovery/rehabilitation is the second phase of substance dependency treatment. It begins when clients have detoxified and are abstaining from substance use. Recovery continues indefinitely.

Psychopharmacology

Medications used in the recovery phase are for the purpose of preventing relapse. Disulfiram (Antabuse) may be prescribed to deter clients from drinking alcohol. It causes a severe, uncomfortable reaction when the client drinks (flushing, throbbing headache, nausea, and vomiting).

Methadone, a synthetic opiate, is used as a replacement for heroin. A regular oral dose is prescribed, which is usually dispensed by a methadone clinic. Clients taking methadone become physically dependent on it (and will have withdrawal symptoms if it is discontinued). The goal is to prevent the risks of intravenous drug use and the dangerous behaviors associated with obtaining heroin (prostitution, burglary, robbery, etc.). Methadone has saved the lives of many former heroin users. Many clients on methadone lead productive lives.

Naltrexone (ReVia) is an opioid antagonist used to treat opiate overdose. It blocks the effects of any opioids used by the client. It has been found to reduce the cravings for alcohol in abstinent clients (Deglin & Vallerand, 2007).

Clonidine (Catapres) is an antihypertensive drug. It is sometimes given to clients with opiate dependence to prevent some of the symptoms of withdrawal. Nurses should take the client's blood pressure before each dose and hold the drug (and notify the physician) if the person is hypotensive.

Cognitive-Behavior Therapy

Other approaches to treatment include cognitive-behavior therapy, in which the client is helped to alter the thinking and behaviors associated with addiction. Family therapy is also used, in which the entire family is counseled to see the combination of unhealthy family behaviors that contribute to the identified client's addiction.

The tasks of rehabilitation/recovery are to:

- Maintain sobriety (abstinence)
- Develop new coping skills
- Make a plan for relapse prevention
- Live life with all its responsibilities, joys, and frustrations

Relapse is common. The best response to relapse is for the person to learn from the experience and to begin recovery again.

Support Groups

Many people with substance abuse and dependency respond well to treatment. The most popular treatment program is Alcoholics Anonymous (AA). This is a self-help program for alcoholics that is based on 12 steps, thus the name "12-step program." Box 12-3 ■ lists the Twelve Steps of Alcoholics Anonymous. AA itself is for alcoholics only. Other 12-step programs are based on their principles. In all these anonymous groups, people with similar problems share experiences, strength, and hope. The groups offer a sense of community and unconditional support.

There are thousands of AA groups. Refer clients to their local telephone book or directory assistance to find Alcoholics Anonymous. There are AA meetings for special interest groups, such as people with dual diagnosis, nonsmokers, women, lesbians, or people who want to focus on religious aspects of recovery. Other 12-step programs include Overeaters Anonymous, Narcotics Anonymous, and Cocaine Anonymous.

Al-anon is a group for family members, especially spouses, of alcoholics. Ala-teen is a similar group for teenage children of alcoholics. Substance dependency is certainly a family illness; these groups have helped many family members.

BOX 12-3

Twelve Steps of Alcoholics Anonymous

We

1. Admitted that we were powerless over alcohol, that our lives had become unmanageable.
2. Came to believe that a Power greater than ourselves could restore us to sanity.
3. Made a decision to turn our wills and lives over to the care of God as we understood Him.
4. Made a searching and fearless moral inventory of ourselves.
5. Admitted to God, to ourselves, and to another human being the exact nature of our wrongs.
6. Were entirely ready to have God remove all these defects of character.
7. Humbly asked Him to remove our shortcomings.
8. Made a list of all persons we had harmed, and became willing to make amends to them all.
9. Made direct amends to such people whenever possible, except when to do so would injure them or others.
10. Continued to take personal inventory and when we were wrong promptly admitted it.
11. Sought through prayer and meditation to improve our conscious contact with God as we understood Him, praying only for knowledge of His will for us and the power to carry that out.
12. Having had a spiritual awakening as a result of these steps, we tried to carry this message to alcoholics and to practice these principles in all our affairs.

Source: Alcoholics Anonymous World Services (1952).

Dual Diagnosis

The term **dual diagnosis** refers to clients who have both a substance use disorder and a serious mental illness. Up to 51% of people with severe mental illnesses also have substance use disorders (El-Mallakh, 1998). These individuals have two separate chronic illnesses, and they have greater functional impairment than the general population of people with substance dependency. Both the mental disorder and the substance use disorder must be treated together. Figure 12-16 ■ shows the frequency of substance use disorders in people with various mental disorders.

Many people self-medicate their psychiatric symptoms with alcohol or drugs. Think about the symptoms of the major mental disorders. Many severely mentally ill people experience impulsiveness, poor judgment, and difficulty anticipating the consequences of their behavior. Now think about the substances of abuse. In the short term they help people forget their problems and make them feel better. Only later will the full consequences of loss of job, family, friends, health, and even life become real. For a person who is living in the moment, substance abuse may seem to make sense. It may seem to be an effective way to solve problems. For people who are unable to plan beyond the current day, problem solving has a different meaning.

Because of the high risk of substance abuse and dependency for the mentally ill, nurses should include assessment

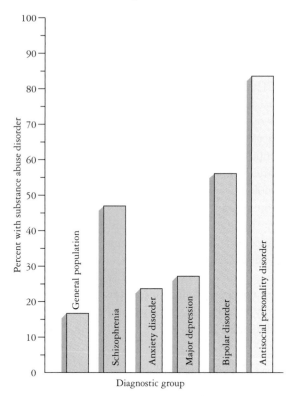

Figure 12-16. ■ Lifetime prevalence rates for substance abuse disorder for people with mental disorders. *Source: Contemporary Psychiatric Mental Health Nursing* by Kneisl/Wilson/Trigoboff, © Reprinted by permission of Pearson Education, Inc., Upper Saddle River, NJ.

of substance use history on each psychiatric client. Substance abuse and dependency should be treated along with the client's mental disorder, rather than trying to treat one after the other is resolved. Mental disorders and substance dependency affect each other.

Substance abuse and dependency complicate the diagnosis and treatment of mental disorders. Psychiatric diagnoses are ideally based on the client's symptoms over time, but acute treatment can be confusing when the client is under the influence of substances. Excessive drinking of alcohol can cause an exacerbation of schizophrenia, depression, or bipolar disorder. Drugs and alcohol complicate the diagnosis of mental disorders. Mental disorders can complicate substance abuse diagnosis and treatment as well.

People with dual diagnoses may benefit from substance dependency treatment that is organized especially for them. People with thought disorders may not fit in socially with other members of therapy groups or may have different issues of concern. For example, schizophrenia causes people to have difficulty taking initiative. People with schizophrenia may have more trouble refusing offers

of alcohol or drugs than the average person would. Special dual-diagnosis AA groups have been organized to meet the needs of people with dual diagnosis.

Substance Dependency Among Nurses

It may seem unlikely for nurses to have problems with substance use because they should know better. In fact, many nurses do use substances. Some reasons our profession is at especially high risk for substance use disorders are as follows:

- Nurses see medications as a solution to problems.
- Nurses have access to drugs at work and to physicians who prescribe them.
- Nurses often believe that they should work even when they are tired or sick, so they may use drugs to increase their ability to continue working.
- Nurses experience pressure, emotional pain, anger, and frustration, which are symptoms that respond to drugs in the short term.
- Nurses think that if they know about drugs and drug abuse, addiction will not happen to them.

When nurses understand substance dependency, they are able to recognize it earlier in their coworkers and themselves. Signs of **impaired nursing** (practicing nursing under the influence of intoxicants) include changes in the nurse's behavior (mood changes, irritability, forgetfulness, isolation from coworkers, inappropriate behavior). Work performance may be affected (multiple medication errors, missed deadlines, sloppy charting, inattention to detail, absenteeism, poor judgment, volunteering to give narcotics to other nurses' clients, excessive wasting of narcotics, client complaints that pain medications are not effective, tampering with drug packaging, going to the bathroom after administering narcotics). The fact that drug use causes practice errors is ironic, because unlike other drug abusers, nurses often begin taking drugs in order to continue working when they are tired (Figure 12-17 ■). The nurse may also have signs of drug use or withdrawal (alcohol on breath, heavy use of breath mints and perfume, red eyes, ataxia, restlessness, anxiety, slurred speech, hyperactivity, tremors, runny nose, family problems that interfere with work).

Substance dependency is a chronic physiological illness that requires treatment. Affected nurses deserve to be diagnosed and treated before they hurt their clients or themselves. If you suspect that a peer is impaired, notify

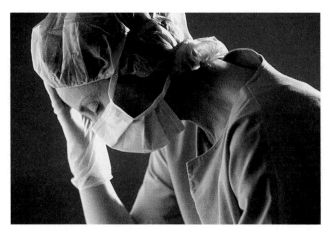

Figure 12-17. ■ Unlike other drug abusers, nurses tend to begin drug use when they feel exhausted, to enhance their ability to work longer and harder. *Source:* Phototake NYC.

a manager or hospital supervisor. The nurse is unlikely to be able to manage the problem alone. Your state board of nursing probably has a nurse monitoring or treatment program that can help affected nurses recover and return to the profession.

In the acute situation, your duty as a nurse is to protect your clients from an impaired nurse. In the big picture of caring for colleagues in the profession, your duty is to help your peers get treatment. The intervention to reach each of these outcomes is the same: tell a supervisor (not just the unit charge nurse for the day), so clients will be safe and the nurse will be treated. A nurse who is so far advanced in substance dependency that s/he is under the influence of substances at work will not be able to stop using just because you say they should. They need treatment. This is no time to engage in denial.

NURSING CARE

ASSESSING

Denial in alcohol-dependent clients was studied in a research project. These clients denied to themselves that they had trouble with alcohol for years after problems developed. Then, for years after they recognized the problem, they continued to deny to others that it existed. They tended to postpone seeking treatment until they had severe chronic health problems (Simpson & Tucker, 2002). This research has implications for nurses. If nurses

assess all clients for substance use problems, these clients can be identified before they are likely to seek help for themselves. Some of these clients may respond positively to the nurse's advice to seek treatment for substance dependency. Confirmation of substance abuse by health professionals can be a powerful tool in the battle against denial.

It is important to assess the substance use history of every client. The nurse can notify the physician of recent use or regular use so appropriate measures can be taken to adjust doses of medications that affect the CNS. Nursing assessment questions are listed in Box 12-4 ■. Note that the substance use assessment does not ask, "Do you drink?" Because alcohol and drug use is associated with strong negative attitudes by society and with guilt by users, the client is most likely to believe that the right answer is "No." People use denial to cope with their substance abuse problems, and they often lie about or underestimate their use. The nurse must present a nonjudgmental attitude and be accepting of clients as people, whether they use drugs or not.

A physical sign of the use of substances that affect the CNS is pupil size. In general CNS depressants tend to constrict the pupils, and CNS stimulants tend to dilate them (a dilated pupil is shown in Figure 12-18 ■). Be careful with this finding, however. Many prescribed medications can also cause pupil changes, and so can the light

---

BOX 12-4

Assessing for Substance Use

This is a screening assessment. A more thorough assessment would be indicated in a substance abuse treatment setting.
- How many cigarettes a day do you smoke?
- How often do you drink alcohol?
- About how much do you drink?
- What kind of drugs do you use that are not prescribed?
- What is your method of use (oral, smoking, inhaling, injecting)?
- Under what circumstances do you drink or use substances?
  or: What leads to your drinking or drug use? (Do you drink for relaxation, fun, something to do with your friends, to help you get through the day, when you are sad, lonely, frustrated, or angry)?
- Have you had any problems because of drinking or drug use (social, job, or legal)?
- When was the last time you used alcohol or any drug, what was it, and how much?

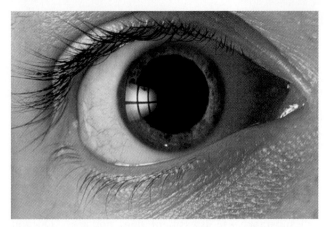

Figure 12-18. ■ Pupil size is one sign of the use of drugs that affect the CNS. Pupil dilation, as shown here, is a sign of use of CNS stimulants. CNS depressants cause pupil constriction. Be careful, though, because other things can also affect pupil size. *Source:* Photo Researchers, Inc.

in the room. Pupil size is one of many signs and symptoms to consider.

Notice the assessment question that asks under what circumstances the client drinks alcohol or uses drugs. This question is trying to determine the purpose the substance serves for this person. People use substances for a variety of reasons. Knowing the reasons increases the nurse's ability to help the client find other choices for coping or entertainment.

A general screening tool for whether a client has problems with alcohol is the CAGE questionnaire (Ewing, 1984). This is a simple tool that identifies which clients need further assessment.

It calls for further inquiry if the client answers "yes" to one of the following questions:

■ Have you ever felt you ought to **C**ut down on your drinking?
■ Have people **A**nnoyed you by criticizing your drinking?
■ Have you ever felt bad or **G**uilty about your drinking?
■ Have you ever had a drink first thing in the morning to steady your nerves or get rid of a hangover (**E**ye-opener)?

Similarly, the nurse can ask direct questions about tobacco use. Box 12-5 ■ lists the five "A"s for assessment and intervention with clients who smoke (Gordon, Williams, & Lapin, 2001). Simply having a conversation with the physician or nurse about quitting smoking or other substance use helps many people to begin the process of quitting. Nurses can be a powerful force for healthy behavior change. Use your power!

BOX 12-5

Five "A"s for Assessment and Intervention with Clients Who Smoke

These should be used at each clinic or hospital visit:
■ **Ask** the client about tobacco use.
■ **Advise** the client to quit.
■ **Assess** the client's willingness to make a quit attempt.
■ **Assist** the client to make a quit attempt.
■ **Arrange** for follow-up contacts to prevent relapse.

DIAGNOSING, PLANNING, AND IMPLEMENTING

Nursing interventions for clients with substance use disorders often relate to three nursing diagnoses: Altered Protection, Deficient Knowledge, and Ineffective Coping. Other nursing diagnoses that commonly apply to people with substance use disorders are:

■ Altered Family Processes
■ Chronic Low Self-Esteem
■ Powerlessness
■ Fear
■ Denial, Ineffective
■ Nutrition, Less Than Body Requirements
■ Risk for Injury
■ Sleep Pattern Disturbance
■ Social Isolation
■ Spiritual Distress
■ Sensory Perceptual Alterations
■ Risk for Violence

Altered Protection R/T Alcohol Withdrawal

■ Take vital signs frequently, at least every 4 hours. If they are elevated (T, P, R, R/T alcohol withdrawal and BP may be involved), medicate with ordered benzodiazepines according to physician's orders. *Benzodiazepines either treat or prevent symptoms of alcohol withdrawal by balancing the CNS stimulation with a depressant effect until the client's CNS can return to homeostasis without alcohol.*

■ Assess for other withdrawal symptoms (anxiety, agitation, sweating, nausea, vomiting, tremors, and ataxia). *Treat with p.r.n. benzodiazepines as above. If withdrawal is so severe that the client has hallucinations or seizures, call the physician immediately. These are symptoms of life-threatening withdrawal.*

- If the client is nauseated, do not push fluids. Offer small amounts of fluids frequently. Offer high-calorie feedings. *Assess for dehydration. Clients in withdrawal are at risk for fluid and electrolyte disturbances. They are also at risk for inadequate nutrition. It is easier for the nauseated client to take foods and fluids in small amounts than in big meals.*
- Assist client with activities of daily living. *Clients experiencing withdrawal are likely to be weak and possibly too tired to do ADLs independently.*
- Maintain a low-stimulation environment for the client. *Clients in withdrawal are experiencing CNS stimulation. They will be more comfortable and less likely to have a seizure if they are in a quiet room with dim lights.*
- Encourage clients to express their feelings. *People with alcohol dependency often have difficulty understanding their own feelings. Expressing them can begin the process of behavior change.*

Deficient Knowledge R/T Lack of Information About Substance Abuse

- Assess what clients know and what they need to learn. Teach them about the process of drug abuse and dependency and how people use drugs for coping, recreation, and company. *When people know what the problem is physiologically and realistically, they can begin to do something about it.*
- Discuss the consequences to the client of substance use. *Because so many people deny the severity of the problem, nurses must be honest about what the consequences are (job loss, divorce, family problems, disease of every body system, etc.). People are more likely to be able to change behavior when they understand the consequences and make the choice to change.*

Ineffective Coping R/T Poor Problem-Solving Skills

- Help plan for new healthy coping strategies to replace substance use. *The client may need to meet new people to make new friends if all his old friends only get together to drink or use drugs. People need alternatives to substance use when they become too **H**ungry, **A**ngry, **L**onely, or **T**ired. (HALT is an acronym for feelings that lead to relapse into drug use.)*
- Help make a list of fun, recreational activities. *Clients may not even know what to do for fun. Be sure the list is realistic and includes the client's preferences (taking a walk, calling a friend on the phone, listening to music, sports, hiking, bike riding, outdoor work, reading, community service,*

spiritual activities, dancing, carpentry, painting, and appreciating nature are a few ideas).
- Help clients identify their resources for various needs and stressful situations (e.g., who could help with a ride to the grocery store or the doctor's office, help care for the cat if the client is in the hospital, or help refill a medication prescription). His/her sponsor from Alcoholics Anonymous may be the one to call if s/he feels like drinking again, or if s/he wants to talk about how hard life is. *A practical list like this may be the thing the client turns to instead of drinking when he has a problem and cannot think of what to do.*

The following strategies for helping people quit smoking may be useful for people who are using other substances as well.

The five "R"s for smokers who are currently unwilling to quit:

- Provide motivational information that is personally **relevant** to the client.
- Discuss the **risks** associated with smoking and the **rewards** of quitting, such as improvements in functioning and self-efficacy.
- Ask the client about **roadblocks** or barriers to quitting.
- **Repeat** motivational strategies at every clinic visit because most smokers need to make repeated quit attempts to be successful (Gordon et al., 2001).

EVALUATING

Look at the outcomes and evaluate whether they were met to evaluate whether nursing interventions for clients with substance use disorders are effective. Desired outcomes include:

- Client will develop a plan for healthy alternatives to substance use for coping.
- Clients will identify resources for obtaining help when they need it (family, friends, Alcoholics Anonymous, social service agencies).
- Client will identify risk factors for relapse and plan for relapse prevention.
- Client will identify and verbalize feelings.
- Client will assume responsibility for own behavior.
- Client will use peer support to maintain sobriety.

DISCHARGE CONSIDERATIONS

When people with substance use disorders are discharged from the hospital, there must be follow-up of their substance use issues. They may benefit from a written list of telephone numbers for counseling resources, drug abuse treatment, or Alcoholics Anonymous. They may need a referral to the social services department for help with discharge planning. The social worker may be able to obtain a referral for treatment on an outpatient basis.

If a client with a substance use history is going to be discharged with psychotropic medications, sedatives, narcotics, or other medications that could interact with drugs of abuse, the potential risks should be discussed with the physician. When a person is not expected to abstain from substance use, the physician must consider this when prescribing medications for use at home.

Remind clients that they are in control of their own behavior. Give clients resources for outpatient support. A promise "never to use again" will not make the person successful. Provide a list of resources for families as well. See the Companion Website for a list of resources for clients and families.

NURSING PROCESS CARE PLAN
Client with Ineffective Coping

The police brought a 27-year-old Latino with a broken leg to the hospital. He was intoxicated and yelling that there was a machine in his body. His medical diagnoses are fractured tibia, alcohol abuse, and exacerbation of schizophrenia. The client lives alone and does not have a job.

Assessment. The nurse did a substance use assessment and found that the client uses alcohol on most days. Lately he has been drinking more, since his television is broken. He can't think of anything he enjoys doing. The client states, "The only time I'm not scared is when I'm drunk." Vital signs are T 99° F, P 100, R 18, BP 128/80. He has an order for Risperdal (risperidone). He says, "I stopped taking the medicine because I don't need it." He cooperates with taking his meds in the hospital.

Diagnosis
- Ineffective Coping

Expected Outcomes. The client will:
- Be compliant with taking his antipsychotic medication.
- Discuss his feelings about alcohol and alcohol dependency.
- List three resources for help when he needs it.

- Plan for three possible alternatives to drinking alcohol when he feels bored or afraid.
- Contact Alcoholics Anonymous while in the hospital to arrange attending a meeting on the day he is discharged.

Planning and Implementation. The nurse will implement the following interventions:

- Spend time talking with the client each shift. *This client has difficulty relating to other people because of his mental disorder. He can benefit from the personal interest of the staff members. He can also benefit from positive role modeling of how to socialize appropriately. Expressing his feelings about alcohol use is the beginning of recovery from alcohol abuse.*
- Discuss the consequences of drinking alcohol with the client. *The client may be having an exacerbation of his mental disorder (schizophrenia) due to drinking and not taking his meds. If he understands the negative effects of alcohol on his life, it will help him decide to stop drinking.*
- Help the client make a list of people who can help him in various everyday situations (refilling his medication prescriptions, driving him to an AA meeting, being available to talk on the phone if he is lonely). *The written list will be available to help him remember his resources when he is at risk for relapse. Using resources on the list (instead of drinking out of fear or frustration) is a method of positive coping.*
- Help the client make a list of alternatives to drinking. These items will be things that the client agrees that he would actually do. They may include going for a walk, watching the TV in the lobby of his apartment building, going to the library, playing a game, listening to music, exercise, drawing, taking a shower, etc. *The client with alcohol dependence may have difficulty thinking of alternatives to drinking. The list will be a reminder of realistic alternatives.*
- Show the client how to find the telephone number of the local Alcoholics Anonymous group in the phone book, and encourage the client to contact them. *People with schizophrenia often have difficulty with motivation and taking initiative. This client is more likely to participate in a group if he is assisted to join.*
- Assist the client to make a list of things he would enjoy doing. The nurse may make suggestions, but the client should choose the enjoyable things. *People with schizophrenia may have difficulty identifying fun activities. Such a list will make it easier for the client to think of something to do when he is independently choosing his activities.*

These enjoyable activities will also become alternatives to drinking.

Evaluation. The client was discharged after 7 days in the hospital. His psychosis symptoms (delusions about a machine in his body) disappeared after 5 days back on risperidone. The outcomes were partially met. He would not discuss his feelings about alcohol. The hospital social worker referred the client to his county mental health clinic where he is in a dual-diagnosis AA group. The clinic has a socialization program where the client can meet other people. He watches TV in the lobby. He is taking his medication and has not had any alcohol since he left the hospital 3 weeks ago.

Critical Thinking in the Nursing Process

1. What are the situations that would put this client at greatest risk for relapse into drinking again?
2. What role did alcohol play in this man's life?
3. What are the additional challenges for this client because he has dual diagnosis (compared with other clients with alcohol dependency)?

Note: Discussion of Critical Thinking questions appears in Appendix I.

Note: The references and resources for this and all chapters have been compiled at the back of the book.

KEY TERMS

Use the audio glossary feature of the Companion Website to hear the correct pronunciation of the following key terms.

abstinence

addiction

blackouts

compulsive substance use

confabulation

cross-tolerance

denial

detoxification

dual diagnosis

impaired nursing

intoxication

relapse

substance abuse

substance dependency

tolerance

withdrawal

KEY Points

- Substance abuse is a maladaptive pattern of substance use despite adverse outcomes. Substance dependency involves continuing to use the substance despite significant substance-related problems, including tolerance, withdrawal, and compulsive use.

- Substance-use disorders affect 20% of adults in the United States, but most of these people go undiagnosed.

- Clients use denial about substance use and so do health professionals.

- The *DSM-IV-TR* lists 11 substances of abuse: alcohol; opioids; sedatives, hypnotics, and anxiolytics; cocaine; amphetamines and similar drugs; hallucinogens; phencyclidine (PCP) and similar drugs; inhalants; cannabis; caffeine; and nicotine.

- The combination of psychotropic medications and alcohol or street drugs can cause increased CNS depression.

- Nurses should assess the substance use history of each client on admission.

- Alcoholism affects the whole family.

- When dual diagnosis exists (a person has both a mental disorder and a substance use disorder), both disorders must be treated together.

- When substance abuse and dependency occur among other nurses and health care professionals, the first responsibility of the nurse is client safety and the second is to seek help for the colleague.

- The goal of substance use treatment is abstinence from substance use and development of skills to replace drug use for coping, enjoyment, or companionship.

- Clients with substance dependency need referral to Social Services for assistance and follow-up after discharge.

- Many people respond well to treatment for substance-related disorders: keep hope alive.

 EXPLORE MediaLink

Additional interactive resources for this chapter can be found on the Companion Website at www.prenhall.com/eby. Click on Chapter 12 and "Begin" to select the activities for this chapter.

- Audio glossary
- NCLEX-PN® review
- Case study
- Study outline
- Critical thinking questions
- Matching questions
- Weblinks
- Video Case: Chris (Alcoholism)

Caring for a Client with Substance Dependency

NCLEX-PN® Focus Areas: Psychosocial Integrity

Case Study: The client is a 41-year-old European American male with alcoholism and Major Depressive Disorder. He is hospitalized in a general psychiatric unit. He was admitted 5 days ago after his daughter visited him in his apartment and found him lying on his bed intoxicated. He said, "Leave me alone. Everyone will be better off without me." He had not eaten in several days and had several empty bottles of whiskey beside his bed. He is thin and underweight for his height. He has medication prescribed for his depression, but he has not taken it since the prescription ran out 3 weeks ago. He had alcohol withdrawal symptoms for the first 4 days of his hospitalization. Now he is feeling better and his vital signs are stable.

Nursing Diagnosis: Ineffective coping

COLLECT DATA

Subjective	Objective
_____	_____
_____	_____
_____	_____
_____	_____
_____	_____
_____	_____

Would you report this data? Yes/No

If yes, to: _____

Nursing Care

_____
_____
_____
_____
_____
_____
_____
_____

How would you document this? _____
_____
_____
_____
_____

Compare your documentation to the sample provided in Appendix I.

Data Collected
(use those that apply)

- Client states, "Drinking helps me forget my problems."
- Prefers to lie in bed but will get up to do ADLs with encouragement
- Eats 90–100% of the food on his meal trays
- Has gained 4 pounds since admission
- Takes all meds given to him in the hospital
- When his daughter visits, he makes only brief responses to her.
- States, "What else can I do besides drink? It is all I know anymore."
- States, "I can quit when I want. I just don't want to quit."
- His affect is blunted and sad.
- He is oriented to person and place. Knows the year and month, not the date.
- States, "Maybe I should go home today. I can take care of myself."

Nursing Interventions
(use those that apply; list in priority order)

- Discuss the consequences of the client's drinking when he is able.
- Spend at least 3 hours each day explaining all the details of alcoholism, the theories of the disease, and potential treatments.
- Help him develop a list of his resources for help.
- Help him develop a list of healthier things he could do when he feels like drinking, to prevent relapse.
- Allow the client to spend the majority of his time in his bed.
- Encourage the client to spend time in the unit's living room where he can be with other people.
- Ask why he wants to go home.
- Reinforce teaching about his disorders and meds at his level.
- Spend time with the client each shift. Talk with him or sit beside him.
- Pressure the client to talk at length about his problems with drinking and depression.
- Ask the client if he has any questions about his medications. If so, provide simple explanations.
- Encourage the client to take his antidepressant medication.
- Ask the client if he has any side effects from his antidepressant medication.

1 A client who has alcohol dependence is admitted to the hospital with a painful injury. What would the nurse expect when planning for pain management for this client? He will:
   1. Need more narcotics, because he is tolerant to CNS depressants.
   2. Try to manipulate the staff to obtain drugs.
   3. Be uncooperative with nursing care.
   4. Be better off if given as little narcotics as possible.

2 An alcoholic client is admitted to the hospital for a fractured humerus. What medication would the nurse expect to give this client to prevent alcoholic encephalopathy?
   1. Demerol (meperidine)
   2. Valium (diazepam)
   3. Thiamine (vitamin B₁)
   4. Dilantin (phenytoin)

3 A client with schizophrenia is also diagnosed with alcohol abuse. What makes it more difficult for this client to stop drinking alcohol than the average client?
   1. Schizophrenia makes it difficult for this client to relate to other people to get help to quit drinking.
   2. He will be unable to respond to alcoholism treatment.
   3. He will be unable to understand any teaching the nurse would provide about alcoholism.
   4. People with schizophrenia prefer to drink alcohol rather than taking psychotropic medications.

4 An outpatient has a new prescription for an antianxiety medication. Which of the following *must* be included in the teaching plan?
   1. Take the drug every 4 hours.
   2. Avoid alcohol while taking the drug.
   3. The drug can cause insomnia.
   4. Avoid driving while taking this drug.

5 The narcotics count has been wrong several times lately. A particular RN frequently volunteers to give pain meds for other nurses' clients. Tonight he has slurred speech when he comes out of the bathroom. What should the nurse do?
   1. Confront the nurse with the suspicion that he is taking narcotics at work.
   2. Wait until the nurse has pinpoint pupils to confirm narcotics use.
   3. Notify the charge nurse that he is an impaired nurse.
   4. Notify the nursing supervisor of the nurse's observations.

6 The nursing diagnosis for a client with substance dependency is Ineffective Coping R/T inadequate problem-solving skills. Select the best nursing intervention for this client.
   1. Explain the signs and symptoms of alcohol withdrawal.
   2. Assist the client to list positive alternatives to substance use.
   3. Teach the client about the side effects of his medications.
   4. Teach the client to never drink alcohol again.

7 A client is suspected of substance abuse with methamphetamines. Which of the following symptoms/signs could indicate a problem with these drugs?
   1. Depression
   2. Skin lesions
   3. Weight gain
   4. Incontinence

8 What question would help the nurse determine the meaning of substance use to the individual client?
   1. "Why are you an alcoholic?"
   2. "How often do you use drugs and alcohol?"
   3. "What symptoms do you have when you use drugs?"
   4. "What circumstances lead you to drink alcohol or use drugs?"

9 A nurse is caring for a client in acute liver failure due to alcoholic cirrhosis. The nurse knows to be alert for signs and symptoms of:
   1. Pneumonia.
   2. Encephalitis.
   3. GI bleed.
   4. Congestive heart failure.

10 The nurse is caring for a client admitted through the ER after a motor vehicle accident. The family cautions the nurse that the client has been an alcoholic for years. What symptoms of the client would make the nurse suspicious that the client is going into alcohol withdrawal? (Select all that apply.)
   1. Depressed affect
   2. Irritability
   3. Hypotension
   4. Elevated pulse and respirations
   5. Confusion

Answers for Review Questions, as well as discussion of Care Plan and Critical Thinking Care Map questions, appear in Appendix I.

Learning About You!

CHAPTER 8 Schizophrenia

It is difficult to put yourself into the disorganized world of the person with schizophrenia. Give the following two exercises a try to allow you to peek into that world. The first demonstrates positive symptoms; the second, disorganized symptoms.

- Write a poem describing what you think it would be like to experience hallucinations or delusions.
- Practice loose association by connecting the following words in sentences the schizophrenic might use: house, flowers, water, walk, flight, move, movies, dark, deer, friend.

CHAPTER 9 Mood Disorders

Everyone has felt happy and sad. At times, you have probably felt very *happy and* very *sad. Because you have felt these emotions, it is easier for you to put yourself into the place of a person experiencing depression or mania than to imagine the world of schizophrenia. Try the following two exercises to allow yourself a glimpse into clinical depression and mania.*

- Remember when you were feeling very sad. Imagine what it would be like to feel ten times worse than that. Then imagine that you could see no end to the sadness. Describe your feelings after this exercise. Thinking about this incident will probably lower your mood. Follow this with a happier exercise.
- Describe in detail a time that you were very happy. Imagine what it would be like to feel ten times better than that. Imagine how living with this continuous "high" would affect your life. Would you want it ever to end? Describe your feelings after this exercise.

CHAPTER 10 Personality Disorders

Remember that this is just for fun. Imagine the following scenario, and then choose how a person with each personality disorder might respond to it.

Scenario: You have just received a telephone bill that shows hundreds of dollars of long distance calls that are not yours. Look at the following responses, and see if you can identify the personality disorder:

1. You put the bill into a basket with other bills that you have never paid.
2. You scream, cry, and call all your friends to tell them about the telephone bill.
3. You call the telephone company and tell them you know it is conspiring with other utility companies to bankrupt you.
4. You call the telephone company and tell them their employees are "incompetent" and demand to speak to your "good friend," the CEO.
5. You call your best friend and ask her what to do.
6. You vandalize the office of the telephone company.
7. You call the telephone company every 15 minutes, demanding that the inaccurate bill be corrected now.
8. You know it's a mistake; you don't have a phone.
9. You are sure this means you are about to get a huge inheritance.
10. You blame yourself for having a telephone and allowing a business to take advantage of you.

Answers to fun quiz

1. Avoidant
2. Histrionic
3. Paranoid
4. Narcissistic
5. Dependent
6. Antisocial
7. Obsessive-compulsive
8. Schizoid
9. Schizotypal
10. Borderline

CHAPTER 11 Anxiety Disorders

Consider this anxiety-producing situation. Decide which of the following coping strategies you would use.

Coping Strategy Choices

A. Active problem solving, adaptive
B. Active problem solving, maladaptive
C. Withdrawal, adaptive
D. Withdrawal, maladaptive
E. Compromise, adaptive
F. Compromise, maladaptive

Situation

You have been asked to participate in a group presentation to your nursing class. Doing the research and write-up is fun for you. However, you are very nervous when you go in front of a group. You are afraid other students will laugh at your anxiety. You would:

A. Call in sick on the day of the presentation.
B. See the school counselor to discuss ways of dealing with social anxiety before the presentation.

C. Tell the instructor that you are paying your tuition to be taught, not to do teaching yourself. Refuse to participate.

D. Tell the other students how nervous you are. Offer to set up, hold the posters, and clean up.

E. Suggest you do all of the research and situation-writing and the other students act out what you have written.

F. Agree to be part of the team by doing the research and situation-writing if the other students will do the actual presentation and then fail to do what you agreed on.

(By the way, A is maladaptive withdrawal; B is adaptive active problem solving; C is maladaptive active problem solving; D is adaptive withdrawal; E is adaptive compromise; and F is maladaptive compromise.)

CHAPTER 12   Substance Abuse and Dependency

As you read the following list of words circle those that cause you an emotional response (positive or negative).

Drinking	Alcoholic	Drunk driver
Drug addict	User	Drugs
Stoner	Meth head	Kegger
Drunk	Lush	Pusher
Medications	Junkie	Doper
Chemotherapy	Speed freak	

How did you learn these responses? Might your feelings about substance use affect your care of clients?

Nursing Care of Clients with Disorders Related to Development

UNIT III

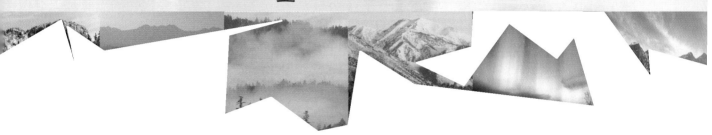

Chapter 13

Disorders in Childhood and Adolescence

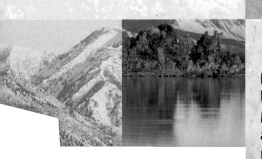

BRIEF Outline

Effect of Mental Disorders on Development

Mental Disorders in Children and Adolescents

Pervasive Developmental Disorders

Attention Deficit and Disruptive Behavior Disorders

Anxiety Disorders

Elimination Disorders

Depression, Psychosis, and Suicide

Self-Concept

LEARNING Outcomes

After completing this chapter, you will be able to:

1. Explain the relationship between developmental level and the client's response to illness.
2. Include a variety of teaching strategies for health teaching of clients with learning disorders.
3. Provide guidelines to parents of clients with attention deficit and disruptive behavior disorders.
4. Provide nursing interventions to promote the self-esteem of clients.
5. Apply the nursing process to clients with disorders diagnosed in childhood and adolescence.

Whether they are healthy or not, children are different from adults. They are immature physically and mentally. They perceive the world and their experiences in a different way. For these reasons, they respond to mental disorders differently from the way adults do. Even when they have the same diagnosis, such as depression, the nurse may observe behavior in children that differs from adult symptoms.

Mental disorders result from an interaction between the genetics a child is born with and the life experiences and stressors that the child experiences. Children who experience hardships and abuse are more likely to grow up with mental disorders. Of course not all children who experience psychosocial stressors and disadvantages develop mental disorders. Many children grow into well-adjusted adults despite many risk factors in their environment and experience. What makes these children immune to the stressors that change other people? The mechanism of their **resilience** (flexibility in a mentally or physically stressful situation and ability to return to normal) is not fully understood. Perhaps a supportive relationship with a member of the community protects the child. Perhaps a positive environment fosters resilience in a child with a genetic predisposition and prevents the disorder. For example, one child with the genetic predisposition for Attention Deficit/Hyperactivity Disorder (ADHD) may live in a stable predictable family and may have minimal symptoms of ADHD. Another child with similar genetics who lives in a chaotic environment will have all the symptoms of the disorder (Keltner, Schwecke, & Bostrom, 2007). Figure 13-1 ■ shows an interactive model of childhood mental illness.

Effect of Mental Disorders on Development

The client's developmental stage at the onset of a mental disorder determines how the disorder affects him or her. We know that children develop according to a predictable pattern (remember Erikson's stages of development?). Chronic medical or mental disorders can affect the development of children.

Mental disorders may make it more difficult for children to achieve developmental tasks. When a child has depression, if she is in the developmental stage of Industry versus Inferiority, she may be unable to participate in group activities with her peers or to accomplish school projects. Both of these are part of her developmental task of Industry. The nurse who understands human development can assess clients for their ability to achieve their individual developmental tasks. The nurse can provide appropriate interventions to promote development. In the case of the school-aged child with depression, the nurse can encourage participation in group activities and create opportunities to complete simple projects to promote the child's development. Figure 13-2 ■ shows a child in the first grade engaging in an age-appropriate development-enhancing activity at a school for disabled children. He is acting out the role of an octopus as he learns about the letter "O."

A mental disorder that begins in childhood may affect the individual's development over a lifetime. For example, a person who begins to suffer from Major Depressive Disorder during adolescence may not be able to achieve the developmental task of Identity versus Role confusion. Without intervention, he may always have role confusion

Genetic Predisposition
- Metabolic Deficiencies
- Nervous System Abnormalities

Interaction Between Genotype and Experience → Child Mental Illness

Life Experience
- Injury/Illness
- Toxic Exposure
- Deprivation/Neglect
- Abuse/Rejection
- Other Major Stressors (e.g., death of a parent)

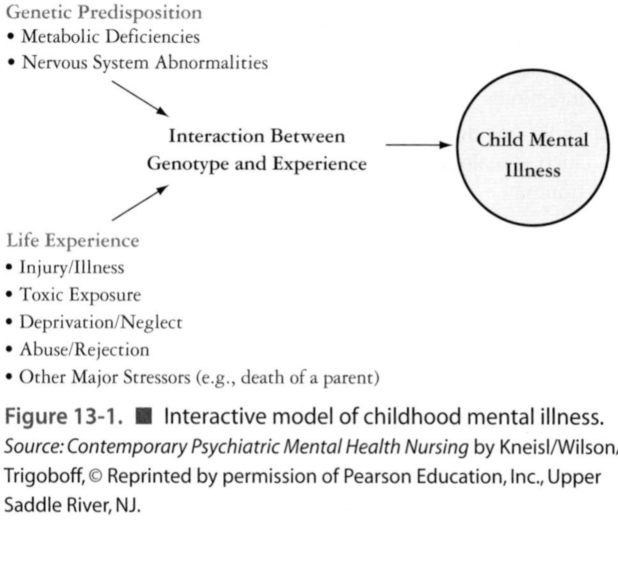

Figure 13-1. ■ Interactive model of childhood mental illness.
Source: Contemporary Psychiatric Mental Health Nursing by Kneisl/Wilson/Trigoboff, © Reprinted by permission of Pearson Education, Inc., Upper Saddle River, NJ.

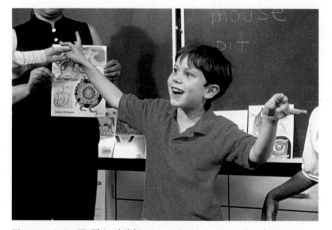

Figure 13-2. ■ This child is engaging in an activity that promotes his development. He is acting out the role of an octopus as he learns about the letter "O." *Source:* Will Hart.

BOX 13-1 NURSING CARE CHECKLIST

Promoting the Client's Development

☑ **Know the developmental tasks of childhood and adolescence** (Trust, Autonomy, Initiative, Industry, Identity) and provide opportunities for clients to achieve them.

☑ **Provide normalizing experiences.**
Provide age-appropriate activities in the treatment setting.
Give children opportunities to choose their play activities.
Reinforce age-appropriate behavior.
Provide opportunity for interaction with peers.
Adapt the environment to make it healthy, pleasant, and conducive to normal interaction with others.

☑ **Promote coping skills.**
Decision making
Stress reduction
Problem solving

and may fail to meet the developmental task of adolescence. He may have difficulty defining personal priorities and choosing a life direction. Because the client was developing normally before the onset of depression, he will probably have achieved the earlier developmental tasks of trust, autonomy, initiative, and industry.

Although physicians must focus on the disease processes of their child psychiatric clients, nurses are more able to focus on clients' developmental needs. This means that nurses can assess clients' developmental level and encourage their development, even when they are in treatment for mental disorders. Development continues throughout life, so the nurse must promote the human development of all clients in all treatment settings.

Development-promoting interventions focus on normalizing experiences, adapting the environment, and promoting the client's coping skills (Hockenberry, 2005). Box 13-1 ■ suggests some ways to promote the child's development while the child is in treatment.

Mental Disorders in Children and Adolescents

MENTAL RETARDATION

Mental Retardation is characterized by significantly below-average intellectual functioning, which begins before the child is 18 years of age. It is accompanied by impairment in adaptive functioning, which is the ability of the individual to cope with the demands of everyday life. Everyday life demands include communication, self-care, relationships, home living, use of community resources, self-direction, functional academic skills, work, leisure, and maintaining health and safety. Mental Retardation can vary in degree from mild to profound (American Psychiatric Association [APA], 2000). Children with mental retardation are seldom treated in psychiatric settings unless they also have psychiatric disorders.

Mental Retardation can result from a variety of causes. In many affected individuals, the etiology is unknown. The major causes of Mental Retardation are listed in Box 13-2 ■.

LEARNING DISORDERS

If a child has lower functioning in academic skills than would be predicted based on the child's learning aptitude, the child may have a Learning Disorder. Learning Disorders are diagnosed when children's achievement in reading, mathematics, or written expression is substantially below expected achievement for their age, schooling, and level of intelligence. Learning Disorders may persist into adulthood (APA, 2000).

Children and adolescents with Learning Disorders may feel demoralized and have low self-esteem. They may have difficulty with social skills. The school dropout rate for those affected with Learning Disorders is nearly 40%.

BOX 13-2

Major Causes of Mental Retardation

■ **Genetics.** Chromosome abnormalities such as Down syndrome and fragile X syndrome; inborn errors of metabolism such as phenylketonuria (PKU); and single-gene abnormalities with variable expression such as tuberous sclerosis

■ **Alterations in embryonic development.** Prenatal damage due to toxins such as maternal alcohol consumption, infections

■ **Problems during pregnancy and the perinatal period** such as malnutrition, prematurity, hypoxia, viral infections, trauma

■ **Environmental influences** such as inadequate nurturing or stimulation

■ **Mental disorders** such as Autistic Disorder and other Pervasive Developmental Disorders

■ **General medical conditions acquired in infancy or childhood** such as lead poisoning, trauma, or infection

Source: Reprinted with permission from the *Diagnostic and Statistical Manual of Mental Disorders, Text Revision*, copyright 2000. American Psychiatric Association.

Adults with Learning Disorders may have difficulty with employment or social adjustment (APA, 2000). Early detection and intervention for affected children give them a better prognosis for learning, self-esteem, and functioning as adults.

Several factors may cause Learning Disorders. These include genetic predisposition, a history of perinatal injury, or a neurological disorder. For many affected people the cause of Learning Disorders is unclear.

Reading Disorder

The most common of the Learning Disorders is Reading Disorder, also known as **dyslexia.** The central feature of Reading Disorder is decreased reading accuracy, speed, or comprehension. In this disorder, reading achievement is substantially below the expectation based on the individual's age, intelligence, and education. Reading Disorder significantly interferes with the affected individual's success in school or with any activities that require reading skills. If the person has a sensory deficit (such as decreased hearing or vision), this diagnosis is not appropriate unless the individual has difficulty with reading in excess of what would be expected because of this deficit (APA, 2000).

When people with this disorder read aloud, their reading often contains substitutions, distortions, or omissions. Both oral and silent reading are slow and contain comprehension errors (APA, 2000). Males are more commonly diagnosed with Reading Disorder. However, the procedures for referring students for diagnosis of Reading Disorder may be biased toward finding more males. Male students who have problems with reading are more likely to have behavior problems than their female counterparts do. Note the reversed letters in Figure 13-3 ■ written by this fourth grade child with dyslexia.

Mathematics Disorder

Individuals with Mathematics Disorder have math ability that falls significantly below what is expected for their age, intelligence, and education. The math disturbance notably interferes with their academic achievement or with activities of daily living that require math skills. If a sensory deficit is present, the math difficulties are more than would usually be associated with the sensory deficit (APA, 2000). The child depicted in Figure 13-4 ■ has a lower level of math ability than expected for his age, although he functions normally in other areas.

Several related skills may be impaired in Mathematics Disorder. Linguistic (language) skills include understanding or naming mathematical terms, operations, or concepts

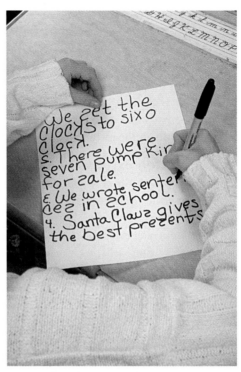

Figure 13-3. ■ Note the reversed letters written by this child who has dyslexia or Reading Disorder. *Source:* Will Hart.

and decoding written problems into mathematical symbols. Perceptual skills include recognizing or reading numerical symbols and clustering objects into groups. Attention skills such as copying numbers or figures correctly, remembering to add in "carried" numbers, and observing operational signs may be affected. Finally, mathematical skills are impaired. Mathematical skills include following sequences of mathematical steps, counting objects, and learning multiplication tables (APA, 2000).

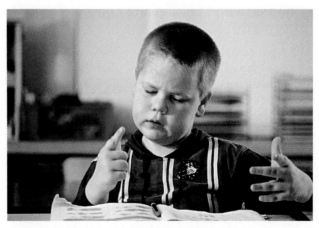

Figure 13-4. ■ This child with Mathematics Disorder functions normally in other areas. *Source:* Ellen Senisi.

Mathematics Disorder may be diagnosed as early as age 5. It may not become apparent until the fifth grade or even later. The age at which math expectations become unreachable depends on the school's expectations and on the child's skills. Some children with Mathematics Disorder and especially high IQ (intelligence quotient) are able to meet school math expectations by using other problem-solving skills in the early grades.

Disorder of Written Expression

Children with this disorder have writing skills below the expected skills for their age, intelligence, and education. The Disorder of Written Expression interferes significantly with academic achievement or activities of daily living that require writing skills. As in reading and math disorders, if affected individuals have a sensory deficit, their writing disability is greater than would be expected due to the sensory deficit alone (APA, 2000).

The Disorder of Written Expression generally causes grammatical and punctuation errors, poor paragraph organization, multiple spelling errors, and poor handwriting. This diagnosis is not used simply for spelling errors and poor handwriting. The disorder is usually apparent by the second grade (APA, 2000).

Developmental Coordination Disorder

In Developmental Coordination Disorder, development of motor coordination is markedly impaired. When children are learning to run, hold eating utensils, fasten clothing, or play games, they are significantly less coordinated than their age-mates. The impairment is significant enough to interfere with school performance or activities of daily living. Impaired coordination is expressed differently in children of different ages. An 8-month-old may have difficulty crawling or sitting, whereas an 8-year-old may have trouble throwing a ball or tying shoelaces. Impaired coordination may resolve or may persist into adolescence or adulthood. This diagnosis is not made if the child has a general medical disorder such as cerebral palsy or a neurological abnormality (APA, 2000).

Nursing Considerations

Teaching or providing information to clients and their families is a major function of nurses. Nurses often ignore the diagnosis of learning disabilities, missing the opportunity to communicate clearly and to teach effectively with children who have special needs in the healthcare setting (Selekman, 2002).

The type of learning disorder the child has suggests the teaching approach. Knowledge of the child's individual learning strengths and challenges helps make teaching effective. The best teaching approach depends on the type of disability (Hockenberry, 2005).

Nurses must adapt their teaching to meet the individual learning needs of each client. This is true when an elderly client has aphasia due to a CVA or when a child has a learning disability. Tips for providing information to children with learning disorders are provided in Box 13-3 ■.

COMMUNICATION DISORDERS

Communication Disorders can involve the child's physical ability to speak, which is the motor (muscular) aspect of speaking. Or, these disorders can involve language, which is the sending and receiving of verbal messages.

BOX 13-3 NURSING CARE CHECKLIST

Children with Learning and Communication Disorders

☑ When a child is admitted to the hospital or clinic, the nurse should ask if the child has any learning or communication problems. If the answer is yes, find out what type of deficit the child has. *Strategies that work best for the child in school and at home can be used for teaching health-related information* (Selekman, 2002).

☑ Provide pictures and diagrams for children with an auditory perceptual deficit. *These children appear unable to follow directions or to comprehend volumes of verbal information. Diagrams, pictures, demonstrations, and written lists are better than verbal teaching strategies for children with auditory perceptual deficit.*

☑ Provide demonstrations and discussions for children with a visual perceptual deficit. *These children have difficulty with reading, putting numbers in the correct order for mathematical problems, or judging distance. They may perceive letters and numbers out of their intended order. They may learn best from demonstrations, discussions, and a verbal approach.*

☑ Provide tools to children with poor coordination. *Children with a deficit in coordination may benefit from using a computer word processor to replace their illegible handwriting. They can be included in physical activities that do not require great coordination. Put them in situations where they can participate and succeed.*

Expressive Language Disorder

Expressive Language Disorder is an impairment of verbal or sign-language communication. The abnormalities interfere with school or occupational achievement or with social communication. The abnormalities may include a limited vocabulary, decreased amount of speech, difficulty acquiring new words, word-finding or vocabulary errors, shortened sentences, simplified grammatical structure, limited varieties of grammar or sentence structures, omissions of critical parts of sentences, use of unusual word order, and slow language development. Language comprehension is usually within normal limits. Most children with this disorder improve dramatically over time. It occurs more often in children with a family history of Communication or Learning Disorders (APA, 2000).

Mixed Receptive–Expressive Language Disorder

Children with this disorder have impairment in development of both receptive and expressive language. The language difficulties interfere with school or occupational achievement or with social communication. People with this disorder have the impairments of expressive language described previously. They also have receptive abnormalities such as difficulty understanding words, sentences, or certain types of words (for example, spatial words such as above, inside, or to the left). The affected child may appear not to hear, not to be paying attention, or to be confused. The child may follow instructions incorrectly, or not at all, and may give inappropriate answers to questions. The child may also have difficulty processing other sounds (APA, 2000). Figure 13-5 ■ shows a child who has an

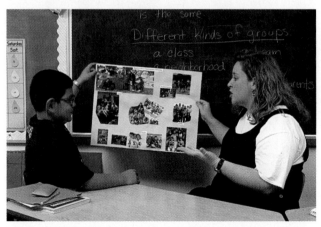

Figure 13-5. ■ A child with a receptive language disorder learns better when pictures are used than he does with verbal teaching. *Source: Will Hart.*

BOX 13-4	CULTURAL PULSE POINTS

Language When Assessing Communication Disorders

Care must be taken when assessing immigrant children or children who speak English as a nonnative language for Communication Disorders. Children should be assessed in their native language to ensure that any abnormality is due to receiving or sending language messages and not due to inadequate acquisition of a new language.

auditory receptive disorder who learns better when pictures are used than he does with verbal teaching.

It can be challenging to help immigrant children who have communication difficulties. Box 13-4 ■ provides information on diagnosing Communication Disorders in nonnative speakers of English.

Phonological Disorder

Phonological Disorder involves a failure to use speech sounds that are expected for the child's age and language. It may include errors in producing sounds or organizing sounds in words, omitting sounds (such as final consonants in words), or substituting one sound for another (such as saying *t* when the word has a *k*). To justify this diagnosis, the speech disorder must be severe enough to interfere with school or job performance or with social communication (APA, 2000). This disorder can be mild or severe, depending on individual factors. It often resolves spontaneously.

Stuttering

Stuttering is a disturbance of normal fluency and patterning of speech that is not appropriate for an individual's age. It includes frequent repetitions or prolongations of sounds or syllables. It may also include pauses in speech, words produced with an excess of physical tension, broken words (pauses within a word), or word substitutions to avoid a problem word. Most people with stuttering recover, usually before age 16. Some continue to stutter into adulthood. More males than females are affected, and the disorder runs in families, suggesting a genetic connection (APA, 2000).

Pervasive Developmental Disorders

There are several Pervasive Developmental Disorders, including Autistic Disorder, Rett's Disorder, Childhood Disintegrative Disorder, and Asperger's Disorder. These disorders are characterized by severe impairment in several areas of development such as communication skills, social interaction skills, or the presence of stereotyped behavior, interests, and activities. These disorders are usually evident in infancy and are often associated with Mental Retardation (APA, 2000).

AUTISTIC DISORDER

Autistic Disorder is the most common of the Pervasive Developmental Disorders. It occurs earlier than the other disorders in this group and is evident before the age of 3 years. This disorder involves three areas of abnormality:

1. **Impaired social interaction** (failure to develop peer relationships, no eye contact or other nonverbal interactive behaviors, no seeking to share enjoyment with others, or lack of social responses)
2. **Impaired communication** (delay or lack of language, stereotyped language, repetition of words said by others, or lack of imaginative play)
3. **Stereotyped behavior** (inflexibility, preoccupation with odd interests such as bus schedules, strict adherence to nonfunctional routines, or repetitive mannerisms such as hand flapping or head banging) (APA, 2000).

Evidence supports multiple causal factors for autism. There is approximately a 5% chance of recurrence in a family that has one autistic child. No single gene has been identified as a cause.

Most children with autism have some degree of developmental delay. Most are unable to live independently as adults. Prognosis depends on intellectual functioning level and development of language skills. Some affected children show improvement in socialization skills as they reach school age. Some experience a major change, either for better or for worse, at puberty. More boys than girls are affected with autism, but girls tend to be more severely affected.

Nursing Considerations

Nurses who care for children with autism must be aware of the major features of the disorder and how to apply this knowledge to individualize their care. People with autism have difficulty relating to others, especially to unfamiliar people.

SHORT-TERM ACUTE CARE. When a child with autism is acutely ill and hospitalized for a brief stay, a goal of nursing care may be to decrease the client's stress level so s/he can cooperate with care. There are several ways to do this:

■ Touch the client as little as possible and even minimize time in the client's room when possible. Clients with autism should have private rooms to decrease excessive stimuli and stress.
■ Encourage parents to visit and to bring familiar objects to the hospital. The child may be able to relate to a familiar object from home.
■ Communicate briefly and concretely with these children. Instead of saying, "Please come over here and sit in this nice blue chair," try "Sit in this chair."
■ Maintain a predictable schedule. Allow the family to repeat their routines from home when possible. Familiar routines are important. Wearing certain pajamas, placing objects in certain exact positions, eating certain food arranged in a certain way, or drinking from a specific cup might be helpful. If the child desires odd yet harmless things such as placing objects in a strange arrangement, the nurse could reduce stress by allowing this.

LONG-TERM CARE ENVIRONMENTS. In the psychiatric or rehabilitation environment, there is more opportunity to promote the child's development. The nurse can help children with autism to reach their full potential by:

■ Encouraging social interactions.
■ Fostering the development of language skills. Figure 13-6 ■ shows a girl communicating with a nonverbal boy who has autism, using his sheets of symbols and pictures.

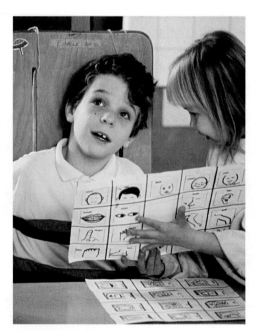

Figure 13-6. ■ A girl tries to communicate with a nonverbal boy with autism using his sheets of symbols and pictures. *Source:* Ellen Senisi.

- Encouraging the development of self-control, including delaying gratification and impulse control.
- Providing opportunities for the development of psychomotor skills (through play and activities of daily living).

ASPERGER'S DISORDER

Asperger's Disorder is another Pervasive Developmental Disorder, yet it is different from Autistic Disorder. Compared to children with Autistic Disorder, children with Asperger's Disorder are less disabled. They have no significant delays in cognitive (thinking) or language development. The disorder is usually apparent between the ages of 3 and 5 years. This disorder is characterized by the following:

- **Severe impairment in social interactions** (impaired nonverbal behaviors, failure to develop peer relationships, lack of sharing enjoyment or interests with others, or lack of emotional sharing)
- **Repetitive and stereotyped behaviors** (rigid adherence to nonfunctional routines, repetitive mannerisms such as hand flapping or rocking, or intense preoccupation with an area of interest such as numbers or music to the exclusion of everything else)
- **Significant impairment in social, school, or occupational functioning** (APA, 2000)

People with Asperger's Disorder may be able to function independently as adults. They continue to have impaired social behavior and have difficulty understanding the feelings of others. Nursing considerations for hospitalized children with this disorder are similar to those for children with autism in the area of socializing and behavior. Because the new environment and social stressors of the hospital may create anxiety, anxiety management may be an important goal for hospitalized children with Asperger's Disorder. These children will develop more language skills than children with Autistic Disorder can.

RETT'S DISORDER

Rett's Disorder is a Pervasive Developmental Disorder observed only in females. The essential feature is the development of multiple deficits following a period of normal functioning. The rate of head growth decreases, previously acquired hand skills are lost, gait is slow and poorly coordinated, and language development is severely impaired. Affected children lose interest in social interaction. The onset of Rett's Disorder is before 4 years, but can be as early as 5 months. The pattern of regression

of development is very distinctive. The disorder persists throughout life, and the loss of skills is progressive. It is associated with severe or profound Mental Retardation (APA, 2000).

CHILDHOOD DISINTEGRATIVE DISORDER

Like Autistic and Asperger's Disorders, Childhood Disintegrative Disorder is more common in males. In this disorder, the child will regress in multiple areas of functioning following a period of at least 2 years of normal development. Most cases are identified between 2 and 4 years of age. The affected child will have a significant loss of skills in at least two of the following areas: language, social skills, bowel or bladder control, play, or motor skills. Usually, skills are lost in all areas. Individuals with Childhood Disintegrative Disorder have the same deficits in social and communication skills as those with Autistic Disorder (APA, 2000).

Critical Self-Check. Children with Pervasive Developmental Disorders are at higher risk for abuse and neglect than other children are. Why do you think this is true?

Attention Deficit and Disruptive Behavior Disorders

There are three relatively common behavior disorders in this group: Attention Deficit/Hyperactivity Disorder (ADHD), Oppositional Defiant Disorder, and Conduct Disorder. Disruptive Behavior Disorders occur in children of all socioeconomic levels.

ATTENTION DEFICIT/ HYPERACTIVITY DISORDER

ADHD is a persistent pattern of inattention and/or hyperactivity-impulsivity that is severe and frequent enough to impair the individual's academic, job, or social functioning (APA, 2000). Box 13-5 ■ provides the *DSM-IV-TR* diagnostic criteria. In the past ADHD was blamed on bad parenting or on children who were not trying to behave in school. It is now known to be a significant brain abnormality.

There is evidence that ADHD is strongly influenced by genetic factors, as indicated by studies of recurrence in families. In families of children with ADHD, 25% of close relatives are affected, whereas the rate of ADHD in the general population is about 5% (National Institute of Mental Health [NIMH], 2006a). Family, school, and

BOX 13-5

Diagnostic Criteria for Attention Deficit/Hyperactivity Disorder (ADHD)

A. Either (1) or (2):

1. Six or more of the following inattention symptoms have persisted for at least 6 months and are maladaptive:
   a. Often fails to give close attention to details or makes careless mistakes in schoolwork or other activities
   b. Has difficulty sustaining attention in tasks or play activities
   c. Does not seem to listen when spoken to directly
   d. Often does not follow through on instructions and fails to finish schoolwork, chores, etc.
   e. Has difficulty organizing tasks and activities
   f. Avoids, dislikes, or is reluctant to engage in tasks that require sustained mental attention
   g. Often loses things that are necessary for tasks or activities
   h. Easily distracted by environmental stimuli
   i. Often forgetful

2. Six or more of the following hyperactivity-impulsivity symptoms have lasted for at least 6 months and are maladaptive:

Hyperactivity
   a. Often fidgets (restless movements) with hands or feet or squirms (wriggles) in chair
   b. Often leaves chair in classroom inappropriately
   c. Runs or climbs in inappropriate situations
   d. Often has difficulty playing or engaging in leisure activities quietly
   e. Often talks excessively
   f. Is more active than expected for age

Impulsivity
   a. Often blurts out answers before questions are completed
   b. Has difficulty waiting
   c. Often interrupts or intrudes on others

B. Symptoms are present before age 7.
C. Symptoms are not only present at school.
D. There must be significant impairment in social, school, or work functioning.

Source: Reprinted with permission from the *Diagnostic and Statistical Manual of Mental Disorders, Text Revision,* copyright 2000. American Psychiatric Association.

peers also have strong influences on the extent of impairment in affected children. Current research on ADHD is focusing on genetics, brain development, and alterations in brain structure and function, especially in brain neurotransmitters (APA, 2000; McCracken, 2000).

The diagnosis of ADHD is becoming more common in girls. This increase is due to more accurate diagnosis rather than to an actual increase in incidence of ADHD in girls. Because they were not diagnosed, girls with ADHD often went untreated. Girls with ADHD are less likely to have disruptive behavior in school, so they were not as likely to be diagnosed as boys with ADHD.

The three major features of ADHD are inattention, hyperactivity, and impulsivity (see Box 13-5). Inattention can make social relationships and school performance more difficult. Affected children may not be able to listen to others, follow directions, or play cooperatively. They have difficulty completing school assignments that require prolonged concentration.

Hyperactivity makes school more difficult. Most school settings require children to sit quietly at a desk for extended periods. Children with ADHD may get up and walk around the classroom at the wrong times. They may disrupt the class by tapping pencils, fidgeting in their seats, swinging their legs, or making other noises.

Figure 13-7 ■ shows how one 5-year-old boy with ADHD felt after sitting quietly in class.

Impulsive children may interrupt others and may not be able to share or wait for their turn. Impulsivity can even put the child in danger. The impulsive child may not consider the consequences of running in the street, riding a bicycle on a railroad track, or climbing to the top of a tree. Figure 13-8 ■ shows a 3-year-old girl with ADHD climbing the hall doorway.

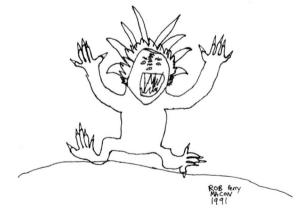

Figure 13-7. ■ This drawing was done by a 5-year-old boy with ADHD after he was required to sit still. *Source:* Courtesy of Rob Perry.

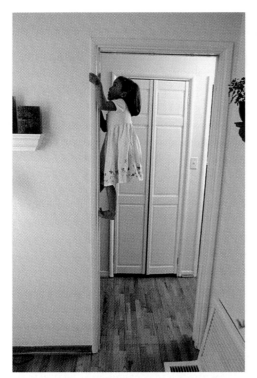

Figure 13-8. ■ A 3-year-old girl with ADHD climbs the hall doorway without concern for her safety. *Source:* PhotoEdit Inc.

Children with ADHD often have difficulty in forming peer relationships and in performing well in school. Children with ADHD are perceived by their teachers and peers to be more aggressive, bossier, and less likable (McCracken, 2000). These children may be rejected by peers and treated sternly by teachers. Affected children, their families, peers, and teachers may feel angry, frustrated, or hopeless.

ADHD is usually diagnosed when the child starts school, although many parents report problems at a much younger age. The behaviors associated with ADHD (impulsivity, short attention, increased physical activity) are all present in normal children. The disorder is only diagnosed when the severity or frequency of these findings is outside the normal range. See Box 13-5 for the diagnostic criteria.

Almost half of children referred to clinics for ADHD also have Oppositional Defiant Disorder or Conduct Disorder. Mood Disorders, Anxiety Disorders, and Learning Disorders are also more likely to occur in clients with ADHD than in the general population (APA, 2000).

Some affected people note a decrease in the severity of symptoms, especially the motor hyperactivity, in late adolescence or early adulthood. The majority continue to have some symptoms of increased activity, inattention, and impulsivity as adults. Most adults develop ways of coping with the symptoms.

Adult ADHD

Many children who have ADHD will continue to have symptoms as adults. Often, adults with ADHD are unaware that they have the disorder. They may believe that they cannot get organized, stick to a job, or keep an appointment. The everyday tasks of daily living such as getting up in the morning, getting to work on time, and being productive on the job can be major challenges (NIMH, 2006a).

The diagnosis of ADHD in adulthood requires that the adult was also affected as a child (ADHD does not begin in adulthood, although it may be first recognized in an individual as an adult). A correct diagnosis of ADHD can bring a sense of relief to people who have had difficulty in school and work for years, and who may have been blamed for not paying attention or trying hard enough. The treatment of ADHD in adults, as in children, usually begins with a stimulant medication; antidepressants are a second-line medication treatment. Education and psychotherapy are also important for adults (NIMH, 2006a).

Collaborative Care

ADHD is a chronic problem that is not specifically curable. Treatment is centered on symptom management. The treatment goal is to manage the inattention, hyperactivity, and impulsivity to allow the child to develop normally and to succeed in school. Figure 13-9 ■ shows children in a classroom situation in which those affected with ADHD is readily apparent. Many reported easy cures promise to treat the disorder with such things as vitamins or diets low in sugar or additives. Nurses should counsel families that most of these promises are not valid (McCracken, 2000).

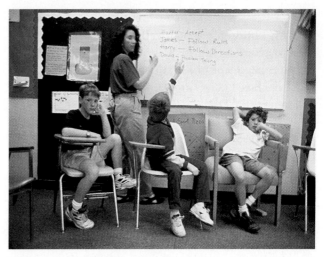

Figure 13-9. ■ Can you tell which of these students has ADHD? *Source:* Aurora & Quanta Productions Inc.

BOX 13-6 **NURSING CARE CHECKLIST**

Attention Deficit/Hyperactivity Disorder with Rationales

☑ **Establish a therapeutic nurse-client relationship.** *Trust facilitates nurse-client communication and is a foundation for all nursing interventions.*

☑ **Assess the problematic behavior for frequency and severity** (tantrums, accidents, acting-out, etc.) *Initial assessment provides a baseline, so the nurse will know where the client started and if the client is making progress.*

☑ **Explain expected behavior.** *The child with ADHD may have difficulty understanding usual social and nonverbal cues that regulate behavior. The child has a better opportunity to adhere to expectations that s/he understands clearly. Many parents have unrealistic expectations for child behavior.*

☑ **Give positive feedback for appropriate behavior.** *Behavior therapy is based on the idea that positively reinforced behavior is more likely to persist. Positive feedback (praise, privileges) will reinforce the desired behavior.*

☑ **Encourage children with ADHD to discuss their feelings, especially the feelings associated with behavior that is problematic.** *Discussing feelings promotes insight (self-understanding). Insight can help the child recognize what leads to the behavior before s/he acts. Verbalizing feelings instead of acting out behavior is a goal of treatment.*

☑ **Help the child to consider alternative behavior** (when you feel like talking when the teacher is talking, you can say to yourself "I'll wait until she's done"). *Cognitive therapy is based on learning new ways to think about problems. A good way to develop new coping methods is to combine cognitive and behavioral approaches: plan new behavior, try it out, and if it works, make it a habit.*

☑ **Keep goals and instructions simple and realistic.** *Unrealistic goals are likely to lead to more frustration and sense of failure. Children with ADHD have difficulty comprehending complicated instructions.*

☑ **If the child has difficulty completing tasks, begin with helping her/him to complete tasks, then progress to prompting, and finally expect the child to complete tasks independently.** *Children with ADHD often do not have experience with successfully completing complex tasks. They will function best if given progressive expectations that increase as their ability to concentrate increases.*

☑ **Divide complicated tasks into smaller parts.** *Smaller tasks are more likely to be completed successfully, which encourages a sense of accomplishment.*

☑ **Plan for breaks in large tasks when the child can be active.** *The child may be able to complete a large task successfully if given opportunities to use excess energy. The goal is for the child to complete the task and experience success.*

☑ **Provide feedback and consequences related to the child's behavior as soon as possible after the behavior occurs.** *The child is most likely to be able to connect the behavior to the consequences if they occur close together. Positive feedback is especially important, because children with ADHD are likely to receive a lot of negative feedback. Sincere positive reinforcement can help to improve self-esteem.*

☑ **Provide a low-stimulation environment.** *Children with ADHD are easily distracted by environmental stimuli. Their ability to concentrate is at its best when external stimuli are at a minimum.*

Many children respond well to treatment. The best client outcomes result from a combination of early detection and treatment, medications, and psychosocial interventions. Box 13-6 ■ provides nursing interventions for children with ADHD, including rationales.

MEDICATIONS. Medications have helped many children and adolescents with ADHD increase their ability to concentrate and reduce their hyperactivity and impulsiveness. Medications provide the child with the ability to respond to other forms of therapy. The most common medication prescribed for the symptoms of ADHD is methylphenidate (Ritalin). The mechanism of action of the stimulant drugs in ADHD is to enhance the activity of brain dopamine and norepinephrine.

Methylphenidate is effective in 70–80% of children with ADHD (Stahl, 2005).

There was some concern that giving children stimulant medications might increase their risk to abuse drugs as adolescents. Biederman (2003) found that the opposite is true. Adolescents with ADHD who were not treated with stimulant medications were found to have a three to four times greater risk to have a substance use disorder than those who were treated with stimulant medications for ADHD. The reason may be that the untreated children are more likely to find maladaptive coping methods when their disorder is not treated effectively. Another hypothesis is that they may look to street drugs as a form of self-medication.

The most common side effects of the stimulant drugs are insomnia and loss of appetite. The insomnia may be

TABLE 13-1

Medications for Attention Deficit/Hyperactivity Disorder

STIMULANTS	SIDE EFFECTS	NURSING CONSIDERATIONS
Amphetamine Sulfate (Adderall) Dextroamphetamine (Dexedrine and Dextrostat) Methylphenidate (Ritalin) Ritalin SR (sustained release) Ritalin LA (long acting) Concerta (long acting) Metadate ER (extended release) Metadate CD (extended release)	Loss of appetite (anorexia), weight loss, insomnia, growth delay Depression if stopped abruptly; decreases saliva production, which promotes tooth decay	Assess for decreased appetite, weight loss, or growth delays; give with meals; appetite suppression is most severe in first few weeks of therapy; give last dose no later than 6 hrs before bedtime to prevent insomnia; do not stop these medications abruptly; teach client importance of good oral hygiene and to rinse mouth with water frequently; do not drink citrus juice within an hour of taking these meds. Assess BP.
Pemoline (Cylert)	Liver damage; interactions: caffeine and ephedrine in cold medicines increase stimulant effect; ascorbic acid increases elimination of amphetamine and dextroamphetamine	Liver function tests should be done on clients taking pemoline. Because of its potential liver toxicity, pemoline should not be used as a first-line treatment for ADHD.
Nonstimulant Atomoxetine (Strattera)	GI distress (constipation, nausea), reduced appetite, weight loss, dermatitis, dry mouth.	Can be taken with or without food. Adults may experience decreased libido.

prevented by scheduling the medication at least 6 hours before bedtime and by having a regular bedtime each night to reinforce the body's **circadian** (day/night) rhythm. Table 13-1 ■ provides information about the drugs used to treat ADHD.

The loss of appetite (anorexia) is worst during the first few weeks of therapy, but persists longer for many children. The child's appetite is lowest when each dose of medication peaks. The nurse can teach the family to provide meals when the medication is at its lowest level. A big breakfast and a substantial snack after dinner would help ensure adequate nutrition. If the medication is ordered three times per day, schedule it with meals. Nurses should assess the growth of children taking stimulant medications for ADHD. If their growth rate slows, inadequate nutrition due to loss of appetite may be the reason.

The first nonstimulant drug for ADHD is now available. Atomoxetine (Strattera), is a norepinephrine transporter (NET) inhibitor. It acts by specifically inhibiting the transport of norepinephrine in the central nervous system. It has been shown to both improve attention and reduce hyperactivity. Atomoxetine is not subject to abuse, because it does not bind to receptors associated with abuse, and is not reinforcing in the same way as stimulant drugs (Gutman & Spollen, 2002).

COGNITIVE-BEHAVIORAL THERAPY. Cognitive-behavioral therapy is used in combination with medications to treat ADHD. Aspects of this therapy are teaching children coping skills, social skills training, and parent training. Parent training helps parents respond productively to their child with ADHD.

To teach new coping skills, the therapist focuses on the child's defective thinking about events and interpretation of others' behavior. Children with behavior disorders often perceive others to be demanding or threatening, when there was no such intent. Possible interpretations of other people's behaviors are discussed in therapy. In role playing, the child tries new ways to cope with stressful events. The child is also encouraged to discuss and examine consequences of her or his own behavior.

Social skills training involves teaching children how other people feel in response to their behavior. When children act impulsively, they probably do not consider another person's reaction. Often the behavior of children with ADHD provokes negative responses from others.

BOX 13-7

Parent Training Suggestions for Child with ADHD

- Set clear limits for behavior
- Give positive reinforcement for desired behavior
- Try time-out for undesired behavior
- Provide feedback as soon as possible after the child's behavior (positive or negative)
- Use a consistent approach from both parents
- Keep instructions simple (say "Put on your socks" instead of "Put on your socks after you comb your hair and brush your teeth")
- Ask the child to repeat instructions to ensure that the child understands what is to be done
- Set realistic short-term goals for behavior ("We will get some ice cream if you do your homework without an argument for 2 days" instead of "We will go to Disneyland if you have good behavior at school every day this year")

When children understand the impact of their behavior on others, they may be motivated to change it. When they try new behaviors that respect others' feelings, they will probably receive positive reinforcement. Role playing, discussion, and positive reinforcement for desired behavior are useful tools.

Children with ADHD are a parenting challenge. Frustrated parents often respond punitively to disruptive, unfocused, or impulsive behavior. Because of multiple negative experiences at home and at school, children with ADHD often feel that they are "bad" or "stupid." In parent training, parents are taught about the nature of ADHD and are given new ways to respond to their child's behavior. Box 13-7 ■ offers some parent training suggestions.

Point systems are a behavioral approach to promoting positive behavior. In this technique, the desired behavior is identified and clearly explained to the child (it might be doing homework, personal hygiene, taking turns, etc.). There might be a list of target behaviors. Whenever the child engages in a target behavior, a token or points are given. The child saves these points and can exchange them or "cash them in" for small rewards such as stickers, playing a favorite game, or a trip to the park. Choosing a reward that motivates the child to change behavior is an important aspect of this therapeutic approach. It is also important to set up the system to make it possible for the child to be successful and to reward the child frequently. Improved self-concept and a sense of accomplishment accompany the repeated experience of success.

CONDUCT DISORDER

Conduct Disorder is a repetitive and persistent pattern of behavior in which the basic rights of others or major societal rules are violated. There are four types of behavior in Conduct Disorder:

- Aggressive conduct that causes or threatens physical harm to other people or to animals
- Nonaggressive conduct that causes property loss or damage
- Deceitfulness or theft
- Serious violations of rules

For the diagnosis of Conduct Disorder to be used, three or more of these behaviors must have occurred within the past 12 months *and* the behavior must cause significant impairment in social, academic, or job functioning. The pattern of behavior is usually present in a variety of settings, such as school, home, and community (APA, 2000).

Children with Conduct Disorder may use bullying or intimidating behavior. They may start frequent physical fights. If severely affected, they might use a weapon that can cause serious harm. They may be physically cruel to people or animals. Physical violence may take the form of assault or rape. Deliberate destruction of others' property may include fire setting or vandalism. Children and adolescents with Conduct Disorder may break promises, avoid debts or obligations, or steal others' things either with or without confronting the victim. They may stay out late at night or spend all night away from home despite parental rules.

There are two subtypes of Conduct Disorder. The childhood-onset type is defined by the occurrence of at least one of the Conduct Disorder behaviors before the age of 10. Children with this type of disorder are frequently aggressive, have disturbed peer relationships, and are likely to have ADHD as well. These individuals are more likely to develop Antisocial Personality Disorder as adults than are children with adolescent-onset type. See Chapter 10 for more information about Antisocial Personality Disorder.

Adolescent-onset type is defined by the absence of Conduct Disorder before the age of 10. These individuals are less likely to be aggressive, have more normal peer relationships, and are less likely to develop Antisocial Personality Disorder as adults. The long-term prognosis for people with the adolescent-onset type is better.

In either type, an individual can have mild, moderate, or severe symptoms. In the mild form, an affected individual may have conduct problems that cause relatively minor harm to others (such as lying, truancy, and staying out after dark without permission). A moderately affected person may steal without confronting the victim or do acts of vandalism. The severely affected person will have conduct that causes considerable harm to others, such as rape, use of a weapon, physical cruelty, or stealing while confronting the victim (APA, 2000).

Conduct Disorder is more common in males. There are also gender differences in the type of behaviors. Males are more likely to be aggressive and to have school discipline problems. Females with the disorder are more prone to lying, truancy, running away from home overnight, substance use, and prostitution. In the majority of people, Conduct Disorder resolves by adulthood (APA, 2000).

Many people with Conduct Disorder perceive that the behavior of others is threatening (even when the other person does not intend to be threatening). They feel that their own aggression is an appropriate response. Children with Conduct Disorder often lack empathy for others as well. Cognitive-behavioral therapy is a good approach to these cognitive errors and is conducted in much the same way as the therapy is used in ADHD.

OPPOSITIONAL DEFIANT DISORDER

Occasional oppositional behavior is common and normal in children. The developmental tasks of the preschool age child or the adolescent may make the behavior of children during these developmental stages seem especially contrary to what parents want. A preschooler frequently saying "No!" or an adolescent disagreeing with her parents are examples of normal behavior. Oppositional Defiant Disorder is not diagnosed unless a child has a pattern of negative, hostile, and defiant behavior that lasts at least 6 months. For this diagnosis, four or more of the following behaviors must be present (APA, 2000). The child often does the following:

- Loses his or her temper
- Argues with adults
- Actively defies or refuses to comply with adults' requests or rules
- Deliberately annoys people
- Blames others for his or her mistakes or misbehavior
- Is easily annoyed by others
- Is angry and resentful
- Is spiteful or vindictive

Affected individuals often perceive their own behavior as justified by the unreasonable demands of others or by the situation that they believe caused their behavior.

Males may have more confrontational behavior than females with the disorder. Oppositional Defiant Disorder is more common in males before puberty and about equal in males and females after puberty. The disorder usually becomes apparent by the age of 8 and has a gradual onset. The disruptive behaviors in this disorder are less severe than those in Conduct Disorder and do not usually include aggression toward people or animals, destruction of property, or a pattern of theft or deceit (APA, 2000).

Anxiety Disorders

Some anxiety is expected in childhood and adolescence. Anxiety becomes a problem when it interferes with normal functioning or the child's ability to reach developmental goals. Anxiety disorders are the most frequently diagnosed mental disorders in childhood and adolescence.

SEPARATION ANXIETY DISORDER

Separation Anxiety is excessive anxiety about separation from the home or parental figures. The anxiety is more severe than expected for the child's developmental level. It lasts for more than 4 weeks, begins before age 18, and causes significant distress or impairment in social, school, or other functioning (APA, 2000).

Diagnostic features from the *DSM-IV-TR* include the following:

- Recurrent excessive stress when separating or anticipating separation from home or parental figures
- Persistent and excessive worry about losing or about harm coming to parental figures
- Excessive worry that something will lead to separation from parental figures, such as being lost or kidnapped
- Persistent reluctance to go to school or other places due to fear of separation
- Fear or reluctance to be alone without a parental figure
- Persistent reluctance to go to sleep without being near a parental figure
- Repeated nightmares about separation
- Repeated complaints about physical symptoms (headaches, nausea, stomachaches) when separation from parental figures happens or is anticipated

Separation Anxiety Disorder occurs in about 4% of children and young adolescents. It may develop after some life stressor such as the death of a relative or pet, illness, immigration, or a move to a new neighborhood. Typically, there are periods of exacerbation when the

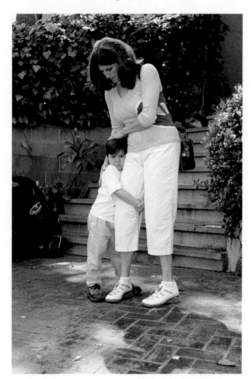

Figure 13-10. ■ This child has separation anxiety.
Source: PhotoEdit Inc.

disorder is most severe, and remissions when it is not a problem (APA, 2000). A child with separation anxiety is depicted in Figure 13-10 ■.

POSTTRAUMATIC STRESS DISORDER

Posttraumatic Stress Disorder (PTSD) affects children differently from the way it affects adults. See Chapter 11 for a more thorough description of PTSD. Although adults tend to relive the extremely traumatic event, children tend to react with behaviors of internalized anxiety.

Preschool-age children with PTSD may demonstrate some of the following behaviors: separation anxiety, repeatedly including the traumatic event in play, irritability, temper tantrums, sleep difficulties, agitated or disorganized behavior, regression, nightmares, withdrawal, or an increase in fears. School-age children may have sleep difficulties, difficulty concentrating, irritability, decreased school performance, thoughts of death, frequent thoughts about the traumatic event, or a sense of dread about the future.

Nurses can help children with disabling anxiety by helping them talk about or work through their anxieties in play. Many children experience regression with severe anxiety. **Regression** is the loss of skills or development

previously attained. For example, after experiencing a natural disaster, a child who was toilet trained may begin to wet the bed. The child may act as if he is younger than he really is. The nurse should accept regression and give the child the emotional support he needs to regain his developmental progress. The nurse may need to provide for the child's most basic physical and psychosocial needs while the child is experiencing severe or panic anxiety. Nurses must also help children have positive experiences, make decisions and choices, and increase their sense of competence to improve their self-esteem and hope for the future.

Children may express their feelings in drawings or through play. Figure 13-11 ■ shows a family drawing by a 6-year-old girl and interprets its possible meanings.

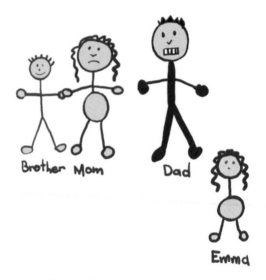

Figure 13-11. ■ Family drawing by Emma, a 6-year old girl. Emma's drawing has a number of distinctive features. She has placed herself at a distance from the rest of the family, suggesting feelings of isolation, rejection, or perhaps fear. The heavy lines around her father's body may indicate that he is seen as aggressive or angry. This interpretation is supported by the father's mouth, which appears to be open as if yelling or showing his teeth. Her brother looks happy, and her mother's downturned mouth looks a bit sad. Emma's drawing of herself is quite small, in contrast to others in the family (especially her brother, who is actually younger and smaller than Emma). Her smallness could indicate some insecurity, low self-esteem, or perhaps a desire to withdraw from the world and not be noticed. She is also missing her mouth and hands. This could imply a sense of inadequacy or powerlessness to act or speak.
Source: Contemporary Psychiatric Mental Health Nursing by Kneis/Wilson/Trigoboff,© Reprinted by permission of Pearson Education, Inc., Upper Saddle River, NJ.

Elimination Disorders

ENURESIS

Enuresis is the repeated voiding of urine into bed or clothes (either involuntary or intentional), which occurs twice per week for at least 3 months. It causes significant distress or impairment in social, school, or other areas of functioning. Enuresis is only diagnosed in children older than age 5, when voluntary bladder control is usually established (APA, 2000).

Most children who have enuresis do not have a mental disorder. It occurs in 5–10% of 5-year-olds, 3–5% of 10-year-olds, and approximately 1% of people over age 15. About 75% of children with enuresis have a first-degree biological relative (parent or sibling) with the disorder. Figure 13-12 ■ depicts a child with enuresis.

Physical causes of incontinence should be considered before the diagnosis of enuresis is made. Untreated diabetes, urinary tract infection, and neurological disorders can cause incontinence.

A child must have a bladder volume of 300–350 ml to hold urine overnight. To assess bladder capacity, the nurse may instruct the child to void into a measuring container after holding the urine as long as possible (Hockenberry, 2005).

Therapeutic techniques for enuresis include the following:

■ Avoiding fluids after the evening meal
■ Bladder training
■ Waking the child up at night to urinate (nocturnal enuresis usually happens during the first third of the night)
■ Providing medications that inhibit urination or bladder contraction
■ Creating a conditioned response to awaken the child with an electrical device when voiding
■ Teaching child and parents about enuresis and the treatment plan
■ Providing consistent support and encouragement for child and parents (Hockenberry, 2005).

ENCOPRESIS

Encopresis is voluntary or involuntary passing of feces into inappropriate places. Usually this is involuntary. Encopresis is diagnosed when a child of at least 4 years of age has passed feces into inappropriate places at least once a month for at least 3 months. When the passage of feces is unintentional, it is often due to constipation, impaction, and retention of stool, followed by overflow. The constipation may develop for psychological reasons, such as fear of defecation in a particular place, anxiety, or oppositional behavior leading to avoidance of defecation (APA, 2000).

Encopresis affects a child's school and social performance. It also causes much stress in the family. Because of the stigma and embarrassment associated with this disorder, families or caregivers may feel that they are the only ones with a problem like this.

The nurse must educate the child and parents or caregivers about encopresis. The first topic for teaching is bowel function. Parents are often surprised to learn that when a child has advanced constipation, the leakage of feces is not under the child's control. It can help families to know that other families also deal with encopresis. Therapy for encopresis must begin with a diagnosis of what is causing the problem, followed by a treatment plan. Treatment approaches include dietary changes, resolving fecal impaction, preventing future constipation, and behavior therapy.

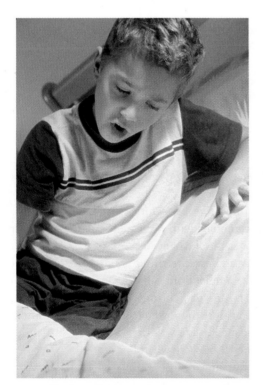

Figure 13-12. ■ Physical causes of incontinence should be investigated before the diagnosis of enuresis is made. *Source:* Phototake NYC.

Depression, Psychosis, and Suicide

CHILDHOOD DEPRESSION

Depression is a major problem in children and adolescents. However, because the symptoms of depression may overlap normal behavior in children and adolescents, depression is difficult to diagnose.

Some depression symptoms in children and adolescents are similar to those of adults, such as sadness, hopelessness, feelings of helplessness, social withdrawal, anhedonia (loss of pleasant feelings), and suicidal thoughts. Children often have difficulty expressing their thoughts and feelings in words, so they are more likely to act out their feelings and concerns. Compared with adults, children more often have somatic (physical) complaints. They might be irritable and aggressive, or dependent and clinging. Their school performance will decline. The depressed child will spend more time in solitary activities.

Adolescents with depression are more likely to have psychomotor retardation (slow movement, loss of energy) and hypersomnia (excessive sleeping). They are also likely to be irritable and possibly even aggressive. Their school or work performance will decrease. One adolescent's experience is described in her own words in Box 13-8 ∎.

The complications of depression in adolescents and children include school failure, substance abuse, sexual promiscuity, running away, aggressive behavior, and suicide. Although the symptoms of depression in young clients are different, the effective treatments are similar to those that work for adults. Antidepressant medications are very effective, especially when combined with cognitive-behavioral therapy.

BOX 13-8

Reality Check on Adolescent Depression

An adolescent with depression said:

"It is hard to describe how bad I felt. My mom thought I was just being lazy, but as I look back on that time, I couldn't get out of bed to go to school. I was failing all my classes. My school counselor thought I was just slacking because I used to be a good student. I was angry, but I don't know why. I had a lot of nightmares. I didn't even want to see my friends. When my mom finally convinced me to see the doctor, it was too late to graduate from high school. Thank goodness for the doctor recognizing my depression, and the antidepressant medication! I graduated from the community college and I have myself back again."

PSYCHOTIC DISORDERS

Psychosis (loss of contact with reality) is a symptom that can accompany several mental disorders, such as bipolar disorder, severe depression, panic anxiety, or schizophrenia. Although the onset of schizophrenia is usually in late adolescence or early adulthood, it occasionally begins in childhood.

The symptoms of schizophrenia begin gradually and vary according to the child's developmental level. The basic abnormality is loss of contact with reality. Schizophrenia in children causes abnormalities in cognition, perception, language, and the emotional life of the child. The most common disturbances are altered language, impaired interpersonal relationships, and abnormal affect (nonverbal expression of emotion).

Treatment includes antipsychotic medications and psychosocial interventions such as social skills training. Children with schizophrenia often respond well to the newer atypical antipsychotic medications. See Chapter 8 for details.

SUICIDE

Suicide is the third leading cause of death among children and adolescents aged 10 to 24. As in the general population, young people are most likely to use firearms, suffocation, or poisoning as the means for suicide (NIMH, 2006b).

---

clinical ALERT

Nurses should be involved in community education about firearm safety. Some families believe that if they teach their children about gun safety, they will be safe even if they have access to loaded guns in their home. The community should be taught about lock boxes for securing guns.

We all know that adolescence is a time of major changes and high emotions. Adolescents have strong feelings. They may have not yet developed mature problem-solving skills. Impulsive behavior is characteristic of children. When combined with inadequate coping skills, impulsive behavior can lead to suicide.

Many adolescents think about suicide. Suicide may seem like a relief from suffering, an escape from humiliation, a means of gaining sympathy, or a way to have revenge against those who have hurt them. Children may think of suicide as a way to punish others. A child might say, "They'll be sorry when I'm dead."

The nursing approach to suicide has three parts:

1. Recognizing the warning signs
2. Responding to the client's needs
3. Preventing suicide

Assess any child with the symptoms of depression for suicidality. Ask the question directly, "Are you thinking about hurting or killing yourself?" This is a hard question to ask, but it makes a big difference. Most people will answer it honestly. Suicide attempts or threats should never be ignored. Unsuccessful attempts at suicide may seem like "just a call for help" or "just trying to get attention." If a child or adolescent is feeling out of control and needs attention, and has so few problem-solving skills that he tries to commit suicide, the person truly needs help immediately (NIMH, 2006b).

A person who has a plan and the means to carry it out is in the most danger. If a child says that he will jump off a mountain but there are no mountains in his area, he is not as likely to complete suicide as another child who says that she will shoot herself with her father's gun, and the father does have a gun. Both children, however, deserve psychiatric evaluation.

Adolescents have four risk factors for suicide (Russell & Joyner, 2001):

- Depression
- Hopelessness
- Substance abuse
- Recent suicide (or attempted suicide) of a family member or close friend

Sexual minority adolescents are about twice as likely to complete suicide as their age-mates. This may be because gay, lesbian, bisexual, and transgender adolescents are more likely to suffer from the four risk factors.

Nurses may be the first professionals to discuss sexual orientation issues with adolescents. In the professional nursing role, the nurse can serve as a support person for these adolescents. Nurses can help this group with education in the schools and community. Education of the peer group is important as well. Gay and lesbian adolescents will be best able to meet their developmental needs in a tolerant and supportive peer group and community. Support groups for students with similar concerns can be helpful. Nurses can provide the education and referral to counseling and group therapy that families need to help them to accept, nurture, and support their children.

Suicide among adolescents taking antidepressant medications has been a topic in the news recently. We have heard that children and adolescents who take SSRI antidepressants to treat depression are more likely than the general population of people their age to kill themselves.

This situation provides an opportunity for nurses and consumers to learn to interpret statistics in the news.

Before reacting to these reports with fear and changing the laws or having the U.S. Food and Drug Association change its warning on package inserts of SSRIs to include a special "black box" of extra warning, people should know the whole story. Nurses should go to reliable sources (the nursing and medical literature) to find whether all the variables that could cause suicide have been considered. Some pertinent facts in this case include the following:

- People with depression are at high risk for killing themselves.
- The risk of suicide is highest from 1 month before treatment to 1 month after treatment; then the risk falls steadily after that.
- Suicide attempt patterns are the same in young people with depression if they start on medications or on psychotherapy (Simon & Savarino, 2007).
- The suicide rates of adolescents with depression who are not treated with medications are higher than those who are.
- In U.S. counties where SSRI antidepressant drugs are prescribed at higher rates, the suicide rates are lower than they are in counties where SSRIs are prescribed at a lower rate (NIMH, 2006b).

An analysis of the information in the reliable professional literature shows that suicide happens when young people are depressed, whether they take medications or not, and if they do take antidepressants, their risk of suicide is decreased. An important implication for nurses and families is that young people with depression should be assessed for suicidal ideation (thinking) frequently, especially for the first month after they start treatment, because it takes that long for drugs to become effective. If their drug is not effective, the provider should be told, so a different drug can be prescribed (Simon & Savarino, 2007).

Self-Concept

The self-concept has three parts (Driever, 1976):

- Body image
- Personal identity
- Self-esteem

Body image is the way a person feels about his or her physical body. Physical features, health or illness, physical function, sexuality, and the way other people respond to the individual affect the individual's body image.

Personal identity is composed of the individual's values, a striving for consistency, and expectations of the self. People have a stronger sense of personal identity when

BOX 13-9

Signs and Symptoms of Low Self-Esteem

- Negative talk about self
- Dislikes own body or appearance
- Persistent guilt or shame
- Feelings of worthlessness
- Feelings of powerlessness
- Passiveness
- Shyness
- Poor attention to personal hygiene

they have chosen values that they believe are important and when they act in a way that is consistent with these values. Acting on one's values is integrity. People tend to act consistently with their expectations of themselves, even if they have low or negative expectations.

Self-esteem is the amount of positive regard or respect that people have for themselves. The ability of a person to adapt to life's challenges is partly dependent on having self-esteem. Self-esteem is also closely related to how significant others respond to an individual. Box 13-9 ■ gives the symptoms of low self-esteem.

Parents, nurses, and others who work with children can promote self-esteem in the following areas (Townsend, 2006):

- *Unconditional love.* Children need to know that they are loved and accepted just as they are by their family and friends.
- *Sense of survival.* Self-esteem is enhanced when people learn from their failures and when they recognize that they are still surviving and are stronger for the experience.
- *Sense of competence.* Everyone needs to feel skilled at something. Knowing that one is doing one's personal best builds self-esteem.
- *Realistic goals.* Failure to achieve goals can undermine self-esteem. A person with unrealistic goals is doomed to failure. Keep goals within the child's reach.
- *Sense of responsibility.* Positive self-esteem results from being assigned responsibilities that a child is able to achieve, especially when others value the child's contribution.
- *Reality orientation.* There are limits on what people can do. Children need to have a healthy balance between what they can possess and achieve and what is beyond their control.

Nursing interventions to promote self-esteem are listed in the following Nursing Care section.

NURSING CARE

Nurses can make a positive difference in the lives of children and adolescents with emotional and behavior disorders. The families of these children can also benefit from nursing interventions.

ASSESSING

Nurses obtain assessment findings about children with emotional and behavior problems through mental status assessment, behavioral observation, family history, social history (socioeconomic status and living situation), and school information. Children offer an assessment challenge. Young children are often unable to explain their feelings in words. Children are likely to act out their feelings, making the observation of behavior an important part of assessment. Although the opinions of parents and other family members are important, nurses must also rely on their own direct observations of their child clients for assessment findings.

A thorough mental status assessment is not a routine part of pediatric assessment. However, it is an important part of nursing assessment in the psychiatric setting, or for a child who has problems with behavior, mood, or emotions. Table 13-2 ■ suggests some data to collect for mental status assessments of children and adolescents with emotional and behavior problems.

DIAGNOSING, PLANNING, AND IMPLEMENTING

Once nursing diagnoses are identified, care is planned to treat each diagnosis in a way that meets the person's individual needs. Some nursing diagnoses that are common to children and adolescents with emotional and behavior problems are:

- Chronic Low Self-Esteem
- Ineffective Coping
- Anxiety
- Powerlessness
- Impaired Verbal Communication
- Risk for Violence: Self-directed or other-directed
- Impaired Social Interaction

Chronic Low Self-Esteem

The nurse may encounter clients with low self-esteem in any nursing setting (see Box 13-9 for the signs and symptoms). Although it takes a long time to develop and to change self-esteem, nurses can help children and their

TABLE 13-2		
Mental Status Assessment of Children and Adolescents with Emotional and Behavior Problems		
ASSESSMENT	QUESTIONS/FINDINGS	RATIONALE
Appearance	Does the child have adequate personal hygiene? How is s/he dressed? Are his or her clothes adequate for the weather, and appropriate for the situation? (A swimming suit would probably not be appropriate in school.)	Appearance can indicate whether adult caregivers are providing adequate care, or if a child has low self-esteem.
Behavior	Is the child's level of activity about what you would expect from a child this age? Is the child acting aggressively? Does the child have strange repetitive behaviors? Has there been a sudden change in the child's behavior?	Persistent hyperactivity or impulsive behavior may indicate ADHD. Aggressiveness is associated with the disruptive behavior disorders. Autism can cause unusual repetitive behavior such as hand wringing or head banging. Illness, abuse, fear, substance abuse, and trauma can cause sudden behavior changes.
Socializing	Does the child play well with others? Can s/he share and take turns? Does s/he feel shy with strangers and comfortable with family?	Disruptive behavior disorders make it difficult for a child to cooperate. ADHD may make the child too impulsive to wait for his or her turn. Normally children are shy around strangers after the age of 6 months. Children with attachment disorder are no more comfortable with their families than they are with strangers.
Thinking	What are the topics the child talks about that the nurse does not suggest first? Can the child solve problems, read, make decisions at an age-appropriate level? Does the child understand the situation? Does the child hear voices (hallucinations)?	Speech is the closest we can come to understanding what people are thinking. Cognitive (thinking) ability affects the child's ability to learn, cooperate with care, and succeed in school. Hallucinations can be caused by schizophrenia.
Speech	Is the rate of speech unusually slow or fast? What is the child's first language? Does the child's speech respond to what others are saying, or is it unusual, repeating the words said by others (echolalia)?	Rapid speech can be caused by anxiety, agitation, or hyperactivity. Depression can cause slow speaking. Communication (and the nurse's assessment) will be less accurate in a nonnative language. Autism can cause echolalia.
Mood	Does the child seem sad, withdrawn, and slow moving? Is s/he irritable and easily angered? Is s/he overly excited? Is s/he thinking about hurting self or others?	A child with depression may be irritable and anxious. If an adolescent seems to be always sad and slow, losing interest in usual enjoyments, s/he may be depressed. The only way the nurse knows if a client is thinking of hurting self or others is to ask.

families begin this process. Some outcomes for children with Low Self-Esteem are that the child will:

- Demonstrate an increased sense of competence.
- Make positive statements about self.
- Demonstrate increased responsibility.
- Try new experiences.

The nurse can encourage the development of a child's self-esteem in several ways:

- Provide opportunities for child to engage in developmentally appropriate activities where s/he can be successful. *Success promotes a sense of competence at the activity. Self-esteem is improved by repeated sense of accomplishment.*

- Keep goals realistic. *Child is more likely to achieve realistic goals and is likely to fail at goals that are not achievable.*
- If the child does not reach the goal, discuss the reason and learn from the experience. Show that you still respect the child as a person. *The child can learn that nobody wins every time, but that there is always a lesson to learn to make us stronger for the next challenge. Respect for people is based not only on success, but also on genuine effort.*
- Teach child to avoid negative self-talk (like "I can't do this" or "I'm stupid"). *Negative self-talk perpetuates low self-esteem.*

- Encourage child to think of positive things about him- or herself. These positive ideas ("I am smart," "I am a hard worker") can be written down and read several times each day. *Positive affirmations promote a change to positive self-talk and positive self-esteem.*
- Role model talking and acting with positive self-esteem. *Children often repeat the behavior of their role models. Role modeling is a way of learning behavior and values.*
- Give the child honest feedback. Avoid flattery or insincere compliments. *Dishonesty undermines trust in the nurse-client relationship and does not promote self-esteem.*
- Demonstrate respect for the child's responsible decisions. *Respect from an adult is a powerful reinforcement.*
- Demonstrate valuing the child's contribution or participation ("Thank you very much for cleaning the table. It looks good."). *The feeling of being appreciated and valued is powerful reinforcement for behavior. Positive reinforcement will increase the chance that the child will repeat the behavior.*
- Offer opportunities for low-risk experiences (playing a simple game or going for a walk with a group of children). *Low self-esteem makes it difficult for children to try anything that might embarrass them.*

Provide Individualized Interventions

No matter what the disorder, children and adolescents are more likely to achieve positive results from nursing interventions when the nurse includes the following points:

- Before nursing interventions are done, know what outcomes you are working toward.
- Make the goals realistic.
- Include the client and family or caregivers in planning and implementing goals.
- Disrupt the client and family's lifestyle as little as possible. (For example, do not schedule medications, appointments, or treatments at home in the morning if the mother works nights and sleeps days.)
- Focus on the child's strengths, not just his or her challenges.
- Be flexible. Especially when children are concerned, flexibility and creativity are the cornerstones of nursing. If one approach does not work, think of a new one.
- Keep hope alive for the child and the family.

EVALUATING

The nurse will evaluate whether the desired outcomes set in the planning phase were met. Some questions the nurse may ask are:

- Is the child interacting in age-appropriate and socially acceptable ways?

- Does the child express positive statements about self?
- Is the child able to express feelings of anxiety?
- Can the child state and use strategies to stop anxiety from increasing?
- Can the child recognize and state choices that are available and within his or her control?
- Did the child cause harm to self or others?
- Can the child state alternatives to violent behavior?
- Is the child establishing a trusting relationship with the nurse?

NURSING PROCESS CARE PLAN
Client with ADHD

Mohammed Said (pronounced "sah-eed") is a 12-year-old sixth grader admitted to the Emergency Department with an asthma attack. He was diagnosed with attention deficit/hyperactivity disorder 5 years ago. His breathing is responding well to nebulized albuterol. Mohammed's mother brought him to the hospital. She and her husband have brought Mohammed to the Emergency Department for asthma rescue treatment six times in the past year. Teaching about how to use his inhalers has been done on each admission.

Assessment

- Respiratory rate is down to 22 from 40.
- Heart rate 110.
- Mrs. Said says, "If you would use your inhalers like you're supposed to, we wouldn't be here now! I am sick of this."
- Mohammed states, "Everything I do is wrong."

The nurse found that neither Mohammed nor his mother knew the difference between his two inhalers (beclomethasone and albuterol). His mother gives him the albuterol inhaler whenever he has severe wheezing. To assess his knowledge, the nurse asked Mohammed to demonstrate how he uses his inhalers. He put the inhaler up to his lips and sprayed it twice without attention to whether he was breathing in or out. He said, "I'm probably doing it wrong."

Diagnosis. The following nursing diagnoses are identified for Mohammed:

- Deficient Knowledge, inhaler use R/T ineffective teaching
- Low Self-Esteem R/T negative parental comments and lack of positive reinforcement

Expected Outcomes. Mohammed will:

- Demonstrate the correct use of an asthma inhaler.
- Describe in simple terms when to use each of his inhalers.
- Identify at least three positive points about himself.
- Accept a compliment by the nurse when he is able to demonstrate correct technique.

Planning and Implementation. The nurse knows from Mohammed's chart that he has ADHD, but nothing about his learning ability except that he is in the correct grade in school for his age and that he has been taught how to use an asthma inhaler many times without learning.

She plans to create a brief teaching plan for Mohammed that is consistent with his best learning style. To determine the best approach, she needs more information. The nurse states to the mother (with Mohammed present), "How does Mohammed do in school? I notice that he has ADHD." The mother answers, "He is always in trouble for not paying attention; he has dyslexia so he goes to a special reading program. He does not like to listen to me or his teacher." The nurse asks Mohammed, "How do you want to learn about these inhalers? What is your favorite way to learn in school?" Mohammed gets up, walks around the room and says, "I can't remember what the teacher says. I like science best because we can see the pictures in the lab book, and do the experiments."

Based on the above, the nurse will:

- Teach Mohammed how to use his asthma inhaler by demonstration and return demonstration, and send home a handout with the process in pictures.
- Teach Mohammed and his mother in simple terms the uses of beclomethasone (corticosteroid to reduce inflammation and prevent asthma attacks, used twice each day) and albuterol (a bronchodilator that dilates airways, which is used only as a "rescue inhaler" when he is wheezing and his breathing feels tight).
- Write instructions for his mother in simple terms about when he should use his inhalers.
- Praise Mohammed for successes in his behavior.
- Talk briefly with Mohammed about changing his self-talk from negative to positive.

Evaluation

- Mohammed was able to demonstrate the correct method for inhaler use.
- He was able to explain that the beclomethasone (the blue inhaler) should be used every morning and every night and the albuterol (brown) inhaler should only be used when he is wheezing.
- His mother and the nurse praised him for successfully learning about his inhalers.
- When asked to state good things about himself, he was not willing to try this. His mother said that he is good at learning about his asthma and he smiled.
- The nurse talked briefly about self-talk, but Mohammed did not seem to be paying attention.

Critical Thinking in the Nursing Process

1. What is the relationship between Mohammed's knowledge of inhaler use and his use of the Emergency Department?
2. Why did Mohammed learn how to use his inhalers on this hospital visit when he did not in the past?
3. What factors probably led to Mohammed's difficulty paying attention to the nurse's teaching about self-talk?

Note: Discussion of Critical Thinking questions appears in Appendix I.

Note: The references and resources for this and all chapters have been compiled at the back of the book.

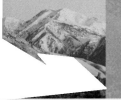

 KEY TERMS

Use the audio glossary feature of the Companion Website to hear the correct pronunciation of the following key terms.

body image

circadian

dyslexia

encopresis

enuresis

personal identity

regression

resilience

self-esteem

KEY Points

- Children and adults react differently to mental disorders.
- Children often express their feelings through behavior.
- Mental disorders make it more difficult for children to achieve their developmental tasks.
- Some people are more resilient and less prone to mental disorders, even when they have many stressors.
- Children with behavior disorders often interpret the behavior of others as demanding or threatening when there was no such intent.
- Impulsivity can put the child in danger.
- The goal for students with learning disorders is to understand their learning challenges, and to learn to cope with or compensate for them.
- Medications have helped many children and adolescents with ADHD increase their ability to concentrate and reduce their hyperactivity and impulsiveness.
- The nurse is responsible for client and family teaching about the stimulant medications used to treat ADHD, and assessment of side effects such as insomnia and loss of appetite.
- Children and adolescents respond best when their families are engaged in their treatment plan.
- Nurses should consider clients' preferred learning method when doing health teaching.

- Any child with the symptoms of depression should be assessed for suicidal thinking or a suicidal plan.
- Firearms are the leading method for suicide in the United States, even among children.
- Low self-esteem is common in children with mental disorders. Nursing interventions can help children build self-confidence and self-esteem.

 EXPLORE MediaLink

Additional interactive resources for this chapter can be found on the Companion Website at www.prenhall.com/eby. Click on Chapter 13 and "Begin" to select the activities for this chapter

- Audio glossary
- NCLEX-PN® review
- Case study
- Study outline
- Critical thinking questions
- Matching questions
- Weblinks
- Video Case: Xavier (Autism)

Caring for a Client with Noncompliance

NCLEX-PN® Focus Area: Safe, Effective Care Environment

Case Study: Wen Charles is a 15-year-old male with ADHD. He was admitted to the hospital pediatric unit with a fractured pelvis, which he sustained when he fell from the roof of his house. His mother states that he has been especially impulsive since he has been off his Ritalin for the past 4 days. He ran out of his pills because he took too many of them last week. Wen states that he wanted to have plenty of energy to stay awake to work on a school project. So, he took extra Ritalin. The physician has evaluated his medication needs and decided to continue the methylphenidate HCl (Ritalin) prescription.

Nursing Diagnosis: Noncompliance with medication regimen

COLLECT DATA

Subjective	Objective
_____	_____
_____	_____
_____	_____
_____	_____
_____	_____
_____	_____
_____	_____

Would you report this data? Yes/No

If yes, to: _____

Nursing Care

_____
_____
_____
_____
_____
_____
_____
_____

How would you document this? _____
_____
_____
_____

Compare your documentation to the sample provided in Appendix I.

Data Collected
(use those that apply)

- 5'6", 150 lbs
- Client states, "I was just trying to do a good job on the school project."
- Client's mother states, "I'm afraid he's becoming a drug addict. This isn't the first time he has done this."
- Pelvic pain is under control (2 on a 1–10 scale).
- Peripheral pulses in lower extremities are present bilaterally.
- Client states, "I feel up on some days and down on other days."
- Client states, "Everybody is always telling me what to do."
- Client's mother states, "I let him be responsible for taking his medications, but I wonder if I should take back the responsibility. He is not taking them safely."
- Client states, "I want to be in charge of myself."
- Client has two younger sisters.
- Physician's order: Ritalin 20 mg twice a day, PO

Nursing Interventions
(use those that apply; list in priority order)

- Tell the client that he will not be able to take this medication when he is discharged due to his drug abuse.
- Ask the physician to change the prescription to a drug without side effects.
- Assess the client's knowledge about his medication, desired effects, side effects, and dosing schedule.
- Teach him what he does not know about his medication regimen (treatment plan).
- Tell the mother to take control of the medications at home.
- Reinforce teaching about the safe use of Ritalin with the client and his mother.
- Explain that he is not a drug addict.
- Tell the client to stop taking the medication if he has a loss of appetite.
- Let the family decide who takes responsibility for giving the medication.
- Measure the client's VS once every hour while he is in the hospital, due to potential side effects of medication.
- Tell the client that his injury is likely a result of not taking his medication as prescribed.
- Tell the client that he is responsible for his own behavior.
- Tell the mother that it is her fault that this child is not taking his medication correctly.
- Ask the client and his mother if they have any questions.
- Teach the client to avoid tyramine-containing foods while he is taking Ritalin.

1 A child with decreased reading accuracy, speed, and/or comprehension is said to have:
1. Dyslexia.
2. Mathematics Disorder.
3. Disorder of Written Expression.
4. Developmental Coordination Disorder.

2 A 9-year-old child with dyslexia has been admitted to the hospital unit with a new diagnosis of Diabetes Mellitus, Type 1. He would learn best about his condition by:
1. Booklets.
2. Having him read aloud to the nurse from educational materials about dyslexia.
3. Demonstrations and verbal explanations.
4. Diagrams and written lists.

3 The mother of a 10-year-old child with diagnosed Expressive Language Disorder approaches the school nurse to ask questions about her child's future. The nurse's best response would be:
1. "The disorder will not get any worse, but it will not improve either."
2. "I am sorry, but the disorder will get worse as your child gets older."
3. "This is as good as he will ever be."
4. "This disorder will improve dramatically as your child gets older."

4 A mother talks with the nurse about her 5-year-old son who stutters. She has a 2-year-old daughter and wonders if she will have the same problem. The best response by the nurse would be:
1. "Stuttering does tend to run in families, but it is more common in males than females."
2. "It is definitely a genetic disorder, so your daughter will probably stutter as well."
3. "She will stutter as well following her older brother's example."
4. "You have nothing to worry about. Girls do not stutter."

5 A 6-year-old child with autism has been admitted to the hospital with pneumonia. The child insists on having a bedside commode, a rocking chair, and a regular chair lined up in a certain order by her bed. She frequently moves from one object to another. The best nursing response to this behavior would be to:
1. Insist that the child use the bathroom in her room, and remove the bedside commode.
2. Offer to rock the child frequently.
3. Allow the child to keep the objects in her room in the order she desires.
4. Check on the child every 15 minutes.

6 A 2-year-old female has been admitted to the pediatric unit with severe diarrhea and vomiting. The mother tells you that the little girl seems to be regressing in her development. Her head is smaller than other 2-year-olds. She can barely walk now and has difficulty picking up and stacking blocks. The nurse suspects that the little girl has:
1. Autism.
2. Rett's Syndrome.
3. Asperger's Disorder.
4. Childhood Disintegrative Disorder.

7 Because of their side effects, medications given for the treatment of Attention Deficit/Hyperactivity Disorder should be given:
1. At bedtime.
2. On an empty stomach.
3. No later than 6 hours before bedtime.
4. Only on school days.

8 A 14-year-old female has been admitted to the orthopedic unit with a severely fractured femur. She is in traction. The client has signs and symptoms of Separation Anxiety Disorder. She is constantly on her call light asking when her mother will be there. She refuses to go to sleep at night unless her mother is there by the bed. She wakes up often with nightmares that something has happened to her mother. The nurse's best response to this behavior is to:
1. Set limits on when the parents can visit.
2. Assess for escalating anxiety, and be accessible to the client at that time.
3. Remind the client that visiting hours are over at 9 P.M., and her mother may not stay beyond that time.
4. Do not respond to the anxious behavior, as this will reinforce it.

9 A 17-year-old client has been admitted to the gynecology unit with pelvic inflammatory disease after a history of repeated sexually transmitted diseases. She admits to the nurse that she is sexually promiscuous to "get back at her father" for years of abuse. She says, "I guess now I will just have to kill myself. There's no other way." The nurse's best response to this statement would be:
1. "Do you have a plan for killing yourself?"
2. "It can't be that bad. You'll get yourself back on track."
3. "Does your mother know about the abuse?"
4. "Have you reported your father to the police?"

10 The best way to assess mental health problems in a young child (3 to 5 years of age) would be to:
1. Accept the parents' assessment of the child's behavior.
2. Talk to the child.
3. Compare the child to Erikson's developmental stages.
4. Observe the child at play.

Answers for Review Questions, as well as discussion of Care Plan and Critical Thinking Care Map questions, appear in Appendix I.

Chapter 14

Eating Disorders

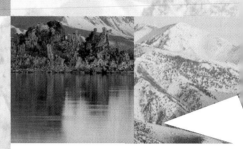

BRIEF Outline

Anorexia Nervosa

Bulimia Nervosa

Binge Eating Disorder

Males with Eating Disorders

Causes of Eating Disorders

Collaborative Care

Obesity

LEARNING Outcomes

After completing this chapter, you will be able to:

1. Examine your own attitudes about eating and eating disorders.
2. Describe subjective and objective symptoms of eating disorders.
3. Help families plan strategies for preventing eating disorders in their children.
4. Apply the nursing process to the care of clients with eating disorders.

Before you begin to care for clients diagnosed with eating disorders, take a look at your own attitudes about eating and body weight. Food and eating have meanings far beyond nutrition. Contemplate the following questions. How do you feel when you see an extremely thin person? What are your feelings about severely obese people? How does your body compare to the people you see in advertising and entertainment? How do you feel about your own body? How do you feel when you have a big holiday meal with your family? What do you eat when you are under stress? Do you ever have problems that chocolate or ice cream can solve?

These questions relate to personal attitudes about eating and body weight. Beliefs about the meaning and importance of issues like these are conveyed through our culture. We learn our standards for beauty and our attitudes about food as we learn the values and behaviors of our culture.

When nurses bring their personal opinions and feelings with them to work, these feelings can affect client care behavior. Maybe you feel that thin people are weak physically and should be protected from demands placed on them. Maybe you feel that obese people are weak emotionally and should be challenged to strengthen their personality.

Critical Self-Check. One of your peers is a nurse who does not like to care for people with eating disorders. She says, "They caused their own problems. Why don't they just get over it?" How should you respond?

Attitudes that cause the nurse to judge the client in advance can be detrimental to client care. It is important for nurses to examine their own attitudes, to ensure that they do not have biases about eating and weight that interfere with their ability to care for clients objectively and professionally.

People who have eating disorders suffer deeply both emotionally and physically. These disorders cause low self-esteem, self-hatred, fear, hopelessness, and risks for a variety of physiological problems (Figure 14-1 ■). People with eating disorders often also have other mental disorders such as anxiety disorder, substance abuse, and depression (Spearing, 2001). Eating disorders can be fatal. Caregivers should not underestimate the significance of these disorders.

There are certain adversities that happen in childhood that put people at risk for eating disorders or weight problems as adolescents and young adults. These childhood experiences include the following (Johnson, Cohen,

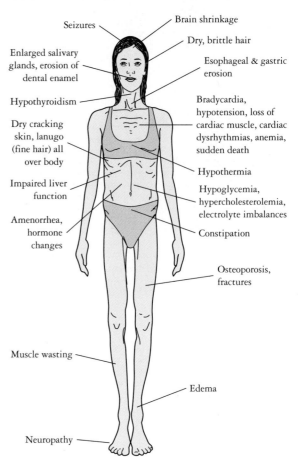

Figure 14-1. ■ Medical complications of eating disorders.

Kasen, & Brook, 2002) (these are risk factors not predictors of individual cases):

- Physical neglect
- Sexual abuse
- Low paternal affection, attention, or time spent with the child
- Poverty
- Low paternal education

Anorexia Nervosa

An individual who has Anorexia Nervosa refuses to maintain a minimally normal body weight, is intensely afraid of gaining weight, and has a significant disturbance in the perception of the size and shape of her/his body (Figure 14-2 ■ depicts such a woman). Women with Anorexia Nervosa have **amenorrhea** (no menstrual periods). The suggested standard for determining underweight is less than 85% of normal for the individual's age and height (American Psychiatric Association [APA], 2000a).

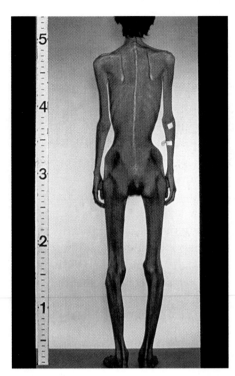

Figure 14-2. ■ Anorexia Nervosa so severe that this woman is near death. *Source:* Custom Medical Stock Photo, Inc.

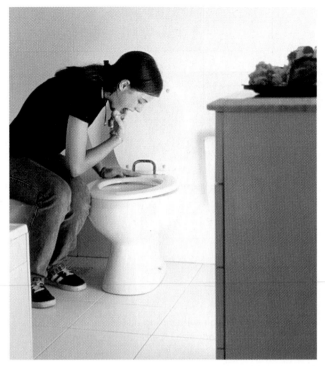

Figure 14-3. ■ Teenage girl with eating disorder forces herself to vomit to avoid gaining weight. *Source:* Photo Researchers, Inc.

People with Anorexia Nervosa usually accomplish weight loss by severely restricting their food intake. They often begin by excluding what they think are high-calorie foods and progress to a very limited diet. Other methods of weight loss include **purging** (self-induced vomiting) or abuse of laxatives or diuretics (demonstrated in Figure 14-3 ■). They have an intense fear of gaining weight, even when they are **emaciated** (excessively thin, wasted). **Cachexia** is another term sometimes used to describe these clients with extreme muscle wasting. Box 14-1 ■ provides the diagnostic criteria for Anorexia Nervosa.

Distortion of how they perceive their body size and shape is another characteristic of people with Anorexia Nervosa (Figures 14-4 ■ and 14-5 ■). Some people feel overweight, even though they are thin. Others know they are thin, but are concerned that parts of their bodies, especially the abdomen, thighs, and buttocks, are too fat. The self-esteem of people with Anorexia Nervosa is closely tied to body shape and weight. Weight loss is seen as an improvement and a sign of extraordinary self-control. Weight gain becomes an unacceptable failure of self-control. Some people with the disorder admit that they are thin, but they typically deny the serious medical implications of their condition (APA, 2000a). The mortality rate

BOX 14-1

Diagnostic Criteria for Anorexia Nervosa

A. Refusal to maintain body weight at or above a minimally normal weight for age and height. This means weight loss leading to maintenance of body weight less than 85% of that expected.

B. Intense fear of gaining weight or becoming fat, even though underweight.

C. Disturbance in the way in which one's body weight or shape is experienced, undue influence of body weight or shape on self-evaluation, or denial of the seriousness of the current low body weight.

D. Amenorrhea (absence of at least three menstrual periods in a woman after puberty)

There are two subtypes of anorexia nervosa:

■ **Restricting Type** with weight loss through dieting, fasting, or excessive exercise

■ **Binge-eating/Purging Type** in which the individual has regularly engaged in binge eating or purging (or both) during the current episode. Purging involves self-induced vomiting or abuse of laxatives, diuretics, or enemas. Some people with anorexia nervosa binge and purge and others purge after eating small amounts.

Source: Reprinted with permission from the *Diagnostic and Statistical Manual of Mental Disorders, Text Revision,* copyright 2000. American Psychiatric Association.

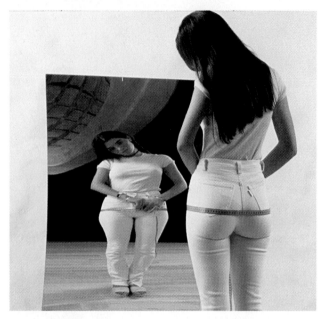

Figure 14-4. ■ People with eating disorders have a distorted perception of their body size. *Source:* Custom Medical Stock Photo, Inc.

of Anorexia Nervosa is 5–10%. Review the physical complications of eating disorders in Figure 14-1.

The term *anorexia* is an inaccurate name for this condition. It means "loss of appetite." In fact, people with Anorexia Nervosa continue to have a normal sense of hunger and appetite.

Usually the affected person is brought to the attention of healthcare providers by parents. Because of clients' denial or lack of insight, the parents may be better sources of information about the client's symptom history. Be sure to follow your institution's policy about confidentiality and disclosure of client information before discussing the client's condition with her parents. The parents may provide information to the nurse, but the nurse must be careful about what information is given to the parents without the client's consent.

Ninety percent of individuals who have Anorexia Nervosa are female. Onset before puberty is rare. It typically begins in mid to late adolescence (14–18 years of age), and rarely starts after age 40. Some people recover

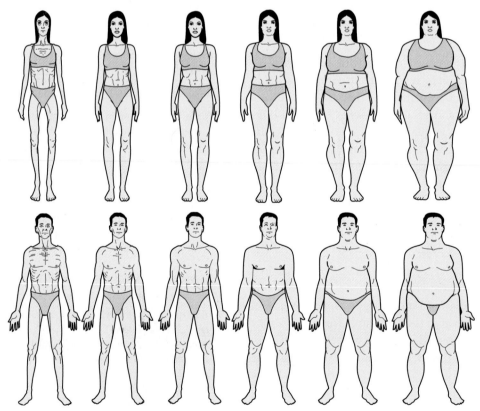

Figure 14-5. ■ Assessing body image. A drawing such as this can be used in several ways. (1) Clients can be asked which image best represents them. This assesses the accuracy of the client's body image. Anorexic clients often believe themselves to be larger than they really are. (2) Clients can be asked which image best represents the ideal for them. This assesses whether a client has a positive (image is similar to the client's own body) or a negative (dissimilar image) body image. *Source: Contemporary Psychiatric Mental Health Nursing* by Kneisl/Wilson/Trigoboff, © Reprinted by permission of Pearson Education, Inc., Upper Saddle River, NJ.

completely after a single episode. Others have a fluctuating pattern including weight gain followed by relapse. Still others have a chronically deteriorating course over many years (APA, 2000a).

Obsessive-compulsive features, whether related to food or not, are often associated with this disorder. Most affected people are preoccupied with thoughts of food. They may collect recipes or hoard food. These symptoms, as well as depression, may be due to the physiological effects of malnutrition. People with Anorexia Nervosa may have concerns about eating in public, a strong need to be in control of their environment, inflexible thinking, perfectionism, limited social spontaneity, feelings of ineffectiveness, lack of initiative, and strained emotional expression. Many have a personality disorder as well. Those with the binge-eating/purging type are more likely to have other impulse control problems, to abuse alcohol or drugs, to have changeable mood, to be sexually active, to have a greater frequency of suicide attempts, and to have Borderline Personality Disorder (APA, 2000a).

Bulimia Nervosa

Bulimia Nervosa is more common than anorexia. The essential features of this disorder are binge eating (as in Figure 14-6 ■) and inappropriate compensatory methods to avoid weight gain. The self-evaluation of individuals with Bulimia Nervosa is excessively influenced by body shape and weight. The binge eating, which is usually followed by self-induced vomiting, occurs at least twice a week (APA, 2000a).

A **binge** is defined as eating in a limited period of time (usually within 2 hours) an amount of food that is definitely

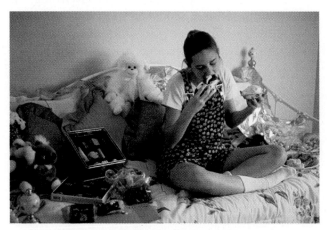

Figure 14-6. ■ A cycle of binge eating followed by self-induced vomiting is associated with Bulimia Nervosa.
Source: Omni-Photo Communications, Inc.

larger than most individuals would eat under similar circumstances. Snacking through the day does not constitute a binge. The food typically includes high-calorie, high-carbohydrate foods such as cakes and ice cream. Binge eating is characterized more by the amount of food eaten than by the specific type of food. A binge may or may not be planned in advance, and the food is usually eaten rapidly (APA, 2000a). An episode of binge eating is characterized by a feeling of loss of control. People are often ashamed of their eating behavior and usually binge secretly. A binge may be triggered by a sad mood, a stressful event, hunger from dieting, or feelings about body image, appearance, or weight. The binge may temporarily relieve the stress or low mood, but shame and self-criticism recur.

The most common method of compensating for binge eating is purging by self-induced vomiting, usually by stimulating the gag reflex. Clients report that the vomiting relieves the sense of physical discomfort and decreases the fear of gaining weight. Some people with Bulimia Nervosa abuse laxatives and diuretics after binge eating. A few misuse enemas after bingeing.

People with Bulimia Nervosa may exercise excessively in an effort to lose weight. Exercise becomes excessive when it significantly interferes with other important activities, when it occurs at inappropriate times or in inappropriate settings, or when the individual continues to exercise despite injury.

For people with Bulimia Nervosa, body shape and weight are the most important factors in determining their self-esteem. People with bulimia are usually within the normal weight range, although they may be slightly above or below it. Box 14-2 ■ supplies diagnostic criteria for Bulimia Nervosa.

There is an increase in the incidence of depression and anxiety in people who have Bulimia Nervosa. Substance abuse, especially of alcohol or stimulants, is also increased in this group. So is the incidence of Borderline Personality Disorder. Ninety percent of individuals with Bulimia Nervosa are female. Bulimia Nervosa usually begins in late adolescence or early adult life. The course may be chronic or intermittent, and the symptoms of many individuals decrease over time.

Binge Eating Disorder

The diagnosis of Binge Eating Disorder is currently under study. It is characterized by episodes of binge eating without the compensatory behaviors used in bulimia (vomiting, laxatives, enemas, excessive exercise).

BOX 14-2

Diagnostic Criteria for Bulimia Nervosa

A. Recurrent episodes of binge eating, which are characterized by both of the following:
   1. Eating, in a limited time (2-hour period), an amount of food that is definitely larger than most people would eat during a similar period of time under similar circumstances.
   2. A sense of lack of control over eating during the episode.
B. Recurrent inappropriate compensatory behavior in order to prevent weight gain, such as self-induced vomiting; misuse of laxatives, diuretics, enemas, or other medications; fasting; or excessive exercise.
C. The binge eating and inappropriate compensatory behaviors occur, on average, at least twice a week for at least 3 months.
D. Self-evaluation is unduly influenced by body shape and weight.

There are two types of bulimia nervosa:

- **Purging Type.** During the episode of bulimia nervosa, the person has regularly engaged in self-induced vomiting or the misuse of laxatives, diuretics, or enemas.
- **Nonpurging Type.** During the episode the person has used other inappropriate compensating behaviors for the binge eating (such as fasting or excessive exercise), but has not regularly engaged in self-induced vomiting or the misuse of laxatives, diuretics, or enemas.

Source: Reprinted with permission from the *Diagnostic and Statistical Manual of Mental Disorders, Text Revision,* copyright 2000. American Psychiatric Association.

As in Bulimia Nervosa, people with Binge Eating Disorder experience marked distress during and after the binge eating episodes. They have feelings of loss of control over the binge eating. They are also concerned with the possible effects of the bingeing. As in bulimia, large amounts of food are consumed quickly, when the individual is not hungry. The individual eats until uncomfortably full, eating alone due to shame, disgust, and guilt about overeating. Unlike people with bulimia, people with Binge Eating Disorder do not regularly purge or abuse laxatives, diuretics, or enemas. To justify this diagnosis, the individual must binge at least twice a week for 6 months (APA, 2000a).

People with Binge Eating Disorder tend to be overweight, whereas people with bulimia are often normal weight or slightly overweight. People with Binge Eating Disorder often report that their eating or weight interferes with their relationships with other people, their work, and their ability to feel good about themselves. They tend to have more self-loathing, disgust about body size, depression, anxiety, and physical complaints than people of the same weight who do not have the disorder. Females are approximately 1.5 times more likely to have this disorder than males. It typically starts in late adolescence or the early 20s. The first episode may occur after a stressful event (APA, 2000a).

Males with Eating Disorders

Ten percent of the people with eating disorders are male. The diagnostic criteria for the disorders and the treatment for them are the same as for women. One difference is that males with eating disorders are more likely to be involved in athletics. Males sometimes begin an eating disorder through an effort to "make the weight" for a sport such as wrestling. Males are more likely than females with eating disorders to be obese before the eating disorder begins, and they are less likely to have guilt feelings about episodes of binge eating and purging (Ricciardelli, Williams, & Kiernan, 1999).

Men with eating disorders tend to suffer from depression and alcoholism at a greater rate than do men without eating disorders. The psychosocial problems of men and women with eating disorders are similar (Woodside et al., 2001).

People with eating disorders often have difficulty trusting others, whether they are male or female. It can be difficult for adolescent males to express their feelings about eating-related problems. Because of this, it is especially important for the nurse to establish a trusting nurse-client relationship.

Pressure is increasing on adolescent males to measure up to an ideal male physique as depicted in advertising, the movies, and by professional athletes (many of whom are pressured to use anabolic steroids). If this process continues, the incidence of eating disorders in males may also rise.

Causes of Eating Disorders

What causes eating disorders? This is a good question. An increased incidence among family members suggests a genetic influence. A strain of rats has been discovered that has a recessive gene for obesity. This discovery shows that body size or fat content can be inherited. These Zucker rats are shown in Figure 14-7 ■. A biological influence is also suggested by the fact that reduced serotonin (which causes depression) lessens the sense of satiety (fullness) and increases food intake. Depressive symptoms are common in people with eating disorders.

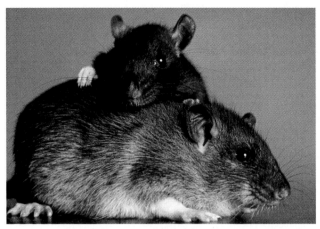

Figure 14-7. ■ This family of rats has a recessive gene for obesity. Some offspring inherit the disorder and others do not. *Source:* Phototake NYC.

Psychological theorists suggest that early separation conflicts, a sense of helplessness, difficulty interpreting feelings, intolerance of high emotion, and fear of maturity may predispose a person to an eating disorder. Women who binge report low mood, shame, guilt, and great fluctuations in self-esteem (Greeno, Wing, & Shiffman, 2000).

Environmental factors and experiences may predispose a person to having an eating disorder. Sexual abuse increases the chance that women will develop bodily shame and guilt, body disparagement, and disordered eating (Petrie & Tripp, 2001).

Control issues have been proposed as a possible contributor to Anorexia Nervosa. The idea is that the person feels a loss of control over the life environment (perhaps from a perfectionist family with unreachable expectations). The person seeks control and satisfaction where s/he can find it, in refusing food. Control of their environment is important to nurses also. Box 14-3 ■

BOX 14-3

Control Issues for Nurses

The nurse's responses to clients with eating disorders can interfere with client care when:

- ■ Feeling overwhelmed by the client's problems, the nurse sets overly rigid rules for the client in order to have some control.
- ■ The nurse, feeling powerless to help the client, becomes resentful and angry with the client.
- ■ The nurse sees other staff feeling frustrated with the client and creates a hidden alliance with the client instead of working with the staff to improve client care.

---

suggests some ways that control issues can affect nursing care.

The behavior theorists believe that children learn how to relate to food early in life. They may learn that when nurturance is not available from the people around them, food can provide a certain satisfaction and sense of calm and composure. Learning to use food as a coping mechanism or substitute for affection can lead to obesity. A behavioral approach to anorexia suggests that avoidance of eating relieves anxiety. Behavioral treatment would include practicing and learning new ways to manage anxiety.

Parents who overemphasize athletic performance, reward slimness, or express disapproval of overweight people are placing their children at risk. Parents who model unhealthy eating behaviors also put their children at risk, because children learn the behavior that they see. Some examples of unhealthy eating behaviors are overeating under stress, not eating when under stress, and using food as rewards.

The expectations of perfection and maintenance of a slender body shape increase the incidence of eating disorders in certain groups. This pressure, and the competition with others to be the best or thinnest, may be the force behind the increased incidence of eating disorders in people who participate in gymnastics and dance (especially ballet). Figures 14-8 ■ and 14-9 ■ show gymnast Christy Henrich at the Olympic trials and then a few years later, just before she died from an eating disorder at age 22.

Cognitive theorists propose that eating disorders are due to cognitive distortions (distorted thinking). People with Anorexia Nervosa tend to **catastrophize,** meaning they consider a small event to be a big catastrophe. For example, "If I gain a pound, my clothes won't fit." They also tend to use dichotomous thinking, which is similar to black-and-white thinking. For someone with dichotomous thinking, something is either all one way or all its opposite. Examples are, "If I am not thin, I will be hugely fat," and, "If I eat anything, I will lose control and gain a hundred pounds." Cognitive therapy focuses on changing the distorted thinking.

People learn their feelings about food and eating as they learn about their culture. Eating can symbolize parental nurturing. It symbolizes celebration and holidays. It can also symbolize loss of control. Box 14-4 ■ discusses the cultural connection with eating disorders as proposed by Perez, Voelz, Pettit, and Joiner (2002).

Eating disorders involve attitudes and coping mechanisms that are perceived by clients as important parts of

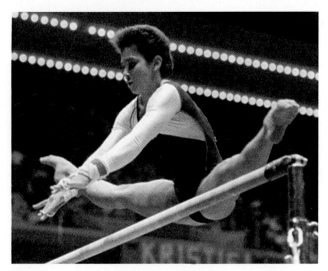

Figure 14-8. ■ Gymnast Christy Henrich performs at the Olympic trials. *Source:* AP Wide World Photos.

How Culture Affects Body Image

Fifty years ago, the perception of feminine beauty still included plump, voluptuous breasts, thighs, and buttocks. In the unindustrialized world, well-fed people are still considered healthy and beautiful. Culture in the industrialized countries has recently developed a vision of beauty that involves extreme thinness. Women are represented in advertising and entertainment that have an almost unattainable standard of body shape. Three percent of women in industrialized nations will have an eating disorder sometime in their lives. As a result of the globalization of Western culture, the incidence of eating disorders is increasing in all racial and ethnic groups in the industrialized world.

themselves. Therefore, maladaptive eating patterns are very difficult to change. Many people with eating disorders feel threatened by the idea of therapy. They are unable to see alternatives to their behavior that will allow them to cope with their stressors. For these reasons, eating disorder treatment is challenging. It requires long-term effort by clients, their families, and the healthcare team. A combination of strategies should be used to treat eating disorders.

Collaborative Care

The desired treatment outcomes for eating disorders are as follows (APA, 2000b):

- Healthy eating patterns
- Normal body physical function (lab values, organ function, body weight at least 85% of typical weight for age, BMI less than 25)

MEDICATIONS

Medications have not been found effective for the general treatment of eating disorders. Some clients respond to antidepressant medications, especially TCAs in low doses, and SSRIs such as fluoxetine (Prozac). These drugs have been used successfully to decrease the mood and obsessive-compulsive symptoms and to prevent relapse in some people with eating disorders. However, the effects appear to be short term (Zhu & Walsh, 2002). Olanzapine (Zyprexa), an antipsychotic medication, has been used to treat the bizarre body-image distortion in Anorexia Nervosa, and because it has a side effect of weight gain.

COGNITIVE-BEHAVIORAL THERAPY

A variety of therapeutic approaches to eating disorders are used. Cognitive-behavioral therapy has been used successfully with clients who have Bulimia Nervosa. It has been shown to reduce binge eating and purging. Because of frequent extensive family involvement, family therapy is a popular technique for treatment of Anorexia Nervosa. A major obstacle to treatment is that insurance companies frequently either do not cover or underfund eating disorder treatment.

Ideally, eating disorders are treated on an outpatient basis, because when lifestyle changes are needed, clients

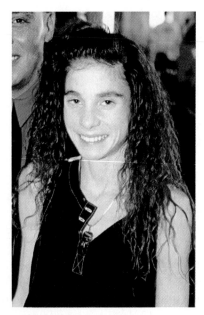

Figure 14-9. ■ In this photo Christy shows signs of her illness. It was taken shortly before she died at age 22 from anorexia. *Source:* Getty Images Inc.—Hulton Archive Photos.

are more successful when they can practice their new behaviors at home. Outpatients have more autonomy, which is important in these disorders. However, there are times when hospitalization is required. Clients who have life-threatening fluid and electrolyte imbalances, organ failure, or complete inability to eat must be hospitalized. Tube feeding and total parenteral nutrition have been used in the short term to treat acute malnutrition.

Obesity

Obesity is not considered a mental disorder. Many people with obesity are mentally healthy. However, obesity is covered here because it causes a great deal of physical and emotional suffering, and many of the people it affects are nurses.

The Office of the U.S. Surgeon General reports that the risks of overweight or obesity may soon cause as much disease and death as cigarette smoking. Overweight in an adult is determined by **body mass index** (BMI). BMI is defined as weight in kilograms divided by the square of height in meters. Another way to calculate it is: weight in pounds multiplied by 705 and then divided twice by height in inches (this is easier with a calculator). Overweight is diagnosed when BMI is between 25 and 29.9, whereas a BMI of 30 or greater indicates obesity. The risk of death increases as the BMI goes above 30. Twenty-five percent of American adults are obese (Blackburn & Bevis, 2003). Figure 14-10 ■ shows a man having his skin fold thickness measured, which is another fat assessment technique.

Many overweight people have a group of major risk factors that constitute a condition called metabolic syndrome. The metabolic syndrome includes:

- Abdominal obesity
- Abnormal serum lipids (increased triglycerides and decreased high-density lipoprotein)
- Elevated blood pressure
- Insulin resistance
- Increased clotting of the blood

This syndrome is caused by improper nutrition and inadequate exercise. The syndrome significantly increases cardiovascular risks, such as heart disease and stroke. Weight loss is the key therapeutic objective. Even modest weight reductions (5–10% of initial body weight) cause significant clinical improvements (Blackburn & Bevis, 2003).

Obesity obviously has adverse effects on physical health. It also affects mental health. Some people with

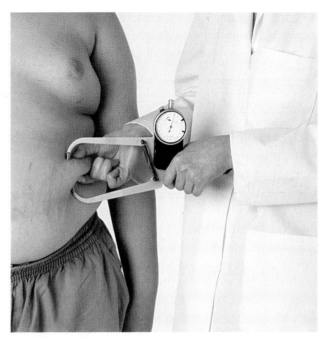

Figure 14-10. ■ Calipers measure the skinfold thickness that estimates the client's body fat percentage. *Source:* Dorling Kindersley Media Library.

obesity experience low self-esteem, poor body image, depression, and anxiety. Some feel guilt and self-disgust. People with compulsive eating behavior overeat for emotional rather than physical reasons. Food may offer the same relief from anxiety or stress that companionship and nurturing from others might provide. Food becomes a mechanism for coping with stress.

CAUSES

Obesity has a similar profile to the eating disorders. It runs in families. This is probably due to a combination of predisposing factors and learned behavior. It has behavioral aspects (people learn to overeat because they receive some reinforcement from food) and cognitive components (distorted thinking). Cultural and social factors also lead to obesity. People are increasingly turning to sedentary recreational activities (electronic entertainment). Fast food is readily available, and yes, thanks, I will have fries with that.

COLLABORATIVE CARE

To lose weight, more energy must be spent than is consumed on a daily basis. The chance of success in long-term maintenance of weight loss is improved with the following (Blackburn & Bevis, 2003):

- Realistic weight loss goals (5–10% of initial body weight)

- Change in eating patterns to include less of high-calorie, low-nutrition foods, and more of nutrient-dense, low-energy foods, such as fruits and vegetables
- Social support
- Structured meal plans, to avoid misunderstanding and measurement errors in food amounts
- Record of eating, to keep it conscious
- Moderate physical activity on most, if not all, days

These lifestyle changes make a lot of sense. The problem is with actually doing them. Lifestyle changes are notoriously difficult. Nurses can help by being role models of healthy behavior, and by acknowledging the difficulty of the challenge. Acknowledge that our culture values thinness and physical appearance and not inner qualities and strengths (Figure 14-11 ■ shows an example of the American standard of beauty), but it does not have to be that way (National Eating Disorders Association, 2007). There is hope. Change is possible, but recognize the challenge, and give the client a lot of support. Once a client begins a regular exercise program, the increased sense of well-being will be very rewarding.

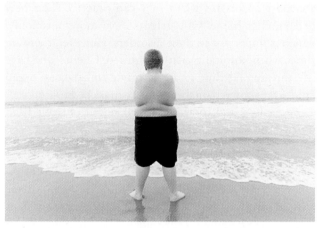

Figure 14-12. ■ The stigma against obesity leaves many people alone. *Source:* Getty Images Inc.—Stone Allstock.

The stigma against obese people is strong. People are rejected for jobs and housing, stared at, bullied, mocked, and humiliated (Figure 14-12 ■ shows an obese boy alone at the beach). Some people with obesity are trying to form a social network that will allow obese people to connect with others who understand their feelings and accept them as they are, and to advocate for the fair treatment of people of all sizes. They formed the National Association to Advance Fat Acceptance. Figure 14-13 ■ shows two members on break from the Association's convention.

Collaboration among healthcare providers and parents to help parents instill attitudes that will make children resilient against eating disorders is probably the best way to prevent eating disorders. The National Eating Disorders Association has 10 strategies for parents to use

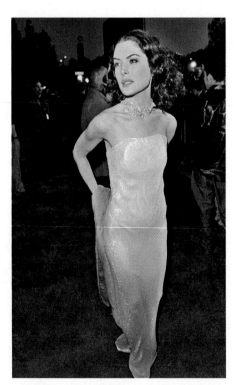

Figure 14-11. ■ Actress Lara Flynn Boyle represents a standard of beauty at the Blockbuster Awards in Los Angeles. *Source:* AP Wide World Photos.

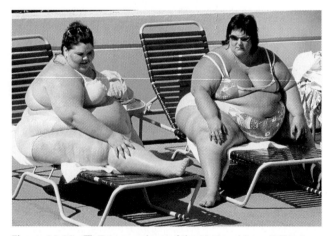

Figure 14-13. ■ Two members of the National Association to Advance Fat Acceptance take a break from the national convention. *Source:* PhotoEdit Inc.

to prevent the development of eating disorders in their children (Levine & Smolak, 2006):

1. Consider how your attitudes about your own body have been shaped by sexism and weightism. Then teach your children about how people come in different shapes and sizes and the nature and ugliness of prejudice. Make an effort to maintain positive and healthy attitudes and behaviors because you are a powerful role model for your children.

2. Examine closely your dreams and goals for your children. Are you overemphasizing beauty and body shape? Avoid sending a message that says: "I will love you more if you lose weight, don't eat so much, look more like the slender models in ads, fit into smaller clothes, etc." Decide what you can do to reduce the teasing, criticism, blaming, staring, etc. that reinforce the idea that larger or fatter is "bad" and smaller or thinner is "good."

3. Learn about and discuss with your sons and daughters the dangers of trying to alter one's body shape by dieting, the value of moderate exercise for health, and the importance of eating a variety of foods in well-balanced meals eaten at least three times a day. Avoid calling foods "bad, dangerous, fattening, good, safe, good or low fat." Be a good role model of self-acceptance, eating, and exercise.

4. Make a commitment not to avoid activities (such as swimming, sunbathing, dancing, etc.) simply because they call attention to your weight and shape. Refuse to wear clothes that are uncomfortable or that you don't like but wear simply because they divert attention from your weight or shape.

5. Make a commitment to exercise for the joy of feeling your body move and grow stronger, not to purge fat from your body or to compensate for calories eaten.

6. Practice taking people seriously for what they say, feel, and do, not for how slender or "well put together" they appear.

7. Help children appreciate and resist the ways in which television, magazines, and other media distort the true diversity of human body types and imply that a slender body means power, excitement, popularity, or perfection.

8. Educate boys and girls about various forms of prejudice, including weightism, and help them understand their responsibilities for preventing them.

9. Encourage your children to be active and to enjoy what their bodies can do and feel like. Do not limit their caloric intake unless a physician requests that you do this because of a medical problem.

10. Do whatever you can to promote the self-esteem and self-respect of all of your children in intellectual, athletic, and social endeavors. Give boys and girls the same opportunities and encouragement. Be careful not to suggest that females are less important than males, such as by not making males do housework or childcare. A well-rounded sense of self and solid positive self-esteem are the best antidotes to dieting and disordered eating.

NURSING CARE

ASSESSING

The assessment of a client with weight loss or gain should begin with subjective information about the client's experience. Imagine that we have two very thin adolescents in the clinic. One states that she is just fine and could only be improved by a little more weight loss. The second client might say, "I've been so hungry, and I've been eating and drinking everything in sight, but I'm still losing weight." The first client may have Anorexia Nervosa, and the second may have untreated type 1 diabetes. Let's not forget that there are general medical conditions that cause weight gain and loss.

Other subjective data to collect includes information about the client's body image. A picture like the one in Figure 14-5 is useful for assessing whether a client has a realistic body image. A distorted image of the thin self as obese is very common in Anorexia Nervosa, but not in bulimia or Binge Eating Disorder. The client's perception of her/his body and attitudes about eating will also demonstrate whether the client has cognitive distortion (distorted thinking) related to body shape and weight.

Another important subjective assessment is about how the eating disorder serves the client. Does it take the focus off unhealthy family dynamics? Does it give the client control in a chaotic situation? Does purging relieve anxiety? Does binge eating give the client some momentary comfort (before the shame and embarrassment)? Although this information is important for the client's insight, it is difficult to discover.

Objective findings include the ever-popular vital signs and weight. Expect the provider to order lab values that indicate the client's nutritional status, and whether an eating disorder has affected organ function. A well-documented baseline assessment is important to provide a point of comparison for evaluating the client's progress in treatment.

Weighing clients with eating disorders can be problematic. Clients may go to great lengths to make it appear that they have gained or maintained weight. Clients have awakened during the night to drink large volumes of water, stuffed their socks with coins, put on extra clothing, and concealed heavy items in their clothing. The nurse's problem-solving skills will be helpful here.

DIAGNOSING, PLANNING, AND IMPLEMENTING

Some common nursing diagnoses for clients with eating disorders include:

- Imbalanced Nutrition: Less Than Body Requirements
- Imbalanced Nutrition: More Than Body Requirements
- Ineffective Coping
- Disturbed Self-Esteem
- Powerlessness
- Disturbed Body Image

Desired outcomes for clients with eating disorders are that the client will:

- Establish healthy eating patterns (without binge eating or purging).
- Maintain body weight at least 85% of desired weight for age and height.
- Maintain a body mass index less than 25.
- Verbalize positive comments about self separate from physical appearance.
- Describe a realistic image of own body.
- Demonstrate a sense of self-efficacy (power over one's own outcomes) by establishing realistic personal goals.

Ineffective Coping

Clients with eating disorders virtually always have ineffective coping skills. They may demonstrate self-destructive behaviors (starving, purging, bingeing, or other self-harm), inability to ask for help, poor impulse control, inability to meet their basic nutritional needs, inability to change their behaviors, denial of illness, or insufficient problem-solving skills. The nurse chooses appropriate interventions for individual clients.

- Encourage the client to express feelings. *Clients with eating disorders often have difficulty expressing their feelings. Verbal expression of feelings can reduce anxiety and decrease the need for purging behavior. Practice with*

expressing feelings helps the client learn to recognize own feelings.
- Discuss feelings the client has before binge eating or purging. Keeping a journal of feelings provides a record of how the client's feelings occur and change. It can help the client develop insight. *If the client is able to recognize the feelings or situations that precede bingeing or purging behavior, s/he may be able to stop before engaging in these behaviors.*
- Help the client explore alternate ways of responding to feelings of frustration, anger, or anxiety that do not involve food. *If the client can identify and plan to use behaviors to relieve anxiety that do not involve food or purging (such as talking with a friend), s/he will have a healthy alternative when the trigger feelings arise. It is important to separate feelings from food.*
- Encourage the client to eat with others. *Eating with other people will take the secrecy out of eating and provide role models for normal behavior. This is very stressful for clients with Anorexia Nervosa.*
- Help the client explore personal strengths that are not related to eating or appearance. *The client's self-concept can be improved by discovering personal strengths. It is important for the client with an eating disorder to recognize that appearance does not define the character of a person.*

Imbalanced Nutrition: Less than Body Requirements

The client may demonstrate weight loss, abuse of laxatives or diuretics, binge eating, purging, compulsive eating, or malnutrition.

- Provide a safe environment. *Safety is the first priority. If the client is in physiological danger from malnutrition, the treatment team must begin with the goal of maintaining adequate nutrition.*
- Help the client to develop a daily meal plan that meets her/his nutritional needs. Consult with the dietitian. *The client has been focused on food and may be an expert on the calorie content of foods. However, the client will need specific information about healthy meal planning. The dietitian specializes in the area of healthy nutrition and meal planning and is an important resource for nurses and clients.*
- Spend time with the client after meals. Discuss the client's feelings. *When the client has developed the habit of purging after eating, s/he may have intense feelings of anxiety after meals. The presence of the nurse is supportive. The client who overeats may have intense feelings of guilt when eating. The client can discuss feelings with the nurse, helping with insight development. The presence of the nurse eliminates*

the secrecy associated with eating and purging and makes purging impossible. The presence of the nurse is distracting from the client's focus on purging. The treatment team may decide to restrict access to the bathroom after meals.

- Engage the client in a distracting activity after meals. *A distracting activity such as walking, talking, or playing a card game can help take the client's focus off purging or gaining weight and can provide the client with practice in doing healthy activities as an alternative to purging.*

- Help the client identify situations and feelings that trigger binge eating or purging. Encourage the client to notify the nurse when these feelings arise, then discuss problem solving with the client. *The goal is for the client to understand her/his feelings and to stop the urge to engage in unhealthy behavior, ultimately replacing it with healthy alternatives. The nurse can support the client as s/he works through this process.*

- Be nonjudgmental in your interactions with clients, even when their behavior is inappropriate. *Clients with eating disorders already have feelings of low self-esteem, guilt, and shame. The role of the nurse is to help the client develop healthy behavior, not to punish the client for poor judgment.*

EVALUATING

Evaluation of the effectiveness of the nursing interventions is an ongoing part of the nursing process. The client's body weight goals will be to maintain body weight at least 85% of typical weight for age, with a body mass index (BMI) less than 25. The behavioral goal is healthy eating patterns, including balanced nutrition without binge eating or purging. The cognitive goals are that clients will have a realistic self-perception, and a positive self-esteem separate from their physical appearance.

DISCHARGE CONSIDERATIONS

Nurses can play a leading role in teaching about healthy eating behaviors. Some strategies the nurse may use are provided in Box 14-5 ■.

NURSING PROCESS CARE PLAN
Client with Bulimia Nervosa

Katie Clark is an 18-year-old female being seen for the first time in the eating disorders clinic where you work as a nurse. Katie is accompanied by her mother who describes Katie's eating habits as "disgusting." Edna Clark states that she found Katie in the kitchen last night "stuffing her face with everything in sight." Then she heard Katie vomiting in the bathroom. Edna looked in Katie's bedroom. She found boxes of laxatives and several enema bottles. There were also boxes of over-the-counter diuretics and herbal preparations for weight loss and prevention of fluid retention. Katie said she needed the medications to keep her from gaining weight.

BOX 14-5	NURSING CARE CHECKLIST

Strategies for Preventing Eating Disorders

- ☑ Address our cultural obsession with slenderness as a physical, psychological, and moral issue.
- ☑ Help children develop self-esteem in a variety of areas that transcend physical appearance.
- ☑ Discuss the roles of women and men in our society, beyond their appearance.
- ☑ Ask parents to examine their own attitudes about food, and think about how these attitudes affect the way they handle food with their children.
- ☑ Encourage parents to learn to identify their child's hunger behavior, loneliness behavior, and need for nurturance. Stress that they should respond to each need appropriately (not with food for all needs). Encourage them to learn the difference between hunger for food and hunger for affection.
- ☑ Allow children to determine their feeding needs: let go of the need for "cleaning the plate."
- ☑ Do not make insulting remarks about overweight people.
- ☑ Teach that parents should not overemphasize success (expecting perfection) in athletics.
- ☑ Be a good role model for healthy eating. Eat a variety of nutritious foods. Avoid overeating under stress or not eating at all when under stress.
- ☑ Make it clear that thinness is not the same as happiness.

During her mother's outburst, Katie sits quietly in a chair with her head down. When you ask Katie to describe what has been going on with her, she says, "It's all true. I try so hard to lose weight, but I have this uncontrollable urge to just eat and eat; then I have to get rid of it. I hate myself. I have no self-control. If I gain weight, people will make fun of me like they do my Aunt Charlotte."

Assessment. She tells you that all her life she has been compared to her Aunt Charlotte, who is quite obese. Whenever she does something her mother doesn't like, her mother says, "Oh, you are just like your Aunt Charlotte." She sees herself becoming another Aunt Charlotte.

When asked what triggers her to start a binge, she states that when she becomes anxious or upset she binges. Her mother watches everything Katie eats, so she usually binges at night while her mother is asleep. Last night, she was laying awake thinking about her appointment for today and became "nervous." Then she got up and began to eat. Her mother found her, and said, "Do you want to look like your Aunt Charlotte?" Katie was ashamed of her actions and went into the bathroom to induce vomiting. Katie tells you she feels powerless to control her situation. She says she uses laxatives and diuretics regularly to keep her weight down. Sometimes, she gets so anxious that the only thing that helps is "lots of food." You ask her about her self-esteem. She sees it as related directly to her weight and appearance. Katie feels like her thoughts about her weight are beginning to "consume" her, and she wants help. She says, "I want to go to college and have a life outside of thoughts about food and weight. I'm tired of this roller coaster."

Her vital signs are BP 110/76, P 70, R 12. She is 5940 and weighs 122 pounds, which is average for her small frame. Looking in her mouth you notice some discoloration of some of her teeth, which could be due to enamel erosion from stomach acids when she is purging. She complains to you about frequent episodes of "heartburn."

When you talk to the mother alone, she tells you that she is very concerned about Katie. She says she has always tried to stress eating restraint with Katie. Edna's sister Charlotte is "disgusting" to her, and she sees a lot of Charlotte's personality in Katie. She's afraid that Katie will become a "laughing stock" like Charlotte. "I don't want that for my child."

Diagnosis

- Ineffective Coping R/T lack of skills
- Chronic Low Self-Esteem Disturbance R/T perceived lack of self-control

- Powerlessness R/T a perceived lack of control over her thoughts and behavior

Expected Outcomes. The client will:

- Identify at least five sources of stress and anxiety in her life.
- Develop a list of five adaptive ways to cope with the identified sources of stress and anxiety.
- Identify at least three positive attributes that she possesses.
- Identify at least two new techniques she will try when she experiences the urge to binge and purge.
- List supportive people she can talk to when she feels like bingeing or purging.

Planning and Implementation

- Maintain an open communication with Katie, actively listening to her and validating her feelings.
- Encourage Katie to keep a journal about her feelings. This will help her identify what circumstances precipitate the stress and anxiety that results in the bingeing and purging response. Have her make a list of these situations, and discuss them with her. Dealing with a situation before it escalates may assist her in changing her behavior.
- Assist Katie to develop positive coping techniques. Find out what has worked for her in the past. Find out who she considers to be in her support system. Does she have a special teacher, youth group leader, supportive peers, a school counselor whom she trusts?
- Suggest that she attend the support group for people with bulimia that is sponsored by the eating disorders clinic. Sharing feelings and coping techniques with others who have similar experiences will let Katie know she is not alone.
- Recommend that the mother participate in a family member support group as well as individual and family counseling. Since her behavior is obviously stress provoking for Katie, she needs assistance to recognize her negative behaviors and what changes she can make.
- Assist Katie to develop a list of positive affirmations about herself that she can post on her bathroom mirror. She should read these when she gets up in the morning and before she goes to bed at night. This will help to replace Katie's negative self-talk with more positive thoughts about herself.
- Encourage Katie to eat in a social environment, not alone and not in secret. Suggest she have a designated

friend to be with her during and after meals to support her in her struggle to avoid bingeing and purging.

- Have Katie make a list of other things she can do instead of eating when her stress and anxiety become too much for her. Perhaps calling a friend, taking a walk, or writing in her journal could be outlets for her. She needs to develop a list of what works for her.
- Encourage her to identify her feelings when the need to eat overcomes her. Is she hungry? Angry? Bored? Anxious? Lonely? Sad? Taking the time to identify her feelings will allow her to consider her next actions and change her patterns of response.
- Praise Katie for all of her successes, and show your support when she expresses her failures. Always remain nonjudgmental.

Evaluation. Katie comes to the Eating Disorders Clinic twice a week, once to meet with a counselor and once to attend the support group. Her mother also comes to the clinic for family counseling, and her relationship with Katie has improved. She no longer compares Katie with Aunt Charlotte or anyone else. She expresses appreciation for Katie as the person she is. Katie still finds herself becoming anxious before a class presentation, a date with a new boy, or taking an exam, but she has better control over her responses to the stress. When she wakes up in the middle of the night, she picks up her journal and starts writing instead of heading to the kitchen to eat. She occasionally relapses and binges and purges, but instead of doing this two or three times a week, she does it only once or twice a month. Her weight is stable, and she expresses more contentment with herself.

Critical Thinking in the Nursing Process

1. Should Katie's Aunt Charlotte be involved in Katie's plan of care?
2. Why should the nurse be nonjudgmental when working with this client?
3. What can the members of an eating disorders support group do for Katie that the nurse cannot?

Note: Discussion of Critical Thinking questions appears in Appendix I.

Note: The references and resources for this and all chapters have been compiled at the back of the book.

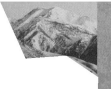
 KEY TERMS

Use the audio glossary feature of the Companion Website to hear the correct pronunciation of the following key terms.

amenorrhea

binge

body mass index (BMI)

cachexia

catastrophize

control issues

emaciated

purging

KEY Points

- Eating disorders are serious and can be fatal.
- Eating disorders affect physiological as well as psychological function.
- People with eating disorders have ineffective coping skills.
- As Western culture extends across the world, eating disorders are increasing in industrialized countries.
- The cultural attitude that extreme thinness defines beauty and symbolizes success and self-control contributes to the occurrence of eating disorders.
- Obesity is becoming more common and causes increased cardiovascular risks, arthritis, poor self-esteem, and mortality rates.
- There are strategies for preventing eating disorders.
- There is hope for people with eating disorders. Effective therapy exists.

 EXPLORE MediaLink

Additional interactive resources for this chapter can be found on the Companion Website at www.prenhall.com/eby. Click on Chapter 14 and "Begin" to select the activities for this chapter.

- Audio glossary
- NCLEX-PN® review
- Case study
- Study outline
- Critical thinking questions
- Matching questions
- Weblinks
- Video Case: Tamora (Anorexia Nervosa)

Caring for a Client with Obesity
NCLEX-PN® Focus Area: Health Promotion and Maintenance

Case Study: Ruby Red is a 38-year-old European American woman admitted to the general hospital for a total knee arthroplasty (replacement) 2 days ago. She is also obese. Ms. Red is concerned about her health, self-image, and recovery from surgery. She would like help to lose weight. She has tried weight-loss diets in the past with no long-term success.

Nursing Diagnosis: Nutrition, imbalanced: More than body requirements

COLLECT DATA

Subjective	Objective
_____	_____
_____	_____
_____	_____
_____	_____
_____	_____
_____	_____
_____	_____

Would you report this data? Yes/No

If yes, to: _____

Nursing Care

_____
_____
_____
_____
_____
_____
_____
_____
_____
_____

How would you document this? _____
_____
_____
_____

Compare your documentation to the sample provided in Appendix I.

Data Collected
(use those that apply)

- 5950 tall, 190 lbs
- Client states that she eats when she feels nervous.
- Client states that she frequently overeats in the evenings.
- BP 128/84
- Friends bring candy to hospital for client.
- Client prefers to wear loose clothing.
- Client has two children.
- She has been married to her current husband for 3 years.
- It is very painful for client to ambulate.
- Client asks, "Is there a pill that will make me lose weight?"
- Client states that her physician has never talked with her about losing weight.

Nursing Interventions
(use those that apply; list in priority order)

- Discuss with the client her reasons for wanting to lose weight.
- Work with dietitian to determine realistic goals, and to plan an eating program based on the food guide pyramid.
- Tell the client that she should start doing aerobic exercise as soon as she is discharged from the hospital.
- Teach the client about the relationship between dietary intake, calorie burning by exercise and metabolism, and weight.
- Encourage client to accept herself as a person, just as she is, and to lose weight for her health and well-being.
- Discuss strategies for dealing with feelings in other ways than overeating.
- Discuss cues for eating that are not related to hunger.
- Tell the client that she should never eat sweet foods.
- Encourage increasing physical activity at the client's ability level.
- Set realistic goals for weight loss, including a discussion of the expected increases and decreases of weight due to hormonal changes and dietary and physical fluctuations.
- Encourage adequate fluid intake.
- Teach the client's husband to monitor her daily intake and to reward or criticize her based on her progress.
- Discuss the use of food as a comfort measure.

When a question includes the client's feelings, they are probably important. Select the answer that shows that you know the importance of recognizing client feelings and treating the client with respect.

1 A person with an eating disorder might present with which of the following signs and symptoms?

1. Tachycardia and hypertension
2. Hyperglycemia and hyperthyroidism
3. Bradycardia, hypotension, and dry, cracking skin
4. Fever and excessively oily skin

2 The mother of a client who is in the hospital approaches the nurse with concerns about her daughter. She tells the nurse that her daughter has started fasting and exercising to the point of not wanting to attend school, so that she may work out. Her daughter is obsessed with her body and thinks she is overweight when, in fact, she is underweight. The nurse's best response to the mother would be:

1. "Your daughter is going through a normal adolescent phase. It is nothing to worry about."
2. "It's not serious unless you see that she is also abusing laxatives and vomiting after meals."
3. "Your daughter may have an eating disorder, and she needs an immediate assessment before she endangers her overall health."
4. "Your daughter may have an eating disorder, but I do not think she's at the point where she needs any medical intervention. Just be alert to her condition."

3 The nurse would expect which of the following responses to continuous weight loss from an individual with Anorexia Nervosa?

1. Disappointment in the failure to maintain control of her body
2. Concern for her overall physical health
3. Fear of death
4. Improvement in her feelings about herself, because she is maintaining self-control

4 When caring for a client with conditions such as anorexia and bulimia, the nurse should also assess for signs of which personality disorder?

1. Borderline
2. Narcissistic
3. Histrionic
4. Passive-aggressive

5 The nurse is caring for a client who has Anorexia Nervosa. Which of the following behaviors, often associated with this disorder, would be of most concern?

1. Being sexually provocative
2. Expressing suicidal ideations
3. Manipulating the staff
4. Having friends sneak alcohol or drugs in to her

6 A mother approaches the nurse in the eating disorders inclient clinic with concerns about the probability of the success of the treatment for her daughter. The nurse's best response would be:

1. "Treatment of eating disorders is very successful. Your daughter will be out of here within the week."
2. "The behavior seen in eating disorders is very difficult to change. Your daughter will require long-term therapy even after she leaves our facility."
3. "As long as your daughter follows all of our rules, she will progress quickly toward a cure."
4. "We use only behavior modification therapy here and have found it to be very successful in treating eating disorders."

7 Which of the following drugs would the nurse expect to use to treat the body-image disturbance and weight loss associated with Anorexia Nervosa?

1. Olanzapine (Zyprexa)
2. Fluoxetine (Prozac)
3. Amitriptyline (Elavil)
4. Lorazepam (Ativan)

8 A 200-pound, 64-inch tall woman has a body mass index (BMI) of:

1. 18.2
2. 34.4
3. 22.1
4. 32.4

9 Which of the following would be a good strategy for parents to adopt to prevent eating disorders in their children?

1. Post a photo of a well-proportioned role model on the refrigerator to encourage healthy eating.
2. Encourage children to eat all that is on their plates to emphasize healthy eating habits.
3. Have special food treats available and use them only as rewards for good behavior.
4. Eat a variety of nutritious foods.

10 In assessing a client with Anorexia Nervosa, the nurse might find evidence of which other medical complications? (Select all that apply.)

1. Impaired liver function
2. Amenorrhea
3. Constipation
4. Renal impairment
5. Hypothermia

Answers for Review Questions, as well as discussion of Care Plan and Critical Thinking Care Map questions, appear in Appendix I.

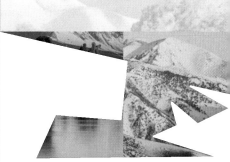

Chapter 15

Dementia and Cognitive Disorders

BRIEF Outline

Delirium

Dementia

LEARNING Outcomes

After completing this chapter, you will be able to:

1. Explain the differences between delirium and dementia.
2. Identify clients with cognitive disorders.
3. Describe the problem behaviors of clients with cognitive disorders.
4. Apply the nursing process to clients with cognitive disorders.
5. Discuss the impact on the families of clients with cognitive disorders.

Cognitive disorders are disorders that distort one's thought processes. They are not traditionally considered mental diseases. However, they are included in this text because many of the signs and symptoms of cognitive disorders are similar to those found in mental illness. Cognitive disorders were formerly referred to as *organic brain disorders*. (Some older medical professionals still refer to them that way.) The *DSM-IV-TR* changed this classification because other mental disorders can have organic, or physical, components, too. The *DSM-IV-TR* classifies cognitive disorders under "Delirium, Dementia, and Amnestic and Other Cognitive Disorders" (American Psychiatric Association [APA], 2000).

This chapter will discuss delirium and dementia, especially dementia of the Alzheimer's type, because these are the most common cognitive disorders you will encounter as a student and as a nurse.

Delirium

Have you ever been confused from a high fever or following a concussion? You might have become restless and mumbled words that made no sense. You might not have known where you were. If so, then you have experienced delirium. **Delirium** is a temporary condition that may alter the level of consciousness. It may affect a person's ability to focus thoughts, recall past events, understand and use language, or have an accurate perception of environmental stimuli (APA, 2000). Delirium may potentially cause other complications and consequently increase the rate of morbidity, so early recognition is important. Unrecognized and untreated delirium may progress to the point where clients require a long-term care facility or full-time home nursing care after discharge. Box 15-1 ■ provides a more detailed description of the diagnostic criteria.

Delirium may be confused with dementia, as the signs and symptoms are similar. Consequently, if a person is already diagnosed with dementia, symptoms of delirium may be ignored and attributed to the dementia process (Vogel, 2005). Table 15-1 ■ lists the differences between the two.

Delirium usually develops more quickly than dementia. It can result from a medical condition (APA, 2000). It may also result from a psychological response to a sudden change in one's living situation, such as relocation from home to an unfamiliar setting. Nursing home staff often report a temporary confusion in clients who are moved even from one room to another.

BOX 15-1

Diagnostic Criteria for Delirium Due to a General Medical Condition

A. Disturbance of consciousness with reduced ability to focus, sustain, or shift attention.

B. A change in cognition (such as memory deficit, disorientation, language disturbance) or the development of a perceptual disturbance that is not better accounted for by a preexisting, established, or evolving dementia.

C. The disturbance develops over short period of time (usually hours or days) and tends to fluctuate during the day.

D. There is evidence from the history, physical examination, or laboratory findings that the disturbance is caused by the direct physiological consequences of a general medical condition.

Source: Reprinted with permission from the *Diagnostic and Statistical Manual of Mental Disorders, Text Revision*, copyright 2000. American Psychiatric Association.

CONDITIONS THAT CAUSE DELIRIUM

Many conditions may cause delirium. Box 15-2 ■ lists the most common causes. When a diagnosis of delirium is made, it is extremely important for physicians to evaluate all evidence of confusion in the elderly to rule out reversible causes. It would be sad to deliver the devastating news to family members that a relative has dementia when the relative actually has a treatable medical condition. In such situations, appropriate care could result in a total reversal of cognitive losses.

In addition to diagnostic tests, the client should have a complete psychological evaluation. Some severely depressed individuals have been diagnosed with Alzheimer's disease.

CASE EXAMPLE

An elderly gentleman was admitted to the nursing home with a diagnosis of Dementia of the Alzheimer's Type. He was aggressive with staff and other clients and would often get into his closet and refuse to come out. He was transferred to a mental health facility. There, the intern documenting his intake data realized that the man's only son had died recently. He recognized that the man was suffering from clinical depression and an ensuing delirium related to grief. He was treated for the depression, and his emotional state improved and his cognitive abilities returned. He was discharged home on medication and resumed a normal life.

Critical Self-Check. What do you think could have happened if the depression had not been recognized and treated?

TABLE 15-1		
Comparison of Dementia and Delirium		
DEFINING TRAITS	**DELIRIUM**	**DEMENTIA**
DSM-IV-TR classification	Yes	Yes
Onset	Develops over short period of time (hours or days)	Gradual (may not be noticed for years)
Etiology	Associated with variety of general medical conditions or psychosocial changes	Unrelated to *general* medical condition or psychosocial changes; may be related to *specific* medical conditions such as HIV or Parkinson's disease
Cognitive changes	Impaired memory, disorientation, language and perceptual disturbances	Impaired memory, disorientation, language and perceptual disturbances
Symptom presence	Symptoms fluctuate	Symptoms do not fluctuate
Behavior	Varies from agitation to withdrawal	May or may not have behavior disturbances
Progression	Temporary if underlying condition is treated	Permanent; progressive, continuous decline in abilities and cognition
Treatment	Ensure client safety; provide the medication or therapy ordered to treat underlying conditions; support client and family	Ensure client safety; respond appropriately to problem behaviors as needed; establish communication techniques; support client and family; administer cholinesterase inhibitors or memantine as ordered

MANIFESTATIONS OF DELIRIUM

Nurses are in the best position to recognize significant change in the client's cognition and behavior. For surgical clients, you will be in a better position to evaluate cognitive changes if you are fortunate enough to care for the client both preoperatively and postoperatively. Take the case of an elderly gentleman who was admitted to the hospital several days before physicians determined that surgery

BOX 15-2	
Conditions That Can Cause Delirium	

GENERAL MEDICAL CONDITIONS

Metabolic disorders
    Untreated hypothyroidism
    Adrenal gland hyperfunction (Cushing's syndrome)
Nutritional disorders
Malnutrition
    Pernicious anemia (Vitamin B_{12} deficiency)
    Folic acid deficiency
Metabolic states
    Acid-base imbalance
    Electrolyte imbalances
Hypo- or hyperglycemia (low or high blood sugars)
Dehydration
Infections
    Urinary tract
    Respiratory
    High fever

Hypoxia (inadequate oxygen levels)
Any form of trauma
Fall—fractures
    Postoperative state
    Head trauma
Sensory impairment such as vision or hearing losses
Pain
Terminal illness
Elderly (over the age of 65 years)

SUBSTANCE-RELATED CONDITIONS

Drug reactions or interactions
Drug or alcohol intoxication
Drug or alcohol withdrawal

PSYCHOSOCIAL CONDITIONS

Grief
Relocation to an unfamiliar environment

was needed. Preoperatively, the client was quiet, cooperative, and mentally clear. One day postoperatively, he pulled out his IV, his NG tube, and his Foley catheter. He was combative with the staff, totally disoriented, confused, and uncooperative. When the client's Phenergan (an antiemetic medication) was discontinued, his mental state returned to its preoperative condition. This is an example of a **substance-induced delirium.**

Because many surgical clients enter a facility on the day of surgery, nurses do not often see preoperative baseline behavior for comparison. Therefore, the nurse has to rely on comments from the client's family or friends about changes in the client's cognitive abilities.

Early symptoms of delirium might also include anxiety, distractibility, and sleep disturbances. The condition may progress to a full delirium within 1 to 3 days; then it may resolve in a few hours or may continue for hours to days (APA, 2000). One client was admitted to the nursing home due to confusion that developed while he was hospitalized for a fractured leg. The confusion did not clear up, and after a few weeks, the family took him home. In a familiar environment, surrounded by family, his delirium eventually disappeared, but it took several months for this to happen.

More severe symptoms of delirium might mimic psychosis. Clients may experience hallucinations, delusions, language disturbances, and agitation. Anxiety or variations in mood may be mistaken for psychotic disorders.

Fluctuation in symptoms (see Box 15-2) distinguishes delirium from other possible mental disorders (APA, 2000).

Delirium may manifest itself in three subtypes: hyperactive, hypoactive, and mixed (Vogel, 2005). Table 15-2 ■ provides a comparison of these types. Symptoms vary depending on the type of delirium the client develops.

At-Risk Clients

Nurses need to be aware of which clients are at the greatest risk for developing delirium during their stay in a healthcare facility. Delirium is a startlingly common experience. The incidence of delirium in clients admitted to the hospital with a medical illness is between 10% and 30%. If clients are elderly, 10–40% will experience delirium during the course of the hospital stay; 60% of nursing home residents who are 75 years and older are expected to experience delirium during their stay (APA, 2000). In addition to the elderly, other clients who are considered at risk for developing delirium in the hospital are postoperative clients like the one mentioned previously and clients with central nervous system conditions such as meningitis. Incidence for these clients could be as high as 50% (Vogel, 2005). Eighty percent of terminally ill clients develop delirium as they approach death (APA, 2000). Having multiple illnesses, multiple medications, or being a child may also be risk factors. Clients who are in the ICU are particularly vulnerable to the development

TABLE 15-2		
Comparison of the Three Subtypes of Delirium		
HYPERACTIVE	**HYPOACTIVE**	**MIXED**
Agitation	Quiet confusion	Emotional lability (showing wide range of emotions)
Disorientation	Disorientation	Fluctuation between hyperactive and hypoactive symptoms
Delusional, possibly related to disorientation and memory impairment	Subdued and apathetic	
Visual and auditory hallucinations possible	Disturbance in levels of consciousness, sleeping in daytime and awake during night	
May be misdiagnosed as a psychotic disorder such as schizophrenia or a worsening of an already present dementia	May be misdiagnosed as depression, catatonia, or dementia or not recognized at all	Difficult to diagnose due to changes in presentation of symptoms

Source: Adapted from Vogel, C. (2005). Clearing up the confusion about delirium. *NurseWeek, 6*(12), 17–19; and Gleason, O. (2003, March 1). Delirium. *American Family Physician.* Retrieved June 3, 2007, from http://www.afp.org/afp/20030301/1027.html.

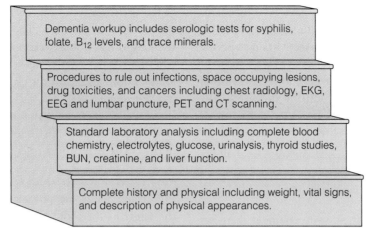

Dementia workup includes serologic tests for syphilis, folate, B_{12} levels, and trace minerals.

Procedures to rule out infections, space occupying lesions, drug toxicities, and cancers including chest radiology, EKG, EEG and lumbar puncture, PET and CT scanning.

Standard laboratory analysis including complete blood chemistry, electrolytes, glucose, urinalysis, thyroid studies, BUN, creatinine, and liver function.

Complete history and physical including weight, vital signs, and description of physical appearances.

Figure 15-1. ■ Levels of biologic assessment for elders. *Source: Contemporary Psychiatric Mental Health Nursing* by Kneisl/Wilson/Trigoboff (p. 650), © Reprinted by permission of Pearson Education, Inc., Upper Saddle River, NJ.

of delirium due to sleep and sensory deprivation. Having too much stimulation or too little stimulation within the environment may worsen delirium once it has developed (Gleason, 2003). Elderly clients with both a medical illness and an already diagnosed dementia are at the highest risk for developing delirium when hospitalized (Vogel, 2005). Confusion, rather than fever, may be the earliest sign of an infection in the elderly who are already immunocompromised. Although nurses should have the best opportunity to recognize clients who are developing delirium, many do not, especially if certain risk factors are involved. These often-overlooked risk factors are in clients who have the hypoactive form of delirium, who are older than 80, who have visual impairment, or who already have a diagnosis of dementia (Vogel, 2005).

According to the *DSM-IV-TR*, the following comparisons may be made between dementia and delirium. Memory impairment is common to both disorders, but in delirium, it is accompanied by a disturbance in consciousness as well. Another difference is the time of onset. In delirium, onset may be rapid; in dementia, the onset is gradual. Delirium symptoms may fluctuate during a 24-hour period, but dementia symptoms do not. It is also important to note that a client can have delirium on top of an already existing dementia (APA, 2000).

COLLABORATIVE CARE

The response to delirium truly requires a team approach. Nurses, physicians, and nursing assistants should be involved in the hospital setting; social workers and activity directors should also have input into the overall plan of care in the long-term care facility.

Diagnostic Tests

When you study the conditions that can cause delirium, it is obvious that there are a number of diagnostic tests that can be performed to determine if a physiological, or medical, condition is indeed the problem. Figure 15-1 ■ shows the levels of biological assessment for elders.

The blood tests that need to be done should include:

Complete blood count and differential, to identify
- Anemia
- Vitamin B_{12} or folic acid deficiency
- Dehydration
- Bacterial infection; some viral infections

Thyroid panel, to identify hypothyroidism

Plasma ACTH and plasma cortisol and a dexamethasone suppression test, to identify Cushing's syndrome

Albumin level, to identify malnutrition

Arterial blood gases, to identify
- Acid-base imbalances
- Blood oxygen levels

Electrolyte panel, to identify any electrolyte imbalances

Blood sugars, to identify hypo- or hyperglycemia

Drug screen as needed, to identify
- Presence of any mind-altering drugs
- Presence of alcohol

Urine tests may aid in diagnosing a urinary tract infection or the presence of alcohol or other drugs. A spinal tap can determine the presence of blood or microorganisms, which could indicate medical conditions causing the confusion. However, this is considered a very invasive procedure and is ordered only as a last-resort measure when other diagnostic tests have been inconclusive. Radiological exams might include CT scan, MRI, and PET scan (where available) to observe brain structure and physiology. An EEG might be done as well and will generally show abnormally fast or generalized slowing of electrical brain activity (APA, 2000). A slowing of the background rhythm might be found in delirium or dementia unless the delirium is related to alcohol withdrawal (delirium tremens), in which case the EEG shows rapid activity (Gleason, 2003).

History

An accurate history is important to determine if there has been a recent fall or head injury. Since **polypharmacy** (the use of many drugs) is a common practice among elderly clients, it is important to know which drugs and how much a client is taking. The list of medications must include over-the-counter drugs including herbal supplements, which some clients may not mention in a drug history unless the nurse specifically asks. Cognitive dysfunction can result from the drug interactions or from a specific drug, such as digoxin, reaching a toxic level in the client. Clients, especially the elderly, may also have a different, unexpected reaction to a drug (*idiosyncratic reaction*).

Alcohol abuse may be a problem that a client keeps well hidden until hospital admission. Going into an alcohol withdrawal state is inevitable for a hidden alcoholic who loses access to alcohol. This can produce a substance withdrawal delirium. Take the case of a 50-year-old truck driver who was admitted to the ICU following a very bad motor vehicle accident. On regaining consciousness in the ICU, he became extremely agitated, pulling out his tubes and actually knocking over supplies and equipment. He kept trying to "put on the brake" with his foot. His family was surprised that he was going through alcohol withdrawal, as they hadn't even suspected a drinking problem.

Other Screening Tools

In addition to a thorough physical assessment and complete history, the mental status of the client needs to be evaluated. The *Folstein Mini-Mental State Exam* is one test and will be discussed later in the chapter. Its best use is to administer it at various times during the course of the delirium to assess improvement in the client's mental state (Gleason, 2003). It is often the nurse who administers this test. Other screening tools include the *Confusion Assessment Method (CAM)*, the *Delirium Rating Scale (DRS)*, and the *Memorial Delirium Assessment Scale (MDAS)*. The DRS and the MDAS measure the severity

of the delirium (Gleason, 2003). The CAM detects only the presence of delirium. The CAM has several versions: the long version, short version, and one developed for use with nonverbal clients on ventilators in the ICU. The long version screens for the clinical features of delirium as they correlate to the *DSM-IV* criteria for diagnosis; the short version looks at only the four areas that are considered most reliable in distinguishing delirium from other forms of cognitive impairment (Waszynski, 2007).

Physical or Chemical Restraints

Physicians may order physical or chemical restraints for the safety of the confused client. However, the statistics suggest that these do not always improve safety. Physically restrained clients are eight times more likely to die than those who are unrestrained, and 47% of restrained clients sustain injuries while struggling to free themselves from the restraints (Napierkowski, 2002). The immobility produced increases the client's risks for developing decubitus ulcers, constipation, and pneumonia. The nurse should also remember that restraints themselves can cause confusion in addition to causing anger, depression, and combativeness (Napierkowski, 2002). Chemical restraints may also increase confusion due to medication side effects.

There are specific requirements for the use of physical restraints. The Joint Commission on Accreditation of Healthcare Organizations (JCAHO) and the Centers for Medicare and Medicaid Services (CMS) provide guidelines in their standards of care for healthcare facilities to minimize the use of restraints (Napierkowski, 2002). Restraints should be used only if the client is a danger to self or others, or if restraining the client is the only way to complete the necessary nursing care.

The CMS guidelines specify the following (Napierkowski, 2002):

- Restraints should not be used for staff convenience or client discipline.
- The client's family should be included when developing a plan of care and involved in any decision to use restraints. (The facility should notify clients and family members of restraint policies at the time of admission.)
- Restraints must be specifically ordered as to type and time and never be "p.r.n."
- Restraints may be applied in an emergency after careful evaluation of the situation, but the physician should be contacted and an order received within 1 hour of the application of the restraint.

- Restrained clients need continual monitoring and reevaluation as to the continued need for the restraint. No more than 4 hours should go by before the adult is reassessed.
- Documentation should be all-inclusive as to circumstances, type, length of time used, and evidence of client monitoring during use.

The healthcare facility should have specific rules and policies for treatment of the client in physical restraints. As with all clients, the nurse should be aware that using a restraint should be the last resort after other least restrictive alternatives have been tried. It is usually the nurse who requests a restraint order from the physician, although the American Nurses Association itself supports a restraint-free approach to client care. A nurse may apply a physical restraint in an emergency, such as a sudden attack on another client or staff, but the nurse must immediately begin to contact the physician to report the behavior and obtain an order.

Chemical restraints likewise have guidelines for use. In a nursing home, there must be documentation each time a psychotropic medication (medication that affects the mind) is given. In addition, psychotropic medication orders must be reviewed routinely by the physician to determine whether the medication could be discontinued or the dosage reduced. Whether the client is in the hospital or nursing home, the nurse should be aware that psychotropic medications could add to the client's confusion and also intensify the danger of falls by increasing the client's unsteadiness. The drugs most often ordered for the hyperactive form of delirium are the antipsychotics. Loxapine (Loxitane), haloperidol (Haldol), risperidone (Risperdal), and olanzapine (Zyprexa) have all been utilized. Studies show that the newer antipsychotic drugs such as Risperdal and Zyprexa are effective and have fewer side effects for the elderly client (Rathier & McElhaney, 2005). Using both physical restraints and chemical restraints on a client is considered a double restraint and is not allowed in most facilities.

NURSING CARE

ASSESSING

First of all, the nurse needs to be acutely aware of each client's cognitive abilities. Any change from the client's normal status needs to be reported immediately to the physician. Remember, delirium often appears as a *sudden* change in the client's behavior. If a client who has just begun a new medication suddenly behaves like a different person, the change may be due to the medication. Other things the nurse might assess would be a change in the client's lab reports such as a sudden increase in the client's BUN (blood urea nitrogen) or a rise in the ammonia level (often found in clients with cirrhosis of the liver). Both of these lab findings could result in behavior changes. Do not rule out the possibility of a new infection that could be developing as well. Always keep in mind those clients who are most at risk for developing delirium.

DIAGNOSING, PLANNING, AND IMPLEMENTING

Possible nursing diagnoses for delirium include the following:

- Risk for Injury
- Disturbed Sleep Pattern
- Self-Care Deficit: bathing/hygiene; toileting; dressing/grooming, feeding
- Acute Confusion
- Impaired Memory
- Disturbed Thought Processes
- Sporadic Wandering
- Impaired Verbal Communication

Outcomes would be identified based on the specific nursing diagnoses. A care plan would include an appropriate time frame for the following outcomes to make them measurable; the time frame would depend on the actual client situation. For example:

- Client will remain free of injury from falls.
- Client will perform oral and hair care with assistance.
- Client will remain on unit.
- Client will call daughter by correct name.

Promote Client Safety

Safety, communication, and acute confusion issues should be foremost in the care provided for the client with delirium. If the client is extremely agitated in the hospital, family members may be encouraged to stay with the client. If this is not possible, many hospitals hire sitters just to be in the room observing the client and signaling for help as needed. Student nurses are often considered for these sitter positions!

Clients suffering with delirium have numerous behaviors that put them at risk for injury. They may be agitated, restless, and disoriented. They may wander. Their judgment abilities may be impaired. For example, a client with delirium might forget what the call light is for or how to use it and try to get out of bed without asking for help. This could result in a fall and possible fracture. The client may pull out a Foley catheter, causing trauma to the urethra. S/he might wander away from the unit and not remember how to get back.

To help prevent falls, check on the client at least hourly. An electronic alarm on the chair or bed, such as the "RN-On-Call," can be beneficial. This device can be placed under the client in either location. If the client starts to rise, an alarm sounds at the nurses' station, so help can reach the client before a fall occurs. In nursing homes, many clients who tend to wander wear a "Wanderguard" bracelet that trips an alarm if the client approaches an exit.

Placing frequently used personal items close to the client may prevent the client from reaching and falling. Call lights should always be within reach and the bed in its lowest position. In nursing homes, legs may be shortened on the bed to make it closer to the floor; foam pads may be placed next to the bed to cushion falls; mattresses may even be placed directly on the floor to prevent falls. Side rails are considered a restraint. They should be left down unless the client requests or gives you permission to raise them or the physician has specifically ordered them. Review the healthcare facility's policy on side rails.

Provide Diversions

Often distracting the client and redirecting attention may help with agitation; giving clients something to occupy their hands may work. We've had clients fold linen (often at the nurse's station where we could monitor them continually), a repetitive task that is not overwhelming. Soothing music may help. Provide physical activity as the client can tolerate. Walking may relieve some agitation. Family members can provide clues as to some favorite quiet activities (jigsaw puzzles, checkers, playing cards) the client has enjoyed in the past.

Monitor and Document Use of Restraints and Client Behavior

If a physical restraint is used, the client should be checked every 15 minutes and the restraints removed every 2 hours. When the restraint is removed, the client should be repositioned, taken to the toilet or offered a bedpan, and given fluids. The skin under the restraint should be assessed and massaged as needed. The least restrictive restraint should be used whenever a restraint is needed. The type of physical restraint must be specifically ordered by the physician.

Documentation of chemical restraints is extremely important. It must occur each time a psychotropic medication is administered. The documentation record must contain an exact description of the client's behavior and the frequency of the behavior.

Critical Self-Check. What does agitation mean to you? If you saw the documentation that a client was agitated, what picture would come into your mind?

An example of *poor* documentation of client behavior would be "Client was agitated." *Good* documentation might be "Client has been pacing the halls and pulling at his gown for 2 hours. He states he 'hates everyone' and threatened another client with his fist." Since everyone's mental picture of agitation will vary, the second description gives the reader of the documentation a clearer picture of the behavior that prompted the use of the chemical restraints.

Documentation should also state what conservative interventions were attempted *before* the psychotropic medication was given. For example, the nurse might have walked a client to the sunroom and back, taken the client to the bathroom, turned on quiet music, or offered a cold drink.

Orient the Client to Reality

To respond to the acute confusion of the client with delirium, all staff should consistently use **reality orientation.** There are several simple ways to do this:

- Have a calendar in the room and mark off each day as it passes.
- Have a digital clock in the room.
- Call the client by name and introduce yourself each time you enter the room.
- Provide a reality orientation board that lists the day, date, season, and expected weather for the day.

Communicate with clients in a clear, calm manner. Use simple words and short sentences. If the client does not seem to understand you the first time you say something, repeat what you said at least two more times using the same exact words. You might have to act out your words as you say them. All staff need to be consistent in communication approaches.

Involve the families. Have them bring familiar objects in from the client's own home. Just the presence of family may help to increase the client's sense of security and lessen the confusion (Gleason, 2003).

Simplify and Clarify the Environment

It often helps to remove nonessential items from the client's room and allow more space between client beds if the room must be shared. Private rooms are much more client-friendly for the client suffering with delirium. Speak in lay person's terms to the client instead of using the "medicalese" language that s/he might misinterpret. Provide enough light including a night light and control as much excess noise as possible. Make sure clients who wear glasses have them on and that clients with hearing aids have them in (Gleason, 2003). It also helps if the glasses are clean and the hearing aids have batteries that are working. (We had a female client who we thought was developing delirium when actually her hearing aid battery needed replacing!)

EVALUATING

Evaluating a client with delirium requires keen observation and listening skills. The family can be a valuable resource in reporting improvements or increased problems. Communication among caregivers is essential. Specific cognitive gains or losses should be documented clearly in the client's chart.

Dementia

Dementia is commonly defined as a progressive, irreversible loss of cognitive functioning that impairs a person's ability to function in social or occupational situations. Dementia describes a group of symptoms; it is not a specific disease itself (Mace & Rabins, 1999).

The *DSM-IV-TR* does not assign a prognosis to the condition but focuses on the pattern of cognitive defects. The American Psychiatric Association describes dementia as being *progressive*, *static*, or *remitting*. It must be severe enough to impair social or occupational functioning and must be clearly identifiable as a decline from a previously higher level of functioning (APA, 2000). Box 15-3 ■ provides a more specific description of Dementia of the Alzheimer's Type.

All dementias are characterized by multiple cognitive deficits. Unlike delirium, in dementia there is a progressive decline in cognitive function as the disorder worsens.

BOX 15-3

Diagnostic Criteria for Dementia of the Alzheimer's Type

A. The development of multiple cognitive deficits manifested by both
  1. *Memory impairment* (impaired ability to learn new information or to recall previously learned information)
  2. One (or more) of the following cognitive disturbances:
     a. *Aphasia* (language disturbance)
     b. *Apraxia* (impaired ability to carry out motor activities despite intact motor function)
     c. *Agnosia* (failure to recognize or identify objects despite intact sensory function)
     d. Disturbance in executive functioning (e.g., planning, organizing, sequencing, abstracting)
B. The cognitive deficits above each cause significant impairment in social or occupational functioning and represent a significant decline from a previous level of functioning.
C. The course is characterized by gradual onset and continuing cognitive decline.
D. The cognitive deficits in Criteria A1 and A2 are not due to any of the following:
  1. Other central nervous system conditions that cause progressive deficits in memory and cognition (e.g., CVA, Parkinson's disease, Huntington's disease,

subdural hematoma, normal-pressure hydrocephalus, brain tumor)
  2. Systemic conditions that are known to cause dementia (e.g., hypothyroidism, vitamin B_{12} or folic acid deficiency, niacin deficiency, hypercalcemia, neurosyphilis, HIV infection)
  3. Substance-induced conditions
E. The deficits do not occur exclusively during the course of a delirium.
F. The disturbance is not better accounted for by another Axis I disorder (e.g., Major Depressive Disorder, Schizophrenia).

Criteria will include whether or not there are clinically significant behavioral disturbance:

  Without Behavioral Disturbance
  With Behavioral Disturbance

There are two subtypes for Dementia of the Alzheimer's Type:

  With Early Onset: if onset is at age 65 years or below
  With Late Onset: if onset is after age 65 years

Source: Reprinted with permission from the *Diagnostic and Statistical Manual of Mental Disorders, Text Revision,* copyright 2000. American Psychiatric Association.

In order to diagnose dementia, memory impairment plus one other evidence of cognitive dysfunction must be present. These dysfunctions include **aphasia** (deterioration of language function), **apraxia** (impaired ability to perform motor activities even though motor abilities and sensory functions are intact), **agnosia** (failure to recognize or identify familiar common objects despite having intact sensory functions), or a **disturbance of executive functioning** (inability to think abstractly or to use critical thinking to plan, initiate, sequence, monitor, and stop complex behavior) (APA, 2000).

Dementia of the Alzheimer's Type involves the parts of the brain that affect thoughts, memory, and language, thus causing the symptoms listed previously. Figure 15-2 ■ gives a more comprehensive description of behavioral changes associated with specific areas of brain damage.

TYPES AND CAUSES OF DEMENTIA

The *DSM-IV-TR* identifies at least 12 different types of dementia. Dementia of the Alzheimer's Type, or Alzheimer's disease, is the most common and is the focus of this chapter.

Alzheimer's disease (AD) was first identified by Dr. Alois Alzheimer in 1906 on a 51-year-old woman. At that time, he thought the disease was a dementia found only in younger clients, so he called it presenile dementia. Now we know that the disease can occur in any age group but is more common in those over 60 years of age. It is estimated that 4.5 million people in the United States have AD. It is categorized as late-onset and early-onset with 65 years being the dividing point (Petersen, 2002).

Many studies have been done to pinpoint the exact etiology of Alzheimer's disease. There are still no definitive answers to the question of cause, although there are a number of hypotheses. (You have probably heard the old theory of aluminum cookware being the culprit!) Scientists now believe that the cause of the disease is not one but several factors acting together to produce disease.

Risk Factors

Scientists do agree on a number of factors that put a person at risk for developing Alzheimer's disease. The most common *definite* risk factor is a person's age. The number of people with the disease doubles every 5 years beyond age 65. By the age of 85, chances of developing Alzheimer's disease increases to 50% (Shankle & Amen, 2004).

Another *definite* risk factor is family history, especially if the family member is a first-degree relative such as a

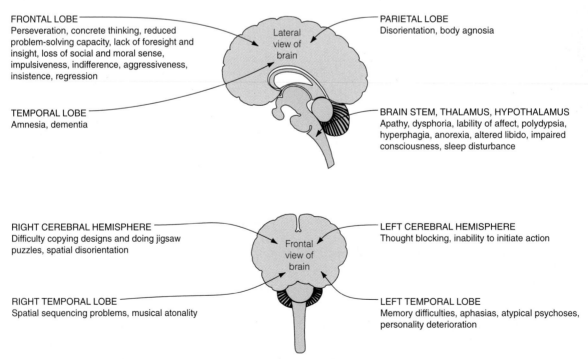

Figure 15-2. ■ Behavioral changes related to specific areas of brain damage. Damage to each part of the brain results in specific alterations and deficits in client behaviors and skills. *Source: Contemporary Psychiatric Mental Health Nursing* by Kneisl/Wilson/Trigoboff (p. 240), © Reprinted by permission of Pearson Education, Inc., Upper Saddle River, NJ.

parent or sibling. Those with a first-degree relative with AD are 1.5 to 2 times as likely to develop the disease as those where there is no family history (Kuhn, 1999). Five percent of Alzheimer's disease cases are called *early-onset familial AD*, a rare type of the disease that usually occurs between the ages of 30 and 60. Three definite genetic mutations are linked to this early-onset form of the disease (Gruetzner, 2001). Studies differ as to whether there is a genetic component to late-onset AD, but most scientists agree that heredity makes certain people more susceptible to the disease.

Other *definite* risk factors that have been proposed include history of Down syndrome, history of head trauma, and low educational status and occupational level (Kuhn, 1999). Being diagnosed with Mild Cognitive Impairment (MCI) is now known to greatly increase one's risk of developing dementia. Clients with this diagnosis need to be evaluated and monitored closely as this diagnosis increases one's chances of developing AD later on (Shankle & Amen, 2004). It is estimated that almost half the clients diagnosed with MCI will go on to develop AD within 5 years (Valeo, 2006). According to the Alzheimer's Association, MCI is difficult to diagnose but often represents a stage in between normal aging function and dementia. Studies are being conducted to determine if donepezil (Aricept), a medication used in the early stages of AD, can delay the development of AD in a client who has been diagnosed with MCI (Valeo, 2006). Some neurologists believe that diet, physical exercise, genetics, as well as mental activity play a role as well in the development of AD after the diagnosis of MCI. The Alzheimer's Association has developed a 1-hour workshop called "Maintain Your Brain" to encourage the continuation of mental activities on into old age (Alzheimer's Association, 2005).

Being female is a *possible* risk factor. Even when you consider that women live longer than men and that advanced age is a risk factor, women still have a greater chance than men of developing the disease (Petersen, 2002). Other *possible* risk factors include history of small strokes, history of Parkinson's disease, African American heritage, environmental toxins, high-fat diet, lack of exercise, and stress. Risk factors that are under investigation include studying a correlation between AD and hypertension, high cholesterol, and smoking. Dr. William H. Thies, Alzheimer's Association vice president, indicates that these studies prove that "what is good for your heart is good for your head" (Alzheimer's Association, 2005).

A newer theory being studied is a link between AD and diabetes. The theory is that impaired brain cell functions and cell death result from the way the brain cells use sugar. People with diabetes who have very poor blood sugar control have the greatest risk of developing dementia. Therefore, scientists see a great need to detect borderline diabetes early in order to proactively deter the advancement into actual type 2 diabetes and possible dementia. Current research is being conducted to determine the effect of the antidiabetic drug rosiglitazone (Avandia). It is hoped that the drug might prevent the development of AD by reducing the inflammatory responses to the presence of the amyloid beta protein occurring in AD (Alzheimer's Association, 2006a).

Etiology of AD

Chromosomes 21, 14, 1, and 19 all contain genes that can be related to the development of AD, especially the early-onset variety (Petersen, 2002). (Abnormalities in chromosome 21 are also found in Down syndrome.) Of these, the most significant abnormality seems to be linked to a certain type of gene, located on chromosome 19, that controls the production of apolipoprotein (ApoE). ApoE is a protein that transports cholesterol in the blood. The genes responsible for the production of ApoE are $ApoE_2$, $ApoE_3$, and $ApoE_4$. One of these types of genes is inherited from each biological parent. People with the gene known as $ApoE_4$ have a higher risk of developing AD than people with the other types. However, not everyone with the $ApoE_4$ gene develops Alzheimer's disease (Petersen, 2002). While the other genes lead to early-onset AD, inheriting variants of the $ApoE_4$ gene increases one's chances of developing late-onset AD and may also lower the age of onset (Petersen, 2002).

Although scientists have been unable to discover the ultimate cause of Alzheimer's disease, they do know what they find in the brain of people who have been autopsied following death from the disease: the presence of **beta-amyloid plaques** and **neurofibrillary tangles.** Figure 15-3 ■ shows a microphotograph of neurofibrillary tangles and senile plaques. The beta-amyloid plaques are the buildup of fragments produced when certain enzymes in the body act on amyloid protein. You might compare this to the buildup of old wax on floors or furniture. Eventually, you have a dirty, gummy substance that no longer lets the beauty of the wood shine through. In much the same way, the brain of the person with Alzheimer's disease is covered with plaques that no longer allow the brain to function normally, and the ability to "shine" is lost.

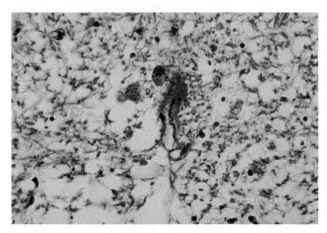

Figure 15-3. ■ Neurofibrillary tangles and beta-amyloid plaques are seen in this microphotograph using a silver stain of the hippocampal cortex in a client with Alzheimer's disease. *Source:* Visuals Unlimited.

The neurofibrillary tangles are composed of another protein called *tau*, which is part of the neurons' (nerve cells') internal support system. In AD, the tau changes, pairs up with other threads of tau, and becomes tangled. Communication between neurons ceases, transportation of nutrients to the cells declines, and the cells die. Imagine if you had tangled electrical wiring with spots that were fused together. You would not be able to conduct a current from the electrical outlet to the equipment you wanted to operate. In just the same way, these tangles eliminate clear pathways in the brain. Clear thoughts are not able to emerge when the brain is full of tangles. The tangles and plaques usually appear in the areas of the brain that are most important to memory, with plaques on the outside and tangles inside the neurons. Studies continue to determine whether the tangles and plaques cause AD or are the result of the disease process.

Another finding has been the deficiency of the neurotransmitter acetylcholine. This chemical substance is a messenger of the nervous system. When it is lacking, not all messages can be transmitted. Again, it is unclear whether acetylcholine deficiency is a cause or an effect of the disease process.

Other hypotheses about the cause of AD consider inflammatory processes within the brain or the presence of free radicals. (*Free radicals* are unstable, freely moving molecules that are "waste products" resulting from oxidative processes within the body.) The theory is that the immune cells of the body see the plaques or damaged neurons in the body as foreign substances. When they try to remove them, an inflammatory process develops. The inflammatory process precipitates an overproduction of free radicals, and so the cycle continues (Petersen, 2002).

Some scientists have suggested that loss of estrogen after menopause makes women more susceptible to the disease as they age. Estrogen is thought to protect the brain from AD. Another suggestion is the presence of plaques triggers excessive calcium entering the neurons and killing the cells (Petersen, 2002).

SYMPTOMS AND STAGES

Alzheimer's disease is a disease of slow change. As a nurse or nursing student, your care of these clients will be determined by which stage of the disease your clients have and which symptoms they demonstrate. The Alzheimer's Association has identified the 10 warning signs of Alzheimer's disease (Box 15-4 ■).

The *DSM-IV-TR* does not stage the disease but lists several cognitive impairments as signs and symptoms. Although impaired memory is a symptom in all stages of AD, the other cognitive impairments do not all appear at the same time in this disorder. For a visual reinforcement of the stages and symptoms of AD, you might want to see the movie *The Notebook*, based on Nicholas Sparks's touching novel.

There are various ways to stage Alzheimer's disease, using from three to seven stages. This text presents the stages of *early, middle,* and *late* used by the Alzheimer's Association. The progression of symptoms in a woman called "Edith" will give you a clearer picture of what you might expect as you care for clients in each stage of the disease.

Early Stage

In the early stage of the disease, symptoms may go unnoticed by family or friends, especially if the client is living alone. A close loved one in the home may notice a few minor things but dismiss them as being a normal part of aging. Spouses have also been known to "cover up" the confusion of the affected spouse, so that other family members are unaware of the condition. The early stage usually lasts from 2 to 4 years. (Antidementia medications may prolong this stage.) During this stage of the disease, there is a gradual memory loss, especially for short-term memory. Clients may become confused about directions and decisions. They may become lost if they go out and so stay home more. They lose spontaneity. They do not try to learn new things (Alzheimer's Learning Institute, 2001). The person may be vaguely aware of memory problems and compensate by avoiding new situations and places and staying with familiar things and routines (Petersen, 2002).

BOX 15-4

Ten Warning Signs of Alzheimer's Disease

1. **Memory loss.** Frequently forgets assignments, colleague's names, or a business associate's telephone number, any recently learned information and does not remember the information later.
2. **Difficulty performing familiar tasks.** May have difficulty planning or completing every day tasks such as preparing a meal, may forget to serve it after it is made, may not remember even preparing the meal. May forget how to place a telephone call or how to play a game.
3. **Problems with language.** May forget simple words or substitute unusual words, making sentences incomprehensible. May describe an item by what it's used for rather than by its name.
4. **Disorientation of time and place.** May become lost on their own street, not knowing where they are, how they got there, or how to get back home.
5. **Poor or decreased judgment.** May dress inappropriately, wearing several shirts or blouses on a warm day or little clothing in the cold. May show poor judgment

such as giving away large sums of money to telemarketers.
6. **Problems with abstract thinking.** May have unusual difficulty performing complex mental tasks such as balancing a checkbook; may forget completely what the numbers are and what needs to be done with them.
7. **Misplacing things.** May put things in inappropriate places such as an iron in the freezer or a watch in the sugar bowl.
8. **Changes in mood or behavior.** May exhibit rapid mood swings from calm to tears to anger for no apparent reason.
9. **Changes in personality.** Personality may change drastically, becoming extremely confused, suspicious, fearful, or dependent on a family member.
10. **Loss of initiative.** May become passive, sitting in front of the TV for hours or sleeping more than usual; may not want to do usual activities and require cues and prompting to become involved.

Source: Adapted from Alzheimer's Association. (2007). *Ten warning signs of Alzheimer's.* Available: http://www.alz.org/alzheimers_disease_symptoms_of_alzheimers.asp. Used with permission.

CASE EXAMPLE

Consider our client, Edith. Edith lived alone in an older apartment building where she had previously been very self-sufficient. She walked to a nearby grocery store, caught the bus to go shopping, did her own laundry in the apartment facilities, wrote letters, cooked for herself, and enjoyed being with and talking to people. She never turned down an invitation to go out. As the disease began to take hold of her, she stayed in more and more. She turned down social opportunities, saying she had to stay in to write her children. When her children called to find out why she hadn't written, she said she had been too busy going out. Numerous half-finished letters were found in her apartment. It was evident that she had lost her train of thought and just stopped writing. She stopped going to the apartment complex's laundry facilities and began washing her clothes in the bathtub. Sometimes, she would just put her dirty clothes back into her drawer or hang them back up in the closet. Her apartment started looking disheveled and she no longer could remember how to cook much except chili and a lemon cake. She had someone else manage her checkbook and pay her bills. She just signed her name.

Middle Stage

The middle, or second, stage of the disease is usually the longest. It may last from 2 to 10 years after the diagnosis. During this stage, memory loss and confusion

increase. The client starts to have difficulty recognizing close family and friends. The client may wander, becoming particularly restless in late afternoon or early evening. S/he might have difficulty organizing thoughts or thinking logically. The client might experience hallucinations, delusions, or illusions as found in mental illnesses already discussed. S/he may behave inappropriately in public or make inappropriate comments.

An **illusion** is a misinterpretation of environmental stimuli. This is a special problem for the client with AD because of already existing perceptual problems. Distance perception is distorted, making a bathtub look like a bottomless pit. The intercom or a radio appears to be a disembodied voice that the client with AD cannot quite comprehend. For example, if clients are watching television, they may not be able to distinguish between what is on the television and what is in their living room. They may become frightened that strangers have entered their home.

Clients may *confabulate*. This means that if they do not know the answer to something, they will make up an answer that sounds logical rather than admit their confusion. They may dress inappropriately, sometimes wearing underwear on top of outside clothing (Alzheimer's Learning Institute, 2001).

CASE EXAMPLE

Consider our client, Edith, in the middle stage of the disease. When Edith's daughter suspected there was something wrong, she invited her mother to come for a visit. On the first night, Edith got up in the middle of the night and urinated in the bedroom trash basket, thinking it was a toilet. She brought summer clothes and no coat for a visit in November. When her daughter moved her from her old home to a new apartment close by, Edith needed daily supervision. When Edith saw herself in the mirror on her door, she did not recognize herself. She told her daughter there was a child living behind the door. Edith sometimes spoke to her daughter as if her daughter were Edith's mother or sister. She called her granddaughter her niece. When she was waiting her turn in the doctor's office, a woman walked in wearing a brightly colored blouse. Edith asked her, "Did you just get back from the circus?" When asked why she had poured water into a jar of instant coffee, she replied, "I didn't. The coffee just melted." The daughter realized it was time for Edith to receive full-time care when Edith cut the cord of her electric blanket because she could not unplug it. (Fortunately, it was not turned on.)

Late Stage

The late, or third, stage of the disease may last from 1 to 3 years. In this stage, the client is disoriented to self and family. Communication becomes a problem, as speech may become more and more nonsensical. The client loses the ability to do any self-care and may not even remember how to use a toothbrush or comb. Some clients may experience **hyperorality** in this stage; that is, they revert back to the infantile behavior of putting everything into their mouths. They become totally incontinent. Clients need to be fed and may even forget how to swallow. They are susceptible to choking, pneumonia, and other infections. Seizures may occur. Some clients just lie in bed in the fetal position. The culmination of this stage, of course, is death.

CASE EXAMPLE

Edith maintained a pleasant demeanor throughout her disease. She laughed inappropriately when she could no longer think of words to say. She had to be dressed, fed, and changed. She died from a stroke less than 10 years from when she was diagnosed.

ALTERED BEHAVIORS ASSOCIATED WITH AD

As you can see from the preceding paragraphs, a pattern of problem behaviors begins to emerge as the client progresses in the disease. Six of those behaviors will be discussed here: wandering, sundowning, refusal to bathe, paranoia, language disturbances, and catastrophic reactions.

Wandering

Wandering is a common manifestation of the confusion that results from AD. It can include pacing up and down, aimless walking, or leaving the home, hospital unit, or nursing facility (Petersen, 2002). Persons may wander because they start to take a walk, forget where they are going, and cannot find their way back home. What started out as a purposeful behavior becomes random, as they search for familiar landmarks. Another reason clients may wander is that they are looking for something they think they have lost. Clients may wander from room to room in the nursing home. If a staff member asks them what they are looking for, the common response will be, "I've lost something." When pressed for what the "something" is, most clients will say, "I don't know. I just know it's gone." It has been suggested that these clients know that something meaningful is now missing from their lives and are searching to regain it. What they do not realize is that what they have lost are their cognitive abilities. Other reasons to wander might include physical discomfort (such as having to go to the bathroom), searching for home or family, or just plain boredom from lack of stimulation (Schweiger & Huey, 1999).

Sundowning

Sundowning is a term used to describe the increased confusion noted in clients with AD in the late afternoon or evening. This behavior might manifest itself as an escalation in pacing and irritability. One suggested reason for this behavior is that the client with AD has perceptual problems. With a dimming of light, those perceptual problems worsen. The environment is filled with shadows; objects are not clear; and what the client thinks he or she sees may be frightening. Another suggestion is that the client is tired by that time of day and does not handle stress as well. Any external stimuli may seem overwhelming and may result in the pacing and irritability so often seen.

Refusal to Bathe

Refusal to bathe or refusal to do any of the activities of daily living (ADLs) might also become a problem behavior. You probably look forward to your bath or shower as a pleasant experience; the client with AD may see it as threatening. Clients with AD often lack depth perception. Just as a bathtub may look like a bottomless pit, a faucet or showerhead may look like a strange, threatening object coming at them. The client does not understand anymore what they are and what they do. Also, the client may associate bathing with being wet, cold, and uncomfortable. The client may be overwhelmed with the number of actions needed to accomplish the bath.

> **Critical Self-Check.** Take a few minutes and write down the steps you take when having a bath or shower. There are probably 30 or more. Now imagine that you do not care about cleanliness, have impaired motor abilities, and do not understand what is happening to you. What would it take to get you into the bathtub?

In addition to being fearful, consider that some old habits, such as personal modesty, may still be ingrained in clients with AD, despite the fact that many memories have been forgotten. Therefore, having someone else assist them in removing their clothing and getting into the bathtub or shower may be the reason for refusal and a combative episode.

> **Critical Self-Check.** How would you react if a total stranger approached you and began removing your clothing to assist you into the bathtub?

Although the caregivers routinely assist clients with activities of daily living, poor short-term memory may make them look like strangers. Clients with AD may strike out at the caregiver and refuse to take a bath at all. Similar refusals to get dressed for the day or get undressed for bedtime may also result.

Paranoia

Paranoia, or suspicious thinking, is almost inevitably a problem behavior exhibited by clients with AD. Clients with AD often accuse family members of stealing from them. For instance, a client named Lois who still lived at home stated, "That girl came in here and stole my sheets." The "girl" was her daughter who came in weekly to change the beds and take the dirty laundry home to wash. Clients with AD may also hide items to protect them from being stolen. With poor short-term memory, they then forget where they put them and may accuse others of taking them.

CASE EXAMPLE

Ruth, a resident of a long-term care facility, could not find her dentures and accused another resident of taking them. In helping Ruth to look for them, the staff member had to consider what item in the client's room might look like a denture cup. Finally, the missing dentures were found pushed down into a jar of cold cream!

Language Disturbances

Language disturbances begin in the early stages of Alzheimer's disease and progress to the late stage where total *aphasia* (no speech) may occur. In the early stages, this might manifest as inability to find the right words. The client begins a sentence and then struggles to find the word needed to complete the thought. The client may sometimes describe an item by its function. For example, a "glass" might be "that thing you put water in when you want to drink." Clients may use invented words (**neologisms**) when they cannot think of the right one. They might use "briarbush" for hairbrush, or a word that does not even resemble the word they are trying to remember. They often giggle nervously when they cannot recall a word.

Clients may also ask the same question or repeat the same word over and over as well as repeat the same actions. This repetitive speech or behavior is called **perseveration.** It can be irritating to the caregiver who is constantly answering the same question or listening to the same word. It does no good to say, "I just answered that. Don't you remember?" Clients do not remember or they would not be asking the question again.

As the disease progresses, clients with AD seem to lose words in the reverse order of how the words were learned. For example, a 2-year-old begins speech by naming objects, or nouns; then verbs are added; and short sentences are formed. Adjectives, adverbs, and prepositions come later to form more complex sentences. Clients with AD lose speech in reverse order. They lose adjectives, adverbs, and prepositions first, and nouns last. They may revert all the way back from complex sentences to single words. Frustration may build for the client and for the caregiver, as communication becomes more difficult, and the client cannot express his/her needs in the language that the caregiver can understand. Other problem behaviors may escalate when verbal communication ceases. Think about a 2-year-old who has a temper tantrum because you cannot understand what s/he wants.

In the final stages, clients may not speak at all. However, it is impossible to predict how much they understand.

CASE EXAMPLE

In one instance, Agnes, who had been aphasic for 1 year, was admitted into the nursing home. Tom, her husband of 50 years, had been caring for her at home. Tom came daily to the nursing home to feed her each meal. During her stay, Tom had a heart attack and was taken to the hospital. After 2 days of Tom not being there, Agnes looked at her nursing assistant and said, "Where's Tom?" The nursing assistant answered her question, and the client never spoke again. The staff had no explanation for those two words!

Catastrophic Reactions

Catastrophic reactions may occur at any time during the course of the disease. They are usually described as an explosive response that is totally out of proportion to the situation that caused it. Behaviors that you might see include screaming, crying, using loud profanity, hitting, spitting, kicking, and so on (you get the picture). Clients with AD have difficulty controlling emotional behavior because of physiological changes in the brain. The part of the brain that allows judgment and critical thinking is not functioning properly, so the client cannot control the inappropriate behavior. Clients with AD have difficulty processing multiple stimuli. They have trouble communicating. When faced with too many requests, too many questions, too many choices, they may respond catastrophically, screaming or striking out at the closest person or object. Clients may also be **emotionally labile.** (Moods may change for no apparent reason.) Clients may cry excessively or laugh at nothing, especially when faced with a situation that they do not understand.

Sometimes, it is possible to predict what situation or person will trigger the catastrophic reaction; other times, it is not. Reviewing each situation as it occurs, including precipitating events or persons, may help the caregiver to avoid the problem behavior in the future. Interventions for difficult AD behaviors are discussed in the Nursing Care section later in the chapter. Figure 15-4 ■ shows a man who is responding with catastrophic anger being supported by his caregiver wife.

COLLABORATIVE CARE

The care of the AD client involves a multitude of team players. In addition to the physician and nurse, the social worker, activity director, sometimes physical therapist or occupational therapist, the speech therapist, and the certified nursing assistant compose the treatment team. Family members and the client, when possible, need to be part of the team as well.

The critical first step is to diagnose the condition as accurately as possible. Because the signs and symptoms of delirium and dementia are so similar, the physician needs to eliminate all of the possible treatable causes of a delirium

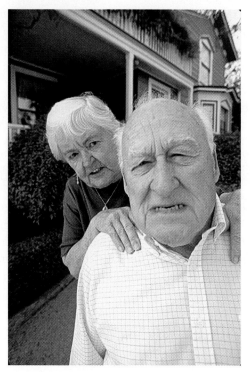

Figure 15-4. ■ Man showing catastrophic anger and his caregiver wife. *Source: PhotoEdit Inc.*

problem. The tests mentioned under delirium are conducted to rule out reversible conditions. The physician will also refer to the criteria (Box 15-3 in this chapter) set up in the *DSM-IV-TR* as part of the diagnosis process.

A complete physical exam is usually conducted and may include questions related to the memory process. It is important that family members are present to hear the questions and answers or that the family members are accessible to validate the answers given by the client. Very often the client will make up answers to cover up for the poor memory; someone unfamiliar with the client might assume these answers are accurate. Remember our client Edith. When the doctor was conducting her physical exam, he asked her where her children were born. Edith replied, "Oh, we lived in so many places, it's hard to remember." Actually, the family had lived in only two places when the children were born. Edith's answer sounded plausible but was untrue.

Although an MRI or CT scan may show some deterioration in the brain (shrinkage in the structure of the brain associated with memory), neither test can *prove* the condition is truly Alzheimer's disease. Another test that is currently being promoted as more definitive is the PET scan, which may help with earlier diagnosis and treatment of AD (Brindle, 2005). Images produced by the

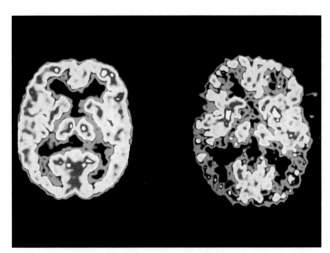

Figure 15-5. ■ Normal PET scan on left with active red and yellow areas signifying normal metabolic rates. Alzheimer's PET scan on right with abnormally large areas of blue signifying abnormally low metabolism in the parietal and temporal lobes. *Source:* Photo Researchers, Inc.

PET scan can show the presence of beta-amyloid protein in the brain of clients with AD (Alzheimer's Association, 2007b). Figure 15-5 ■ shows an example of the PET scan of a client with Alzheimer's disease.

ApoE genotyping is a genetic test that may be used to assist in confirming only the late-onset AD (Brindle, 2005). In addition to the laboratory tests and radiologic studies, the client's mental status is also examined. As mentioned earlier, the physician may simply ask the client random questions during a physical exam to determine the client's cognitive abilities and the extent of memory impairment. If the client is being admitted to a healthcare facility, a structured brief mental status exam may be administered. There are a number available. The Mini-Mental State Examination (MMSE) developed by M. F. Folstein is one of the most commonly used exams (Box 15-5 ■). It tests the client's orientation, language ability (usage, comprehension, reading, and writing), math ability, and short-term memory. The examiner provides a subjective estimation of the client's level of consciousness. When administering this test, the nurse needs to consider the client's educational level as well (Naylor, Stephens, Bowles, & Bixby, 2005). A perfect score on this test is 30, but anything over 24 is considered within the normal range.

Clients who pass the MMSE with a borderline score, that is, anything around 23 or 24, may also be tested with the Brief Dementia Severity Rating Scale (BDSRS), which may be more definitive in identifying clients with

---

BOX 15-5

Mini-Mental State Exam

Orientation to Time
  "What is the date?"
Registration
  "Listen carefully. I am going to say three words, You say them back after I stop.
  Ready? Here they are . . .
  HOUSE (pause), CAR (pause), LAKE (pause). Now repeat those words back to me."
  [Repeat up to five times, but score only the first trial.]
Naming
  "What is this?" [Point to a pencil or pen.]
Reading
  "Please read this and do what it says." [Show examinee the words on the stimulus form.]
  CLOSE YOUR EYES

Source: Reproduced by special permission of the Publisher, Psychological Assessment Resources, Inc., 16204 North Florida Avenue, Lutz, Florida 33549, from the Mini Mental State Examination, by Marshal Folstein and Susan Folstein, Copyright 1975, 1998, 2001 by Mini Mental LLC, Inc. Published 2001 by Psychological Assessment Resources, Inc. Further reproduction is prohibited without permission of PAR, Inc. The MMSE can be purchased from PAR, Inc. by calling (800)331-8378 or (813)968-3003.

---

cognitive losses (Naylor et al., 2005). The Confusion Assessment Method (CAM), referred to in the section on delirium, is sometimes used during the mental assessment for diagnosing AD. A newer mental status exam is called the Mini-Cog, and it is composed of a three-item recall and a clock-drawing test. It can be used in all healthcare settings and, unlike the MMSE, results are not skewed by education, language, or culture (Doerflinger, 2007).

The diagnosis usually is reached when the physician has ruled out all other causes. Then, the doctor may say that the *probable* diagnosis is Alzheimer's disease. Statistics show that this ruling out process is 90% accurate (Brindle, 2005). To date, the only absolute confirmation of the disease is by autopsy.

Medications

Although there is no cure for AD, researchers have discovered medications that may prolong the early to middle stages of the disease. These medications are in the family of the **cholinesterase inhibitors** and are referred to as antidementia drugs. As mentioned earlier, clients with AD have reduced amounts of a chemical messenger (neurotransmitter) called acetylcholine. Cholinesterase inhibitors prolong the time that the body has use of acetylcholine. They do this by inhibiting the action of acetylcholinesterase, a natural enzyme that destroys acetylcholine in the body. Fifty percent of clients using the cholinesterase inhibitors show some improvement with the drugs (Alzheimer's Association, 2007e).

Many clients with AD who use cholinesterase inhibitors have improved cognition, behavior, and functioning (Gray-Vickrey, 2002). However, the brain produces less and less acetylcholine as Alzheimer's disease progresses, so there is a smaller amount of the neurotransmitter available to the drug. Table 15-3 ▪ provides a comprehensive review of the current medications.

The first cholinesterase inhibitor that was available was tacrine (Cognex) in 1993. Currently, it is not mar-

keted by the drug company and seldom prescribed, because it is associated with serious GI disturbances and liver toxicity (Brindle, 2005). Tacrine also must be given four times a day, a disadvantage if the client resists taking medications.

The newer cholinesterase inhibitors are donepezil (Aricept), rivastigmine (Exelon), and galantamine (Razadyne). The most common side effects of these drugs are nausea, vomiting, anorexia, and diarrhea. These drugs increase the risk of stomach ulcers and are therefore given with caution in those clients who are currently taking NSAIDS. All have the potential for causing bradycardia and should be used with caution in those clients already taking medications to slow the heart or those who have a tendency toward bradycardia.

TABLE 15-3

Drugs Used in Treatment of Alzheimer's Disease

DRUG	ACTION	USUAL DOSE AND FORM	SIDE EFFECTS	NURSING CONSIDERATIONS
Tacrine (Cognex)	Cholinesterase Inhibitor	Capsule form 10 mg 4X/day; may be increased by 4 mg/day every 4 weeks to reach max. of 40 mg 4X/day	Nausea, diarrhea, liver damage, GI bleeding, bradycardia	Monitor cognitive functions. Monitor heart rate daily. Monitor liver enzymes. Use NSAIDS with caution. Give with food.
Donepezil (Aricept)	Cholinesterase Inhibitor	PO tablets and orally dissolving tablets (ODT) 5 mg daily; may be increased to 10 mg daily after 4–6 weeks	Nausea/vomiting, diarrhea, headache, bradycardia	Monitor cognitive functions. Monitor heart rate daily. Use NSAIDS with caution. Note the drug interactions possible. Give at bedtime. Allow ODT to dissolve on tongue, and then follow with glass of water.
Rivastigmine (Exelon)	Cholinesterase Inhibitor	Capsules and oral solution 1.5 mg twice a day; may increase by 3 mg/day every 2 weeks until a maximum of 6 mg twice a day given	Nausea/vomiting, weight loss, upset stomach, muscle weakness	Monitor cognitive functions. Monitor for GI disturbances. Remind client that smoking may decrease blood levels of drug. Use with caution with NSAIDS. Educate client and caregiver on proper use of oral solution syringe. Give with food.
Galantamine (Razadyne)	Cholinesterase Inhibitor	Tablet, extended-release capsule, oral solution 4 mg twice a day; may be increased every 4 weeks until a maximum of 12 mg twice a day is reached. Extended-release capsules are given 8 mg/day in single dose and may be increased every 4 weeks to reach a maximum of 24 mg/day.	Nausea/vomiting, weight loss, diarrhea, bradycardia	Monitor cognitive functions. Monitor heart rate daily. Monitor for GI disturbances. Give with morning and evening meals. Give extended-release capsules in AM with food. Encourage client to drink 6–8 glasses of water daily.

(continued)

TABLE 15-3				
Drugs Used in Treatment of Alzheimer's Disease (continued)				
DRUG	**ACTION**	**USUAL DOSE AND FORM**	**SIDE EFFECTS**	**NURSING CONSIDERATIONS**
Memantine (Namenda)	N-methyl-D-aspartate (NMDA)-receptor antagonist	Tablets and oral solutions 5 mg daily; may increase weekly until a maximum dose of 20 mg/day (10 mg twice a day) reached.	Dizziness, headache, constipation, confusion, anemia	Monitor cognitive functions. Monitor hemoglobin and hematocrit. Educate the client and family about the possibility of falls due to dizziness. Give oral solution with syringe provided.
Vitamin E	Nutritional supplement	400 to 800 IU twice a day as supplement to cholinesterase inhibitor	No significant problems noted with low dosages; nausea and cramping with high dosages	Educate clients about the blood-thinning effects of Vitamin E. Clients on warfarin (Coumadin), aspirin, or gingko biloba supplements could see an increase in bleeding tendencies.

Source: Adapted from Brindle, J. (2005). Meeting the challenges of Alzheimer's care. *RN, 68*(1), 29–34; Deglin, J., & Vallerand, A. (2007). *Davis's drug guide for nurses* (10th ed.) Philadelphia: F. A. Davis; and National Institute on Aging. (2006, December 14). Alzheimer's disease medication fact sheet. Retrieved June 3, 2007, from http://www.nia.nih.gov/Alzheimer's/Publications/medicationsfs.htm.

Galantamine has a benefit of facilitating the release of more acetylcholine and enhancing cholinergic neurotransmission. Donepezil is the only one that is given once a day. Scientists are currently working on a rivastigmine transdermal patch that could be applied once a day, delivering a continuous dose of the medication. This would be particularly beneficial for those clients who are resistant to taking oral medications. Although the cholinesterase inhibitors have been traditionally recommended for mild to moderate AD, in 2006, the FDA approved donepezil (Aricept) as being effective for severe AD as well.

A different type of drug, memantine (Namenda), was approved by the FDA in October 2003 and was available by prescription in January 2004. It is the first antidementia drug designed specifically for moderate to severe Alzheimer's disease. This drug protects the brain's nerve cells from excess amounts of the neurotransmitter glutamate, which is overproduced in clients with AD. When glutamate attaches to brain-cell surfaces, it allows calcium to flow into the cell freely, causing further cell destruction. Memantine prevents this destructive event from occurring. In clinical trials, memantine was used alone or with the anticholinesterase inhibitor, donepezil, with excellent results. Memantine is given twice a day and has few serious side effects.

There are currently 100 drugs in clinical trials to determine their effectiveness in the treatment of AD. One of these drugs, tramiprosate (Alzhemed) has reached phase three of the clinical trial, which indicates that it has almost successfully completed the testing needed before being submitted to the FDA for approval. It is designed to prevent amyloid from forming and being deposited on the brain and to repress the inflammation associated with the buildup of the amyloid protein (Alzheimer Research Forum, 2007). Other promising drugs being tested are nefiracetam (Translon) and CX516 (Ampalex), which are both in phase two of the clinical trials (Brindle, 2005). Scientists continue to look for a vaccine that would actually prevent the disease.

Other medications for clients with AD do not promote cognitive functioning but control the problem behaviors of combativeness and agitation, depression, paranoia, and delusions. These drugs might be antipsychotic, antianxiety, or antidepressant drugs. A strong warning is now included in the use of the antipsychotics. Olanzapine (Zyprexa), risperidone (Risperdal), and quetiapine (Seroquel) are to be used cautiously in elderly clients with psychotic symptoms related to dementia. These drugs increase the risk for death of these clients due to cardiovascular problems. The other difficulty with using these antipsychotics is that they block acetylcholine receptors, reducing the amount of a neurotransmitter already diminished in AD. Cognitive losses may actually accelerate (Petersen, 2002). The following are some of the more commonly used drugs:

Antipsychotics
    haloperidol (Haldol)
    olanzapine (Zyprexa)
    risperidone (Risperdal)
    quetiapine (Seroquel)
Anxiolytics (antianxiety)
    alprazolam (Xanax)
    buspirone (BuSpar)
    lorazepam (Ativan)
Antidepressants
    bupropion (Wellbutrin)
    fluoxetine (Prozac)
    sertraline (Zoloft)
    paroxetine (Paxil)
    citalopram (Celexa)

Box 15-6 ■ discusses the use of complementary and alternative therapies for clients with AD. None of the herbals is regulated by the FDA.

Anti-inflammatory drugs such as ibuprofen (Motrin), naproxen (Anaprox/Aleve), and indomethacin (Indocin) have been proposed as protectants against the early onset of AD (Gruetzner, 2001). The newer anti-inflammatory drugs, the COX-2 inhibitors such as celecoxib (Celebrex), are safer on the stomach and kidneys than the NSAIDs and may eventually also be recommended to treat early AD or to slow the onset of the disease

As seen from Table 15-3, vitamin E, an antioxidant, is recommended by the Alzheimer's Association after many research studies found its efficacy in treating clients with AD, either alone or combined with a cholinesterase inhibitor. Researchers have found that the death of brain cells in people with AD may result from the presence of free radicals (unstable, freely moving molecules released during the body's daily physiological processes). In preliminary studies, vitamin E has been shown to slow the rate of decline in clients in the middle to late stages of AD. One study found that vitamin E delayed AD progression by almost 1 year (Shankle & Amen, 2004). Combining it with daily vitamin C, another antioxidant, makes it even more effective.

Supportive Treatments

Other treatments for clients with AD are mainly supportive. As you can see from the progression of the disease, clients need to be protected from their own lack of cognition and

---

BOX 15-6

Complementary/Alternative Therapy for Clients with AD

Among complementary and alternative medications currently being investigated for use in AD are the following:

1. Dehydroepiandrosterone (DHEA) is also known as prasterone. It is produced in the adrenal glands and is a precursor of the sexual hormones, androgens, and estrogens. It is used in AD to improve cognitive function and memory. It should not be used in clients with any cancers that are hormone related, such as breast or prostate cancer, or in clients with diabetes.
2. Gingko biloba is an herb with both anti-inflammatory and antioxidant properties. Research studies have found it effective in improving cognition, ability to perform ADLs, and social behavior. Gingko biloba does have some anticoagulant properties, so clotting time for the client is increased. It should not be used if the client is taking aspirin or other anticlotting agents.
3. Huperzine A, an extract from a Chinese moss plant, has properties similar to the cholinesterase inhibitors (Alzheimer's Association, 2007e). It is as potent as the prescription drugs already described. However, as with other herbals, it is over-the-counter and not regulated by the FDA for purity and quality. It should not be used with any of the prescribed cholinesterase inhibitors, as it could produce a drug toxicity.
4. Coenzyme Q10 (ubiquinone) is an antioxidant occurring naturally in the body. It can also be produced synthetically. A safe dosage has not yet been determined.

---

judgment. They need a safe environment. They need assistance with all of the activities of daily living and eventually will need total care. Families may need respite from the 24-hour job of caring for the client with AD.

Therapists and Support Staff

In the early stages of the disease, physical therapists might be enlisted to assist with mobility problems. Occupational therapists may be able to provide suggestions for simplifying tasks, such as cooking and cleaning. They also may provide suggestions for diversionary activities.

Social workers or chaplains may work with the families who are struggling with the diagnosis of AD for their loved one. Often, social workers are involved in or lead caregiver support groups. Speech therapists may assess the swallowing abilities of the client and suggest ways to prevent choking. Certified nursing assistants provide most of the hands-on care in long-term care facilities; they need education and practice in the most appropriate ways to respond to the behaviors of the client with AD.

The activity director or activity assistants on Alzheimer's units or in adult day-care facilities may make the difference in the lives of those clients affected with AD. Activities help to maintain a sense of physical well-being and may divert clients from other unacceptable behaviors. Activity staff members are trained to provide experiences that allow clients with AD to be successful. A client may not be able to bake a loaf of bread alone but may be able to add one ingredient to the dough that will be placed in a breadmaker to make bread for the unit. In addition to giving the clients something productive to do, the smell of bread baking on the unit may bring back many pleasant memories of home. Taking walks, going on van rides with others, simple games, and exercises are valuable activities in the lives of clients with AD. Even when clients with AD have reached the advanced stage of the disease, they may respond to human touch. Often, activity staff members will provide soft music for the client while doing hand or foot massages. It is a simple sensory stimulation action that can be soothing for the client who is essentially unresponsive. The use of aromatherapy is another nonpharmacological method used to reduce the agitation sometimes found in AD—combining the essential oils in a lotion base and then applying it to faces and arms combined the soothing effects of the aroma with the sensory stimulation of touch (Resnick, 2003).

The American Therapeutic Recreation Association (ATRA) has developed guidelines to integrate recreational therapy into the treatment of those clients with AD who also exhibit either aggression or passivity. The premise is that this behavior results from the clients' unmet needs. Recreational therapists who are especially trained in this technique are able to assess and develop a treatment program to meet these unmet needs. They provide meaningful activities that allow the client to be successful and restore some of the independence the client once exhibited (Buettner & Kolanowski, 2003). Unfortunately, licensed recreational therapists are found only in specialty rehabilitation hospitals and units and not in the regular long-term care facilities where most clients with AD find themselves.

Reminiscence Therapy

Facilitating *reminiscence* (remembering) with the client who is in the early stages of AD can be valuable for family, staff, and client. Often long-term memory is better preserved than short-term memory, so this activity is likely to produce a response. **Reminiscence therapy** is therapy in which topics are introduced in an attempt to bring back related memories. The reminiscence session might focus on one particular topic where staff members provide items related to the subject. For example, bring in a pair of shoes, pictures of shoes, a poem or song about shoes, and then ask the client, "Tell me about your favorite pair of shoes." In other cases, staff members just ask the client about his/her past, sometimes after helpful hints from family members. In one study, uncooperative clients with cognitive disorders became more compliant and involved if they were given the opportunity to reminisce (Conroy & Nottoli, 1999). Family members may want to tape some of these sessions to capture memories that will eventually be lost. If a client is in a long-term care facility, family members are often asked to bring in photograph albums, family photos for the wall, and scrapbooks to provide a basis for reminiscence times.

Validation Therapy

Validation therapy was devised by Naomi Feil, a social worker, in 1963. She described the therapy as an "empathetic method for communicating" with clients suffering with AD (Feil, 1993). It is a means to affirm, or validate, a person's individuality and abilities (Fazio, Seman, & Stansell, 1999). It may be used to respond to repetitive questions and behaviors. Instead of attempting to orient the client with advanced AD to reality, in validation therapy, the caregiver enters into the client's reality. By orienting to the client's reality rather than forcing the client to adapt, the nurse may prevent a catastrophic reaction. The nurse *validates* (gives value to) AD clients and their beliefs.

CASE EXAMPLE

Take the example of Clara, an elderly AD client who continually came to the nurse's station asking what time the bus was leaving. A nurse who was not familiar with validation therapy kept answering, "This is a nursing home. It is not a bus station. There is no bus coming." The client would leave and then return periodically with the same question, getting more frustrated each time she came to the desk. The nurse also became irritated at being asked the same question and having to continually "orient" the resident to reality. Finally, a nursing assistant said to the resident, "You know, Clara, it is very late, and there are no more buses running tonight." Clara looked relieved, went back to her room, and let the staff assist her into bed. She did not return to the nurses' station.

Another technique of validation therapy is to give the client a chance to imagine going home, seeing their children, or seeing their parents. For example, when a client becomes upset about not being able to go home, just saying, "You must miss your home very much. Tell me about it," is a way for the AD client to "travel back home" without ever leaving the facility.

Creative Therapies

Pet therapy, music therapy, and art therapy are other techniques that have been utilized with AD clients with some success. Clients with AD also respond positively to visits from children if the situation is not too overstimulating for them. It is wise to avoid having a lot of small children, loud music, and many visitors at once. Keep activities calm and simple.

Family Support

Alzheimer's disease is a truly devastating disease for the client as well as the family. The family needs to be just as much a part of the plan of care as the client. Encourage family members to become part of an Alzheimer's support group, whether the client is remaining in the home or entering a nursing care facility. The more information family members have about the disease, the more they can accept the behavior changes that exist and that will occur. In the nursing home, family members are invited to participate in quarterly nursing care planning meetings. The LPN/LVN charge nurse usually conducts these meetings. Family members can hear of the progress the client is making as well as any problems the staff is having. Often the family member may contribute information about the client's past that might explain current behavior. Staff members had a frequent problem with one client in a long-term care facility frequently going outside to have a bowel movement. Family informed the staff that the client had been a shepherd in his earlier days, and the outside was the only place he had to relieve himself! This did not help the staff's consternation, but it did help them to understand the behavior! Family members may also have worthwhile suggestions for successful ways to manage some client actions.

NURSING CARE

ASSESSING

The first step in gathering data for the assessment is to determine whether the client has the ability to participate. You must gather data about the client's cognitive abilities carefully and check its accuracy. In the early stages, some AD clients can answer simple questions. They respond to close-ended yes-or-no questions the best. Others might be beyond this stage by the time you are assessing them. In any case, confirm the information you receive from the client with the client's family or close friends, or obtain that information directly from them. Remember confabulation is often used by clients with AD to cover up their confusion. They will rarely say, "I don't know." What sounds like a plausible answer to you might be far from the actual truth.

Observe clients closely. Note whether they are dressed appropriately and use good hygiene. Be aware of any difficulties in language. Do they lose their train of thought easily? Do they use the wrong words? Do you notice any perseveration or confabulation? Are they oriented to time, place, and person?

If clients are able to answer, ask questions about medical diagnoses they might have, and obtain a list of medications they are currently taking including over-the-counter medications and supplements. It is advisable to have the family bring in the client's medications, so you can see them yourself. Family members are probably the best ones to question about the ability of clients to perform their own activities of daily living, pay their bills, shop, and so on. Family members can also describe any personality changes or unusual behaviors they have noticed. Have clients started hoarding things or accused others of stealing from them? Have they left the house and gotten lost? Have they become incontinent? Have they demonstrated behavior that showed a lack of good judgment? Do they sleep more or less? Have they begun to isolate themselves from others?

All of these answers and observations will aid in establishing appropriate nursing diagnoses for the client. It is also important to observe the caregivers. They may be beginning to suffer from caregiver role strain if they have been caring for the client for some time without respite. Clues to caregiver role strain might include an unkempt appearance of the caregiver or irritability with the client during the interview. In one case, we noted the smell of alcohol on the caregiver's breath at 10 o'clock in the morning. Caregivers might mention their extreme fatigue, insomnia, or weight loss, or they may appear apathetic. Caregivers may require nursing interventions as well. It is interesting to note that depression appears in 20% of clients with AD, but in close to 50% of those who are caregivers of clients with AD (Brindle, 2005). Figure 15-6 ■ depicts a caregiver suffering from depression.

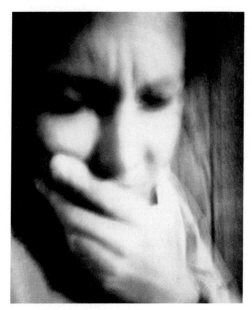

Figure 15-6. ■ Caregivers of clients with AD often suffer from depression. *Source:* Getty Images, Inc.-Taxi.

DIAGNOSING, PLANNING, AND IMPLEMENTING

Many nursing diagnoses apply to the client with AD. Some of the more common ones are:

- Chronic Confusion R/T organic impairment
- Disturbed Sleep Pattern R/T decreased daytime activities and change in environment
- Self-Care Deficit: bathing/hygiene R/T cognitive impairment
- Risk for Injury R/T cognitive impairment, poor balance, perceptual problems, and poor judgment
- Impaired Memory R/T organic changes
- Wandering R/T cognitive impairment

Anxiety and Ineffective Individual Coping are more common early in the disease, because the client still has enough cognitive ability to understand the diagnosis and perceive what the future will bring. Confusion and Impaired Memory are present throughout all stages of AD. During the late stages of AD, nursing diagnoses related to impaired motor function, incontinence, self-care, and communication increase.

Goals or outcomes for the AD client must be realistic. Nurses should try to help the client maintain contact with reality as much as possible for as long as possible. Sample outcomes for the AD client include the following:

- The client will answer three yes-or-no questions appropriately on my shift.

- The client will sleep 6 hours uninterrupted at least four times by the end of this week.
- The client will wash own face with minimum assistance by the end of this week.
- The client will not fall on my shift.
- The client will be able to locate his room at least once a day during the next week.
- The client will not leave the facility unattended during my shift.

These goals are examples of simple, measurable, and realistic outcomes for the client with AD. Talking to the current caregivers for clients will give you the best picture of what clients can actually do and what they can potentially accomplish at this point.

Address Problem Behaviors

Many of these nursing diagnoses relate to problem behaviors discussed earlier in this chapter. Suggested interventions for each of these behaviors are provided in Box 15-7 ■. The chronic confusion of clients with AD may manifest itself in any of the problem behaviors discussed earlier.

Show Interest

Recognize that all behavior is meaningful to the client, whether you understand its meaning or not. Indicate to the client that you are interested in him/her and want to understand. This involves making eye contact with the client and taking time to really watch and listen. This is also where validation can be used. For instance, being home for the children after school is often a concern for female clients. You are validating the client's feelings and emotions when you recognize how disappointed she is that she cannot be home to fix the children an after-school snack. Be creative in finding a reason why the children won't be coming home right now, then have the client describe the after-school snacks she used to prepare. If there is a way the client can fix a simple snack to serve to other residents, assist her with this.

Protect Against Falls

The leading cause of injury-related deaths among those clients 65 years and older are falls, and clients with AD are very susceptible to these incidents. Clients with AD often suffer from muscle weakness; deficits in balance, vision, and gait; impaired physical mobility (present in 89% of clients with dementia who are living in long-term care facilities); depression; and cognitive impairment. Other factors that add to the risk include medical conditions and medications (Alzheimer's Association, 2007a).

BOX 15-7	NURSING CARE CHECKLIST

Interventions for Problem AD Behaviors

Wandering

☑ Try to determine why the client is wandering: toileting needs, hunger, thirst, fear, stress, looking for a lost item, seeking a former relationship (going to work, looking for an old neighborhood). If you can determine the reason, you should try to meet the need. Toilet the client; provide food or drink; validate feelings of fear, reassure, and provide an environment where the client feels safe; mentally take the client back to his/her job or old neighborhood by having him/her describe it for you. Allow the client to wander if it is safe to do so. Walk with the client. Remove clutter and provide clear pathways. In the nursing home or hospital, provide the client with an electronic alarm, such as a Wanderguard bracelet or an RN-On-Call unit, so that an alarm sounds if the client rises or nears an exit. Place a stop sign where you do not want the client to go. Distract the client with other activities. In the home, install motion detectors. Add deadbolt locks to the inside of outside doors and place them high or low. Disguise doors to dangerous areas. Register the client with the Safe Return program of the Alzheimer's Association (Rowe, 2003).

Sundowning

☑ Keep the home or unit in the nursing home well lit at all times. Decrease environmental stimuli in the evening, for example, turn down or turn off the television or radio. Provide opportunities for exercise during the day, so the client is tired in the evening. Do not offer foods with caffeine in the evening. Offer a light snack (Alzheimer's Association, 2007a).

Refusal to Bathe

☑ Determine the reason for the refusal: fear because of lack of understanding; lack of good motor coordination to accomplish the actions needed; unpleasant memories; uncomfortable having someone in the bathroom; lack of interest in personal hygiene. Reassure if fear is the reason. Be calm and matter-of-fact. Offer assistance. Make sure there are devices in the bathroom to assist with balance and coordination, for example, grab bars on the tub and strips to prevent slipping in the tub. Follow the client's old routine of tub or shower and time of day. Have everything prepared ahead of time, for example, have bath water already run at a comfortable temperature, have towels ready, change of clothes in place, bathroom warm and comfortable. Tell clients it is time to take a bath; do not ask them if they want a bath or if they are ready to take a bath. Simplify the bathing routine as much as possible. Try singing favorite songs as a distraction. Encourage the client to smell the soap or shampoo to increase the enjoyment of the bath. If all else fails, consider using a sponge bath or towel bath with non-rinsing soap (Petersen, 2002).

Paranoia

☑ Understand that this is not a behavior the client can control; it is part of the confusion of the disease. They have no other explanation for their losses than to think someone is taking things from them. Do not argue with the client about their suspicions. Offer to help the client look for lost items. Make a list of frequently sought items and their location. Try diversionary tactics to get the focus off of the lost items. Respond to the emotion of the client, not the behavior. Validate their feelings on confusion and helplessness. Do not take the accusations personally if the client thinks you are the one stealing. Be calm and reassuring. Consider keeping duplicates of items the client frequently hides (Petersen, 2002).

Language Disturbances

☑ To respond to language difficulties, you must work on your listening skills, verbal skills, and nonverbal skills. Listen attentively. Because the client is having difficulty expressing himself/herself, it is even more important to listen without distractions. Maintain eye contact, and show interest in what the client is saying. Encourage and reassure clients who are having difficulty. Decide how important it is to correct a client when a mistake is made. If the client usually takes a correction well and even laughs at a mistake, go ahead. However, if corrections tend to anger the client, it is not worth it (Petersen, 2002). Try to find meaning in what was said. Do not argue. Try to help clients out by supplying the word you think they are looking for. If you cannot come up with the word, ask the client to describe it or point to it (Mace & Rabins, 1999). Before beginning a communication, introduce yourself to the client as appropriate. Always approach from the front. Call the client by name. Speak slowly, calmly and clearly, and use short, simple sentences. Give clients time to respond. If clients do not understand, repeat what you have said exactly for two more times before changing the message wording. You may have to accompany your verbal communication with visual cues and gestures. We know a nursing assistant who always carried her toothbrush in her pocket, so she could demonstrate toothbrushing to her clients as she explained the process to them. Sometimes, writing things down will be received more easily than speaking. Always treat clients with dignity and respect and speak to them as adults, not children. Clients with AD seem to pick up on a demeaning tone of voice and a disapproving facial expression very quickly. Use humor when possible, be patient and cheerful (Alzheimer's Association, 2003).

Catastrophic Reactions

☑ Understand that these behaviors are responses that the client with AD cannot help. The best response is to prevent the reaction from occurring. When you are familiar with the client, you begin to understand what types of circumstances precipitate a catastrophic reaction. The Mayo Clinic recommends using the ABC approach in AD care to prevent the reoccurrence of problem behaviors. This method has the caregiver look at the cause, or **a**ntecedent, of a behavior. Then review the response, or **b**ehavior, that was precipitated. And, lastly, look at the **c**onsequences of the behavior. Too often, caregivers focus on the consequences of the behavior rather than the antecedent. If we know what will trigger certain behaviors, then we should be able to prevent the behavior and consequences from occurring (Petersen, 2002). For instance, if seeing your keys always invokes a catastrophic reaction from a client with AD, because it is a reminder that s/he is in a locked unit and has lost independence, then keep your keys out of sight. It will differ with each client. Keeping to a routine will help to avoid some of these reactions. Keep things simple. Do not hurry the client. Provide activities where the client can be successful to avoid the frustration of failure. Make sure the client is well rested, as catastrophic reactions seem to occur more often when the client is fatigued. If a catastrophic reaction does occur, maintain a calm approach. If it is possible, let the client walk, but remain close and try to distract from the out-of-control behavior (hostility or anxiety) by pointing out familiar and comforting surroundings or people. Discussing grandchildren or showing a photo of a grandchild may help. Position yourself so that you are between the client and an exit if hostile behavior might be redirected toward you. Watch the client's eyes for indication as to where the behavior might be leading (Brindle, 2005). Remove the client from the precipitating event, object, or person as quickly as possible. You might need to call in a quiet, calm coworker to help. Gentle touch and calming techniques may work to reduce the agitation *after* the outburst, but be aware that touch during the catastrophic reaction might result in the client swinging at you. As you learn about the client, you will learn the best techniques for calming him/her (Brindle, 2005). Above all, you need to remain calm and in control yourself. The client feels out of control and insecure during these times and needs caregivers who can provide structure and security.

Being continually aware of the environment will go a long way toward protecting the client from injury. You always have to consider that perception of stimuli might be altered for the client with AD. For example, in one long-term care facility, new tile was laid on the floor of the Alzheimer's unit. After the tile was down, the clients were afraid to come out of their rooms. If they did venture out, they took huge steps to get over the tile. In looking at the pattern on the floor, it was finally obvious to the staff that the dark tiles around the border of the floor were the problem. With altered perception, the dark tiles appeared to be a deep hole that clients were afraid of falling into; thus, they avoided leaving their rooms. You will see clients with AD take giant steps to avoid stepping on a string or small item on the floor. This is dangerous when you consider that they might have poor motor function and poor balance. It is the nurse's job to recognize danger for the client with AD. For example, wet floors are a major problem when clients do not realize what it means to be careful. Make sure that clients have on nonslip-soled shoes; if clients refuse, socks with nonslip treads might work. There is nothing more slippery than plain socks on a tile floor!

This can be more of a challenge if you are working in a home situation where there can be a multitude of obstacles. Educate family members on keeping walking paths in the home clear of obstacles, such as electrical cords, oxygen tubing, and small rugs. Encourage the installation of handrails or grab bars where appropriate. Improve lighting by using fluorescent bulbs; keep night lights on in the bedroom and bathroom (Alzheimer's Association, 2007a).

Remove Unsafe Materials

A medication cart or open cleaning cart left unattended on the Alzheimer's unit is a prescription for disaster. Items left unintentionally at the client's bedside may be disastrous as well. For example, a staff member might leave a washcloth on the bedside table of a client in the terminal stages of AD. If the client is experiencing hyperorality, the staff member might find the entire washcloth in the client's mouth on returning to the client's room. The client could choke to death if the staff member does not return in time. All plants used in an Alzheimer's unit or yard need to be evaluated for their poison potential. Poinsettias are common gifts to clients during the Christmas season, but are really not safe items to be left on an Alzheimer's unit.

Monitor Clients' Whereabouts

Electronic alarms such as the Wanderguard bracelets and RN-On-Call, mentioned in the section on delirium, are useful here as well. Before the advent of such items, a gentleman with AD walked out of the long-term care facility where he resided, got into the unlocked automobile of a staff member, and released the brake. The car rolled back into the street. Luckily, another staff member pulled up at that time and was able to prevent a disaster from happening. The lack of good judgment by the AD client can put the client in harm's way if staff or caregivers are not attentive and alert at all times. This is one of the reasons why caregivers in the home become so burned out. Care of a person with AD is a "24/7" job, and it takes its toll on the mind and heart of the caregiver.

> **Critical Self-Check.** Imagine you are caring for your mother with Alzheimer's disease in the home. Your mother wanders at night, going through the house, turning on lights and turning on the gas on your old gas stove. One night she walks outside in the snow wearing just her nightgown. You cannot sleep for fear she will get hurt or do something to injure the family. You do not want to lock her in her room. What will you do?

Show Respect

In all of your interactions with clients with AD, remember the person behind the disease, and treat clients with dignity and respect. They may not be very dignified walking down a hall with nothing on but a coat and hat, or spitting at you when you try to feed them something they do not like. Remember that they have a disease that robs them of the ability to control that type of behavior. You, however, are responsible for how you respond.

EVALUATING

It is often the case with the AD clients that expected goals are set too high and need to be revised. Maybe the interventions used by the staff did not work. If it is a new client, maybe the staff has just not hit on the interventions that will work with that particular client. Textbooks suggest many interventions for the behaviors of the client with AD. However, it is up to the staff to determine which interventions work with which clients,

and which *staff members* work best with which clients and also which staff members work well in the Alzheimer's unit *period*. Clients with AD need to have successes. As the disease progresses, these become fewer and fewer. Nurses and other staff need to recognize the strengths of each client and set goals that are attainable.

DISCHARGE CONSIDERATIONS

The caregiver cannot be left out of any planning done for the client with AD. This is especially important if the caregiver decides to keep the client at home. (Sometimes, caregivers will decide on this course of action after they have had some respite with the client in long-term care.) Notice Peter, the caregiver, in the care plan that follows. Like so many other caregivers, he is suffering from the strain of caring for a loved one with AD.

As long as the caregiver has help, the strain of caring for the client with AD does not feel so overwhelming. Having assistance in the home is the key to avoiding caregiver role strain. Attempting to care for the client alone leads to burnout, depression, and sometimes resentment toward the client (Alzheimer's Association, 2007a). Respite is a rest or break from the usual routine of caring for the client. It can be for a brief period such as an hour or two or can be for several weeks. Respite care can be provided by paid caregivers or volunteers, family or friends, a long-term care facility, or a day-care facility. The caregiver needs to be able to get out of the house periodically while feeling that his/her loved one is safe. The caregiver can use this time to grocery shop, go to the senior center for activities, or do something he or she really enjoys doing. Some caregivers actually place the client in a facility, so they can take a much needed real vacation. Families who are immigrants to this country, or who are not from the dominant European-American culture, may have different psychosocial issues related to elder care. (Box 15-8 ■ provides information about cultural issues in elder care.)

The nurse might put the caregiver in touch with the local Alzheimer's Association. If there is not an office nearby, the nurse could locate the phone number for the AD support group in his area. A local nursing home can usually provide this information. The support-group members often have names of competent caregivers who can give respite.

Adult day-care facilities, where available, can provide respite for the caregiver while offering a structured environment in which the client can socialize and enjoy activities with others who have AD.

<table>
<tr><td>

BOX 15-8   CULTURAL PULSE POINTS

Cultural Issues in Elder Care

The type of support given to the elderly by their families is partly dependent on cultural expectations. Larger numbers of elders from European American families are cared for in nursing homes than are elders from other ethnic and cultural backgrounds. Elders of diverse families may be cared for in the home for several reasons:

■ Care in the home is less expensive.

■ Caring for the elder at home is consistent with cultural values.

■ Language barriers make it difficult for families to know about services, and for elders to cope with long-term care placement.

■ Large extended families may have mechanisms for sharing the care.

In the United States many families are trying to live in two cultures. The elder family members may expect to be cared for by younger relatives, who are also expected to be working outside the home. Potential caregivers may be at risk for caregiver role strain if they keep the elder in their home, and for criticism from their community if they do not. The nurse providing culturally sensitive care must help families create a mutually agreed-on plan for elder care.

</td><td>

BOX 15-9

Being a Healthy Caregiver

1. Get a diagnosis as early as possible if you suspect your loved one has a dementia problem. You will be better able to handle the present and plan for the future.

2. Learn what resources are available in your community. Start with the local Alzheimer's Association chapter. Other resources could include adult day-care centers, volunteers for respite, home health care, Meals-on-Wheels.

3. Become an educated caregiver so that you can better understand and cope with the challenging behaviors and personality changes that occur with AD. Learn how to develop new caregiving skills with each stage of the disease progression.

4. Get help, and do not try to do everything by yourself. Ask for assistance if no one offers it. If stress becomes overwhelming, seek professional help for yourself. Join a support group.

5. Take care of yourself. Practice healthful behavior. Eat a nutritious diet, exercise, and get plenty of rest. Use respite services to take time off to go shopping, have lunch with friends, or even take a short vacation.

6. Manage your level of stress. Stress can cause physical problems and changes in behavior. Be aware of your symptoms and consult a physician. Practice relaxation techniques that work for you. Get a monthly massage.

7. Accept changes as they occur. People with Alzheimer's disease will change, and so do their needs. You may have to seek care beyond what you can provide at home. Investigate available care options ahead of time to make the transition easier.

8. Do legal and financial planning. Consult an attorney and discuss issues related to durable power of attorney, living wills and trusts, future medical care, housing, and other key considerations. If early in the disease, the person with AD should be part of this process. Involve others in the family as well.

9. Be realistic. The progression of Alzheimer's disease is inevitable and beyond your control. Give yourself permission to grieve for the losses you experience. Keep a sense of humor and focus on positive moments. Remember, it is okay to laugh, not at the person with AD, but with them and the situation.

10. Give yourself credit, not guilt. You're only human. Occasionally, you may lose patience and, at times, be unable to provide all of the care the way you'd like. Remember you're doing the best you can, so give yourself credit.

Source: Adapted from "Be a Healthy Caregiver." *Colorado Chapter Newsletter* of the Alzheimer's Association. Winter, 2006.

</td></tr>
</table>

A home health nurse is often the person to see signs of caregiver burnout in the caregiver. The nurse should educate caregivers on the signs of burnout, so that they can recognize them in themselves. Signs of burnout include:

■ Loss of interest in taking care of oneself

■ Loss of interest in caring for the client

■ Turning to alcohol or medication for relief

■ Yelling at or treating the client roughly

■ Isolating oneself from friends and other family members

The Alzheimer's Association has prepared a list of suggestions for a caregiver to remain healthy. Box 15-9 ■ lists 10 appropriate ways to remain healthy as a caregiver.

Ineffective Family Coping might also be a nursing diagnosis identified for the caregiver. Caregivers may stay awake trying to keep loved ones from getting lost or injuring themselves. They eventually become less vigilant as physical illness or mental exhaustion takes over. A good outcome for this diagnosis would be the following:

■ The family will install different locks on the outside doors, so that the client will be unable to open them from the inside.

Figure 15-7 ■ illustrates the complete care needed by clients with dementia.

The Alzheimer's Association is aware of the impact of culture on care of the client with dementia. It has developed a set of 10 steps to educate caregivers about incorporating cultural values into the understanding and care of ethnic elders. Box 15-10 ■ contains these guidelines.

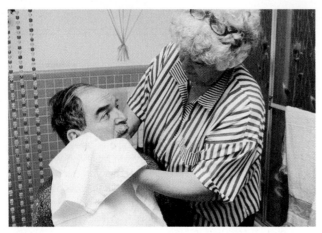

Figure 15-7. ■ Caring for someone with dementia is an enormous burden. Support groups and respite programs provide assistance. *Source: Mental Health Nursing* by Fontaine, K. Reprinted by permission of Pearson Education, Saddle River, NJ.

BOX 15-10

Ten Steps to Providing Culturally Sensitive Dementia Care

■ Consider each person as an individual, as well as a product of their country, religion, ethnic background, language, and family system.

■ Understand the linguistic, economic, and social barriers that individuals from different cultures face, preventing access to healthcare and social services. Try to provide services in a family's native language.

■ Understand that families from different cultures consider and use alternatives to Western healthcare philosophy and practice.

■ Do not place everyone in a particular ethnic group into the same category, assuming that there is one approach for every person in the group.

■ Respect cultural differences regarding physical distance and contact, appropriate eye contact, and rate and volume of voice.

■ Cultivate relationships with families over time, not expecting immediate trust in and understanding of the Alzheimer's Association.

■ Consider the family's background and experience in determining what services are appropriate.

■ Consider the culture's typical perceptions of aging, caring for elderly family members and memory impairment.

■ Understand that a family's culture impacts their choices regarding ethical issues, such as artificial nutrition, life support and autopsies.

■ Regard the faith community for various cultures as a critical support system.

Source: Reprinted by permission from the Alzheimer's Association. (2007). *Diversity.* Available: http://www.alz.org/Resources/Diversity/downloads/GEN_EDU_10steps.pdf. Used with permission.

CASE EXAMPLE

A 75-year-old Chinese American man was diagnosed with Alzheimer's Disease. He has chronic confusion, total self-care deficit, impaired skin integrity, and incontinence of both urine and stool. He has been living in the home of his son, daughter-in-law, and their three young children. None of the other siblings have stepped forward to assist with his care, as it is expected that the eldest son will care for the elderly parents. The elder has become too difficult to care for in the home due to his wandering at night and turning on the gas stove. He accuses the son of stealing from him and hiding his belongings. The family feels that dementia and its resultant delusional behavior is a form of mental illness and therefore has been hiding it from others in the community. They would like to place the father in a nursing home but feel that they would no longer be fulfilling their family obligation and would cause shame and "loss of face" for the family. They believe that members of the Chinese American community would criticize them for failing to provide adequately for the elderly parent. The son has asked the physician to tell their father and other siblings that he recommends placement in a nursing home, which he does. The client is reluctant to go, but the physician reassures him that he will have healthcare professionals caring for him 24 hours a day. The physician also counsels the other siblings concerning the amount of care the elder has required, much of which they were unaware. All of the family is encouraged to participate in the plan of care for the elder and invited to be part of his daily life in the long-term care facility. Staff have gone out of their way to include the family in his care, to educate them about AD, and reassure them about the care being provided. The family no longer feels guilt or shame and are relieved that the elder is now receiving the care they can no longer provide.

The caregiver needs to ease his/her mind about the client wandering outside. There are other things to keep the client safe inside. First of all, the caregiver should register the client with the Safe Return program of the Alzheimer's Association. This program allows people to register clients who wander. It also has a 24-hour help line to facilitate the return of lost clients with dementia. The program requires that a photo, wrist measurement, and phone numbers of local law enforcement agencies be on file with their office. The Alzheimer's Association will then send an identification bracelet for the client and clothing identification tags. If the client becomes lost, a call to the toll-free number of the help line will ensure a rapid response in the recovery process (Rowe, 2003).

Providing safety within the home is also important. The Alzheimer's Association suggests assessing the home for possible hazards and removing those as much as possible.

This might involve disguising the entrance to various areas of the home that might be dangerous, such as the door to the basement stairs. Installing deadbolt locks that are either high or low on the inside of the outer doors will make it difficult to wander out of the house. Even simple motion detectors may be installed inside the home (Rowe, 2003).

Putting childproof devices on cabinets and doors where harmful substances might be another action that should be taken. The house should be well lit at all times. Clutter and area rugs should be removed. Any household appliance that could be dangerous for AD clients to use on their own should be locked away. (Remember Edith and the electric blanket!)

The refrigerator should be cleaned out often, so that all foods are fresh and wholesome. All houseplants should be assessed for safety. Some plants are poisonous and could be another source of harm if the client decides to taste a flower or a leaf. By removing as many harmful objects as possible, the caregiver can relax a little and enjoy the client's company without worrying about safety issues.

The client with Alzheimer's disease is a challenge for any caregiver, whether the client is in the home, day care, or long-term care facility, or whether the caregiver is a family member, friend, or paid staff member. The main focus for nurses is to provide for the safety of the client and the support of the family. Keeping educated on the latest information about Alzheimer's disease and other dementias is of paramount importance to the nurse who wants to provide the best care possible for her/his clients.

NURSING PROCESS CARE PLAN
Client with Middle-Stage AD

Blanche Smith is a 70-year-old female with middle-stage Alzheimer's disease. Her 75-year-old husband has been caring for her at home with the help of his 45-year-old daughter. Unfortunately, the daughter moved out of state. Mr. Smith has finally made the painful decision to place Blanche in a long-term care facility; she will move there next month. Blanche wanders the house day and night. Many times, she asks him who he is and what he is doing in her house. Although they have been married 50 years, she thinks he is there to harm her. She has called the police on more than one occasion. When she managed to get out of the house yesterday, she wandered several blocks before he found her. She became so hysterical when he tried to bring her home that the neighbors came

out to see what the problem was. Blanche is having trouble thinking of the word she wants to use and may call objects by names she has made up. She asks him the same question over and over, and it is irritating to him. Then he becomes angry with himself for getting irritated. He is not getting enough sleep and is tired all of the time. He has been unable to hire anyone to help him to watch Blanche even while he goes to the store. Long-term care seems the only solution. He wants Blanche to be safe, and he wants to rest.

Assessment. On admission, Blanche is well-dressed and clean. She is accompanied by her husband, Peter, who is very attentive to her needs. She refers to Peter as her friend and says that she is 25 years old and single. She says she has no children. Blanche recognizes her own name. She does not know what day this is and does not know where she lives. She is often distracted during the interview. She starts sentences and then stops in mid-thought and giggles. Her speech is hesitant, and she sometimes uses the wrong word or makes up a word. Peter tells the nurse that he has had to take over the household chores. Blanche can no longer cook, but she helps Peter in the kitchen. She is occasionally incontinent of urine when he misses the signs and does not take her to the bathroom. He assists Blanche with bathing, but sometimes she fights him. He reports that she wanders around the house at night and has gotten lost in the neighborhood. He admits to being very tired.

Diagnosis. Although there are many nursing diagnoses that can be identified from the case study, the following would have the highest priority:

- Disturbed Sleep Pattern
- Self-Care Deficit: bathing/hygiene
- Self-Care Deficit: dressing/grooming
- Self-Care Deficit: toileting
- Chronic Confusion
- Risk for Injury
- Impaired Verbal Communication

For Peter, two nursing diagnoses apply:

- Caregiver Role Strain R/T loss of daughter's help and being unable to find additional assistance with wife's care
- Ineffective Family Coping R/T wife's erratic behavior and fear for her safety

Expected Outcomes. Goals/outcomes for Blanche include that:

- Client will not be injured.

- Client will answer three yes-or-no questions appropriately each day.
- Client will communicate at least one need a day either verbally or nonverbally.

Planning and Implementation.   Interventions for these three nursing diagnoses will be integrated, since they are all related to the client's cognitive impairment.

- The nurse brings Blanche and Peter to Blanche's new room and introduces her to her roommate. She suggests to Peter that he should bring in some familiar objects for Blanche to place in her room. *Having a scrapbook, photograph album, and some pictures for the wall will help the staff in reminiscence with Blanche. Bringing in her favorite chair and familiar comforter for her bed can ease the transition into a new location.*
- The nurse also suggests that Peter bring in a large calendar and a digital clock that will be easy for Blanche to read. She asks Peter to bring in a photo of Blanche when she was a young woman. *Since Blanche identifies herself as a young woman, this picture—placed outside her door—will help her find her new room more easily. Since Blanche's favorite color is purple, the nurse will place a purple bow next to Blanche's photo to help her to identify her new room.*
- The nurse will communicate to the staff about Blanche's tendency to wander. *Since the unit is locked, Blanche will not have to wear a Wanderguard bracelet. However, staff will be aware of Blanche's tendency to wander in and out of other residents' rooms. This could be a source of catastrophic reactions with other residents if Blanche is in the room uninvited and rummaging through their belongings. This could result in injury to Blanche if the staff is not watchful.*
- The nurse asks about favorite activities and learns that Blanche loves to walk outside, likes music, enjoys helping Peter prepare a meal, and can still play Bingo. *All of these facts will give the staff examples of diversionary activities that can be used with Blanche when her behavior intrudes upon others.*
- Staff will be aware when floors are wet or when there are articles on the floor that need to be picked up. Clutter will be avoided. The unit will be kept well lit when it starts to get dark outside, so Blanche can still see to walk.
- The staff will communicate with Blanche in simple sentences. When Blanche does not understand what is said, the directions will be repeated to her, using the same words at least two more times. The staff will avoid using negatives when speaking to Blanche. *It is better to say "Turn around here" than "Do not go there." The second phrase takes more processing because of the negative word "not."*
- Staff will limit Blanche's choices, so she is not overwhelmed. *It will be easier for her to choose between a red dress or a blue dress than to decide on a whole outfit to wear.*
- When Blanche has difficulty remembering a word, staff will supply it for her, then use the word in a sentence to see if that is what she meant to say. The nurse assured Peter that staff will always approach Blanche from the front and will not touch her until she sees them. They will speak in a calm manner. *These interventions will help Blanche feel safe and will prevent catastrophic reactions.*

Evaluation.   After 2 weeks, Blanche has adjusted to her new surroundings. She is happy to see Peter when he arrives. She still thinks he is a friend, but she does recognize him as someone she knows. She is able to show him her room. She plays Bingo every Wednesday and sets the table for lunch every day. She has not been injured and follows directions reasonably well if given step-by-step instructions. Staff members take the time to listen to her and help her with her communication. Peter hears Blanche laugh for the first time in months when a staff member has a hard time guessing what object she wants. It is obvious that Blanche feels more at ease in this environment than she did at home where the expectations of her behavior were different. Here she can be herself, and not have to struggle with who she used to be.

Critical Thinking in the Nursing Process

1. What factors were involved in Peter's decision to place Blanche in a nursing home? If he had chosen to keep Blanche at home, what adaptations would he have had to make?
2. Discuss the choices of the nursing diagnoses that were considered the most important. Do you agree with those choices? Why or why not?
3. If you were educating Peter on the middle and late stages of Alzheimer's disease, what information do you think would be the most important for him to know?

Note: Discussion of Critical Thinking questions appears in Appendix I.

Note: The references and resources for this and all chapters have been compiled at the back of the book.

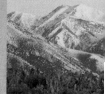

Chapter Review

KEY TERMS

Use the audio glossary feature of the Companion Website to hear the correct pronunciation of the following key terms.

agnosia

aphasia

apraxia

beta-amyloid plaques

catastrophic reactions

cholinesterase inhibitors

delirium

dementia

disturbance of executive functioning

emotionally labile

hyperorality

illusion

neologisms

neurofibrillary tangles

perseveration

polypharmacy

reality orientation

reminiscence therapy

substance-induced delirium

sundowning

KEY Points

- Cognitive disorders distort one's thought processes. Delirium is a cognitive disorder that is reversible if the underlying cause is treated. Dementia is a cognitive disorder that is progressive and irreversible. Impaired memory and confusion are symptoms of both disorders.

- Depression may sometimes be mistaken for a cognitive disorder.

- Delirium and dementia both involve a team approach to care with physicians, nurses, therapists, social workers, activities directors, and nursing assistants becoming involved.

- There are 12 identifiable types of dementia, but Dementia of the Alzheimer's Type is the most common, affecting 4.5 million Americans.

- Scientists have not found the definitive cause for Alzheimer's disease but have discovered definite and possible risk factors. The older one becomes, the more susceptible s/he is to developing AD.

- A diagnosis of Alzheimer's disease is reached by ruling out other disorders. It can only be definitively diagnosed by autopsy.

- The structure of the brain of the AD client at autopsy shows beta-amyloid plaques, neurofibrillary tangles, and a deficiency of the neurotransmitter acetylcholine.

- There are three basic stages of AD: early, middle, and late. The longest stage is the middle stage. From beginning to end, the course of the disease may be from 5 to 17 years.

Symptoms vary and worsen as the disease progresses through each stage.

- There is no cure for AD. Cholinesterase inhibitors prolong the early and middle stages. Scientists are working on other medications and vaccines. Other care is supportive.

- The focus of care is on protecting the client with AD from danger and on providing assistance with all activities of daily living.

- Reminiscence therapy may assist the client with AD to recall distant memories; validation therapy gives value to the client's beliefs.

- The family of the client with AD needs support and attention as well.

EXPLORE MediaLink

Additional interactive resources for this chapter can be found on the Companion Website at www.prenhall.com/eby. Click on Chapter 15 and "Begin" to select the activities for this chapter.

- Audio glossary
- NCLEX-PN® review
- Case study
- Study outline
- Critical thinking questions
- Matching questions
- Weblinks

Caring for a Client with Delirium
NCLEX-PN® Focus Area: Physiologic Integrity

Case Study: Arthur Song is a 78-year-old retired farmer who is hospitalized for a change in his mental status. He had a CVA (brain attack) 5 years ago and recovered most of his function. He is still slightly weaker on the right side, but was independent with ADLs and alert and oriented until 2 days ago. He sees a neurologist about his stroke rehabilitation, a urologist for his prostate problem, and an internist for his general medical care. On admission to the hospital, he is oriented to person only, not to place or time. His wife states that this morning he did not know who she was.

Nursing Diagnosis: Acute confusion

COLLECT DATA

Subjective	Objective
_____	_____
_____	_____
_____	_____
_____	_____
_____	_____
_____	_____

Would you report this data? Yes/No

If yes, to: _____

Nursing Care

_____
_____
_____
_____
_____
_____
_____
_____

How would you document this? _____
_____
_____
_____

Compare your documentation to the sample provided in Appendix I.

Data Collected
(use those that apply)

- The neurologist prescribed several medications.
- The internist prescribed several medications.
- The urologist prescribed several medications.
- Client had sudden onset of change in mental status.
- His symptoms are inconsistent; sometimes he is oriented, sometimes not.
- History of smoking, until 30 years ago
- Wife states that client takes several over-the-counter medications for nasal congestion, GI upset, and occasional headaches.
- Client states, "I don't know what to do."
- Client is unable to bathe himself, which he could do before this episode.
- Client eats a high-salt diet at home.
- Right grip is weaker than left.
- His hobby is woodworking.

Nursing Interventions
(use those that apply; list in priority order)

- Orient the client to reality.
- Make a list of all the medications the client is taking, prescribed and over-the-counter.
- Tell his wife to prepare for nursing home placement.
- Begin bladder training to prevent incontinence.
- Assist the client with ADLs while he is acutely confused.
- Teach the client memory-enhancing strategies.
- Tell the client's wife that because he is sometimes oriented, he is probably not sick, and is doing this for attention.
- Place frequently used personal items near the bed within easy reach.
- Use simple words and sentences.
- Restrain the client in bed to prevent falls.
- Introduce yourself each time you enter the room.
- Encourage a family member to stay with the client when possible.
- Teach the client about unit policies.

Pay attention to the location in the question. The correct nursing action may vary if the client is at home or in a clinic, hospital, or long-term care facility. For example, hallucinations may represent a life-threatening situation if they are associated with acute delirium of alcohol withdrawal in the hospital. Hallucinations in a client with schizophrenia in a clinic may be reason for a medication adjustment.

1 When the nurse notices a change in cognition of a new postoperative client, the nurse's first action would be to:

1. Notify the physician.
2. Begin assessing him/her for possible causes.
3. Withhold the client's pain medication until the physician arrives.
4. Send a urine specimen to the lab for a culture.

2 A client has been diagnosed with delirium related to his recent onset of pneumonia. His wife asks the nurse how long the confusion will last. The nurse's best answer would be:

1. "It will definitely be resolved by the time he leaves the hospital."
2. "As soon as the pneumonia begins to clear up, the confusion will clear up as well."
3. "As soon as he adjusts to being in the hospital, the confusion will disappear."
4. "All clients with delirium react differently. It could be anywhere from several days to several months."

3 Which of the following characteristics differentiates delirium from dementia?

1. In delirium, onset is gradual; in dementia, it is sudden.
2. There is no memory impairment in delirium.
3. In delirium, symptoms may fluctuate during a 24-hour period; in dementia, they do not.
4. Aphasia is present only in dementia, not in delirium.

4 A client with delirium is constantly trying to climb over the side rails. The most appropriate response of the nurse would be to:

1. Medicate the client with an antianxiety drug.
2. Suggest to the family that a family member might want to sit by the client's bed to keep him calm.
3. Restrain the client with a vest restraint until the physician can be notified.
4. Leave the side rail down.

5 A confused client who picks up a toothbrush and begins brushing her hair might be described as having:

1. Agnosia.
2. Aphasia.
3. Apraxia.
4. Disturbance of executive functioning.

6 The daughter of a client, newly diagnosed with Alzheimer's disease, asks the nurse if she will develop the disease as well. The nurse's best response would be:

1. "There is no hereditary component to Alzheimer's disease."

2. "You are no more likely to develop the disease than anyone else."
3. "Having a parent with the disease increases your risk to 1.5 to 2 times that of the general population."
4. "Just being a female is a definite risk factor."

7 A nurse is caring for a male Alzheimer's client who refuses to get out of the bed of another client who is ready to get into it. The nurse says, "Please get up." When the client does not move, what should the nurse do next?

1. Repeat, "Please get up."
2. Say, "I asked you to get out of this bed. It's not yours."
3. Pull the cover off of the client, and help him into a sitting position.
4. Say, "If you do not get out of this bed right now, you will not get any dessert at dinner tonight."

8 A female client walks toward the nurse shaking her fist and says, "You have been hiding my things. Where did you put my purse?" The nurses' best response would be:

1. "You know I would not hide your things."
2. "Do not shake your fist at me. I work here."
3. "You seem upset. Let me help you look for your purse."
4. "I am too busy to be hiding your things. I saw another resident in your room earlier. Perhaps she took it."

9 A female client will not take her bath unless she can bring her doll with her. What would the nurse do?

1. Insist she leave the doll on her bed. Reassure her that it will be okay.
2. Take the doll from Millie and give it to her roommate to take care of until Millie returns.
3. Open a dresser drawer and put the doll into it before you leave the room.
4. Let her bring the doll.

10 A female client is standing at the door of the locked Alzheimer's unit pulling on the doorknob and crying, "My children are due home from school any minute now, and I need to get home for them." The nurse's best response would be:

1. "Your children are all grown up. You do not need to go home."
2. "This is your home now. Your children live far away."
3. "Tell me about your children."
4. "You are 75 years old. Your children grew up a long time ago. Don't you remember?"

Answers for Review Questions, as well as discussion of Care Plan and Critical Thinking Care Map questions, appear in Appendix I.

Learning About You!

CHAPTER 13 Disorders in Childhood and Adolescence

Review Erikson's psychosocial theory on a personal level. In each of the stages up until your present age, consider how your environmental experiences helped you to achieve success. (Do not forget to consider the negative as well as the positive experiences you might have had.) What do you think contributed to your resiliency? If you had had a genetic tendency toward a mental disorder, is there any experience that might have adversely affected your mental health?

>   Infancy (birth to 18 months): trust versus mistrust
>   Early childhood (18 months–3 years): autonomy versus shame and doubt
>   Late childhood (3–6 years): initiative versus guilt
>   School age (6–12 years): industry versus inferiority
>   Adolescence (12–20 years): identity versus role confusion
>   Young adulthood (20–30 years): intimacy versus isolation
>   Adulthood (30–65 years): generativity versus stagnation

CHAPTER 14 Eating Disorders

As this chapter emphasizes, a person's total self-concept, that is, body image, self-esteem, and personal identity, are closely related to the development of eating disorders. It is important for nurses (or student nurses) to get in touch with their own attitudes about those areas of life. Take a few minutes and consider your own self-concept. You need to know what you are bringing into the clinical setting.

Body Image

Describe how you see your body. Decide what you would change about your body if you could. Overall, are you satisfied or dissatisfied with how you look? Did eating or weight come into your answers at all?

Self-Esteem

What do you see as your strengths? How would you describe your ethical/moral standards? Does your appearance affect your self-esteem? Would you describe your self-esteem as positive or negative? Who helped you develop your self-esteem? How? What kinds of things threaten your self-esteem? How do you protect yourself against the threat? Do you see yourself as having an influence in the lives of others? How can you help to shape a positive self-esteem in others?

Personal Identity

Describe yourself in objective terms, for example, your age, race, occupation, height, weight. Describe your qualities or traits, for example, your usual behaviors, feelings, moods. Are there any of those things you would like to change? Do you have a role model? Did your weight or eating habits enter into your description of yourself? How do you think other people might describe you? How do you react to people who are obese? How do you react to people who are severely underweight? How do you think your reaction to people affect their personal identities?

CHAPTER 15 Dementia and Cognitive Disorders

Take this simple matching quiz for fun. A sign or symptom of delirium or dementia is on one side and an example of the resulting behavior is on the other.

Signs/Symptoms	Description/Example
1. Confabulation	A. Hearty laugh followed by loud sobs and tears
2. Disorientation	B. "Why are those men in uniforms in my living room?"
3. Sundowning	
4. Confusion	C. "Where is my wallet?" "Where is my wallet?" "Where is my wallet?"
5. Perseveration	
6. Illusions	D. "It's getting dark. There are shadows all around. Who is that? I'd better keep moving, so he can't get me."
7. Emotional lability	
	E. "How old am I? I am 18. I just graduated from high school."
	F. "Where am I? What day is this? Who are you?"
	G. "I must get home now. My children will be coming home from school, and I need to be there."

Answers

1 (E) 2 (F) 3 (D) 4 (G) 5 (C) 6 (B) 7 (A)

Special Topics in Mental Health Nursing

UNIT IV

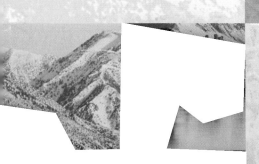

Chapter 16

Violence and Abuse

BRIEF Outline

Violent Families

Child Abuse

Elder Abuse

Legal Issues in Family Violence

Sexual Assault and Rape

Language Matters

Violence in the Healthcare Workplace

LEARNING Outcomes

After completing this chapter, you will be able to:

1. Identify clients at risk for family violence.
2. Apply the nursing process to clients experiencing family violence.
3. Identify clients who are at risk for becoming violent in the healthcare setting.
4. Apply the nursing process to clients at risk for aggression.
5. Describe ways to provide for the safety of staff and clients.

The World Health Organization (WHO) spent 3 years studying violence all over the world. Their Report on Violence and Health indicates that 1.6 million people lose their lives each year to violence. For every person who dies as a result of violence, many more are injured and suffer from a range of physical, reproductive, and mental health problems. According to the follow-up review of progress based on this report, violence in one form or another affects almost every individual at some point in time during his/her lifetime (WHO, 2007).

The WHO defines **violence** as the intentional use of physical force or power, threatened or actual, against another person, against oneself, or against a group or community, that either results in or has a high likelihood of resulting in injury, death, psychological harm, abnormal development, or deprivation (WHO, 2007).

The definition encompasses violence between individuals, as well as suicidal behavior, and collective violence, such as armed conflict. In addition to physical acts, it includes intimidation and threats and the various psychological and developmental consequences to individuals, families, and communities. The report uses an "ecological model" to explain the multifaceted nature of violence (Figure 16-1 ■).

The first level in the ecological model identifies biological and personal history factors that influence how individuals behave. It explores the person's likelihood of becoming a victim or perpetrator of violence. The person being subjected to abuse is a victim during the abuse. Afterward s/he is a survivor. In nursing care, we emphasize the ability of the person to survive and overcome the abuse. A **perpetrator** is a person who inflicts violence on another. Examples of factors that affect the risk of violence include personality disorders, substance abuse, experiencing abuse, and history of aggressive behavior (WHO, 2002).

The second level looks at relationships, such as families, friends, peers, and intimate partners. It explores how these relationships can increase the risk of being a victim or perpetrator of violence. For example, if a child grows up in a family in which violence is tolerated, s/he is more likely to be either a victim or perpetrator of violence (WHO, 2002).

The third level explores the community contexts in which social relationships occur, such as schools, workplaces, and neighborhoods. It identifies the characteristics of these settings that can contribute to the risk of violence. Community examples include population density, tolerance of the community to drug trade, and high levels of unemployment (WHO, 2002).

The fourth level in the ecological model looks at the broad societal factors that create a climate in which violence is encouraged or discouraged. These include the availability of weapons and social and cultural norms. Pertinent cultural norms include attitudes that give priority of parental rights over child welfare, the attitude that suicide is an individual choice rather than a preventable act of violence, male dominance over women and children, and support of the use of excessive force by police. Societal factors affecting violence also include economic, educational, and social policies that help to maintain economic or social inequality between groups in society (WHO, 2002).

The overlapping rings in the model represent how factors at each level strengthen or modify factors in the other levels. For example, a person with a history of abuse is more likely to act violently in a community that tolerates violence than in a more peaceable environment. No single factor explains why an individual behaves violently. Violence is a complex problem rooted in the interaction of biological, social, cultural, economic, and political factors. The ecological model also suggests that in order to reduce and prevent violence, it is necessary to act across several different levels at the same time (WHO, 2002). The first section of this chapter covers violence among individuals and in families. The second part covers violence in the healthcare workplace. Box 16-1 ■ presents some WHO examples of how actions across the different levels of the ecological model can prevent violence.

Violent Families

Children are shaped by their childhood experiences. Some are exposed to positive experiences and parents who are usually good role models. Some are exposed to parenting models of abuse, neglect, exploitation, and victimization. How will this latter group learn to parent their own children?

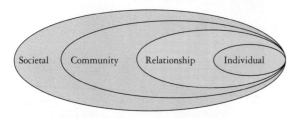

Figure 16-1. ■ WHO ecological model for understanding violence. *Source:* World Health Organization. (2002). *World report on violence and health.* Geneva: Author. Used with permission.

BOX 16-1

WHO Recommendations for Violence Prevention in a Society

- Address individual risk factors and take steps to modify individual risk behaviors.
- Influence close personal relationships and work to create healthy family environments, as well as providing professional help and support for dysfunctional families.
- Monitor public places such as schools, workplaces, and neighborhoods and take steps to address problems that might lead to violence.
- Address gender inequality and adverse cultural attitudes and practices.
- Address the larger cultural, social, and economic factors that contribute to violence and take steps to change them, including measures to close the gap between the rich and poor and to ensure equitable access to goods, services, and opportunities.

Source: World Health Organization. (2002). *World report on violence and health.* Geneva: Author.

Family violence is violent behavior that occurs among people who are related or who are members of the same household. It includes physical and emotional abuse and neglect of children, abuse between adult intimate partners, and elder abuse. It is a cruel irony that the social group that is supposed to provide love and support is also the most violent group to which most people belong. Behaviors that would not be accepted between strangers, coworkers, or friends are often tolerated in families (Fishwick, Parker, & Campbell, 2001).

IDENTIFYING PEOPLE AFFECTED BY FAMILY VIOLENCE

Family violence occurs across all socioeconomic groups. Race does not indicate who is at risk for family violence. It occurs in all races at about the same rate. Batterers and victims may be of any age. They can be doctors, nurses, librarians, lawyers, or alligator trainers.

Nurses will not find family violence by looking for a type of person. Behavior is the indicator. The basis of violent behavior is the establishment of a powerful control over another person usually through the promotion of a climate of fear. The abuser believes s/he is entitled to control the other person through whatever means necessary (Berlinger, 2001).

When healthcare providers try to create a stereotype of a violent family, the tragedy is that people who do not fit the stereotype are missed and therefore are denied treatment. Could the chairman of the board's wife with the

black eye who said she fell down the stairs really be battered? Yes, and she needs a nurse or other healthcare provider to recognize it.

Gender

Approximately 1.3 million women and 835,000 men in the United States are assaulted annually either physically or sexually by a present or former spouse, intimate partner, or someone they are dating; 25–30% of women will be assaulted by an intimate partner during their lifetime (Kovach, 2004). Although men are affected, the overwhelming majority of family violence is perpetrated by men against women and children. Figure 16-2 ■ shows a male threatening a woman and child with his fist.

Same-Sex Battering

People in homosexual relationships can also be violent. Statistics show that intimate partner violence in same-sex relationships occurs at the same rate as in heterosexual relationships. It has similarities to heterosexual intimate partner relationships in that it crosses age, race, lifestyle, and socioeconomic lines; escalates over time; victims often stay despite the ongoing abuse; and the basis for the abuse is power and control (American Medical Association [AMA], 2000). Because of the stigma against homosexuality,

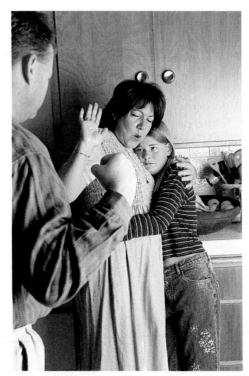

Figure 16-2. ■ Abusive male threatening woman and child with his fist. *Source:* PhotoEdit Inc.

people in same-sex relationships are less likely to report or seek help for the abuse (AMA, 2000). There is a higher prevalence of abuse among homosexual males than females, and resources are limited for male victims (Kovach, 2004). In the United States, there are approximately 2,000 shelters for intimate partner violence; only 21 of these offer services to men (Kovach, 2004).

CHARACTERISTICS OF VIOLENT FAMILIES

Violent families have some things in common. Multigenerational transmission of violence means that violent parents often had violent parents themselves. Children learn their behavior patterns in their families by taking their parents as role models. Although parents usually do not act in entirely positive or negative ways toward their children, the more children are exposed to a particular parenting style and quality of experience, the more they internalize that style and manifest it in their own parenting attitudes and practices (Bavolek, 2000).

Just as violence persists from one generation to the next, so does poor family functioning. When parents have never learned how to be nurturing to children, or what to reasonably expect from children at different developmental levels, or how to cope with life's frustrations and challenges in a healthy way, they are more likely to neglect their children or to continue the legacy of inadequate family functioning (Moss, Lynch, Hardie, & Baron, 2002).

Children who witness violence learn aggressive behavior. They also come to see violence as an option for coping with frustration or anger. Child abuse and abuse of intimate partners both show a repeating pattern in families.

Risk Factors

Statistics indicate that there are numerous risk factors that may be found in the families in which abuse is present. According to WHO's latest report, alcohol and substance abuse, mental illness, and economical inequalities increase the risk for most types of violence (WHO, 2007). Age, marital status, and employment seem to play a major role in intimate partner abuse. Younger women between the ages of 17 and 28 have the highest rate of intimate partner violence. This is compounded if the woman is single, separated, or divorced; pregnant; abuses drugs or alcohol, or is in a relationship with someone who does; was abused as a child; has a partner who is unemployed and if the combined income is low (Kovach, 2004; Walton-Moss & Campbell, 2002).

Social Isolation

Social isolation is another common characteristic of violent families. Because there are legal and social consequences for violent behavior, violence in the family becomes the family secret. Even if there is never a spoken rule to "keep the secret," family members are told in many subtle ways that they should not tell. Secrecy is one factor that accounts for the underreporting of family violence. The abuser often discourages family members from having friends or socializing outside the family. The abuser's wife may not be allowed to work outside the home. Social isolation occurs in child abuse, intimate partner abuse, and elder abuse.

Abuse of Power

In all forms of family violence, the abuser has some power or control over the victim (child, partner, or elder). The abuser may have financial and social control. The abuser is usually the one in control of the whole family, making all the decisions, spending the money. The abuser blames the victim for family problems and even for the abuse itself. If the abuser senses any indication of victim independence or disobedience, violence usually escalates.

The abuse of power resulting in domestic violence can take many forms, and these tend to overlap. Rarely does a violent relationship involve only one type of abuse (Walton-Moss & Campbell, 2002). Some examples include the following (Kovach, 2004):

- *Physical.*   Inflicting physical injury, withholding access to resources necessary to maintain health, or forcing alcohol or drug use, tying down or restraining
- *Emotional.*   Undermining the victim's sense of self-worth by intense criticizing, insulting, ridiculing, intimidating, belittling, name-calling
- *Sexual.*   Forcing sexual contact without consent, intentionally hurting someone during sex, forcing someone to have sex without protection from pregnancy or sexually transmitted diseases, making degrading sexual comments
- *Psychological.*   Arousing a sense of fear by threatening to hurt or abandon the victim, showing extreme possessiveness or jealousy, maintaining control over finances or isolating the victim from others

Alcohol and Drug Abuse

Substance abuse has been associated with family violence. Although families with a parent who abuses substances are more likely to experience violence, the relationship is not a simple cause-and-effect. Beware of concluding that

BOX 16-2

Reality Check on Family Violence

Quotes are from the people involved. Each quote is from a different situation:

- "If only I hadn't talked back. Dad wouldn't have killed my dog. Poor dog. I'm so sorry."
- "I was just trying to scare you. It was just because I was drunk, you know? I wouldn't have hurt you so bad if I was sober."
- "If only I had kept my mouth shut. He wouldn't have hit me."
- "Mom said: 'Hush, or he'll hit you again.'"
- "I shouldn't have smiled at my uncle that first time he put me on his lap. Maybe he wouldn't have touched me like that. I should have tried harder to stop him, and I hate myself."
- "She asked for it."
- "If you tell, I'll just do this to your sister."
- "Now that he is dead I'll never forgive myself. The last time we saw him in the ER his dad said he fell off his skateboard again, like he said he had four other times. I should have known it was abuse."

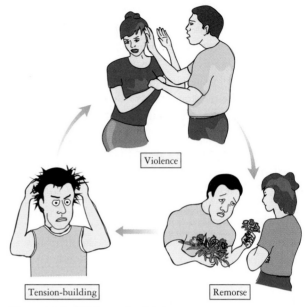

Figure 16-3. ■ The cycle of violence.

alcohol causes people to batter their families. Everyone who uses drugs and alcohol is not violent toward their families. Being drunk is not a valid excuse for violence. Abusers often use excuses for their behavior, such as, "I hurt them because I was drunk." If drinking caused people to be violent, why do they not hit the bartender or the police officer who gives them a traffic ticket? People have learned that they can control their partners or children with violence and that, to some extent, our society condones it. Box 16-2 ■ gives some quotes from people involved in violent situations.

Cycle of Violence

A pattern has been identified in family violence behavior. The tension-building phase may last for months or years, beginning with verbal criticism and belittling that progresses to the first incident of physical violence, which may last anywhere from 2 to 24 hours (Kovach, 2004). This first episode of violence is followed by sincere remorse on the part of the abuser. The abuser apologizes, says it will never happen again, and does something nice for the person s/he hurt. This remorseful time is also called the "honeymoon period." The abused wife believes that it will never happen again. Then the tension begins to rebuild. The abuser is irritable, jealous, or argumentative. The tension-building phase ends with another

violent episode, after which the abuser is sorry again. The cycle then repeats itself. Because the problem of family violence worsens over time, the violent incidents become closer together. Eventually the remorseful episodes fade away and all that remain are tension and violence. Figure 16-3 ■ illustrates the cycle of violence.

Intimate Partner Violence

Ninety-five percent of the abuse between intimate partners is by men abusing women. An estimated one of every three women has experienced violence from an intimate partner at some time in her life (Hastings, 2001). Figure 16-4 ■ shows man readying himself to hurt intimate partner.

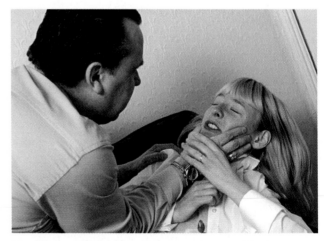

Figure 16-4. ■ Abusive male preparing to punch intimate female partner. *Source:* Alamy Images.

As in other forms of family violence, partner-abuse victims tend to conceal their abuse. More than half of all women seen in emergency departments are abused by their intimate partners, although most do not give an honest reason for their injuries (Hastings, 2001). Interestingly enough, it is more often that female victims of abuse visit the emergency room for something other than the injuries related to abuse. The fear and stress that being a victim of intimate partner violence (IPV) generates often leads to chronic conditions such as headaches, backaches, and anxiety. These are often the focus of the ER visit, not their injuries (Kovach, 2004). Physically, victims of IPV are often prone to GI problems such as irritable bowel syndrome, urinary tract infections, and sexually transmitted diseases. Mental effects are more likely to be depression and posttraumatic stress disorder (Kovach, 2004). The American Medical Association and American Nurses Association both advocate that all women being seen in a healthcare facility should be routinely screened for IPV (Kovach, 2004). Even when health facility staff members ask every woman if she is abused, many cases are not detected.

Because victims of partner abuse tend to be secretive, nurses must rely on their assessment skills to detect the likelihood of partner abuse. Some of the indicators of partner abuse that a nurse may assess include:

- Multiple injuries in various stages of healing; these can include unexplained bruises, burns, lacerations particularly if they are located in areas usually covered by clothing (Kovach, 2004)
- A story about the injury that is not consistent with the damage (such as a report of falling down stairs when a spiral humerus fracture can only result from twisting of the arm)
- Embarrassment about unexplained old injuries; appears evasive, anxious, or depressed (Berlinger, 2001)
- Has postponed obtaining treatment for the injury (Berlinger, 2001)
- Fear in the presence of the abuser, and trying to conceal the fear
- No friends, distant relationships with family
- Concerns about keeping the partner from being angry
- Partner not leaving the client alone with anyone; partner may appear uncooperative or domineering and may answer all the questions for the client; partner may also appear overly concerned for the welfare of the client (Berlinger, 2001)

When these cues to abuse are present, the nurse assesses further by asking the client specifically about abuse. Remember that the client is the one who decides how she

will respond, and whether she is able to receive help at this time. Studies have shown that the woman is most receptive to seeking help for her situation right after the abuse has occurred and before the abuser has entered the honeymoon phase of the violence cycle (McFarlane et al., 2004). However, the nurse cannot control another person's behavior. It is not the nurse's responsibility to rescue the woman or to convince her to bring charges against her partner (Berlinger, 2001). If possible, the nurse should avoid using words such as *abused* or *battered* or any other term that might be interpreted as judgmental by the client (Kovach, 2004). If the client denies any abuse or the need of help, the nurse must respect that decision but can still give her information about shelters and other resources. One reason women stay in abusive relationships is that they do not know they have choices. Nurses can treat this problem with information even in a brief emergency department or clinic visit. The information you give to the client on a small, wallet-sized card might be a seed that grows into action later when she is ready. However, you need to make sure that she feels safe in taking this information home if there is the chance that it might be seen by the abuser and be the source of more violence (Kovach, 2004).

WHY DO WOMEN STAY WITH ABUSIVE PARTNERS SO LONG?

On the surface it seems obvious: If a woman is being emotionally or physically abused by her partner, she should leave him. Her children are witnessing violence, learning both how to be violent and how to be victims. So, why does she stay? There are many reasons that it is very difficult for women to leave.

- He threatens to kill her if she leaves (30–50% of all women killed in the United States are killed by a partner as they try to leave [Hastings, 2001]).
- She is economically dependent on him and has no job skills (the abuser isolates his partner and won't let her out to work).
- Fear of losing custody of the children (only recently is a history of partner abuse being used as a factor in child custody decisions).
- She has no place to go (he has isolated her from friends).
- Lack of information about her choices (she does not know where to obtain information, advice, or help).
- She probably has low self-esteem and fear of being alone (she's not sure she can make it on her own; he has been telling her she is worthless for years).
- She believes that batterers are not held responsible for their behavior (she has seen this happen).

BOX 16-3

Myths and Facts About Domestic Violence

Myth: Perpetrators of domestic violence abuse their partners because they are under a lot of stress or unemployed.
Fact: Stress or unemployment does not cause people to abuse their partners. Domestic violence happens in all socioeconomic groups, not just in the unemployed. If stress causes violence, why do perpetrators only abuse their families? They learn that they can achieve what they want (power and control) through the use of force, without facing serious consequences.

Myth: People abuse their partners because of alcohol or drug abuse.
Fact: Alcohol or drugs do not cause people to abuse their family members, although they are often used as an excuse. Substance abuse does increase the severity of violent episodes. Requiring abusers to attend only substance abuse treatment will not stop them from battering their partners or children.

Myth: Victims of domestic violence like to be beaten.
Fact: Survivors of domestic violence have been characterized as masochistic women who enjoy being beaten. There is no evidence for this notion. Survivors of abuse desperately want the abuse to end. They engage in various survival strategies to protect themselves and their children. Taking a beating to keep the batterer from beating the children may be one survival strategy, but the victim does not enjoy it.

Myth: Victims of domestic violence never leave their abusers, and if they do they get into other abusive relationships.
Fact: Most survivors of domestic violence leave their abusers. It may take a number of attempts to permanently separate because abusers use violence, financial control, or threats about the children to compel victims to return. Lack of community support may force victims to return. The risk of future violence may increase when the victim leaves. Although some victims enter into other abusive relationships, there is no evidence that this is the experience of the majority.

Source: Center for Substance Abuse Prevention. (2004). *It won't happen to me: Alcohol abuse and violence against women (for those who are concerned about the issue).* Substance Abuse and Mental Health Services Administration, Washington, DC: Author. Accessed August 28, 2007, from http://pathwayscourses.samhsa.gov/vawc/vawc_intro_pg1.htm.

- Denial. She thinks: "He is sick and needs me" or "His true self is when he is sorry" (instead of "He is a criminal and should be in jail").
- She suffers from severe depression that may accompany the abuse and does not have the energy to take any action (Berlinger, 2001).
- She may experience religious, cultural, or societal pressures to stay (Berlinger, 2001).
- She has developed good survival skills but not assertiveness skills (she knows how to stay but not how to go).

Box 16-3 ■ compares myths and facts about domestic violence.

Working with survivors of family violence is another area where nurses must look at their own attitudes. Would you feel angry with a woman who came into the emergency department injured by her partner, who planned to return to live with him? Some nurses do, and this judgmental attitude can affect their professional functioning.

Critical Self-Check. Consider the situation of a mother who is afraid to leave her abusive partner. She has no job, skills, or friends. What would it be like to think that living with abuse is better than taking the chance of being alone in the world?

Nurses can make a difference for battered women. Begin by believing them when they tell you they were abused, and accept these clients as people no matter what they decide to do. Acknowledge the client's experience by validating that "abuse is a very common problem," so the client knows she is not alone. Establish a trusting relationship. The therapeutic use of your self is effective in crisis situations like this. Figure 16-5 ■ shows an abused woman visiting with a nonjudgmental counselor.

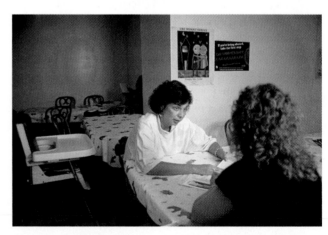

Figure 16-5. ■ Abused woman seeking help from nonjudgmental counselor. *Source:* Pearson Education/PH College.

Other interventions are discussed in the Nursing Care section of this chapter.

Child Abuse

Child abuse or maltreatment can take the form of physical, emotional, or sexual abuse or of physical, emotional, and medical neglect to someone younger than 18 years of age. Children who witness family violence are also victims.

Almost 1 million American children annually are the victims of child abuse. The latest statistics break down the proportions of abused children as follows (Anbarghalami, Yang, Van Sell, & Miller-Anderson, 2007):

- 62.4% are neglected
- 17.5% are physically abused
- 9.7% are sexually abused
- 7% are emotionally or psychologically abused
- 2.1% are medically neglected

Physical abuse of children can take the form of severe corporal punishment. Figure 16-6 ■ shows a child who was punished by being whipped with an electrical cord.

Such punishment is often associated with not knowing what can reasonably be expected of children at different

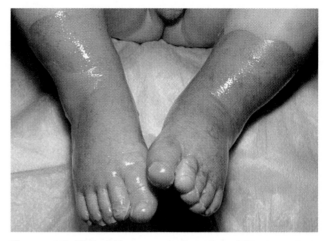

Figure 16-7. ■ Scald burns on the feet of a toddler. *Source:* Roy Alson, PhD, MD FACEP, FAAEM.

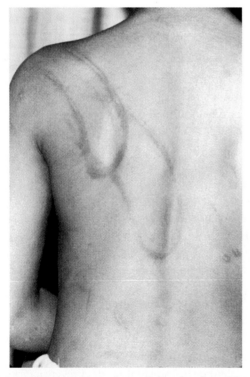

Figure 16-6. ■ Boy with marks made by a beating with an electric cord. Sometimes the type of abuse can be determined by the characteristics of the wounds on the victim. *Source:* Robert A. Felter, M.D.

stages of development. For example, a 1-year-old may be punished for crying, or an infant for soiling diapers. Head trauma (sometimes from shaking) is the leading cause of death and disability among infants and children who are abused. Intentional injuries to children can also take the form of hitting, shaking, cutting, burning, choking, hair pulling, or other injuries.

Nurses must consider abuse when a child's injuries are not consistent with the explanation given. The toddler who is brought to the emergency room with scald burns on the feet should raise suspicion in the healthcare provider if the caregivers report the child accidentally turned the hot water on while in the tub while the child is screaming about the "hot pot" (Figure 16-7 ■).

The child's behavior may be withdrawn, overly aggressive, or show delay in reaching developmental tasks. The abused child may have multiple injuries in various stages of healing. The child may have a history of multiple emergency department visits or visits to a variety of healthcare providers. The abusive parent may speak for the child and may not want to leave the child alone with the nurse, for fear that the child will tell what happened.

Emotional abuse includes verbal assault such as demeaning the child, blaming, screaming, and insulting. Constant conflict and chaos may be present in the home. Parents may withhold affection and nurturing, possibly because they are unaware of how to provide them. Emotional abuse usually accompanies other forms of abuse or neglect. Parents who abuse their children may be emotionally immature. They may lack the skills to meet their own emotional needs, let alone the needs of their children. Emotional abuse may manifest itself in many ways in the child: withdrawal, anger, learning difficulties, nervous habits such as thumb-sucking or nail-biting, or conduct disorders that might be seen in antisocial or destructive behaviors (Mulryan, Cathers, & Fagin, 2000).

Sexual abuse involves sexual acts (fondling, penile penetration, insertion of fingers or other objects, masturbation, exposure of perpetrator's genitalia, oral-genital contact, exposure of victim to pornography) performed by an adult, for the gratification of the adult, on a child under age 18. Another type of sexual abuse is exploitation, which involves using a child to produce pornography. The majority of sexually abused children know their abuser; a parent or caregiver is involved in about half of the cases (Mulryan et al., 2000).

Most cases of child sexual abuse are undetected. This is in part due to family secrecy. Victims are carefully influenced not to tell. The perpetrator may threaten the victim with death, beating, or loss of his love if she tells. He may tell her that if she tells anyone, he will do the same thing to her sister. The fact that child abuse is so much more common than healthcare providers and law enforcement know is partly due to denial by professionals because of the taboo of incest. Father-daughter incest is the most common form of reported child sexual abuse. Siblings can also be perpetrators of incest. If a diagnosis of sexual abuse is suspected, siblings should also be considered as possible perpetrators. When the evidence is ambiguous, healthcare providers may not want to think about the problem. Another reason for underdiagnosis of child abuse is that, if it is reported and the child was not abused, the family and the child may suffer considerably from the stigma of this charge and the legal process involved. Healthcare providers may be afraid to take this chance.

The child survivor of sexual abuse who has not told anyone about the abuse may be taken to a healthcare provider with nonspecific symptoms such as sleep disturbances, abdominal pain, enuresis (bed-wetting), encopresis (fecal incontinence), or phobias (Anbarghalami et al., 2007). The child may experience the following signs and symptoms: sexually transmitted disease, vaginal or rectal bleeding or discomfort, pregnancy, recurrent urinary tract infections, sexual acting-out, premature knowledge about sexual behavior, social withdrawal, low self-esteem, decrease in school performance, insomnia, or aggressive behavior. Most cases of child sexual abuse are discovered when the child finally tells someone of the abuse (Anbarghalami et al., 2007).

Neglect is failure to provide for the physical, emotional, medical, or developmental needs of a child. Sometimes neglect is due to the lack of knowledge and resources, or to personal issues of the parent or other caregiver such as immaturity, mental health problems, or substance abuse (Mulryan et al., 2000). Medical neglect might be due to religious or cultural beliefs. Sometimes the abuse is intentional. Neglect includes abandonment of a child, inadequate supervision, failure to provide health care, failure to seek timely treatment for injury or illness, abusive emotional treatment, not sending a child to school, or putting the child's safety at risk. Neglect is the most common type of child abuse.

It is not only active physical battering that causes lifelong problems. Neglect can also be destructive to children over time, even more than physical abuse is. Both abuse and neglect increase the likelihood of certain mental disorders and issues such as depression, posttraumatic stress disorder (PTSD), other anxiety disorders, difficulty trusting others, substance abuse, and antisocial behavior. The odds of future delinquency and adult criminality are increased by 29% in children who survive family violence (Widom & Maxfield, 2001).

PREVENTION OF CHILD ABUSE

Prevention is a powerful tool against family violence. Does it really work to teach the public preventive behaviors that promote their health? The answer is "Yes!" Alcohol-related traffic deaths have decreased as a result of several national campaigns to increase public awareness. Have you seen "Designated Driver" or "Mothers Against Drunk Driving" spots on television or in magazines? Their campaigns put a human face on the tragedy of alcohol-related traffic crashes. These education programs save lives. Demonstrations of protestors to break the cycle of violence are there to educate the public about the dangers of an abused child growing up to be an abusive parent (Figure 16-8 ■).

Prevention programs for child abuse build on family strengths. Strategies include parent education, home visitation, and parent support groups. Prevention programs help parents to develop parenting skills; understand age-appropriate discipline; understand the benefits of nonviolent discipline; and learn to meet children's emotional, physical, and developmental needs. Prevention programs can also help parents learn to identify their own needs for support or respite. Box 16-4 ■ provides some tips on how to be a nurturing parent.

BOX 16-4

Tips on How to Be a Nurturing Parent

We can all take steps to improve our relationship with our children. Try these:

- Help your children feel loved and secure.
- Make sure they know you love them, even when they make mistakes.
- Encourage them.
- Praise their talents.
- Spend time with your children doing things you all enjoy.
- Seek help if you need it:

Talk to someone (friend, neighbor, family member, clergy, teacher, nurse, physician, counselor).
Get counseling.
Take a parenting class.

- Be a role model for solving problems without violence, shouting, or insults. Take a problem-solving approach with your partner and children.
- Know what your children are capable of doing at different ages so your expectations are reasonable.
- Take a break. Get a babysitter. If you can't afford one, take turns with another parent: you take a turn watching theirs and they take a turn watching yours.

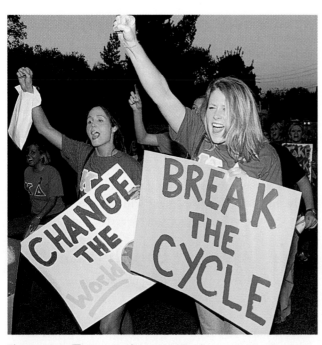

Figure 16-8. ■ Women demonstrating in a protest, trying to break the cycle of domestic violence. *Source:* AP Wide World Photos.

Elder Abuse

Elder abuse is the abuse or neglect of an older adult. It can occur at home or in a long-term care facility. It can be perpetrated by a family member or another caregiver. Just like with children, the abuse may have different forms, and the elder may be subjected to more than one type (Gray-Vickrey, 2004). The abuse may be physical or emotional; it may be neglect or financial abuse or material exploitation (Gray-Vickrey, 2004). The cases of spousal abuse of elders overlap the issues of abuse of an intimate partner. It is estimated that between one and two million Americans over the age of 65 have been abused in some form by someone they depended on for care (National

Center on Elder Abuse, 2005). The latest statistics from the Adult Protective Services agencies show the following breakdown (National Center on Elder Abuse, 2006):

Neglect: 57.6% (caregiver neglect, 20.4% and self-neglect, 37.2%)
Emotional/psychological/verbal abuse: 14.8%
Financial abuse or material exploitation: 14.7%
Physical abuse: 10.7%
Sexual abuse: 1%
Other: 1.2%

Elder abuse may include physical force that results in injury, failure to meet basic physical needs for food and water, withholding eyeglasses or hearing aids, confinement, leaving the person alone for long periods, restraining, sexually molesting, or misusing drugs (either misusing the prescribed medications, or forcing the victim to take sedating drugs or alcohol). It may include denying the elder medical treatment, ignoring the victim's emotional needs, or actively abusing the person emotionally with threats, humiliation, or insults. It can also involve misusing someone's property and resources, stealing items from the home to sell, tricking the elder into signing over Social Security checks, or "borrowing" funds that are never returned.

It is important for the nurse to recognize which elders are most likely to be abused. Studies have shown that most abuse occurs in women who are older than 80 who need partial or total assistance with their activities of daily living (Gray-Vickrey, 2004). Often the perpetrator is a family member with whom the elder lives. Adult children are the most common perpetrators of abuse (National Center on Elder Abuse, 2006). Perpetrators may have limited resources for providing care to the elder person, may feel overwhelmed, and may have inadequate coping skills. This is especially true if the elder has a physical or emotional disability due to a stroke, paralysis, Parkinson's or Alzheimer's disease, or are involved in substance abuse, especially alcohol. Being incontinent of either urine or feces or both often results in anger or frustration on the part of the caregiver. Caregivers themselves may have a history of other violent behavior or substance abuse. They may also be retaliating for times in the past when they were abused by the elder person. It might be a continuation of a lifetime of spousal abuse (Gray-Vickrey, 2004).

Abuse in long-term care facilities may have different triggers. It is usually due to stressful working conditions that could include being short-staffed and lack of appreciation for the staff by clients and administration. Inadequate staff education regarding difficult client behaviors and appropriate responses to those behaviors could also be part of the cause. Figure 16-9 ■ shows an elderly woman who suffered multiple bruises on arms and body while living in a residential care facility.

It may be difficult for abused elders to disclose that they are being abused. The same family dynamics that were described under intimate partner violence may occur here. In addition, elders may fear institutionalization if they report abuse by their caregivers.

Because of this, the nurse's assessment skills are especially important. Box 16-5 ■ lists some of the indications

BOX 16-5

Signs of Elder Abuse and Neglect

- Bruises on upper arms bilaterally
- Multiple injuries in various stages of healing
- Any injuries around face, neck, and ears including broken teeth
- Spiral bone fractures, especially arms
- Burns, especially of soles, palms, or buttocks; any sign of rope burns on extremities
- Vaginal injury
- Dehydration
- Malnutrition
- Skin breakdown
- Poor personal hygiene: matted hair, strong odor, dirty clothes, long nails
- No dentures, glasses, or hearing aids, although the client needs them
- Fear of caregiver
- Verbal belittling of elder by caregiver

that an elder may be experiencing abuse. Keep in mind that general medical disorders or old age can cause some of these signs. The presence of one or a few of these signs does not definitively diagnose abuse but, taken in context, they may suggest abuse. If the elder person is cognitively impaired, the assessment will be more challenging and the nurse will rely more on objective signs.

Legal Issues in Family Violence

The laws that regulate the response by the nurse to suspected family violence are passed by state legislatures. Therefore, no single rule governs nursing responsibility.

Most states also require nurses who suspect elder abuse to report to the state agency that provides adult protective services. The long-term care ombudsman for the county could be contacted for suspected abuse within a long-term care facility. The decision of whether to report intimate partner abuse is usually left to the victim, unless the victim is less than 18 or more than 65 years of age. Nurses must be aware of the laws in the states where they practice.

clinical ALERT

All U.S. states and Canadian provinces have mandatory child abuse reporting laws. The telephone number for reporting child abuse is usually under "Child Abuse" in the business white pages of the phone book. You could also call the national emergency child abuse hotline: 1-(800)-422-4453 (1-800-4-A-CHILD).

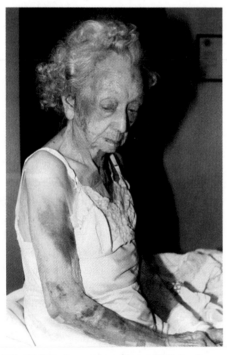

Figure 16-9. ■ Elderly woman with multiple bruises on arms and body inflicted while living in a residential care facility. *Source:* National Association of State Units on Aging.

In cases of family violence, the nurse's documentation is especially important because it is more likely to be used as evidence in court. Documentation by the nurse can corroborate police data. It is considered to be objective, factual information documented soon after the abuse has occurred when facts and appearances are fresh in the nurse's mind (Isaac & Enos, 2001). Documentation should include quotes from the people involved about what happened, and an objective description of the interaction between the victim and potential perpetrator. Describe behaviors without interpretation. For example: "Client cringed and turned away when her husband moved closer to her bed," not, "Client is very fearful of her husband." It goes without saying that the documentation should be legible if handwritten! Sometimes photos of injuries are included in the medical record but only with the client's permission. Any photos should be signed and dated by the attending care provider and photographer (Gray-Vickrey, 2004). Another way to document the injuries is the use of a "body map," which is a diagram of the body allowing the nurse to indicate the location and type of injuries found (Isaac & Enos, 2001). It is not necessary for the nurse to ask the abuse survivor for a detailed description of the abuse. The tasks of full disclosure and in-depth discussion of the abuse are best saved for psychotherapy.

Physical assessment findings that should be documented include (Hockenberry, 2005; Isaac & Enos, 2001):

- Location, size, shape, and color of bruises or other injuries; approximate size and location can be documented on the drawing of a body outline; take photos of injuries with client's informed consent
- Distinguishing characteristics, such as a bruise in the shape of a hand or a buckle; round burns that could be caused by a cigarette
- Symmetry of injury (such as symmetrical bruises on both upper arms)
- Degree of pain, any bone tenderness
- Evidence of past injuries
- General state of health and hygiene
- Client's demeanor/affect (crying, shaking, angry, calm, etc.)

In addition to the physical assessment documentation, it is important for the nurse to document the client's own words and set off the phrases with quotation marks. Do the same for the caregiver's comments. Include what is called "excited utterances" in legal terms; these are statements made by the victim soon after the abuse event while s/he is still in an agitated state of mind (Isaac & Enos, 2001). Record how much time has passed since the abuse occurred.

PERPETRATORS OF FAMILY VIOLENCE

The people who perpetrate violence on their families are often grown-ups who were abused as children. Still, if responding to frustration with violence is learned, then responding in a nonviolent way can also be learned. Like other lifestyle changes, these are difficult yet possible changes to make. Again, violence issues may be affected by differing cultures. Immigrant women can be especially vulnerable to domestic violence (Box 16-6 ■).

Many communities have treatment programs for abusive men. These treatment programs are most effective when the court mandates them, with punishment for noncompliance. Abusive men seldom have the insight to admit and understand their own behavior. The nurse must clarify with all concerned that the responsibility for the violent behavior lies with the abuser. Long-lasting change is more likely if treatment combines both anger management therapy and a program designed to change attitudes toward women (Fishwick et al., 2001).

BOX 16-6   CULTURAL PULSE POINTS

Violence Against Immigrant Women

Domestic violence is thought to be more common among immigrant women than it is among U.S. citizens. There are several reasons: Immigrant women may suffer higher rates of battering because they come from cultures that tolerate domestic violence, or because they have less access to legal and social services than U.S. citizens. They may distrust the legal system, fear deportation, or have a language barrier. A battered woman who is not a legal immigrant, or whose immigration status depends on her husband, is isolated by cultural and legal dynamics that may prevent her from leaving her husband, or even from seeking legal assistance. She may not even be understood if she called 911 or tried to obtain help for food or shelter. According to Leslye Orloff, director of the Battered Immigrant Women Program in Washington, DC, the immigrant factors of stress, economic problems, and cultural issues are not the cause of the abuse, but these conditions create barriers to make it more difficult for the immigrant women to obtain help (Voice of America, 2004).

Nurses must be alert to the possibility of family violence in immigrant families, and arrange for interpreters and referrals to social services as indicated. Newer federal legislation provides the same assistance to battered immigrant women regardless of their legal status as to American citizens; however, if illegal immigrant males are guilty of domestic violence, they may be deported (Voice of America, 2004).

In the case of elder abuse or neglect, the primary concern of the elder client may be fear of institutionalization in a nursing home. Sometimes it is necessary to remove the client from the home, and to prosecute the offender. When admitted to a nursing home, this client will have significant psychosocial needs, including grief, anxiety, and powerlessness. When the abuse is the result of caregiver ignorance or caregiver role strain, it is sometimes possible to keep the elder in the same home, with social services for clients and caregivers. The abusive or neglectful caregiver may benefit from education about the needs of the client and how to meet them, counseling, respite-care services, or therapy for mental disorders or substance dependency.

Sexual Assault and Rape

Sexual assault and **rape** refer to any forced sexual contact without consent. Consent is the critical issue. Sexual contact with a minor is considered a crime, regardless of the issue of consent. Minors are not legally able to provide consent for sexual intercourse because of their immaturity and vulnerability.

The statistics are staggering. In America, someone is sexually assaulted every 2½ minutes; one in six women and one in 33 men in America are victims of sexual assault (Rape, Abuse & Incest National Network, 2005).

Rape is a crime of violence, rage, and power, not sex. The motivations for raping women or men are similar: to humiliate, control, or dominate the victim. Survivors of rape often state that they are never the same again. They can never trust in their safety or be as carefree as they were before this kind of an assault.

It was not until the 1970s in the United States that marital rape was considered a crime. Before that time, if a man attacked and forced sexual penetration on a woman he was committing rape, unless the woman was his wife. Currently, marital rape is a crime in every state. Sixty to 80% of all rape victims are raped by a spouse, partner, relative, or friend. As many as 70% of rapes may go unreported, even though rape is a felony. Women are less likely to report rape when they know their attackers (Smith & Kelly, 2001).

RAPE TRAUMA SYNDROME

Rape Trauma Syndrome is a nursing diagnosis for the group of symptoms that develop after a forced violent sexual attack, or attempted attack. It includes an acute phase of disorganization of the survivor's lifestyle and a

---

BOX 16-7

Symptoms of Rape Trauma Syndrome

- Sleep disturbances, nightmares
- Denial, guilt, self blame
- Disorganization
- Fears, anxiety, phobias
- Humiliation, embarrassment
- Low self-esteem, feelings of worthlessness
- Changes in relationships with family and friends
- Powerlessness, helplessness
- Inability to make decisions
- Sexual dysfunction
- Loss of appetite
- Low mood
- Substance abuse
- Physical trauma initially, then physical symptoms (either specific or vague) may persist

---

long-term process of reorganization. Box 16-7 ■ lists the symptoms of Rape Trauma Syndrome. The desired outcomes for clients with this diagnosis are that in the short term the client will resolve the crisis related to the trauma, and begin the process of grief resolution. The long-term outcome is that the client will resume usual social relationships and lifestyle.

Language Matters

Let's talk about how we talk. Language matters because it communicates our attitudes. When we refer to people who have experienced violence as *victims,* we suggest that they are powerless. When we use the term *survivors,* we imply that these people have experienced a hardship and outlasted it. They have survived. When we refer to people who are in the healthcare system for care related to family violence, we will use the term *survivors*, and our goal as nurses will be to empower these survivors to work through their grief and trauma, put the abuse behind them, and move on to new healthy lives.

NURSING CARE

ASSESSING

Our cultural attitudes make it difficult for nurses to assess for abuse and sexual assault. Both clients and healthcare providers are reluctant to discuss these issues. Because abuse is so common, and yet so emotionally charged, it is important for the nurse to be nonthreatening and to establish trust with clients, to allow them to talk about it. It is also important that the nurse and client have total privacy. If the client does not feel safe and supported, s/he might be afraid to be honest (Berlinger, 2001). The nurse should explain to the family that privacy is needed to conduct an examination. It is helpful if the healthcare facility has a privacy policy that is posted in the waiting room where the nurse can refer to it (Berlinger, 2001).

It may help to ask broad questions to find sexual abuse history, such as "Has anyone ever forced you to have sex when you didn't want to?" followed by "Would you tell me more about that?" (Fishwick et al., 2001). Every woman should be asked about abuse. Some will be offended, but some will say: "Yes. Thank you for asking. Can you help me?" This is why we ask.

To assess for physical abuse, the nurse might say: "We see a lot of injuries like you have. Sometimes they are from someone hitting the woman. How did this happen to you?" or "I don't think you walked into a doorknob. Did somebody hit you in the eye?" In this assessment the nurse does not want to suggest that the "correct" answer is that the client was abused, but to suggest that it is believable and acceptable for the client to disclose the abuse if it occurred.

DIAGNOSING, PLANNING, AND IMPLEMENTING

When the client has disclosed that s/he is a survivor of family violence or sexual assault, the nurse's first action must be active listening. Now that the client is willing to disclose the abuse, s/he is likely to benefit from discussing it with a nonjudgmental listener (Fishwick et al., 2001). Once again, the therapeutic use of self is an important nursing intervention.

Some common nursing diagnoses for survivors of violence include:

- Posttrauma Syndrome or Rape Trauma Syndrome
- Ineffective Coping
- Powerlessness
- Risk for Other-Directed Violence
- Risk for Suicide
- Situational Low Self-Esteem
- Disturbed Sleep Pattern
- Spiritual Distress

Nurses working in any setting may encounter clients with Posttrauma Syndrome, which is a sustained maladaptive response to an overwhelming traumatic event, such as family violence or sexual assault. It may last for a short time or persist for years.

The nursing assessments that lead to the diagnosis of Posttrauma Syndrome include:

- Flashbacks or reexperiencing the traumatic event
- Nightmares, insomnia, and other sleep disturbances
- Anger, guilt, anxiety
- Fear, which may be related to people or situations that remind the survivor of the trauma
- Difficulty expressing feelings
- Difficulty experiencing feelings of love, empathy, or happiness
- Difficulty in relationships
- Substance abuse
- Physical symptoms that may be specific to the trauma or nonspecific, such as abdominal pain, nausea, or headache

The desired outcomes for the client who has Posttrauma Syndrome are that the client will:

- Discuss the traumatic event.
- Express feelings directly.
- Establish a balance of sleep and activity.
- Demonstrate reduced anxiety, fear, guilt, and anger.
- Report a decrease in physical symptoms.
- Identify support systems to help with coping.
- Demonstrate increased ability to cope with stress.

The nurse may choose from the following interventions designed to treat Posttrauma Syndrome:

- Establish a trusting nurse-client relationship. *Trust is the foundation for beginning work on personal and grief issues such as those experienced after trauma. Clients may have additional difficulty establishing trust after being traumatized. Trusting the nurse is a good step toward normalizing relationships with others.*
- Encourage the client to express feelings about the traumatic event, especially negative feelings such as anger. Journaling (or other writing), talking with the nurse or a friend, and crying are some ways to express emotions. *Identifying and expressing feelings help the client begin to resolve the grief and anger associated with the traumatic event. People understand their own feelings better when they have expressed them verbally.*
- Take an accepting, nonjudgmental approach to the client. *The client may have strong negative, angry feelings and may feel that these feelings are frightening or even inappropriate. When the nurse is nonjudgmental, the message to the client is that the client's feelings are acceptable. Acceptance of the client also helps reduce the client's feelings of self-blame.*

■ Give the client an opportunity to discuss the event with others who have survived violence. *People with similar experiences understand the associated feelings best. Others who have survived violence, such as members of a rape survivors support group, may be able to help the client identify problems and plan coping mechanisms to deal with them. Sharing with others who have an experience in common can be a powerful tool for recovery.*

clinical ALERT

Many nurses have personal histories of family violence or sexual assault. To have objective professional relationships with clients who are survivors or perpetrators of violence, these nurses must resolve issues about their own abuse. Nurses must heal before they can help others heal.

■ Do client and family teaching as indicated, for topics such as Posttrauma Syndrome, community resources, parenting groups, survivor groups, shelters, and laws pertinent to family violence. *The client is more empowered if s/he is informed.*

■ Discuss coping strategies and assist the client to create a list of resources that s/he can realistically use. *After a crisis, the client may be more open to changing coping behavior. The nurse's suggestions for new ways to cope or new resources to use are more likely to be accepted by the client when s/he is open to change. The client may be unaware of services even in the town where the client lives. A list of resources for use when the client is ready can be very helpful. Realistic options are the only ones the client can use.*

EVALUATING

After the nurse has intervened with a client who has experienced violence or abuse, the nurse will evaluate whether the desired outcomes are met. The client who is a survivor of violence should be able to discuss the traumatic event, expressing feelings directly. Survivors should be able to balance sleep and activity. They should be able to identify resources for help with coping, and to demonstrate reduced anxiety and increased ability to cope with stress.

Violence in the Healthcare Workplace

This section covers the care of clients who are angry, aggressive, or agitated. These clients may be in any healthcare setting. Some situations relate specifically to clients hospitalized in the psychiatric setting.

As we will discuss in more detail in the next chapter, anger is a normal feeling in response to frustration. It can be productive and adaptive when it motivates a person to change behavior or to battle injustice, but it can also be destructive or maladaptive. When anger is not rationally based, or when the client is acting out angry feelings toward other people, it can be dangerous. **Aggression** is forceful physical or verbal action, which can be dangerous in the healthcare setting. **Dangerousness** includes actions that have a high risk of harming self or others.

Violence in healthcare settings results from clients and occasionally their family members who feel frustrated, vulnerable, or out of control. Nurses and aides who have the most direct contact with clients are at the highest risk. Violence may occur anywhere in the hospital environment, but it is most frequent in psychiatric units, emergency departments, waiting rooms, and geriatric units. The nursing-home rate of injury and illness is more than double the rate in industry as a whole. The injuries to nursing-home employees include blood-borne pathogen exposure, ergonomic injuries, falls, and infections, as well as workplace violence (National Institute for Occupational Safety and Health [NIOSH], 2002).

CAUSES OF VIOLENT BEHAVIOR

Biological Factors

Some scientific evidence suggests that brain chemistry, brain damage, genetics, and environmental factors may lead to aggressive tendencies and violent actions. A predisposition to violence may be the result of genetics and brain chemistry and then shaped into an abusive pattern by the psychological environment of one's younger years. A serotonin deficiency has been linked to impulsive aggressive behavior. Negative influences may be softened by good parenting and pharmacological treatments (Wilkinson, 2003).

The frontal lobe of the brain regulates the ability to plan, solve problems, and control impulses. If it is damaged (such as in head trauma), the client may have impulsive behavior with aggressive outbursts. Poor impulse control is an important aspect of some violent behavior. An impulsive act is one that is not premeditated. It is action done without consideration of consequences. When a client has poor impulse control, s/he may act out violently without warning. Figure 16-10 ■ shows the areas of the brain that are associated with violent behavior.

Temporal-lobe epilepsy may cause emotional outbursts. Tumors of the limbic system can cause personality

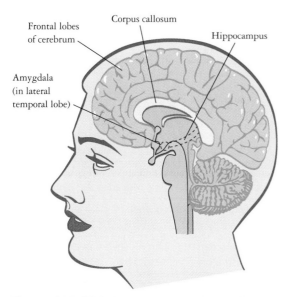

Figure 16-10. ■ Brain structures associated with aggressive behavior. *Source: Contemporary Psychiatric Mental Health Nursing* by Kneisl/Wilson/Trigoboff, © Reprinted by permission of Pearson Education, Inc., Upper Saddle River, NJ.

changes, including irritability and poor impulse control. In current research, brain neurotransmitters are being linked to aggressive behavior.

Cognitive Factors

Cognitive theory explains how a person's **attributions** (the meaning a person places on an event), expectations, and self-talk connect experiences with aggressive reactions.

CASE EXAMPLE

Consider the case of Ken and Maxine. They were both driving to work on Monday morning. Ken was thinking: "These idiot drivers! They'll make me late for work." Maxine thought: "The traffic is heavy this morning." A car stalled ahead of them, delaying traffic. Ken sped up and dangerously passed a line of cars on the right, swearing as he sped by. Maxine waited in the line of cars. She turned on her radio to listen for a traffic report, and then to listen to music. Ken and Maxine had different attributions of the same event. Ken thought the other drivers were mean or stupid, or maybe even wanted to make him late. Maxine attributed the slowdown to inevitable heavy traffic. Ken's violent behavior and Maxine's information-seeking behavior resulted from their cognitive (thinking) reaction to the situation. Attributions play an important role in anger arousal (Rickelman, 2003).

The way people talk to themselves, called *self-talk*, is affected by the meanings they attribute to their experiences. This self-talk affects the person's perceptions and emotional reactions to events. If a nurse accidentally mixes up the medications of two clients, one client may think: "Nurses are so stupid. She doesn't care if she kills me." The other may think: "Accidents happen. The nurse was probably busy." The self-talk affects how these clients will respond emotionally, and whether they will become angry.

Social Learning Factors

When people are exposed to violence in their families of origin, and then grow up to abuse their own children, the social learning theory is that their behavior was learned. Observing role models or experiencing positive reinforcement for behavior results in social learning.

Children may learn through television programs, movies, and video games that violence pays social and material rewards. Some children are exposed to these media and are only mildly stimulated by them. Other children feel very drawn to the violence portrayed in the media. The reaction of people to violence in the media and in the real world is complicated. The perpetual dilemma of nature versus nurture applies to the etiology of violence, too (Figure 16-11 ■).

COLLABORATIVE CARE

Goals of the treatment team in any healthcare setting include the safety of clients and staff. The healthcare environment can be designed to increase safety. The National Institute of Occupational Safety and Health (2002) has recommendations for environmental design

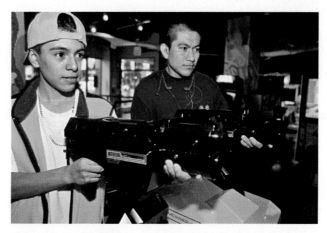

Figure 16-11. ■ Children may learn violence while engaging in violent video games. *Source:* The Image Works.

TABLE 16-1	
Safe Healthcare Workplace Environment: NIOSH Recommendations	
RECOMMENDATION TO INCREASE WORKPLACE SAFETY	**RATIONALES**
Develop emergency signaling, alarms, and monitoring systems.	Allows staff to summon help. Prevents staff from being isolated with violent client.
Install security devices such as metal detectors to prevent armed persons from entering the facility.	Metal detectors are proven to reduce the number of guns, knives, and Mace-type sprays brought into healthcare facilities.
Use good lighting in hallways and parking lots. Install cameras and mirrors in areas with reduced visibility.	Attacks are reduced in lighted areas and areas with good visibility. Potential attackers are made visible with adequate lighting.
Provide security escorts to parking lots at night.	Staff are less likely to be confronted when they are with a security guard.
Design waiting areas to be comfortable for clients and visitors who may have a delay in service.	Waiting areas are at increased risk for violence. Crowding, discomfort, and frustration increase the risk.
Provide staff restrooms and emergency exits.	A secondary exit promotes safe escape without confrontation of potentially violent person. Perpetrator may hide in restroom to confront staff.
Install deep service counters or bullet-resistant glass enclosures in reception areas and pharmacies.	Pharmacies are robbed for money and drugs. Reception areas are at increased risk for violent behavior.
Arrange furniture and other objects to minimize their use as weapons.	If furniture is lightweight, without sharp edges, or attached to floor, it is less likely to be a dangerous weapon.
Design staffing patterns to prevent personnel from working alone and to minimize client waiting time.	It is more dangerous for employees to be alone. Waiting increases frustration.
Restrict the movement of the public in hospitals.	The environment is under better control when access by the public is limited to pertinent areas.
Provide all workers with training in recognizing and managing assaults, resolving conflicts, and maintaining hazard awareness.	Knowledge is power.

and administrative controls for increasing employee safety. These are outlined in Table 16-1 ■.

Limit Setting

Limit setting occurs when the staff decides on boundaries of appropriate behavior and clearly set these limits with clients. The purposes of these limits are safety and client learning of appropriate behavior, not punishment of the client. Another goal is to provide the client with the security of limits and the knowledge that s/he will not be allowed to harm self, others, or property.

Anger Management

Anger management is a therapy that comes from cognitive-behavioral theory. In anger-management groups clients learn what anger is, how to identify it in themselves, the events or cues that come before anger outbursts, how to think differently about the cues that formerly caused anger, and how to use alternative nonviolent behaviors.

Some clients automatically experience anger due to a variety of stimuli that others would not find threatening. In anger-management therapy, these clients learn how to think differently about these situations (to "reframe their cognitive response") so they can respond with more genuine emotions, such as fear or frustration. This reframing of client thinking is called *cognitive restructuring*. When clients know themselves well enough, they can begin to change their attributions. They can stop the automatic anger and move instead into a problem-solving frame of mind. The goal of anger management is for the client to use cognitive problem solving rather than emotional reactions to respond to problems.

Verbal Interventions

The principle of "least restrictive intervention" (see Chapter 8) applies to the management of client behavior. The treatment team begins by talking to the client. Box

Caring for Client at Risk for Aggressive Behavior

☑ Speak slowly, and in a normal tone of voice. *Elevated voice may appear threatening to the client.*

☑ Give simple concrete directions, such as "Mr. King, go to your room." *The agitated client may be overstimulated with internal stimuli of psychosis, or may be overwhelmed by events and feelings. Simple directions will be easier to process. Clear directions reduce misunderstanding.*

☑ Acknowledge the client's feelings, such as "It looks like you're having a hard time" or "You must be disappointed." *The client may not feel so isolated if the nurse validates his feelings.*

☑ Communicate that you expect the client to be in control, for example: "Put the book down. I know you can do this." *The client's own self-confidence may be increased by the nurse's confidence in him or her.*

16-8 ■ supplies guidelines for verbal interventions for the angry client. The sequence of interventions from least to most restrictive is as follows:

■ Verbal interventions
■ Redirection of the client (to her/his room or away from the area where behavior is escalating)
■ Medications
■ Seclusion or restraint

Medications

Clients learn more about impulse control or behavior management if they are allowed to manage their own behavior with only verbal interventions from the staff. Sometimes clients are too agitated and are unable to manage their anger even with verbal cues from the staff. They are then asked to remove themselves from the stressful situation. If they are not able to do this, or if redirection is not effective, medications may be necessary.

The physician will choose the medication based on the client's reason for agitation. If the client has psychotic symptoms, an antipsychotic drug such as haloperidol (Haldol) or risperidone (Risperdal) will be used. If the predominant symptom is anxiety, an antianxiety agent is the best choice. Lorazepam (Ativan) is often the benzodiazepine of choice because it acts quickly. A mood-stabilizing agent such as lithium or carbamazepine (Tegretol) will

be used in addition to a benzodiazepine if the client is experiencing mania. Moderately aggressive clients have also responded to the anticonvulsant drugs divalproex sodium (Depakote) and phenytoin (Dilantin) even though they were not experiencing mania (Wilkinson, 2003). If the client demonstrates an impulsive aggression, using the antidepressant category of selective serotonin reuptake inhibitors such as fluoxetine (Prozac) may be effective (Wilkinson, 2003).

Some nurses question the use of benzodiazepine drugs for anxiety. Their idea is that people need to learn how to manage their own behavior. They believe an antianxiety drug takes away a client's opportunity to learn this lesson. They argue that drugs may even become the client's preferred coping mechanism. Actually, in an acute situation of severe anxiety or agitation, when the client is unable to cope effectively, antianxiety drugs are indicated to maintain safety of the client, other clients, and the staff. The use of medication is appropriate when it is used after other interventions have failed, within the principle of least restrictive intervention.

Seclusion and Restraint

In the inpatient psychiatric setting, seclusion in a room alone or physical restraints may be used as security measures. These approaches were once widely used in psychiatry. Secluding or restraining clients was even considered a form of treatment. Over the years clients have been injured and have even died while they were restrained or secluded. Even without physical injury, the process causes a loss of dignity. The client's human rights can be abused. Current thought is that seclusion and restraint are not treatments. They should only be used as security interventions to protect the safety of the client or others.

There are strict and clear regulations set by the Health Care Financing Administration (Center for Medicare and Medicaid Services) about the circumstances under which a client may be restrained or secluded. Although a nurse may initiate restraint in a behavioral emergency that threatens the safety of the client or others, a physician or other licensed independent practitioner must write an order within an hour. Adults may be restrained for a maximum of 4 hours, adolescents and children age 9–17 for 2 hours, and children less than age 9 may be restrained for a maximum of 1 hour. Clients in seclusion or restraint must be under constant observation by staff.

NURSING CARE

ASSESSING

The client's history is an important part of the nursing assessment. Several aspects of client history increase the likelihood that a client will have violent behavior. If the nurse is aware of the client's history, plans can be made to prevent violence before it happens. These predictors of violence are:

- History of violent behavior (strongest predictor)
- Untreated psychosis, especially if accompanied by paranoid delusions
- Substance abuse
- Age and gender—young adult men are most likely to act out violent behavior, although untreated psychosis can cause both men and women to be violent; young males have been known to bring guns into school, anywhere from elementary school age through high school (Figure 16-12 ■)

When a client has poor impulse control, s/he may act out violently without warning. Most of the time, however, client behaviors indicate that aggressiveness is escalating. The behaviors that indicate a risk for violence include:

- Loud voice
- Dilated pupils
- Clenched fists
- Pacing

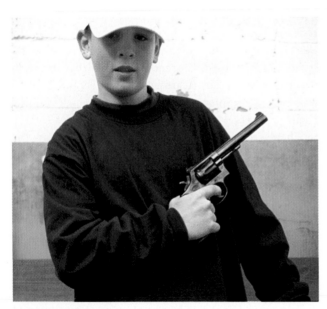

Figure 16-12. ■ Boys have been known to take guns to educational institutions from elementary school to high school.
Source: The Stock Connection.

- Suspicion/paranoia
- Threats of violence
- Sarcastic comments
- Clenched jaws
- Angry facial expression

DIAGNOSING, PLANNING, AND IMPLEMENTING

The most pertinent nursing diagnosis is Risk for Other-Directed Violence. Clients may also experience Anxiety, Ineffective Coping, and Risk for Self-Directed Violence.

The desired outcomes for clients at risk for aggressive behavior are that the client will:

- Not harm self or others.
- Verbalize feelings of frustration or loss of control to nurse.
- Discuss feelings of fear, anger, anxiety, and frustration, and alternate nonviolent ways to cope with them.
- Reframe thoughts that lead to anger or aggression.

The nurse may choose from among the following interventions for clients at risk for aggressive behavior:

- Position yourself safely. Stand just outside the client's personal space (arm's length), on client's nondominant side. Use an open posture with your hands in sight. Keep client in your sight. Put yourself between the client and the door (Pryor, 2006). Instead of facing the client directly, turn your body slightly to the side. *These positions minimize the aggressive client's opportunity to hit the nurse, or to trap the nurse in the client's room. If the client does strike out, the nurse will be injured less by a hit to the side rather than the front of the body.*
- Encourage the client to express feelings. *Often clients with aggressive behavior do not understand their own feelings. Verbalizing feelings can help the client develop insight.*
- Work with the client on cognitive restructuring (changing self-talk from aggressive themes to problem-solving approaches). *Cognitive restructuring helps the client change automatic aggressive behavior to a problem-solving approach to life events.*
- Avoid defensiveness or behavior that can be interpreted as aggressiveness. Act confidently, not aggressively. *If the client says, "I didn't get breakfast and I'm going to beat up everybody on this unit," the nurse should take a problem-solving approach to the client's feelings. The nurse should not try to justify why the client did not receive breakfast. If he is hungry, get food for him. If he feels forgotten, let him know that he is important. Keep your voice within normal range, so you do not appear aggressive.*

Having a sense of confidence, not one of controlling the client, will promote cooperation instead of aggression.

- Be a role model for a problem-solving approach to conflict. For example, if the client refuses to take his medications, listen to his reasons first, discuss any problems, and then tell him the consequences of his choice. Encourage the taking of medication without coercion. *Clients can learn new problem-solving behaviors by the nurse's example. Compliance is increased when the client decides to comply, instead of being tricked or forced. It is important for the nurse to be trustworthy. Clients become defensive when nurses are authoritarian.*

- Help the client to identify cues for anger, or events that trigger angry responses. The client may want to work on this through journaling. *When the client can identify what leads to anger, s/he can begin to prevent the angry behavior. Journal writing helps many people who are working on insight development.*

- If you are afraid, get help. *Trust your own sense of the situation. Client care is teamwork. Clients are less likely to be aggressive when more than one staff member is present.*

- Praise the client for successful attempts to use alternatives to aggression. For example, the nurse could say, "I saw you go outside to play basketball when Charlie was yelling at you. Good way to avoid a fight." *Positive reinforcement encourages new behaviors to persist.*

EVALUATING

When the nurse is evaluating the plan of care for a client at risk for aggressive behavior, several issues should be considered. Did the client avoid harming anyone, express feelings, learn new strategies for avoiding aggressive behavior, and actually try to use the new strategies? If so, the client's goals are reached.

The most difficult and important of these desired outcomes is actually trying new behavior. Behavior change is difficult and a long-term goal, so nurses will often need to refer clients to services for counseling or anger-management groups in the community for continued work on coping behavior. Consult with the social services department at your facility for local referral information.

NURSING PROCESS CARE PLAN
Client in an Abusive Relationship

Jill Donovan, a 24-year-old white female, has been admitted to your medical-surgical unit with a possible gallbladder attack (cholelithiasis). She is accompanied by her husband, Jeff, who appears very concerned and attentive to her needs. He rarely leaves her side.

Assessment. When you arrive to collect data on Jill for the assessment, Jeff does not want to leave her room and argues with you about the necessity of your examining Jill alone. Jeff finally leaves but reassures Jill that he will be waiting "right outside the door" if she needs anything. Jill answers your questions quietly using as few words as possible. She says she is a "stay-at-home Mom" of a 2-year-old with little time for outside activities. The pain she is experiencing now began last night after a high-fat meal. Her physician was concerned that it was her gallbladder and wanted to admit her for possible surgery after a battery of tests. Her husband really didn't feel that was necessary but finally relented when the pain was so severe she could not stand up.

When you ask her about the bruises on her skin, she becomes evasive. She tells you that she is "clumsy" and is always bumping into things. She says that she bruises easily. When you ask to see her arms, she holds them out after adjusting the sleeves of her gown to cover the upper arms. You also notice bruising on both shoulders. When you palpate her abdomen for tenderness, you see additional bruising on her abdominal area. When you listen to her posterior lung sounds, you see bruising on the right flank. She attributes the many bruises to a recent fall down the steps at home when she tripped over her daughter's toy at the top of the steps. She giggles nervously about being a "klutz" and doesn't know how her "wonderful husband" puts up with her. "He's just so perfect. I really don't deserve him. He makes all the decisions and handles all of our money. I have such a good life. I rarely have to do anything except take care of our daughter." As you start out the door after the assessment, Jeff is coming in. He goes straight to Jill and begins to straighten her cover. You overhear him ask her if the nurse had upset her in any way and if everything was all right. Jill confirms the conversation with the nurse as being nonthreatening.

Diagnosis. You report your data to the RN charge nurse who initiates the care plan. Because of the suspicion of physical and psychological abuse, you both decide that the most pertinent diagnosis would be:

- Posttrauma Syndrome

  Other diagnoses that might be appropriate would be:

- Pain, Acute R/T possible inflammation of gallbladder AEB client statement

- Chronic Low Self-Esteem R/T personal vulnerability AEB negative comments about self, unwillingness to report abuse, and passive demeanor
- Ineffective Coping R/T spousal abuse AEB inappropriate use of denial as a coping mechanism

Outcome Identification. Outcomes would be established as pertinent to the nursing diagnoses. The following are examples for each of the above:

- The client will state pain of 3 on a scale of 1 to 10 thirty minutes after pain medication administered.
- Client will state one of her positive traits daily during hospitalization.
- Client will admit that she is being physically and psychologically abused before discharge.

Planning and Implementation

- As a first step, you should gain Jill's trust by establishing a therapeutic nurse-client relationship. Seek a time when you can be alone with Jill, such as during a bath or when Jeff leaves for a meal, to question her directly. Tell her that her injuries seem inconsistent with her story and ask, "Who did this to you?" *Asking her about the injuries in front of the husband will increase Jill's fear and may make Jeff more apt to retaliate against her after discharge. The nurse tries to make it easier for the client to disclose the truth without telling the client what to say.*
- Even if Jill continues with denial, you can still provide her with information about shelters and other resources. Information might be printed on a small card for her wallet. *If she is fearful of Jeff finding it and questioning it, a telephone number only might be given to Jill and identified as that of a women's support group for young mothers.*
- Emphasize that abuse is a common problem to reassure her that she is not alone in her situation. Report suspicion of the spousal abuse to your supervisor and the hospital social worker. *Although all states have laws requiring reporting of suspected child abuse, and most states require the reporting of suspected elder abuse, there are few laws that require the reporting of spousal abuse. This reporting is left up to the survivor of family violence. The social worker for your facility should be aware of the laws in your state involving abuse.*
- Document your findings of client's injuries including location, size, and shape. Document any interactions that you observe between the client and her husband

that would be suggestive of abuse. Do not interpret the behavior, but describe it accurately and objectively. *Clear description without interpretation is crucial, because information may be used in court.*

- Assess the level of pain regularly and provide pain relief, including medication and comfort measures.
- Promote her self-esteem. Actively listen to her concerns. Teach her to replace her negative self-talk with positive. Praise her successes. *A trusting relationship with the nurse promotes self-esteem.*
- Determine her strengths and how she has coped with stressful situations in the past. Let her know of her options without expressing your opinion. *Jill needs to know her options so she can make adaptive choices for effective coping.*
- Treat Jill with dignity and respect, and withhold judgment if she stays in her abusive situation. *It takes, on average, five to seven attempts for an abused woman to leave her abuser. Direct support from the nurse may empower her to leave sooner.*

Evaluation. To evaluate your success, look toward each expected outcome to see if you were able to reach them. Was Jill safe from injury during her hospitalization? Was her pain under control? Did she share ideas about positive traits she saw in herself? Did she admit she was a survivor of spousal abuse? If you were not successful in helping Jill to achieve any of these outcomes, reassess the problem and outcome, and determine whether or not other interventions might be successful.

Critical Thinking in the Nursing Process

1. How would you feel about a client who was obviously being abused and denied the situation? Would your feelings interfere with your objective treatment of the client?
2. How would you respond to the husband who might be the perpetrator of violence against your client?
3. If nothing was resolved by the time of discharge, describe your feelings and whether or not you would pursue any further avenues for this case.

Note: Discussion of Critical Thinking questions appears in Appendix I.

Note: The references and resources for this and all chapters have been compiled at the back of the book.

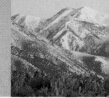

Chapter Review

 KEY TERMS

Use the audio glossary feature of the Companion Website to hear the correct pronunciation of the following key terms.

aggression

attributions

dangerousness

elder abuse

emotional abuse

neglect

perpetrator

physical abuse

rape

sexual abuse

sexual assault

violence

KEY Points

- Violence is a complex problem rooted in the interaction of biological, social, cultural, economic, and political factors.

- Family violence occurs in families from all socioeconomic groups, races, and cultures.

- It is a cruel irony that the social group that is supposed to provide love and support is also the most violent group to which most people belong.

- Violent parents often had violent parents themselves.

- Abusers often keep their partners socially isolated, abuse the power they have over their families, and coerce the victim to keep the abuse secret.

- There is a repeating pattern of family violence called the "cycle of violence."

- Substance abuse does not actually cause family violence, but it is related. Abusers under the influence are more violent. They often use substance use as an excuse.

- There are effective strategies for preventing family violence and sexual assault.

- Children, intimate partners, and elders are the groups most likely to experience family violence.

- Rape is a crime of violence, rage, and power, not sex. The motivations for rape are to humiliate, control, or dominate the victim.

- All states have mandatory child abuse reporting laws.

- In the case of elder abuse or neglect, the primary concern of the elder client may be fear of institutionalization in a nursing home. If this client is admitted to a nursing home, s/he will have significant psychosocial needs for the nurse to address including grief, anxiety, and powerlessness.

- Nurses can make a difference for survivors of violence.

- Nurses who are survivors of violence themselves must resolve their own issues before trying to intervene professionally with other survivors.

- People who work in the healthcare environment are at risk for violence. There are effective strategies to prevent it.

- Anger-management groups teach people how to use cognitive restructuring to change the way they respond to stress.

 EXPLORE Media Link

Additional interactive resources for this chapter can be found on the Companion Website at www.prenhall.com/eby. Click on Chapter 16 and "Begin" to select the activities for this chapter.

- Audio glossary
- NCLEX-PN® review
- Case study
- Study outline
- Critical thinking questions
- Matching questions
- Weblinks
- Video Case: Sara (Posttraumatic Stress Disorder)

Caring for a Client Who Is Agitated
NCLEX-PN® Focus Area: Safe, Effective Care Environment

Case Study: Edward Clay is a 55-year-old male European American client who was admitted to the hospital for surgery 2 days ago. He also has schizophrenia. The surgery went well, and his condition is stable. Last night he started to develop anxiety and did not sleep well. This morning when the nurse entered his room, Mr. Clay shouted, "Get me out of here! The demons are after me!" The physician was called and will come to the unit in approximately 15 minutes.

Nursing Diagnosis: Risk for other-directed violence

COLLECT DATA

Subjective	Objective
_____	_____
_____	_____
_____	_____
_____	_____
_____	_____
_____	_____
_____	

Would you report this data? Yes/No

If yes, to: _____

Nursing Care

_____
_____
_____
_____
_____
_____
_____
_____
_____

How would you document this? _____
_____
_____
_____

Compare your documentation to the sample provided in Appendix I.

Data Collected
(use those that apply)

- Client is restless, first moving around in bed, then walking around his room.
- History of hypertension
- His fists are clenched.
- His voice is loud.
- The client has a history of pushing a caregiver in the group home where he lives.
- The client states, "They are trying to dry me to death."
- T 99.8 °F
- Client states, "I don't know what to do."
- Client is looking around, as if he can see things that are not present in the room.
- Client is 5'4" tall.
- Client is a vegetarian.

Nursing Interventions
(use those that apply; list in priority order)

- Ask the client for a thorough description of his medical history.
- Act calmly and confidently.
- Talk in a quiet tone.
- Leave client in his room and close the client's door until the physician comes.
- Ask the client if he wants a drink of water.
- Stand near the door in the client's room.
- Stand out of the client's reach.
- Tell the client that the doctor is coming in about 15 minutes to see what she can do to help him.
- Reassure the client that he is safe in the hospital.
- Tell the client that if he tries to hit you, you will call the police.
- Tell the client that you are the nurse, and you are here to help.
- Ask the client if he needs anything.
- Call the hospital security guard to help restrain the client to his bed.
- Tell the client, "I think you should go back to bed until the doctor comes."
- Tell the client, "Quit acting this way, or you will get into trouble with the doctor."

1 A client states that her partner frequently calls her names and criticizes. She then says, "At least I am not being abused like some women." The nurse's best response would be:

1. "That is certainly preferable to being beaten up."
2. "It is important that we realize our limitations so that we can improve our situation."
3. "Although there is no physical violence, emotional abuse can be just as devastating to one's self-esteem."
4. "It is important to be satisfied with your life situation."

2 Which of the following statements best describes violence?

1. Violence can be traced to one particular factor in an individual's early life.
2. Violence is a complex problem that can be related to an interaction among biological, social, cultural, economic, and political factors.
3. Violence is more often related to a person's biological and personal history than to anything else.
4. Violence is caused by weapons in the home.

3 A client suspects that his daughter is being physically abused. Then he states, "But that can't be right. She's married to a prominent physician." The nurse's best response would be:

1. "Family violence occurs across all socioeconomic groups. Tell me why you feel your daughter is being abused."
2. "Abuse is much more common in lower socioeconomic groups."
3. "Physicians are interested in promoting health. Your son-in-law is (probably not) an abuser."
4. "I would find that hard to believe as well."

4 A client states that she has just ended an abusive relationship of 15 years. She asks if the behavior patterns of her 11-year-old son, who witnessed and was the recipient of physical abuse, will be affected in later life. The nurse's best response is:

1. "As long as you got out of the relationship before he turned 18, there should be no problem."
2. "He will forget the situation the farther removed he is from his earlier circumstances."
3. "If he is not showing any signs of being abusive himself by now, chances are good that he will not be affected."
4. "Children may learn behavior patterns from the parent they choose as a role model. Witnessing violence can often result in aggressive behavior for the child."

5 A battered client states, "My husband is very sorry. He told me it will never happen again." The nurse's best response is:

1. "Being sorry after an episode of violence is common. Unless he gets help with his anger, this could happen again."
2. "I'm happy he realized that his response was wrong. I hope, for your sake, this is the end of it."
3. "Once the perpetrator admits his error, that is usually the end of the violence."
4. "You are fortunate that the violent behavior occurred only once in your marriage."

6 A 4-year-old is admitted to the pediatric unit for a fracture. This is the third time this year he has been hospitalized. The nurse suspects physical abuse. The nurse's legal responsibility is to:

1. Tell the parents someone is abusing their child.
2. Immediately report your suspicions to the proper authorities based upon your state's laws.
3. Report your suspicions and let your supervisor handle it.
4. Care for the child while hospitalized. Any reporting of suspicious injuries should be left up to the physician.

7 Which of the following behaviors would suggest that a child was being sexually abused?

1. A 5-year-old asks you where babies come from.
2. A 10-year-old boy asks you about whether or not he will begin bleeding like girls do every month.
3. A 10-month-old infant girl develops recurrent herpes lesions in her mouth.
4. A 4-year-old girl wants to play doctor with the 4-year-old boy who lives next door.

8 The nurse is evaluating an 80-year-old male for admission to a long-term care facility. His home is filthy. The man has not shaved and has unbrushed teeth and dirty fingernails. The nurse's response to the situation would be to:

1. Admit the client into the long-term care facility as soon as possible.
2. Suggest the daughter-in-law bathe the client before bringing him to the facility.
3. Ask the client who has been caring for him. Refer further questions about his appearance to the caregiver.
4. Report the neglect and abuse to the appropriate state agency responsible for community elder care.

9 An appropriate short-term outcome for clients experiencing Rape Trauma Syndrome would be:

1. Client will resume usual social relationships and lifestyle.
2. Client will identify and testify against the perpetrator.
3. Client will begin the process of grief resolution.
4. Client will refuse to discuss the rape incident as evidence of self-protection.

10 A client in the psychiatric unit walks toward the nurse shaking his fist and threatening loudly. Which of the following nursing interventions would be appropriate? Indicate all that apply.

1. Move outside the client's personal space. Stand between the client and the door.
2. Obtain assistance in restraining the client while you medicate him with a psychotropic drug.
3. Speak slowly and in a normal tone of voice.
4. Walk toward the client confidently and tell him you will not be intimidated by his threats.
5. Give the client simple, concrete suggestions as to what he should do.

Answers for Review Questions, as well as discussion of Care Plan and Critical Thinking Care Map questions, appear in Appendix I.

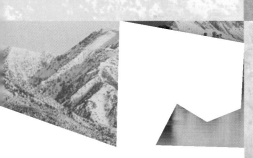

Chapter 17

Psychosocial Issues in General Client Care

LEARNING Outcomes

After completing this chapter, you will be able to:

1. Identify the psychosocial needs of clients in the general medical setting.
2. Apply the nursing process to meet the psychosocial needs of clients outside the psychiatric setting.
3. Apply the nursing process to the spiritual needs of clients.

Illness or hospitalization can be very stressful. The stress can be difficult for people to manage with their usual coping skills. As a result, people are often at their worst when they are sick or hospitalized. Sometimes clients direct their feelings of anger and frustration at nurses, which can be very hard to take. Nurses may feel unprepared to meet their clients' challenging psychosocial needs. In addition, nurses may have more tense interactions with clients due to the advent of the nursing shortage and the reduction in the amount of time that the nurse has to spend with each client (Childers, 2003).

Nursing practice is holistic, meaning that we treat the whole client, not only his or her disease process. All people have both physical and psychological needs. When we do the best job of nursing, our clients' physiological and psychosocial needs are both addressed. However, in a busy nursing practice, it is easy to focus only on the client's medical illness. Remember that a person with schizophrenia can have a bladder infection, and a person with congestive heart failure can have anxiety or spiritual distress. We all have body, mind, and spirit dimensions that make up our whole selves (Figure 17-1 ■).

Sometimes nurses are very good at meeting clients' physiological needs, but have more difficulty with their psychosocial ones. This chapter will provide some strategies for meeting the psychosocial needs of clients in the general medical setting.

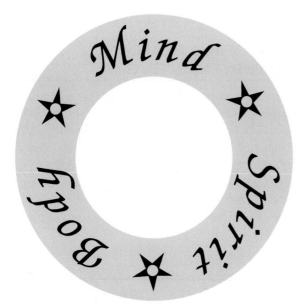

Figure 17-1. ■ ■ Dimensions of a person. All are included in holistic nursing care.

Critical Self-Check. Tom is a nursing student who likes science and nursing skills. He dislikes psychosocial stuff, and thinks there is too much of it in nursing school. He wants to work where he can avoid clients' psychosocial issues. What should Tom do?

Anxiety

In Chapter 11 we discussed anxiety disorders, which are actual mental disorders characterized by anxiety. In this chapter we are covering the type of anxiety that occurs commonly in everyday life, especially in hospitalized people.

Mild anxiety can actually be an asset to clients by making them more alert and ready to learn. It does not require any specific intervention by the nurse. The nurse may use client teaching to prevent an increase in the level of anxiety.

Many experiences of clients in hospitals or of residents in long-term care lead to anxiety. There may be threats related to biological integrity, including pain, physical symptoms of illness, concern about the outcomes of treatment or diagnostic tests, and even changes in food. The client may have had a previous unpleasant experience in a healthcare facility or with a healthcare provider that affects his/her current behavior. There are threats to emotional security and self-esteem, such as change in family roles, separation from significant others, financial concerns, employment insecurity, loss of professional status, concern about disfigurement from injury or surgery, and even their own mortality. Some are concerned about how they will look in a hospital gown! It is no wonder clients in the hospital are anxious.

Anxiety can also result from experiencing the unknown. Clients may have a vague sense of dread when they do not know what to expect. Nurses can help clients avoid this source of anxiety through client teaching. Even if a procedure is painful, clients tend to tolerate it better if they have guidance by the nurse in advance about what to expect. It is important to orient clients on admission to their units, telling them what is expected of them and what they can expect from the staff. Showing clients how to call the nurse is a critical part of this teaching. Keeping a client informed about when procedures are to be done, when test results will be ready, and when the doctor will make rounds seem simple but will do wonders to alleviate client anxiety.

The client who already has multiple stressors is more likely to experience increased anxiety in the treatment setting. Anxiety is caused not so much by the event as by how an event is perceived by the client, what else is happening in the client's life, and what skills and resources the client has to cope with all the current issues. The nurse should keep in mind that the majority of so-called difficult clients are motivated by fear (Childers, 2003).

The nurse may observe behaviors that anxious clients use to manage their anxiety. They include:

- *Acting out*, which is expression of anxiety as angry or agitated behavior
- *Somatization*, or expressing anxiety as physical symptoms or disturbed body functions (such as headache or stomachache)
- *Withdrawal*, which is retreating from the source of anxiety, or becoming immobilized
- Active problem solving

Because everyone has experienced anxiety, there are a variety of methods used to cope with it. Some common coping mechanisms are talking about problems with others; participating in physical work or activities; systematic problem solving; avoiding stressful situation; crying or laughing; expressing intense emotions verbally; using humor; praying; sleeping excessively; distracting oneself from the stressful situation with other activities (reading, music, relaxation techniques, or hobbies); and obtaining relief through food, cigarettes, or mind-altering drugs (including alcohol) (Gorman, Raines, & Sultan, 2002; Meisenhelder & Chandler, 2000).

Antianxiety medications are used to treat the anxiety of clients while they are in the hospital when nonpharmacologic methods of treatment are not effective. Hospital and long-term care nurses give these medications frequently and should be familiar with their indications, effects, and side effects.

NURSING CARE

ASSESSING

The nurse begins with an assessment of the client's appearance and behavior. The nurse also asks the client about subjective anxiety symptoms. (The symptoms of anxiety are those of sympathetic stimulation. See Table 11-2 for the different levels of anxiety.) If the client

has mild to moderate anxiety, the nurse can act both to treat the symptoms and to prevent escalation to the higher levels. As the level of anxiety increases, the client's ability to concentrate decreases.

If the client has severe or panic-level anxiety, the nurse must act quickly to promote the client's coping and reduce the level of anxiety. The client with high anxiety will be extremely uncomfortable and will not be able to cooperate with treatment. At the level of panic anxiety the client may feel that death is pending. At this point the client's safety is the foremost concern.

After assessing the client's anxiety level, the nurse should assess the client's usual coping mechanisms. It is difficult to assess this by direct observation, so the nurse may ask: "What usually helps you feel better when you are stressed?" or "When you have a serious problem, how do you solve it?"

To assess the resources the client has for problem solving, the nurse may ask: "Whom can you ask for help when you have a problem?" or "When you need help, who can help you?" Sometimes clients do not have experience with asking for help. In this case, the nurse could ask specific questions to help the client develop an understanding of her/his resources, such as: "If you needed a ride to the doctor's office, what would you do?" "How about if you needed help to buy groceries, or to pick up a prescription?" "Do you belong to any groups?" Clubs, fraternal organizations, unions, and religious groups often have mechanisms for helping their members.

DIAGNOSING, PLANNING, AND IMPLEMENTING

Anxiety is a recognized nursing diagnosis by the North American Nursing Diagnosis Association (NANDA). *Anxiety* is "a vague uneasy feeling of discomfort or dread, accompanied by an autonomic response" (elevated vital signs). Anxiety is caused by an anticipation of danger; it alerts an individual to take measures to deal with a threat (NANDA, 2005).

The desired outcomes for the client with anxiety are that the client will:

- Verbalize her/his feelings.
- Demonstrate decreased symptoms of anxiety: vital signs within normal limits; calm, peaceful demeanor; client statement of relief.

- List alternative ways to deal with stress.
- Practice relaxation techniques to reduce own anxiety level.

Following are some nursing interventions for clients with anxiety, with rationales:

- Have a calm, nonthreatening attitude when interacting with the client. *Anxiety is contagious—it is easily transmitted from one person to another. The client will feel more secure when the nurse is calm. Nurses should also assess their own anxiety level. Nurses can become anxious when working with anxious clients. Nonverbal communication is sometimes more important than the words the nurse speaks. Maintaining a pleasant facial expression and speaking in a calming tone will help to allay anxiety* (Childers, 2003).
- Communicate with the client according to your assessment of the client's anxiety level. *Clients with mild anxiety can be receptive to teaching or complicated communication. Those with moderate anxiety may be able to learn, but their ability to focus may be impaired. Severe anxiety limits the client to brief responses to concrete directions and questions. In panic anxiety, the client's safety is the most important issue.*
- Offer yourself, by spending time with the anxious client. *The presence of the nurse can be reassuring to an anxious client, especially during a procedure or treatment, but also during generalized anxiety.*
- Actively listen to the client's feelings and concerns. Box 17-1 ■ lists behaviors associated with active listening. *Active listening promotes trust. It increases the client's self-esteem, insight, and ability to cope.*

BOX 17-1

Active Listening

Active listening is an important nursing intervention. To listen actively, the nurse:

- Ideally sits at the client's eye level.
- Is free from distraction.
- Uses attentive body language (nodding head, eye contact, paying attention, uncrossed arms).
- Focuses on the client's feelings and concerns, not nursing assessment or other nursing issues.
- Encourages the client to elaborate on feelings and actions, their precursors, and their consequences.

- If the client is severely anxious, do not leave her/him alone. *Severe anxiety may make people fear for their lives. The presence of the nurse can convey reassurance and safety.*
- Acknowledge the client's anxiety and possible fear; encourage the client to verbalize feelings about the anxiety-producing event and other life issues. *Validating the client's feelings may be the impetus for the client to vent frustrations and to begin asking questions that would alleviate fear and anxiety. Verbalizing feelings helps the client understand them. It also helps the nurse assess the client's situation. Listening nonjudgmentally to the client's feelings and answering questions promote trust.*
- Help client explore options for healthy coping responses, including active problem solving. *If the client's anxiety level is mild to moderate, this can be a good time for learning new coping methods. Anxiety can help motivate the client to try new behavior. Relief of anxiety reinforces the client's use of the new coping skill.*

EVALUATING

Ultimately, the goal is for clients to manage their own anxiety with healthy coping skills. If interventions are successful, the nurse's evaluation will show that the client is using healthy coping strategies, anxiety is at a mild to moderate level, and the client relates a decrease in feelings of anxiety.

Client in Crisis

A crisis occurs when an individual's usual coping skills or problem-solving methods are unable to adapt effectively to an event. A **crisis** is an acute, time-limited state of disequilibrium, or imbalance. The individual's ability to function may be affected. Crises are potentially life-threatening events that can motivate people to alter the course of their lives (Cohan & Cole, 2002). Figure 17-2 ■ shows how a crisis can progress into powerlessness and personality disintegration or into new coping skills and a higher level of functioning.

There are generally considered to be three kinds of crises. A *situational crisis* can be the result of:

- Environmental events (death of a loved one, natural disaster, war)

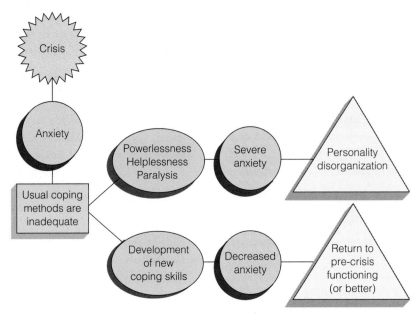

Figure 17-2. ■ Progression of crisis. The progression of a crisis to either successful or unsuccessful resolution depends on what people do when their usual coping mechanisms are ineffective. *Source: Contemporary Psychiatric Mental Health Nursing* by Kneisl/Wilson/Trigoboff, © Reprinted by permission of Pearson Education, Inc., Upper Saddle River, NJ.

- Personal or physical events (diagnosis of severe illness, injury, body disfigurement)
- Social events (death of loved one, separation, divorce)

The second type of crisis is maturational. A *maturational crisis* is triggered by normal transitions in human development. Humans develop through the stages of infancy, childhood, adolescence, adulthood, middle age, and old age. Each developmental stage has its own stressors and tasks. Maturational crises occur when the individual is not able to adapt to the changes required to achieve the new developmental tasks. Examples of maturational crises include inability to adapt to the challenges of starting school, the transition from school to work, or retirement.

The third type is *crisis reflective of psychopathology*, or a mental disorder. This type of crisis is either caused by the mental disorder, or made more difficult to resolve because of the disorder (Townsend, 2002). An example of crisis reflective of psychopathology is the case of Craig. Craig is a 30-year-old man with schizophrenia. He became fearful that the aliens on television were coming to kill him. He ran in terror onto a busy street, where police picked him up and brought him to the hospital.

The number and severity of stressors in a person's life also affect whether this individual will experience a crisis.

If a person already has multiple life stressors, the addition of a new one is more likely to overwhelm the client's coping ability.

There are three core components of crisis intervention theory that are basic to identifying whether a client is in crisis. They are the precipitating event, the client's perception of the event, and the client's usual coping methods (Registered Nurses Association of Ontario, 2006).

If two people experience the same event, one may have a crisis while the other does not. Whether an event becomes a crisis or only a stressor for a certain individual depends on certain risk factors for crisis development. These risk factors include:

- How intensely the person was exposed to the situation. (For example, people who survived the attack on the World Trade Center on September 11, 2001, were more likely to experience a crisis than those who watched it on television.)
- How life threatening the event is (diagnosis of brain cancer vs. diagnosis of appendicitis).
- Preexisting psychiatric disorders (such as depression, schizophrenia, or anxiety disorder that can decrease coping ability).

- Childhood abuse. (This event may result in a catastrophic reaction or less effective skills at coping with life stressors.)
- Poverty (makes fewer resources available).
- Cultural expectations that the individual may not seek help with coping, or culture-based beliefs that a situation is a crisis, which might not be recognized by caregivers of another culture.

Three factors can balance a potential crisis and help a person be successful in reestablishing equilibrium (Aguilera, 1998). They are as follows:

1. **Perception of the event.** How the individual perceives the event is critical to how it will affect the individual. Is the disease a punishment from God? Is it a minor inconvenience? Is it the worst possible thing? Is the event going to change the future?
2. **Situational support.** The availability of people to help resolve the problem is important. Meaningful relationships give support and assistance during a crisis, and aid in its resolution. Lack of supportive relationships can result in low self-esteem, which also makes an event seem more threatening.
3. **Coping mechanisms.** Whether an individual has skills to cope with life changes and stressful events is critical. A crisis may be resolved when the person learns new adaptive coping methods.

Figure 17-3 ■ illustrates balancing factors to prevent crisis.

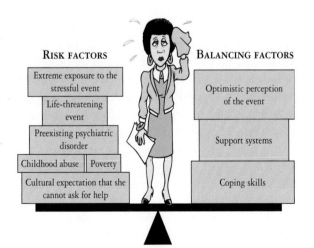

RISK FACTORS

Extreme exposure to the stressful event

Life-threatening event

Preexisting psychiatric disorder

Childhood abuse | Poverty

Cultural expectation that she cannot ask for help

BALANCING FACTORS

Optimistic perception of the event

Support systems

Coping skills

Figure 17-3. ■ Balancing factors to prevent crisis. This person has experienced a stressful event and is off balance. She will have a crisis without some balancing factors.

CASE EXAMPLE

Consider the following cases. Monica was admitted to a long-term care facility. She has a husband, who is supportive emotionally. He accompanied her when she was admitted. One of her coping methods is listening to music when she feels stressed. The staff made it possible for her to listen to music in her room. She was very sad to leave her home, but she did not experience a crisis.

David was also admitted to long-term care due to an inability to care for himself after a fall. He recently ended a relationship with his partner of many years. David always believed that the worst possible thing would be to live in a nursing home. His family does not visit. He lost interest in eating, talks very little, and says that he feels "completely overwhelmed." David is experiencing a crisis.

In these cases of Monica and David, Monica had several balancing factors that helped her avert a crisis. David had multiple stressors and fewer balancing factors, so he ended up in crisis.

NURSING CARE

ASSESSING

The nurse begins the assessment process for clients in crisis with the knowledge of which situations may put the client at risk. Situations likely to result in crisis include the environmental, physical, and psychosocial events just discussed. In the hospital, a significant new diagnosis, a sudden injury, or the potential for a disfiguring surgery may precipitate a crisis. In long-term care, leaving home, loss of a spouse, or sudden loss of functional abilities may cause crises for some residents.

After identifying clients at risk, the nurse collects data about:

- The client's usual coping style (what the client usually does when under extreme stress)
- The potentially crisis-causing event
- Other stressors the client is currently experiencing
- How the client perceives the current event
- The client's support system

DIAGNOSING, PLANNING, AND IMPLEMENTING

Some common nursing diagnoses for clients in crisis include Anxiety (level to be specified), Ineffective Coping, Risk for Self-Directed Violence, and Spiritual Distress.

Humanism assumes that people are capable of personal growth and of influencing and controlling their own lives. Because nurses take a humanistic approach to client care, the goals/outcomes of crisis intervention are that people in crisis will (Kneisl, Wilson, & Trigoboff, 2004):

1. Regain control over their lives.
2. Understand what events led to the crisis.
3. Work toward a resolution of the crisis that will foster the growth and strength of the individual and meet the individual's unique needs.

Nursing can provide the following interventions to reach the above outcomes:

- Keep your communication simple and brief. *The client in crisis probably feels overwhelmed. Simple questions and instructions will make it easier for the client to understand and comply.*
- Identify the client's usual coping behavior. *Assessment of the client's coping skills gives the nurse information about the skill level of the client, and it helps the client develop insight about her/his own skills. The client may be able to see that s/he already has ideas that might work in this situation.*
- Together with the client, identify goals for resolving the problem. Clarify what the client perceives the problem to be. *The client's perception defines what the problem is. The client is likely to be feeling powerless. Involving the client in goal setting increases the client's sense of control and increases the likelihood that the goals will be reached.*
- Encourage the client to discuss feelings. *Verbalizing feelings helps the client understand them and the circumstances that led to the feelings.*
- Acknowledge clients' feelings, such as by saying "This must be difficult for you" or "You must feel powerless." *The acknowledgement of feelings is therapeutic. It helps clients realize that their feelings are understandable.*
- Keep your actions and plans focused on the here-and-now. *The client in crisis is unable to focus on abstract issues or future plans. The goal is to regain equilibrium now.*
- Discuss possible realistic alternatives for action to solve the problem. *The client in crisis is unable to choose alternatives for action. Suggesting choices, which the client will decide to use or reject, puts the client in control and may begin new healthy coping strategies.*
- Help the client identify available resources. *When the nurse helps the client create a list of resources, the list helps the client organize thoughts about who and where the resources are and how to use them in this situation.*
- Assess functional ability and personal safety. Refer as indicated. *If the client's functional abilities are severely impaired, or the client is thinking about suicide, the nurse should refer the client to other health professionals.*
- Help the client "reframe" or redefine the meaning of the stressful event. *The client's perception of the meaning of the event is very important in determining whether the client will be able to cope with it. If the client has an optimistic outlook, s/he is more likely to be able to solve a problem.*

EVALUATING

Everyone experiences occasional crises. The best outcome is for people to learn from these experiences and to grow as a result. The nurse evaluates whether the client has regained control of her/his life, understands what led to the crisis, and is engaging in personal growth by using new coping strategies to prevent future similar crises. These are the measures of success of nursing interventions for clients in crisis.

Critical Self-Check. What does the following saying mean? "Perception is reality."

Angry Clients

People who study to become nurses usually imagine that they will work hard caring for clients, who will in turn kindly appreciate their efforts. This would be justice. It might be nice if clients never became angry, but is that a realistic possibility? Wouldn't it be normal for a person who is told that he will have to remain in skeletal traction for another 3 weeks to be angry? Wouldn't you be angry if you had to repeat a barium enema because the X-rays were lost? Sometimes anger is a logical reaction to life events. This is called *rational anger* (Gorman et al., 2002). During illness and hospitalization, people are confronted with multiple stressors, and their coping skills are challenged. Often clients and their families feel angry as a result of these stressors.

Everyone becomes angry sometimes. Anger is a natural response to frustration, disappointment, or even fear. Angry feelings can motivate a person to seek resolution of a conflict or solutions to problems. Anger is a physiological and emotional warning that should be recognized. It warns against danger or discomfort or loss of control.

CULTURAL PULSE POINTS

Different Ways of Expressing Anger

"I'm not angry, I'm just upset."

Our culture, through our families, teaches us how to express and respond to anger. Anger is complex, and its expressions are many. In some families, loud voices and aggressive behavior are acceptable. Many families teach their children, especially females, to deny, ignore, or reject their own anger. Girls may be taught to pacify and appease others, to give in rather than deal directly with conflict. We learn other more acceptable words to describe our feelings, such as upset, sad, irritated, disappointed. Even acknowledging that we have angry feelings is seen as negative. It is important for nurses to recognize that anger has many different expressions.

Nurses' Unconstructive Responses to Client Anger

Taking the Client's Anger Personally
Example: "My client is so irritable. He won't talk and he's so unfriendly. I think he hates me. I don't want to work with him tomorrow."

Responding Defensively
Example: "If you don't like the way I take care of you, fine, I'll take a different client tomorrow."

Anger is normal as long as it is expressed appropriately. The Cultural Pulse Points Box 17-2 ■ provides some different ways of expressing anger.

Some people learn that when they become angry, people in their environment act differently. When a person's anger results in others trying to please the person, s/he may learn that anger yields a sense of control.

When children from keep-the-peace-at-all-costs families grow up to be nurses, they may not recognize their own anger. Coping with the anger of their clients may be even more difficult. Nurses may take clients' anger personally or have unconstructive responses to client anger (Box 17-3 ■).

CASE EXAMPLE

Consider the case of Althea, LPN. Althea's client had a myocardial infarction. He feels powerless and afraid. When Althea went into his room to take his vital signs he yelled: "Why do you have to keep bothering me? Just leave me alone!" Althea felt hurt, sad, and personally rejected. She left the room.

Nurses sometimes react defensively to a client's anger. Bob, LPN, has a client with a fractured hip. The client is in pain. When Bob brought the client a pitcher of water, the client said: "You had to wake me up didn't you? I am so sick of this hospital!" Bob replied: "You should be grateful that I'm bringing water to you. Next time I'll let you get your own!"

Neither of these nurses is responding to the client's anger professionally or appropriately. Althea's client does not hate her personally. She has no social relationship with this person. Althea's responsibility is to provide the care this client needs, not to be accepted as this client's friend. Instead of feeling rejected, Althea might respond to the client: "I am just here to take your vital signs. We are doing them every hour for the first 4 hours you are here. You seem angry. This must be frustrating." In this case, Althea acknowledges the client's feelings, while reassuring the client that her activities are routine.

Bob's client spoke to him angrily. This client was talking to Bob, but his real frustration was with his injury and his pain. When Bob reacts defensively, his client may feel the need to respond even more defensively. Instead of being defensive, Bob might have said, "It is important to stay hydrated while you're in bed, so I brought water for you. You seem upset; is there anything you need?" A response such as this, acknowledging the client's feelings and offering help, is useful in cases of rational anger (Figure 17-4 ■).

When the client is not able to cope effectively with stressors and engages in angry acting-out behavior, anger takes on a different meaning. Acting out is a sign of ineffective coping and may be a precursor to aggression. When anger goes out of control toward rage, the client may engage in dangerous impulsive behavior. The client who is acting out anger may throw things, pace rapidly and aimlessly around the room or halls, shake fists, stomp feet, shout, or threaten to hurt people.

If the client is rationally angry, the nurse can discuss the source of the client's anger, acknowledge the client's feelings, and discuss solutions if there are any. Every problem does not have a solution, though, and sometimes the best action is to acknowledge this fact. For example, a client may be raging about his impending leg amputation due to tissue necrosis. The nurse cannot solve the problem of the amputation, but may be able to help this client look at the situation in a different way (or to

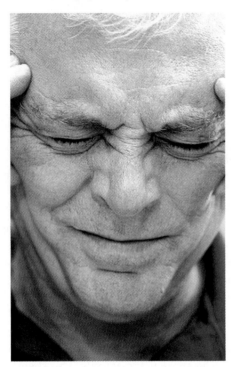

Figure 17-4. ■ Chronic pain might lead to angry behavior.
Source: PhotoEdit Inc.

"reframe the issue"). If the client thought his life would not be worth living with one leg, the nurse might help him list things he enjoys that can be done one-legged, such as playing checkers with his grandchildren, painting, and playing the saxophone. He might be a role model of courage for his grandchildren. Visiting with someone who has already had an amputation and adjusted well might put these activities into perspective for him. These attitudes put the picture of amputation in a different light.

An important approach to angry clients is **limit setting.** The best approach is to tell the client calmly and firmly what the limits are when behavior is inappropriate. When setting limits, do not argue with the client or demand that s/he behave better (Arnold & Hallinan, 2000). The nurse might say in a positive tone of voice: "It is not appropriate for you to raise your voice like that. If you yell, I will leave the room." The nurse's body language should reinforce the words.

Another approach is **redirection.** If a client focuses persistently on an issue that causes her/him to be angry, the nurse should take a problem-solving approach first, then try to change the client's focus. Eliminate anything that might be a trigger for the anger (Arnold & Hallinan, 2000).

CASE EXAMPLE

Michelle, an adolescent client, is expressing anger about her brother Josh not coming to visit. First, the nurse encourages Michelle to communicate her concern to her brother and her parents. Direct communication is an excellent strategy. The nurse also helps her with problem solving about how Michelle's brother can get to the hospital. But, even after making these arrangements and talking about her feelings, Michelle still focuses on her anger. It is time for the nurse to try a distracting activity, such as a walk in the hall or a conversation on another subject, to direct Michelle's attention to another area.

NURSING CARE

ASSESSING

The nurse begins with assessment of the client's appearance and behavior. A flushed face, tightened jaws, flared nostrils, clenched fists or jaw, rigid posture, and rapid eye movements are signs of angry feelings (Arnold & Hallinan, 2000). Tone and volume of voice are also indicators.

Some people express their anger passively. We will cover passive-aggressive behavior later.

When the nurse believes that the client is experiencing angry feelings, the next step is to ask the client. It helps both nurse and client when the nurse can explain what behavior led to the conclusion that the client is angry. The nurse could say, "You are frowning, and you look angry. How are you feeling?" or, "I've noticed that you're raising your voice. Are you angry?" These objective statements might make it easier for the client to become more self-aware and give a clarifying response.

The expression of anger itself does not warrant a nursing diagnosis. It is when the angry client is not coping effectively or is not expressing anger appropriately that the nurse may step in with some nursing intervention.

Anger and irritability can be manifestations of symptoms of alcohol or drug withdrawal. If the client is at risk for withdrawal, assess for this. See Chapter 12 for information about substance abuse.

DIAGNOSING, PLANNING, AND IMPLEMENTING

Common nursing diagnoses for clients experiencing anger are Anxiety, Ineffective Coping, Impaired Social Interaction, and possibly Risk for Other-Directed Violence.

When an angry client is acting out and behaving inappropriately, desired outcomes for nursing care are that the client will:

- Cause no harm to self or others.
- Stop inappropriate behavior.
- Express angry feelings in a safe and appropriate way.

Some interventions that may be useful for clients who are experiencing angry feelings follow:

- Establish a trusting nurse-client relationship with the client. *This might be accomplished by finding common ground with the client, giving the client a time to talk about nonmedical issues, and offering the client some control of the situation if possible (Childers, 2003).*
- If the client has a rational reason for anger, acknowledge that these feelings are appropriate and work on problem solving if it is indicated. *Some angry feelings are appropriate. Clients may feel guilty for being angry due to their cultural background.*
- Discuss with the client the events that lead to anger, including past experiences with hostile or angry behavior (Schultz & Videbeck, 2004). *Discussion of the causes and consequences of angry behavior and of the client's history are insight producing.*
- Help the client plan realistic alternatives to acting-out behavior when s/he feels angry. *Healthy anger management skills can be learned. The client must practice behavior change after talking about it. Only plans that are practical and realistic for the individual will be effective.*
- Give positive reinforcement when the client tries healthy new behaviors. *Positive reinforcement for using new behaviors will encourage the new behaviors to continue.*
- Communicate professionally and objectively. *The client's anger can be contagious to the nurse. The nursing professional should not enter into angry exchanges with clients. When a client is angry, calm, clear, and objective communication is the most effective.*
- Set limits on client behavior, and enforce them consistently. *A client is more likely to comply with rules that s/he understands. Although clients may test the will of the staff to apply rules, overall client compliance will improve when staff members have consistent expectations.*
- Do not take the client's behavior personally. *The client's behavior reflects the client, her or his skills, values, experiences, and pathologies. It does not reflect the value of the nurse as a person!*

EVALUATING

The nursing goals are met when the client is able to recognize feelings of anger and express them appropriately, and then move on to problem-solving behavior. Even though anger is normal, persisting in it indefinitely is not an effective way to cope with life's challenges.

Unhealthy Coping and Communication Skills

Some clients are just more difficult to care for. Sometimes the difficulty is the complex treatment technology. Sometimes the difficulty is the person's complex physiological needs. This section discusses difficulties nurses encounter when clients have unhealthy coping or communication styles or special psychosocial needs.

PASSIVE-AGGRESSIVE BEHAVIOR

Clients who are overtly angry offer challenges to nurses. However, those who express their anger in hidden ways can be even more difficult. Remember the Cultural Pulse Points box that covered the cultural influences to avoid expression of anger? Some people meet this cultural expectation with passive-aggressive, or negativistic, behavior. These clients resent and passively resist demands put on them by others. Instead of an active refusal to do something, the passive-aggressive response would be to procrastinate, forget to do it, or intentionally do a poor job. These clients might complain of being misunderstood or blame their failures on others. People who use passive-aggressive behavior often have a negative outlook. They may be ambivalent about decisions, wavering from one option to its opposite (American Psychiatric Association, 2000).

CASE EXAMPLE

Dan was recently diagnosed with type 2 diabetes and received client education on diabetes management. He said he would follow his treatment plan. His wife reports that he has not adhered to any of the recommendations from the diabetes class. On this admission his blood glucose was extremely elevated. He told the nurse that it is because his wife always fixes too much rice. He stated: "I meant to stay on the diet."

Passive-aggressive behavior can be very challenging for nurses. The client initially seems to agree with health recommendations, yet does not comply. This client does not take personal responsibility for her/his own health or behavior, blaming others when problems arise. Communication with this client can become confused and unhealthy.

BEWARE OF JUDGING NONCOMPLIANCE

Although the example of noncompliance above reflects passive-aggressive behavior, not all noncompliance with medical recommendations is due to client pathology or negativity. There are many reasons for noncompliance. Perhaps the client has not been taking her medication at home, because it is too expensive, and she cannot afford to buy it. Perhaps the recommended dietary changes don't fit in with the lifestyle of the client's family. Maybe the client or family members disagree with the recommended treatment because it goes against some aspect of their culture. Maybe the client does not understand how to comply with the medical recommendations. Maybe the client is still in denial about the diagnosis and therefore, does not follow necessary treatment recommendations.

NURSING CARE

ASSESSING

When a client is noncompliant with recommended treatment, the nurse should engage the nursing process. Begin with an assessment of how the client perceives the instructions. If the client does not fully understand, intervene by teaching. If the client understands the instructions and is not compliant, find out why. The reasons will guide your problem solving. Be sure to consider cultural and financial issues. If you are making dietary recommendations, begin with assessing what the client usually eats. Include foods that the client likes and has at home. Remember that lifestyle change recommendations must be realistic for the client, or they cannot be followed. A newly diagnosed diabetic who has always been a "snacker" needs to have acceptable snacks calculated into his/her diet plan.

When the nurse collects data about passive-aggressive behavior patterns, the nurse is really assessing the client's coping skills. Passive-aggressive behavior is an ineffective way to cope, which brings us to the nursing diagnoses.

DIAGNOSING, PLANNING, AND IMPLEMENTING

The nursing diagnoses of Ineffective Coping, Anxiety, Noncompliance, or Powerlessness may apply to clients who use passive-aggressive coping behavior.

Desired outcomes for these clients are that the client will:

- Verbalize feelings directly.
- Demonstrate adaptive (healthy) coping behavior.
- Identify appropriate problem-solving techniques.
- Adhere to the recommended treatment regimen as prescribed.

Nursing interventions designed to treat Ineffective Coping, Anxiety, Noncompliance, and Powerlessness in clients who use passive-aggressive behavior include the following:

- Encourage the client to discuss genuine feelings and opinions. Pay special attention to helping the client be direct in expressing angry feelings or attitudes of disagreement. *The client who uses passive-aggressive behavior may not understand her/his own feelings. The client usually expresses these feelings indirectly. Expressing them to the nurse develops insight and the new skill of direct communication.*
- Accept the client without judgment. *The client may expect angry feelings to be judged harshly. The nurse's nonjudgmental acceptance can help the client feel accepted and more confident.*
- Give the client opportunities to practice new direct communication skills. *Behavior is more likely to persist when it is practiced, especially if positive reinforcement is received for the new behavior.*
- Include the client as much as possible in decision making about her/his care and treatment plan. *This client may feel like a victim of care instead of a participant.*
- Reassure the client that perfection is not possible. *Sometimes ambivalence is caused by fear that the outcome of a decision must be perfect.*

EVALUATING

The nurse evaluates clients with passive-aggressive behavior by reviewing the outcomes. Is the client stating feelings directly? Is some healthy form of coping being attempted? Does the client understand what appropriate problem-solving behavior is? Does the client engage in problem solving? Positive answers to these questions indicate successful outcomes, even if the steps the client has achieved are small.

Manipulation

Everyone must learn how to have his or her personal needs met. Usually people learn how to cooperate with others for the purpose of meeting their needs. They learn to have empathy and concern for others along the way. On the other hand, sometimes people learn to meet their needs by manipulating others. **Manipulation** is a maladaptive social response. Some characteristics of people who use manipulation are that they (Stuart & Laraia, 2001):

- Treat others as objects
- Are self-oriented or goal-oriented, not other-oriented
- Have relationships that center around control issues

Interacting and caring for clients who use manipulation can be challenging for nurses. Like other people, nurses often resent being manipulated.

CASE EXAMPLE

Consider the case of Les. Les is hospitalized on an inpatient surgical unit recovering from coronary artery bypass surgery. He asked Toni, his nurse, to give him some extra salt packets, because "the food is so bland here." She told him that his doctor ordered a reduced sodium diet, and she can't give him extra salt. He became angry and told her that she is trying to control him and that she is a bad, uncaring nurse. That evening, Les asked Susan, his evening nurse, for extra salt. He told her that Toni gave him extra salt, and that "the doctor said it was OK." Susan was busy and gave Les extra salt packets. He thanked her sincerely and told her that she was very kind, and the only one who understands how hard it is to be a client. Both Toni and the physician later reprimanded Susan. Susan felt betrayed and angry with herself for allowing herself to be manipulated. She was also angry with Les, Toni, and the physician and had a very bad day as a result of the incident.

The client in the above example experienced **splitting,** which means that he tends to see people or situations as either all good or all bad. The good people are the ones who serve his needs. The bad ones are those who don't. He also engaged in a manipulative behavior called **staff splitting.** Staff splitting occurs when the client plays one staff member against another, using staff to obtain extra privileges or services, or to avoid responsibilities. The only way for nurses and other staff to prevent and avoid staff splitting is to work together as a team, to keep communication open, to respond to the client consistently,

and to consult with each other when an individual client seems to be manipulative.

The needs, perceptions, and behavior of manipulative clients foster vicious cycles that continue unhelpful patterns. They provoke negative reactions from others, including their caregivers (Millon & Davis, 1999). Nurses might feel used and keep that feeling even after the behavior ends (Arnold & Hallinan, 2000). This can cause resentment and a desire to have little contact with the client who is manipulative. The nurse needs to remember that the manipulative behavior, like the other behaviors discussed in this chapter, are generally not personal.

Clear limits and consistent expectations promote healthy communication with these clients. When nurses are able to provide structure, with clear boundaries, consistent expectations, and guidelines for self-control, the client's sense of security will be increased, and the need to manipulate will be decreased (Kneisl, Wilson, & Trigoboff, 2004).

When Nurses Encourage Client Pathology

Sometimes the uninformed good intentions of nurses get in the way of client care. A good example of this problem is in pain management. Remember Maslow's hierarchy of needs? Check out Chapter 3 if you need a review. The lowest level of the pyramid is composed of the most basic human needs. One of them is freedom from pain. Another is oxygen.

If a client is hypoxic and the nurse stands on his oxygen tubing, the client will be highly motivated to get air. He might first ask the nurse to get off the tube, but if the nurse stays, he will do what he has to do to get air. He might even push the nurse out of the way if he is desperate. The same is true of pain. If the nurse does not manage the client's pain, the client may try to solve the problem maturely, but will eventually go to unhealthy measures to get the pain relieved. The unhealthy behavior of clients in pain can include withdrawal, hostility, or trying to manipulate the nurse for drugs.

Pain management is a critical client care issue. The nurse must intervene to relieve the client's pain and act as the client's advocate with the physician if the pain persists. Sometimes nurses mistakenly believe that they should minimize the amount of medication a client takes to prevent addiction. Addiction is not a real issue with hospitalized clients in acute pain.

Some clients start out with manipulative attempts to receive pain medications. They present a challenge. With these clients the healthcare team must cooperate (we don't want to be "split"). An effective dose of medication must be determined, and the client must be given the dose regularly, not on a p.r.n. schedule, to minimize motivation for manipulation. The client receives the drug on time, at every scheduled time. If the dose is not effective, the physician can reassess the dose daily. This method meets the needs of the client for pain management and helps solve the problem without staff manipulation.

NURSING CARE

ASSESSING

Assessment of coping behaviors is the source of information for cues to manipulative behavior. Manipulating others is an ineffective coping behavior. When a client is manipulative and splits the staff, an entire unit can be in a state of frustration, with staff angry at each other and the client.

DIAGNOSING, PLANNING, AND IMPLEMENTING

The pertinent nursing diagnoses for a manipulative client include Ineffective Coping, Defensive Coping, and Impaired Social Interaction. The desired outcomes are that the client will:

- Express feelings and needs directly.
- Adhere to limits set by staff.
- Interact with others without rationalizing behaviors, blaming others, or manipulating others.

To reach these desired outcomes, the nurse may choose from the following interventions:

- Speak with the client in a normal (not raised) tone of voice. Use an assertive (not passive or aggressive) approach. Be confident in yourself. *Manipulative clients can benefit from positive role modeling of appropriate assertive communication. Confidence by the nurse instills trust and respect by clients.*
- Set limits (such as no profanity or shouting, no interfering with the care of other clients, adhering to physician's orders, communicating all requests to one staff member each shift, etc.) Choose only the most important issues for the individual. Tell the client about them. Notify all staff of the limits and apply them consistently. *The client must understand the rules in order to follow them. Consistency is the key to compliance. Having too many rules encourages resistance from the client. Set priorities.*
- Be firm, but also caring. *The nurse is setting limits as part of the client's treatment, not as a punishment.*
- Do not allow the client to give gifts to the staff, or to flatter or manipulate some staff to feel that they owe the client favors. *This client should be treated like other clients and is expected to be as responsible as other clients.*
- If the client complains about one staff member to another, refer him back to the person he is complaining about. *Accepting complaints about other staff members is the beginning of staff splitting.*
- Encourage the client to express his feelings and needs directly and appropriately. Reinforce positive attempts at desired behavior. *Direct communication is a desired outcome for this client. Behavior is reinforced by positive reinforcement.*
- Confront the client when s/he attempts to engage in unhealthy communication or coping behavior. *Naming behavior verbally promotes the client's insight about the behavior.*
- Assign consistent staff. *Assigning the same staff can decrease the chance of manipulation and staff splitting. It can also provide a foundation for the client to develop trust in another person, the regular nurse. Trust is difficult for this person.*

EVALUATING

Assess the client's progress continually. Clients who manipulate can affect all the staff on a unit, or even cause difficulty between departments. When the client is expressing feelings and needs directly, interacting with others appropriately, and trying new coping and communication skills that take into consideration the needs of others, the desired outcomes are met.

Chronic Illness

Usually when people think of someone having an illness, they picture the person getting sick, being ill for a while, and then recovering completely. This picture of acute illness is the most common way people conceptualize illness. Even when people have chronic illnesses, such as chronic obstructive pulmonary disease (COPD), they often think and behave like they have no health problems between **exacerbations** (flare-ups) of the disease.

This common misconception of chronic illness helps explain why some clients do not adhere to treatment and preventive strategies when their symptoms subside. Nurses should consider this when they plan client education about lifestyle changes and ways to prevent relapses of chronic conditions. Teaching should include the concept of chronic illness and its course. It should describe the usual episodes of exacerbation and periods of **remission** (a decrease or temporary resolution of disease symptoms). It should focus treatment and lifestyle changes toward preventing exacerbations and prolonging remissions.

Any time a client attempts to make lifestyle changes, stress is involved. Nurses sometimes approach asking clients to change their lifestyle as if they were simply asking them to take a pill.

Critical Self-Check. Let's look at this for a minute. You are a nursing student. You are bright, knowledgeable about health and illness, and motivated to be healthy. Have you ever tried to change any lifestyle activities, such as eating a low-fat diet, exercising most days of every week consistently, eating five servings of vegetables every day, sleeping 8 hours every night, avoiding alcohol, stopping smoking, reducing salt in your diet, avoiding allergens like dust or dogs, losing weight, reducing the amount of stress in your life (be honest, you are in nursing school)? Was it easy to do?

Nurses ask clients to make big lifestyle changes all the time. Realistically, it is not easy to change your habits. These habits are coping mechanisms and part of how we see ourselves.

The nurse can help the process by acknowledging the difficulty of the task when asking a client to make lifestyle changes. The client is more likely to make the health-promoting changes if health professionals suggest the change and explain its importance. Nurses can help by suggesting alternative healthy coping mechanisms, and by referring clients to community support groups. **Keep hope alive!** It will be difficult, but it is possible to change one's habits.

The **chronic illnesses** have several characteristics that increase the risk of psychosocial problems. These characteristics include functional impairment, degenerative course, effects on physical appearance, requirement of regular monitoring and lifestyle change, and potential threat to life. Especially when the client is a child, chronic illness can affect development. (The parents of a child with a chronic illness are also impacted by the condition, which in turn affects family dynamics and may produce more psychosocial problems for the child.) The nurse must work to help people with chronic illnesses achieve developmental tasks. Table 17-1 ■ lists some of the psychosocial issues and nursing diagnoses associated with chronic illnesses.

TABLE 17-1		
Psychosocial Issues Related to Chronic Illnesses		
CHARACTERISTICS OF CHRONIC ILLNESSES	**EXAMPLE ILLNESSES**	**POTENTIAL PSYCHOSOCIAL NURSING DIAGNOSES (EACH OF THESE MAY BE PERTINENT TO SEVERAL CHRONIC ILLNESSES)**
Decreased ability to function	Arthritis, COPD	Risk for Delayed Development, Anxiety, Ineffective Role Performance
Degenerative course	Multiple sclerosis, amyotrophic lateral sclerosis, Parkinson's disease	Powerlessness, Compromised Family Coping, Risk for Suicide, Caregiver Role Strain
Affects physical appearance	Psoriasis, scleroderma	Chronic Low Self-Esteem, Disturbed Body Image
Requires regular long-term monitoring	Diabetes, chronic renal failure	Disturbed Body Image, Ineffective Coping, Powerlessness
Life threatening	AIDS, cancer	Hopelessness, Anticipatory or Dysfunctional Grieving, Ineffective Denial

Psychosocial Needs of Special Populations

PEOPLE WITH AIDS

People who have the human immunodeficiency virus (HIV) or acquired immune deficiency syndrome (AIDS), the advanced form of HIV, have multiple psychosocial issues. The life-threatening nature of the disease brings lifestyle changes, multiple grief issues, issues related to death and dying, functional impairment, numerous medical treatments, and medication side effects. Other psychosocial issues include the social stigma of the disorder, financial challenges, threats to self-concept, and potential for social isolation.

Active listening, promoting adaptive coping skills, and therapeutic use of self by the nurse are effective interventions. Nursing care should also include mental status assessment, because 15–30% of people with AIDS experience dementia (AIDS Dementia Complex, 2005). The early symptoms of AIDS dementia are impaired memory and concentration, uncoordinated motor function, irritable mood, and personality changes.

The healthcare team must collaborate to ensure that clients have adequate resources in the hospital and in the community to maintain their function and to meet their complex needs. Appropriate care for clients with HIV or AIDS requires a healthcare team in the hospital, in the outpatient clinic, and in the community.

When clients with chronic illnesses, disfiguring surgery, substance abuse, life-threatening diagnoses, or challenging health problems are discharged from the hospital into the community, they may be able to benefit from a support group. A support group includes people who all share a common disorder. There are support groups for people with a large variety of disorders. For example, there are groups for people living with AIDS, people who have had mastectomies, children with diabetes, spouses of people with Alzheimer's disease, and people who have multiple sclerosis. The most popular and famous support group is Alcoholics Anonymous. Box 17-4 ■ provides information about how support groups help people.

Spiritual Needs

The mysteries of life and death, good and evil, and pain and suffering generate spiritual questions. *Religion* is an organized system of beliefs concerning the cause, nature,

---

BOX 17-4

Community Care: Support Groups

Support groups are made up of people who share a common challenge who come together to help each other and themselves. They benefit members by:

- Providing support and validation of others in a similar situation
- Decreasing social isolation that can accompany serious or chronic illness
- Empowering members
- Promoting active coping
- Reducing anxiety
- Promoting self-efficacy
- Allowing participants to feel that they have helped others

---

and purpose of the universe. The religions of the world offer various interpretations of these mysteries. Most individuals seek a personal understanding of the meaning of existence at some time in their lives. *Spirituality* is each individual's personal effort to find purpose and meaning in life (Andrews & Boyle, 2003). According to the Joint Commission on Accreditation of Healthcare Organizations, or JCAHO (now known simply as the Joint Commission), this search helps people experience "hope, love, inner peace, comfort, and support" (Joint Commission, 2005). The focus of health care has become increasingly holistic, which has brought back a renewed attention to spirituality (Hicks, 1999). Parish nursing is a specialty nursing field that has evolved to incorporate spirituality into health care. One Jewish nurse who carries along the Book of Psalms on her home visits believes the spiritual aspect of a person is critical to health (Weber, 2006).

Even people who do not have religious beliefs have a spiritual dimension. Insightful nursing requires nurses to know themselves and their own values. Nurses do not need to be fully aware of the meaning of life, but they do need to be aware of their own spiritual direction. The only time holistic care is possible is when nurses can recognize and address the spiritual needs of their clients.

Spiritual issues have their challenges. Nurses who are not religious may believe that spiritual issues are irrelevant to them and are therefore irrelevant to everyone. Devout nurses may feel that their work as nurses is an extension of their religious beliefs. For them, it may be easier to discuss spiritual issues with clients, but preaching, teaching, or persuading clients toward the nurse's own religious beliefs is intrusive and unethical.

Prayer is a communication with a divine being. Fifty-seven percent of Americans report that they pray on a daily basis. Ninety-six percent of elderly Americans use prayer to cope with stress, and prayer is the most frequently reported alternative treatment modality used (Dunn & Horgas, 2000). Research shows that praying can positively affect not only anxiety, but also blood pressure, the course of heart attacks, and migraine headaches (Meisenhelder & Chandler, 2000).

Despite the time crunch found in providing care of the client, nurses need to make time to nurture the spiritual needs of their clients; just being "mindfully present" with clients during any nursing activity can be a spiritual experience (Hemmila, 2002). This connection between a client's spiritual beliefs and positive outcomes of his/her physical condition has been recognized by the Joint Commission and is now included in its performance standards used when surveying healthcare institutions. The Joint Commission now requires that spiritual assessment of clients be included with the overall client assessment in the healthcare facility to determine how spirituality affects the client's care, treatment, and services (Joint Commission, 2005). Minimally, the Joint Commission requires that the facility determine the client's denomination, beliefs, and the importance of spiritual practices.

Joint Commission surveyor Janet Sonnenberg has developed five strategies to address spiritual issues appropriately (Joint Commission, 2003).

1. **Think outside the box.** Proper spiritual assessment is more than finding out about a client's religious affiliation. It includes determining the client's beliefs about the nonphysical, or spiritual, aspects of life. This might result in the caregiver providing the client with time to meditate or encouraging the client to keep personal objects that have spiritual meaning in the room.
2. **Ask about spiritual orientation in as broad a way as possible.** Answers to open-ended questions may provide more information about spirituality than close-ended ones. A good question might be, "What spiritual needs do you have that we could help you meet during your stay here?"
3. **Screen for and assess spiritual suffering.** Spiritual suffering, or distress, might be manifested as despair, guilt, hopelessness, and a lost sense of integrity, or poor self-esteem. This is especially true with life-threatening conditions. In this situation, the nurse may advocate for the client to be referred for counseling from qualified facility personnel.
4. **Educate the assessors.** Education of nursing staff is critical so they can use proper spiritual assessment techniques with clients. Screening for spiritual needs should be part of the initial client assessment. Nurses should be knowledgeable of other spiritual and cultural practices in order to assist clients with meeting their spiritual needs.
5. **Document assessment findings.** The Joint Commission requires that staff document findings related to the spiritual assessment; however, it does not require that the documentation be part of the clinical chart. If spiritual needs have been identified, pastoral care or social work personnel may document in their own records. Having a facility spiritual assessment tool is evidence that staff have evaluated spiritual needs in each client.

NURSING CARE

ASSESSING

How does the nurse know what the client needs? Assessment, of course, is the answer. Every situation does not call for a thorough spiritual assessment, but a basic assessment of spiritual needs must be included. That initial assessment may require that a more thorough assessment be conducted as a follow-up. Because of Joint Commission regulations, facilities may develop their own assessment tool or use one that is already in practice. The Jarel Spiritual Well-Being Scale is a thorough assessment tool that consists of 21 questions regarding the client's spiritual health. Using the mnemonic device of HOPE may guide the assessment by some (Joint Commission, 2005):

Hope
Organized religion
Personal spirituality
Effects on medical care or end-of-life issues

The following questions may help the nurse obtain information about clients' spiritual needs (Mohr, 2003):

1. Is religion or spirituality important to you while you are here in the hospital?
2. Would you like to talk with someone about religious matters?

3. If so, do you have someone in mind, or would you like to see our chaplain?
4. Will you need help from the staff to be able to do any of your religious practices?

The final question makes it possible for the client to tell the nurse about religious practices that may not be known by the nurse. For example, the Muslim client may need to pray five times daily, and may need to know which direction is east (toward Mecca). A Hindu client may need to have a vegetarian diet. A Buddhist or Christian client may want to avoid surgery on a holy day. A Catholic client may want a priest to be called to perform the Sacrament of the Sick. A Native American might want to have the tribal Medicine Man there to perform certain rituals. The nurse is not expected to anticipate all of these needs. But the nurse is expected to know that clients have spiritual needs, and to apply the nursing process to these needs, just as we do to physiological and psychosocial needs. The nurse should be willing to call in whatever spiritual advisor the client requests and ensure the client's privacy when religious rituals are occurring.

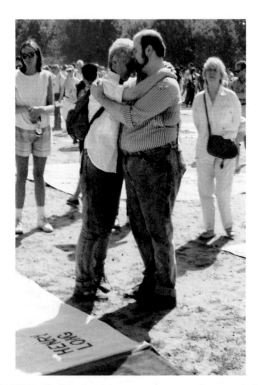

Figure 17-5. ■ Grieving parents embrace as they see their son's name displayed on the AIDS quilt. Grief can be a source of spiritual distress. *Source: Pearson Education/PH College.*

The following experiences can cause spiritual distress: separation from cultural ties, death of a significant other, extreme suffering, serious illness, significant loss, or a challenge to the person's beliefs and value system (Figure 17-5 ■). The nurse may observe that the client is questioning the meaning of her or his life, expressing hopelessness or helplessness, expressing concern about death and its meaning, searching for a spiritual source of strength, or stating that s/he has feelings of intense guilt (Varcarolis, 2000). Seeing religious items in the client's room, hearing the clients speak about "God," or seeing the client reading from a holy book can all be indicators of the client's spirituality.

DIAGNOSING, PLANNING, AND IMPLEMENTING

When the nurse assesses that a client is experiencing the aforementioned symptoms, Spiritual Distress is diagnosed. NANDA defines Spiritual Distress as "disruption in the life principle that pervades a person's entire being and that integrates and transcends biological and psychosocial nature" (NANDA, 2005).

The desired outcomes for clients with spiritual distress are that clients will:

- State that they have meaning in their lives.
- Verbalize a sense of self-esteem and hope for the future.
- Verbalize acceptance of themselves as not deserving of the life-threatening illness or situation, that no one is to blame (Doenges, Moorhouse, & Geissler-Murr, 2002).
- State that they have achieved comfort or a sense of well-being through their spiritual/philosophical practices.
- Discuss their values.

The nurse may help the client achieve these goals through the following interventions:

- Encourage the client to discuss her or his spiritual concerns (concerns about the greater meaning of the event). *Sometimes the client trusts the nurse and is ready to discuss doubts and frustrations with this nurse. A client may or may not desire the consultation of a chaplain or religious practitioner. If the nurse is comfortable with the subject, a conversation may meet the client's need.*

Sometimes the real need is just to discuss life with a trusted person.

- Help the client list his/her resources for support. *Forming a list of supportive people will demonstrate that the client is not alone.*
- Arrange for the client to talk with her or his selected spiritual leader, or the facility's chaplain, if the client desires to do so. *If the client wants to engage in religious practices or wants a religious discussion, the religious practitioner may be the best person to meet this need. Hospital chaplains are educated on how to counsel people of various religions.*
- If the client's distress is related to the diagnosis of an illness, arrange for the client to meet a person who has the same disease who has coped with it in a healthy way, who can act as a role model. *Another person who has coped with the same problems in a healthy way is the best source of information about the "lived experience" of an affected person. The role model will understand what the client is experiencing and has developed strategies for coping that may help the client.*
- Discuss what has given the client consolation or reassurance in the past. *The client is likely to respond to strategies that have been previously successful.*
- Encourage the client to write her or his thoughts and reflections on practical and philosophical issues in a journal. *Journaling helps to identify significant personal issues. It expresses and allows for review of thoughts and feelings about spiritual subjects. Journal writing is an excellent way to develop insight and to explore the deeper meanings of life (Varcarolis, 2000).*
- Refer the client to an appropriate support group in the community. *See Box 17-4 for more information about support groups.*
- Assist the client with spiritual practices if possible. *It is acceptable for the nurse to pray with a client or to read from the client's holy book. Provide religious articles close at hand if the client desires. The Catholic may find comfort in having a rosary close by; the Muslim, a copy of the Koran; the Jewish person, a copy of the Hebrew Bible. Assist clients with bathing and hygiene in preparation for a visit by their spiritual advisor; have the room cleared of unnecessary items.*

EVALUATING

After the nurse intervenes, if the client feels a renewed sense of meaning in life, expresses hope for the future, understands that "bad things can happen to good

people," or is comforted by her or his spiritual practices, then the desired outcomes for spiritual distress have been reached.

Critical Self-Check. Consider the following question: Can a nurse who has no religious beliefs (such as a nurse who is an atheist) deal with the spiritual needs of clients?

NURSING PROCESS CARE PLAN
Client in Spiritual Distress

Gertrude Golden is a 55-year-old Jewish client on the oncology unit who had a mastectomy yesterday.

Assessment. Ms. Golden is alert, oriented, and her vital signs are stable and within normal limits. She has been crying off and on all day. She states, "Why me?" "What did I do to deserve this?" and "There could never be a God who would let this happen."

Diagnosis. The diagnosis of Spiritual Distress is established for Ms. Golden.

Expected Outcomes. The client will:

- Express her feelings about the diagnosis of breast cancer and the mastectomy.
- Discuss her values/beliefs related to the meaning of this experience for her.
- Verbalize acceptance of herself as not deserving this illness, and that no one is to blame.

Planning and Implementation

- Encourage Ms. Golden to express her feelings and values, and actively listen to her.
- Assist the client to identify her resources for support.
- Provide the client with a role model. This would be another woman who has experienced a mastectomy for breast cancer who is coping with her experience in a healthy way.
- Discuss hope with the client. Help her identify goals and things she still has to look forward to in the future.
- Ask the client if she would like to talk with a religious adviser (a rabbi, or the hospital chaplain).

Evaluation. Ms. Golden was able to build a trusting relationship with the nurse and discussed her feelings about cancer and surgery. She stated, "I realize intellectually that this is no one's fault. I was feeling alone and desperate." She responded well to the woman with the mastectomy who came to visit her in the hospital. They even joked and laughed together about bras. She told the client about a support group in the community for women who have had mastectomies. She chose not to talk with a religious adviser. The client's husband is supportive.

Critical Thinking in the Nursing Process

1. How could the nurse find a role model to come in to visit a client like Ms. Golden?
2. Why is it important to realize that it is not helpful to blame anyone for a client's illness?
3. How might a support group help Ms. Golden?

Note: Discussion of Critical Thinking questions appears in Appendix I.

Note: The references and resources for this and all chapters have been compiled at the back of the book.

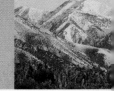

Chapter Review

 KEY TERMS

Use the audio glossary feature of the Companion Website to hear the correct pronunciation of the following key terms.

chronic illness

crisis

exacerbation

humanism

limit setting

manipulation

redirection

remission

splitting

staff splitting

KEY Points

- All people have physiological, psychosocial, and spiritual dimensions. Nurses apply the nursing process to treat problems in all three areas.

- Anxiety can result from experiencing the unknown. Nurses can help clients avoid this source of anxiety through client teaching.

- Anxiety is contagious (easily transmitted from one person to another). The client will feel more secure when the nurse is calm and confident.

- Whether an event becomes a crisis for an individual depends on that individual's perception of the event, situational support, and coping mechanisms.

- Assessing a client's coping style involves finding out what the client usually does when under severe stress.

- Anger is normal as long as it is expressed appropriately.

- Nurses often have difficulty dealing with clients' anger.

- Nurses should not take the feelings or behavior of clients personally.

- There are healthy and effective strategies for responding to clients who use manipulative or passive-aggressive behavior.

- People with chronic illnesses are at risk for more psychosocial problems than are those with acute illnesses.

- Even a nurse who is an atheist can and should learn to meet the spiritual needs of clients.

 EXPLORE MediaLink

Additional interactive resources for this chapter can be found on the Companion Website at www.prenhall.com/eby. Click on Chapter 17 and "Begin" to select the activities for this chapter.

- Audio glossary
- NCLEX-PN® review
- Case study
- Study outline
- Critical thinking questions
- Matching questions
- Weblinks
- Video Case: Julia (HIV)

Caring for a Client Who Uses Manipulative Behavior

NCLEX-PN® Focus Area: Psychosocial Integrity

Case Study: Ray Daniels is a 27-year-old European American man who is admitted to the hospital for orthopedic surgery, which he had 1 week ago. His physical assessment is normal, with no indication of infection or impaired circulation in the surgical leg. The surgeon ordered Demerol 75 mg IM every 4 hours p.r.n. for pain. He states that he needs more pain medications. The staff are upset, angry at each other, and generally frustrated over the care of Mr. Daniels.

Nursing Diagnosis: Ineffective coping

COLLECT DATA

Subjective	Objective
_____	_____
_____	_____
_____	_____
_____	_____
_____	_____
_____	_____
_____	_____

Would you report this data? Yes/No

If yes, to: _____

Nursing Care

_____
_____
_____
_____
_____
_____
_____
_____
_____

How would you document this? _____
_____
_____
_____

Compare your documentation to the sample provided in Appendix I.

Data Collected
(use those that apply)

- Client requests pain medication every hour.
- Client states, "You are the only person who really understands me."
- Client states, "The other nurses never give me enough pain medicine. They don't seem to care."
- Client states, "Will you do me a favor and give it early just this once?"
- Divorced
- Has three children
- Responding well to physical therapy, ambulating with a walker
- Sleeps 8 hours per night in hospital
- States, "I plan to give a dozen roses and $100 to every nurse who takes good care of me."
- BP 120/80, T 98.8 °F (tympanic), P 80, R 12
- Has many visitors
- Works as a construction worker
- Client states, "I am a very religious man."
- Client told the physician that the nurses are not caring for him.
- Client told the nurses that the physician does not like him.
- Peripheral pulses palpable and strong, bilaterally

Nursing Interventions
(use those that apply; list in priority order)

- Assess the client's pain.
- Assign consistent staff to this client.
- Change his medication schedule from p.r.n. to a regular schedule of Demerol 75 mg IM every 4 hours.
- Provide client with antianxiety medication.
- Tell the client that he will be given his pain medication on a schedule every 4 hours. He does not need to ask for it. The physician visits daily and can change the dose then if necessary.
- Offer nondrug pain-relief interventions.
- Tell nursing assistants not to report the client's frequent requests for painkillers.
- Encourage the client to express his feelings.
- Tell the client, "I care about you. I will help you learn how to communicate with us directly. This is a skill you need to develop."
- Have a staff conference about the client and develop a plan of care that everyone follows consistently.
- Include the client in planning.
- If the client complains about staff members, take his concerns seriously and assess each situation objectively.
- Give the client positive reinforcement when he asks for help assertively, without manipulation.

1 A client who has been admitted for diagnostic surgery in the morning tells the nurse he is having difficulty going to sleep because of his fear of what the doctor will find. The nurse's best response to the client would be:

   1. "Everyone is always a little anxious before surgery. I'll see if you have something ordered for sleep."
   2. "I can understand your anxiety. Let's talk about your fears."
   3. "What helps you sleep at home when you have trouble?"
   4. "I really think that you have little to worry about. The physician does not seem that concerned."

2 A client with pneumonia is pacing in his room. He tells the nurse that he thinks he's going to die. "You've got to help me!" His color is good, and his breathing is not labored. The nurse's first responsibility is to:

   1. Provide a safe environment for the client. Remain calm and listen to his concerns.
   2. Make sure that his oxygen saturation is at a therapeutic level. Assess his respiratory status.
   3. Go to the nurses' station to check on orders for an antianxiety medication.
   4. Call the physician to get an order for oxygen.

3 Which of the following clients would be most likely to experience a crisis when faced with a diagnosis of a chronic disease?

   1. A 25-year-old married man with a white-collar job
   2. A 35-year-old female who has had to adjust to a new job, a new marriage, and a move to a new city within the past year
   3. A 70-year-old retired male who lives with his wife of 50 years
   4. A single 55-year-old female who watched her mother slowly die of COPD

4 What intervention would be appropriate for clients at risk for crisis?

   1. Research support groups that are available in the immediate area.
   2. Advocate for antianxiety medication.
   3. Identify the client's past method of coping with stress-producing situations.
   4. Advise the client on better ways to respond to the situation.

5 When a client is in crisis, the nurse should focus on:

   1. The future; remind the client that although things do not look favorable today, time will bring a new perspective to the problem.
   2. The present; the client needs to deal with the current problem now.
   3. The past; remind the client of past successes.
   4. The past and future; avoid a discussion of the current problem until the client is better able to cope.

6 Which nurse is actively listening to a client?

   1. The nurse stands with arms folded in front of his chest.
   2. The nurse uses the time with the client to also straighten the client unit.
   3. The nurse sits at client's bedside with privacy curtain drawn.
   4. The nurse interprets each statement of the client to validate its meaning.

7 If a client is rationally angry because of losing a breast to cancer and is fearful of her husband's response to her, which of the following responses of the nurse would be appropriate?

   1. "I can imagine your anger at your loss. Have you discussed your fears with your husband?"
   2. "Women often feel low self-esteem after losing a breast. Let me find another woman who has had a mastectomy for you to talk to."
   3. "I think you will find that men do not hold the breast in as great an esteem as women think they do."
   4. "Why are you angry? Your cancer is gone, and you will probably lead a long, healthy life."

8 The nurse will know that the client is handling anger appropriately when the client:

   1. No longer demonstrates angry behavior.
   2. Is able to acknowledge his/her angry feelings and then describe how he/she will solve the problem causing the anger.
   3. Is verbally loud with the nurse but not violent.
   4. Tells the nurses that he/she is no longer angry.

9 Which of the following clients is acting in a passive-aggressive way about physical therapy? The one who:

   1. Refuses to go.
   2. Goes but refuses to participate.
   3. Puts off going until the therapist has gone home.
   4. Accuses the physical therapist of enjoying inflicting pain.

10 A client complains to the day nurse about the care he received on the night shift. He says the day nurses are much more caring. The nurse's most appropriate response is:

   1. "I am sorry you feel that way. Let me talk to the night supervisor and have him talk to you about any complaints you have."
   2. "Thank you. We try to do our very best."
   3. "I really do not think you have cause for concern. Our night shift nurses are very competent."
   4. "Would you like me to get the day supervisor for you?"

Answers for Review Questions, as well as discussion of Care Plan and Critical Thinking Care Map questions, appear in Appendix I.

Learning About You!

CHAPTER 16 Violence and Abuse

You are a school nurse in a high school where violence among a group of four sophomores has become a daily issue. Using the WHO recommendations for prevention of violence in society (Box 16-1), construct a framework for dealing with the problem before it becomes a more global one. Consider the following questions.

1. Which other high school staff and/or students would you involve in the plan?
2. How would you assess the individuals involved and the underlying causes of the daily violence?
3. How would the families of the individuals be involved? Who would be the contact person with the families?
4. What steps could be taken within the school to discourage violence? How would you determine whether or not bullying was a factor?
5. How would you proceed to educate yourself and others about cultural and gender issues that might be affecting the atmosphere of violence?
6. Would you involve the local community involved in the high school, for example, other parents, the parent-teacher organization, clergy from area churches?
7. Would law enforcement or social services be incorporated into your plan? If so, how?
8. If the problem were resolved, what plans could be put into place to ensure that an environment of safety would be maintained?

CHAPTER 17 Psychosocial Issues for General Client Care

Determine whether or not the following clients are responding to the situation with angry, passive-aggressive, anxious, or manipulative behaviors.

Behavior

A. Angry
B. Anxious
C. Passive-aggressive
D. Manipulative

Description of Response

1. The client faced with a new diagnosis of cancer becomes flirtatious with her male nurse.
2. The alcoholic client who states, "I could quit drinking if my boss didn't invite me out for drinks after work every night."
3. The client who tells the nurse, "I hold you all responsible for my needing an amputation. You have not taken very good care of me. I'm going to sue, you know!"
4. The client who is a smoker is scheduled for early A.M. surgery and tells his nurse, "If you'll let me go outside for just one smoke before surgery, I'll let everyone know that you're the best nurse up here."

Answers

1 (B) 2 (C) 3 (A) 4 (D)

Appendix I
Answers and Critical Thinking Discussion

Chapter 1

NCLEX-PN® ANSWERS

1. (3) The mentally healthy person realizes the need for relationships with others. Maximum mental health cannot be achieved in isolation. All other answers indicate mentally healthy attitudes.

2. (4) With medication and healthier behavior choices, the person with a chronic mental illness may become mentally healthier. The other statements are all true in regard to mental health.

3. (1) With a multiaxial approach to diagnosis, the *DSM-IV-TR* takes into account psychiatric disorders, general medical conditions, and psychosocial and environmental problems as well as the global assessment of functioning. This provides a basis for holistic assessment of mental illness. The *DSM-IV-TR* is appropriate for mental health issues universally. It classifies mental disorders, not people.

4. (2) The client best fits the description given to the moderate symptoms category. The client is still seeking relationships and jobs but is unable to succeed in those areas. He is beyond the minimal, or mild, symptoms category, as he does not have good functioning in all areas. He has not reached the serious symptoms level, as statement indicates he has friends and obtains employment. He has difficulty maintaining both for long.

5. (3) Major depressive disorder is the most common mental disorder found throughout the world. Alcohol abuse is the second most common, followed by schizophrenia, self-inflicted injuries, and bipolar disorder.

6. (1) The failed experiment in discharging clients from psychiatric institutions or deinstitutionalization resulted in homelessness for many people with mental disorders. Once out in the community, these clients failed to return to community clinics to continue their treatments and medications. Without treatment, the clients failed to recognize their needs for housing, medication, and other medical care and did not seek them.

7. (3) The nurse must act as an advocate for those clients diagnosed with severe mental disorders. Tertiary prevention involves rehabilitation after the resolution of the acute phase of the disease for those clients. The goal is to prevent further disability. Primary prevention begins with preventing mentally healthy people from being affected. Secondary prevention involves identifying and treating people already affected by a mental disorder to prevent negative outcomes. *Active intervention* is not an acceptable psychiatric nursing term for mental health promotion.

8. (2) People with mental illnesses often cannot speak for themselves because of their illness. They may be out of touch with reality, depressed, or otherwise unable to speak about their needs. They may not be articulate, understand their healthcare needs, or be fearful of speaking out, but these are the result of their illness and cannot be taken as separate causative factors.

9. (1) The National Alliance for the Mentally Ill is an advocacy group for the mentally ill and their families. The other organizations are not directly related to mental illness.

10. (1, 2, 3, 5) Although the nurse might not be successful in all these areas, education about treatment options and the need for adequate rest and sleep would be important nursing interventions for a client with these risk factors. Promoting healthy coping behaviors and encouraging a healthy self-concept are other ways the nurse can help with modification of risk factors. The nurse has no influence over genetic predisposition to mental illness.

Chapter 2

NCLEX-PN® ANSWERS

1. (1) Although an expert nurse may incorporate intuition into an ethical decision, the novice nurse does not have enough experience to do so. Ethical decisions should always include the client's personal value system and any other information that would affect the outcomes of the decision. The duty of the nurse cannot be the only basis for the ethical decision-making process.

2. (4) Autonomy gives the client the right to choose what treatment options he wants to follow. By insisting that the client continue with the treatment option, the

nurse has violated that ethical principal. The nurse is using the principle of paternalism, which includes making decisions for others. Beneficence and justice have not been violated here.

3. (1) Protecting the client from harm is called non-maleficence. Following all infection control guidelines when caring for clients is a good example of this nursing ethic. Autonomy, justice, and paternalism do not come into play here.

4. (3) The nurse should not give an opinion to a client or family about what they should be doing. The nurse should express concern for the situation but not express an opinion as to what should be done. Clients and families may need the nurse to assist them in the thinking process to make an educated decision. By asking the family to discuss their options, the nurse is opening the way for the family to walk through the ethical decision-making process thoughtfully.

5. (2) A client who is threatening suicide and already has a plan of action is a definite and immediate threat to himself/herself and meets the criteria for an involuntary admission. A client not taking his/her medication or hearing voices is in no immediate danger but certainly bears further observation and may need admission in the near future. Being placed in a mental health care facility is not an appropriate housing option for a homeless person.

6. (3) The mental health care client has the right to the use of the least restrictive approach to stopping escalating behavior first. In this case, the least restrictive choice would be to approach the client cautiously and talk to him quietly. If this does not work, another option might be necessary. The next step might be seclusion. Depending on the severity of the behavior, restraints or IM medication might follow.

7. (1) The client has not been declared legally incompetent but cannot understand the treatment being ordered due to severe psychosis. It would do no good to explain the therapy to the client. With no legal guardian assigned, the next best option would be to consult the client's closest relative to obtain permission. If there were no close relative, the primary physician may also ask the court to appoint a guardian for the client. If the treatment is critical to the client's well-being, the physician cannot wait until the client is able to understand the necessity of the treatment. He cannot proceed without permission of some type being given.

8. (2) Touching a client without permission is battery. Assault would be threatening to perform an action to which the client has not agreed, thereby causing fear in the client. Malpractice and negligence are both unintentional torts. Giving the enema was intentional.

9. (3) In this situation, medicating the client against his will is the best option because of the immediate need to protect the staff and other clients. With the severity of his escalating behavior, leaving him alone is not an option. Because the client is a new admission, there has not been an opportunity to establish a trusting nurse-client relationship. Jail or physical restraints at this point may agitate the client further, although physical restraints or a seclusion room may be necessary at some point in time as well.

10. (3) This response shows a respect for the client's privacy and upholds the institution's rules for confidentiality. The other responses avoid the issue.

CRITICAL THINKING CARE MAP

Subjective data Client asks, "Why do you want to kill me?" Client states, "You want me to take poison."

Objective data Client expresses delusional thinking that medication is poisoned. Oriented to person, place, and time. Refuses to take his ordered antipsychotic medication.

Report Yes, to the charge nurse.

Interventions Establish trusting nurse-client relationship. Calmly explain that you are the nurse and you are here to help him. Reassure the client that you will not hurt him. Tell him that this is his antipsychotic medication that will help him straighten out his thoughts. It is not poison. You would like him to take it. Act in a cooperative, nonthreatening way. Thank him for his cooperation when he takes the medication.

Documentation 10/08/06 Client expresses delusional thinking that his medication is poisoned. Responds well to nonthreatening, reassuring communication that his medication will help him straighten out his thoughts. Took medication without incident.—Irena Florence, LPN

Chapter 3

NCLEX-PN® ANSWERS

1. (3) The ego, as defined by Freud, is the "I," which develops to respond to the realities of everyday life. The basic instincts and urges comprise the id. The conscience is the super-ego. All of these elements combine to form the total, or holistic, person.

2. (3) The student is using an exercise routine to relieve stress rather than holding on to those feelings that could be physically and psychologically harmful. This is an example of sublimation, where unacceptable feelings are diverted into socially acceptable behavior. Compensation, rationalization, and repression are not represented by this example.

3. (3) Children between the ages of 6 and 12 are working through the task of industry versus inferiority. It is important for children of this age to learn how to cooperate and compete with others, following the rules. The other tasks and statements are not applicable to children in this age group. Children between the ages of 3 and 6 are working through the task of initiative versus guilt and are beginning to develop consciences. Children between the ages of 1 and 3 are working through the task of autonomy versus guilt and might develop shame and doubt when disciplined for incontinence episodes. Children between the ages of 12 and 18 are working through the task of identity versus role confusion and are integrating their personal values with those of society.

4. (1) The success of antipsychotic medication lends support to the biological theory of personality development. The antipsychotics affect the neurotransmitter amounts in the brain, which minimize certain psychotic behaviors. These medications would have no effect if trait, humanistic, or behaviorist theories were the only ones valid in explaining behavior.

5. (3) Desensitization is an approach often used by behaviorists to alleviate phobias by exposing phobic clients to small doses of a feared object in a safe environment. Once clients have been exposed often enough, they may be ready to face their fears. The situation does not meet the definitions of the other choices given. Positive reinforcement involves a reward for a desired behavior. Assertiveness requires a client to respond assertively in situations in which they have been acting passively. Reality confrontation is not an accepted behaviorist term.

6. (2) Administering the drug disulfiram (Antabuse) is a type of behavior modification by negative reinforcement. This is a technique used to change drinking behavior. The belief is that if the client associates alcohol with being violently ill, the behavior will stop. Positive reinforcement would reward the client for positive behavior. This is not the basis for disulfiram use. Assertiveness and desensitization are not applicable here. Assertiveness is used to treat passive behaviors; desensitization is used in the treatment of phobias.

7. (1) The nurse is promoting the trait of self-efficacy. The nurse is empowering clients to be responsible for their own behavior and well-being. Clients may become assertive as a result, but this is not the first trait that will appear. Determinism and dependence are not relevant here.

8. (4) The client in this question is most likely experiencing needs in the safety and security level of the hierarchy. Whenever a client feels insecure, having a staff person present is often reassuring. Finding nonessential tasks for someone to do will ensure the client is not alone. There are no observable physiological needs and self-esteem is not involved. The client may not feel loved at this point, but the need to feel safe and secure is more basic in the hierarchy and needs to be met first.

9. (1) Hildegard Peplau developed the interpersonal theory of nursing. She saw the nurse as a tool in assisting clients to see their options in life's decision-making processes. The other theories mentioned were not used by Peplau. Developmental is associated with Erikson; behavior modification with Pavlov and Skinner; psychoanalytical with Freud.

10. Maslow's hierarchy of needs is organized with the most basic human needs that are the highest priority at the bottom of the pyramid. More basic levels of needs must be met before higher level needs. The hierarchy is structured in this order:

1. Physiological (most basic)
2. Safety and security
3. Love and belonging
4. Esteem and recognition
5. Self-actualization

Therefore, the clients in question would be ranked in this order:

1—The client who needs to be fed is having a physiological need met.

2—The totally dependent client with lowered side rails requires care based on a safety and security issue.

3—The client who has received no visitors or phone calls in 3 days might have issues in the love and belonging realm.

4—The client who is disfigured runs the risk of lowered self-esteem and acceptance based on physical appearances.

5—The client who is seeking to read is advancing into the realm of self-actualization.

Chapter 4

NCLEX-PN® ANSWERS

1. (2) The nurse who accepts the responsibility for the son's failure to set his own alarm is demonstrating codependent behavior. The other behaviors indicate nurses who have set appropriate boundaries and who know that others must take responsibility for their own actions.

2. (1) The codependent helps people avoid the consequences of their actions. Although the nurse may feel as if he is helping the impaired nurse, he is postponing her

recognition of her problem and getting help. The other behaviors indicate a healthy use of boundaries—confrontation, helping others see choices, and accepting praise.

3. (4) Once again, the codependent is helping the client to avoid the consequences of a poor health choice. The nurse is essentially giving the client permission to behave irresponsibly. The nurse who says "no" to an extra shift, the nurse who confronts a client about poor diet choices, and the nurse who empathizes with a client and then offers to discuss appropriate life choices is a nurse who is demonstrating no codependent behaviors.

4. (2) When a nurse experiences a situation where morale and efficiency of staff is affected by the poor performance of one staff member who suffers no disciplinary action, the scene is set for burnout. Nurses in this situation feel helpless and have a loss of control. The other situations are appropriate and facilitate a good work environment.

5. (3) Dissatisfaction with one's work environment could precipitate gossiping and complaining. Negativity promotes negativity among staff members and serves no helpful purpose. The other situations show nurses who have set appropriate boundaries, who demonstrate creativity, and who are rewarded for exemplary care.

6. (2) Getting out and doing something fun away from nursing is a good way to prevent professional burnout. Quitting does not prevent burnout but is the result of burnout that is already blazing. Treating oneself to ice cream after work each day will result in weight gain but will not prevent burnout. Keeping one's feelings about work to oneself will increase the risk of burnout.

7. (3) Asking for help when needed recognizes the fact that nursing is a team profession. Burnout will certainly come quickly if nurses forget that they are not alone in their efforts to care for clients. The nurse should ask for and offer help. Putting others' needs ahead of one's own and working independently as a source of pride are not ways to promote mentally healthy nursing. Leaving notes on time cards is a passive-aggressive technique and is never a healthy response.

8. (2) Always follow the chain of command in problem solving. There will be fewer hard feelings and a healthier work environment. Of course, if nothing is resolved by approaching the person directly involved in the problem, the nurse would move on up the chain to unit supervisor and eventually Director of Nursing. Gathering anonymous complaints and refusing to work are self-defeating responses to problem work situations.

9. (4) Spirituality is a broad term that includes the meaning a person finds in life. This can be nurtured in a variety of ways and does not have to include one's participation in organized religion, although this can be one method of nurturing it.

10. (1, 3, 5) Not eating, negative talk, and alcohol abuse are all signs of burnout in caregivers whether it is in the professional nurse or in family caregivers. The nurse needs to recognize it in self as well as in family members of clients. Recognizing the need for respite and being proud of accomplishments as a caregiver are evidences of positive, healthy attitudes.

CRITICAL THINKING CARE MAP

Subjective data   Client states, "I don't even have time to drink water while I'm at work." Client states, "I feel out of control of my life." Client states that she is losing confidence in her ability to manage her diabetes. Client asks, "What can I do to get my life back?"

Objective data   Client has been hospitalized for a diabetic emergency. She has been having difficulty sleeping while in the hospital. She is 5 ft. and weighs 160 lbs. (overweight for her height)

Report   Yes, to the charge nurse.

Interventions   Encourage the client to express her feelings about diabetes, her work, and her life stressors. Assess the coping methods the client has used in the past. Encourage the client to prioritize the demands on her time. Discuss ways the client can manage her diabetes, at home and at work. Discuss coping strategies. Give the client positive feedback when she does problem solving, expresses her feelings, or has ideas about how to cope with her stressors in a healthy way. Support the client's positive attitudes about her ability to manage her life (her sense of self-efficacy).

Documentation   08/28/06 Client expresses concerns about her ability to manage her diabetes. States she feels out of control of her life. Is having difficulty sleeping in the hospital and states she wants to "get my life back." Strategies for coping with her diabetes, lifestyle changes, and time management were discussed.—Florence Kingstad, LPN

Chapter 5

NCLEX-PN® ANSWERS

1. (3) The sender needs to validate the understanding of the receiver for there to be complete communication. If the receiver has not understood the message, the therapeutic

communication will be lost. All the other statements are true.

2. (4) Empathy is trying to look at the situation from the client's point of view. This is the only answer that indicates that the nurse is attempting empathy. The nurse's comments also facilitate open communication with the client. The other statements express sympathy but are not therapeutic in their approach.

3. (3) To listen actively and attentively, you must give your undivided attention to the sender of the message. If you are thinking about what you are going to say next, you are not doing that. You need to place value on what the sender of the message is saying. You need to indicate attention by verbal or nonverbal signs. This is a nursing skill that requires practice just like all your other skills.

4. (1) Sitting down to communicate with a client indicates an interest and willingness to listen attentively. Being on eye level with the client allows the nurse to communicate nonverbally with the eyes and facial expressions. Standing to communicate gives the impression that the nurse has little time to devote to the interaction and/or that the nurse considers him- or herself on a superior level to the client. Sitting 4 feet away from the client does not allow good eye contact. Folded arms could communicate nonverbally that the nurse is not open to any discussion.

5. (3) Touch is not always associated with comforting and caring by someone who has been abused or by a mentally ill person with a psychosis. Use touch with care. It can be interpreted differently by diverse people. Some cultures consider touch to be intrusive and direct eye contact to be rude. Although the hands can be expressive, the face is the most expressive part of the body.

6. (4) This response indicates caring to a client. The nurse is willing to be available and is unhurried. The client feels no pressure to talk but feels the nurse's supportive presence. Although the other responses validate some of the client's feelings, they do not indicate a willingness to stand by and be supportive without forcing the client to talk. Offering a client a cliché as a support technique is a communication barrier and never therapeutic.

7. (1) Any time the nurse asks the client to describe his/her feelings about a subject, the door is opened for continued conversation. The other choices here could be answered with only one word.

8. (3) The reflection technique uses the client's own words to open up the communication. Although the other choices will aid in continuing the conversation, they are not examples of the reflection technique.

9. (2) This choice gives the power and control back to the client who will be affected by the consequences of the decision. Even though discharge decisions are not the responsibility of the staff nurse, guiding the client to think about the choices is appropriate for the nurse. Giving advice is a barrier to communication.

10. (1) This choice would block further discussion, as the nurse has essentially told the client s/he does not want to discuss the client's feelings and that the client was wrong to even think about it. The other choices open the way for therapeutic interactions.

CARE PLAN HINTS

1. "I'm sorry, Ms. Barefoot. I can't go to your home, but I can help find some resources for you."
2. No, because this is not the nurse's job. The nurse could call in the social worker to help find other resources. Imagine if you went to the home of every client who needed help. In a few years, your caseload would be pretty large.
3. The social worker and discharge planning nurse are prepared to help clients and their families plan for alternate care, such as supervised living arrangements.

CRITICAL THINKING CARE MAP

Subjective data   Client states, "I don't want to bother anyone." Client states, "I just hate myself. I don't know why you want to take care of me." When told that she has a beautiful robe, she states, "This ugly old thing?" When her daughter brought Dorothy's grandson in to visit, she stated, "Why would he want to see me?"

Objective data   Lack of eye contact

Interventions   Establish trusting nurse-client relationship. Encourage client to express her feelings. Spend time with the client each shift to show acceptance. Discuss the use of positive self-talk (changing the automatic negative thoughts about self to positive affirmations of client's commendable qualities). Offer pain medication to client every 4 hours. Help the client identify her own strengths. Discourage negative comments about self. Help client practice asking for what she needs.

Report   No

Documentation   09/27/06 Client states that she hates herself. Reluctant to ask to have her needs met. Not using call light or asking for pain meds. Will work on esteem building with client. Offer pain meds every 4 hours. Encourage to call staff p.r.n.—Ruth Adams, LPN

Chapter 6

NCLEX-PN® ANSWERS

1. (3) Although all the life events could be a source of stress for the client, promotion and recognition at work are positive stressors and would probably not impact his hospitalization. Receiving a ticket for a minor traffic violation is a negative stressor but probably not severe enough to cause additional stress. A recent divorce, however, is a significant negative stressor and the most likely to affect his behavior about his illness and hospitalization.

2. (2) Increased pulse, blood pressure, and respirations are all physiological responses to stress, which can be the result of the client's apprehension over test results. The other conditions mentioned are not part of the expected physiological responses to stress.

3. (3) Continuous stimulation of the sympathetic nervous system can contribute to the development of cardiovascular disease, which can lead to strokes, heart attacks, and kidney disease. Hypoglycemia (low blood sugar), glaucoma (increased pressure in the eye), and chronic obstructive pulmonary disease are not triggered by this continuous stimulation.

4. (1) The client would be more fearful about his hospitalization if his wife had recently died in the same hospital. He would associate the hospital with a deep loss and an uncertain outcome to his own hospitalization. Although his first serious illness and his first hospitalization would be definite stressors for him, they would not hold the same connotation as losing his wife. Missing his son's first soccer game would probably be the easiest situation to accept.

5. (2) The poor, elderly woman would be the best choice, because she has more risk factors for a negative response to stress: age (old), health status (pain and chronic disease), lack of resources (poor). The other clients have fewer risk factors for a negative response.

6. (1) The first step in dealing with stress in an adaptive way is to assess the reasons for the stress. Avoidance, self-blame, and wishful thinking are all maladaptive ways of dealing with stress. They don't provide resolution to a problem.

7. (3) The most therapeutic response would be to validate the client's feelings and then encourage her to talk more about those feelings. Discouraging a discussion of her feelings, giving false reassurance, and changing the subject are all effective ways of blocking further communication about her stress, its sources, and possible resolutions.

8. (2) The client who chooses not to discuss her stress might be in denial about its existence. Seeking out her support system, journaling, and requesting prayer are all effective coping mechanisms for stress.

9. (2) Practicing progressive muscle relaxation including breathing exercises would be effective stress management techniques for someone confined to bed and could produce long-term benefits. Certain herb teas could be effective only momentarily for stress relief. Caring for a cat or dog can relieve stress but would be difficult for a client confined to bed. Practicing aggression would be a maladaptive approach to handling stress.

10. (1, 3, 4) Assessing the client's perception of the immediate sources of his stress would be the first step. Educating him about the types of dialysis available would be appropriate, as some of these can be done at home with assistance and would not require transportation. Helping him to explore these choices would be helpful. If he decides on hemodialysis, which requires transportation, investigating community resources for his required transportation would be another appropriate intervention. Always allowing choices for the client gives him a feeling of control, which is a major stress-reliever. Giving him false reassurance and questioning the physician's recommendation would be inappropriate and could have negative consequences. Advocating for a medication to reduce the client's stress response might be appropriate in the future if cognitive/behavior techniques are not successful but should not be the earliest consideration.

CARE PLAN HINTS

1. Without the active coping approach of contacting the instructors, Casey likely would have received failing grades in the courses. Active coping/problem solving is an adaptive coping method.

2. Anger occupies the focus of clients and makes it difficult for them to think of anything else. Angry clients have to deal with the anger before they can be fully cooperative with their treatment plans.

3. A sudden stressor is harder to cope with than one that develops slowly, because the client has no opportunity to plan for coping in advance.

CRITICAL THINKING CARE MAP

Subjective data   Client states, "I can't handle all of this stress. It is killing me." Client's wife states, "He's not usually so anxious," "His father died last month in a hospital in Mexico," and "He's having trouble at work."

Objective data Elevated pulse, blood pressure, and respirations; rocking his upper body back and forth; clutching the bedspread; pulls away when anyone touches his catheter or IV.

Report Yes. This client needs a lot of help. Nurses can help with coping issues. A social worker can help with his financial concerns and stress management.

Interventions Say to the client, "What do you mean when you say 'the stress is killing me'?" Ask the client, "Besides the fractured pelvis, what other things are stressful for you now?" Assess the client's social support by asking, "Who can help you with these problems?" Say to the client, "You seem anxious when I touch the catheter or the IV. Would you tell me about this?" Say to the client, "Your wife told me that your father died recently. That must be hard for you."

Documentation 08/20/06 Client observed rocking back and forth in bed, clutching his bedspread. States, "I can't handle all this stress. It is killing me." When asked, he reports multiple life stressors, including financial concerns, problems at work and the recent death of his father. Wife is visiting and states that client's anxiety level is unusual. Physician notified. Advocated for social work referral.—M. Shere, LPN

Chapter 7

NCLEX-PN® ANSWERS

1. (3) Research into the etiology of schizophrenia indicates that there is a change in the anatomy and physiology of the brain itself. Because of the stigma of mental disorders, family members often want to blame drug use or other specific events for the illness. Parental relationships, abuse, or illicit drug use may contribute to the symptoms but do not cause the disease.

2. (1) Neurotransmitters are chemicals that conduct impulses from one neuron to the next through the synapse. They do not nourish the neurons but are nourished themselves by one's food intake. They follow the nerve pathways that have already been created. They do not manufacture enzymes.

3. (3) The MRI requires that a client be confined in a closed tube during the test. Although tranquilizers, quiet music, and constant reassurances from staff may be used, this can still be a devastating experience for someone with claustrophobia (fear of closed places). PET, SPECT, and CT scans do not require the same degree of a closed space.

4. (2) There is a definite genetic component to schizophrenia and research has shown there is a higher risk to identical twins of schizophrenic clients than for others in the family. Risks would certainly be greater than for the general public. It would certainly be an issue of concern to someone who is an identical twin.

5. (2) Melatonin is released in response to darkness. In the winter months, when there is more darkness, melatonin may be produced in excessive amounts, which can lead to depression. Cortisol is not affected by darkness and thus is not a cause of seasonal affective disorder.

6. (3) Serotonin, norepinephrine, and dopamine are all decreased in depression. These are the mood neurotransmitters. Antidepressants increase the availability of one or more of these to improve the client's mood and lessen the depression. They do not change any of the brain anatomy, increase the utilization of glucose by the brain, or alter one's genetics.

7. (1) A CT scan utilizes both X-rays and the computer to produce images of the brain as if it were in slices, so that abnormalities, tumors, and so on might be detected. The other choices describe the techniques of the MRI, PET, and SPECT tools.

8. (2) A deficiency in certain neurotransmitters produces the symptoms presented in most types of clinical depression. There is no structural defect. Giving the mother platitudes does not help her to understand the disease.

9. (3) Psychotropic medications are just a part of the treatment regimen for mental disorders. They are usually not effective alone but require that the client receives other treatments, such as counseling, as well. Often the medication makes the client more accepting of other therapies; thus, they are more effective. They do not cure the mental disorder. They may have serious side effects, especially the older medications.

10. (1, 2, 4, 5) Nursing responsibilities during the stabilization phase include all of these except an ongoing review of the client's medical history. This would be a part of the admission process but not an ongoing role in the initial administration of the client's psychotropic medications.

CARE PLAN HINTS

1. Mr. Sanchez is embarrassed because of the stigma against having mental illness.

2. Yes. The consequences of not taking this medication can be life threatening. Most psychiatric medications have side effects that the client must endure to achieve the desired effects. This is a common reason for noncompliance. Research is being conducted to develop drugs with fewer side effects.

3. Probably. This client did not learn about his medication because he was not ready or able to process new information when he was in a manic phase. Medication teaching must often be reinforced.

CRITICAL THINKING CARE MAP

Subjective data   Client asks, "Do I have to take this medication because I am crazy?" Client states, "I hope I will feel less depressed by the time I go home." Client states, "I will be able to quit taking this medication in a few weeks when I feel better."

Objective data   Client is unable to state the potential side effects of fluoxetine. Client is unable to state the target effects of fluoxetine.

Report   No

Interventions   Teach client that depression is a biological illness caused by low levels of neurotransmitters in the brain. Teach client that the target effects of fluoxetine are more energy, improved mood, and improved mental concentration. Teach client that the side effects of fluoxetine are dry mouth, constipation, and increased heart rate. The drug may cause some people to feel anxious. Schedule fluoxetine (Prozac) for every AM, because it can make clients anxious and may affect sleep if taken at bedtime. Instruct client to take fluoxetine in the morning at home. Teach client that the medication may take several weeks to be effective. Instruct client that she should continue taking the medication even when she feels better. Ask the client if she has any questions.

Documentation   10/19/07 1000 Client unable to state target effects or side effects of fluoxetine. Medication teaching reinforced, including actions, side effects, expected onset, and recommendation to take in AM at home. Client states understanding of above information.—Kathy Caton, LPN

Chapter 8

NCLEX-PN® ANSWERS

1. (4) This is a delusion, as it is a fixed idea that is disconnected from any reality. It does not involve a disruption in any of the senses such as a hallucination might do. It does not involve a new word, and there is no event connected to it that a client could misinterpret personally.

2. (1) Flat affect and little speech are the only symptoms here that are negative. Rigid posture, excessive purposeless movements, and inappropriate laughter are all disorganized symptoms.

3. (3) The older antipsychotic medications are more effective in treating the positive symptoms of schizophre-

nia such as hallucinations, delusions, and disorganized thoughts. Anhedonia, flat affect, alogia, and avolition are all negative symptoms. The newer atypical antipsychotics are effective for both negative and positive symptoms.

4. (1) Zyprexa is an atypical antipsychotic. It takes at least 3 weeks to begin to show an effect. It may help the client sleep better or have less anxiety because it is relieving her schizophrenic symptoms, but this is not the purpose of the medication.

5. (3) The nurse's best response would be to encourage the client to discuss her feelings of insecurity. The nurse needs to validate that the client does not feel safe and then have her describe those feelings. Trying to logically explain why the grandmother cannot be there or to gloss over the delusion blocks therapeutic communication. The last statement is reassuring but does not give the client the opportunity to discuss her fear and its source.

6. (2) In milieu therapy, structure by staff is necessary to provide security for clients. The environment needs to be kept simple and safe with minimal stimulation. Clients need to know the staff is in charge and has set limits for them.

7. (2) The client described here is showing an escalation of behavior that could easily erupt into violence and should be watched closely. Intervening before behavior progressed to violence would be appropriate. Other choices are not predictors of upcoming violence.

8. (3) The nurse should never touch or attempt to touch a potentially violent client. Touch can easily be misinterpreted as a threat or as a sexual overture. Try to deescalate the situation with the least invasive means possible. Isolation and restraint should be the last resort.

9. (3) Orthostatic hypotension is a common side effect of the antipsychotic medications; thus, the client should change positions slowly to avoid dizziness and possible falls. The client on these drugs needs to watch fat and calorie intake. Antacids will prolong absorption. Photosensitivity is often a side effect of these drugs, so prolonged exposure to the sun is not recommended.

10. (2, 3, 4) The main focus of psychosocial rehabilitation is to prepare the client for successful reentry into the community. To do so, emphasis is placed on occupational and interpersonal skills.

CARE PLAN HINTS

1. The client could have died from neuroleptic malignant syndrome, which can also cause damage to the kidneys.

2. Almost all the antipsychotics can cause NMS, although the disorder is rare. The newer atypical antipsychotics are less likely to cause it.

3. The symptoms of schizophrenia are likely to recur. The most likely symptoms to recur are psychosis (positive symptoms). The fluphenazine probably did not control any negative symptoms.

CRITICAL THINKING CARE MAP

Subjective data   Client states, "I don't need the medication. I am fine. The doctor is the one who is crazy." Client states, "I'll use this log to fight off the attackers!"

Objective data   History of suicide attempt at age 18. Weight loss of 15 pounds since last hospitalization 9 months ago. Client is dirty and has strong body odor. Client takes the blanket off his bed, rolls it into a log shape and swings it around.

Report   Yes, to charge nurse.

Interventions   Tell the client, "You are safe here in the hospital." Maintain a low-stimulation environment. Tell the client, "This medication will help to straighten out your thoughts. I think you should take it." Communicate simply and calmly with the client. Say, "There are no attackers here." Encourage the client to take a shower.

Documentation   Client is fearful and having delusional thinking. Reluctant to take his medication. Reassured him that he is safe and encouraged him to take his medication to clear up his thought process. Client rolled blanket and swung it around stating, "I will fight off the attackers." Charge nurse notified of this aggressive behavior.—N. Freud, LPN

Chapter 9

NCLEX-PN® ANSWERS

1. (3) The client has a combination of factors that put her at risk for another episode of depression. She has had a previous depressive episode, is female, and has a history of a suicide attempt. With a new baby, she would be experiencing another stressful episode in her life and would be more susceptible to postpartum depression. She should seek professional counseling before deciding to become pregnant. The other answers do not take into consideration the risk factors for developing postpartum depression.

2. (2) By stating that being a new mother is stressful, the nurse has validated the client's feelings. The second part of the statement encourages the client to discuss her feelings with the nurse and gives the nurse the opportunity to explore coping strategies with the client. Because of the high risk for self-injury or infant injury, it would be imperative for the nurse to share the client's thoughts and behavior with other healthcare providers. The other statements minimize or negate the client's feelings.

3. (1) Light therapy is the treatment of choice for SAD. It is the loss of light that seems to precipitate the symptoms. The other treatments mentioned have been unsuccessful in treating this disorder.

4. (4) Anhedonia is the medical term for the inability to experience pleasure and is a common symptom of depression. The other symptoms mentioned are not included in the definition of anhedonia.

5. (3) Clients tend to be quiet about their feelings of depression, so that the physician is unaware of their psychological state. The most common reason for this is the stigma society has placed on mental illness. It is often viewed as a weakness on the part of the depressed person. Physicians could recognize and treat the condition if the client were totally honest during clinic visits. Most physicians are holistic practitioners and do value the psychological health of their clients.

6. (2) The depression may be severe when the client finally requests assistance in dealing with the condition. It will take 2 to 6 weeks for the maximum effect of the medication to be achieved. As nurses, we need to be aware that a client may be at high risk for self-injury during the first couple of weeks of antidepressant therapy, as the client regains some of the energy necessary to make and carry out suicidal plans. The other answers give unrealistic time frames for a therapeutic effect to be reached.

7. (1) ECT has been used for a number of years, but the procedure has been altered and perfected from the early days of its use. It still commonly causes temporary memory loss and mild confusion but is successful in those clients who have not responded to other forms of treatment. It is used only when other first-line treatments have been unsuccessful. Except in rare cases, the memory loss is not permanent.

8. (4) Clients who are in the manic state do enjoy the feelings of high energy and euphoria that they experience in this state. They do not want to lose the "high" by complying with a medication regime. This feeling of being "high" supersedes all other reasons for noncompliance.

9. (4) Clients in the manic state do not respond well to excessive environmental stimuli. The nurse should remove the client from the stimulation by taking him outside as the first line of intervention. Walking with him allows

him to continue his movement and prevents him from attracting negative comments from others at the party. As the nurse walks with the client, s/he should slow the pace down gradually. Talking calmly and softly to the client will assist him with deescalation of the manic behavior. Letting him continue to pace and eat at the party will not defuse his behavior and may result in an altercation with others. Medicating and restraining him are interventions to be used if redirecting his behavior is unsuccessful.

10. (1, 3, 5) These interventions are appropriate when a client is admitted with already identified suicidal ideations. The nurse's primary focus would be to protect the client from self-injury. Asking him to clarify his suicidal thoughts should be part of the initial assessment. Removing items that could be used for self-injury is imperative. The nurse should initiate a no self-harm contract. Although this is not binding for the client, it gives him a feeling of control over his behavior. At no time should the nurse tell a suicidal client that his suicidal thoughts and plans will remain confidential. The entire healthcare team should be aware of any such behaviors. Giving the client privacy on admission makes him feel unsupervised and perhaps unsafe while giving him an opportunity to carry out his plans.

CARE PLAN HINTS

1. Outcome was met. Making choices is giving her control.
2. The outcome was only partially met, probably because it was unrealistic. It might be broken down into smaller goals and given more time. Focusing on one area of self-care needs at a time might be more successful. For example, work on self-feeding until she has accomplished as much as she can with this task, then begin to work on bathing, etc.
3. Having some of Kevin's time, some of other residents' time, and some of family's time means that the client is getting more types of contacts and is less likely to be disappointed if one is not available.

CRITICAL THINKING CARE MAP

Subjective data Client states, "My hands won't stop shaking." Client states, "Would you please read the menu to me? I can't see very well."

Objective data Pulse 108, irregular. When the physical therapist was teaching him to use crutches, the client was too weak to bear his own body weight on his unaffected leg. Refused dinner last evening and breakfast today.

Report Yes, to physician.

Interventions Look in the client's chart to find his baseline vital signs. Hold the lithium dose that is due now. Call the physician to report the presence of symptoms of lithium toxicity.

Documentation 03/08/07 0900 AP 108, irregular. Client has hand tremors, anorexia (refused dinner and breakfast), blurred vision and weakness (unable to bear weight on unaffected left leg). Dr. J. Joy called re: symptoms of lithium toxicity. Orders received to hold lithium, offer PO fluids, and draw serum Li level STAT.—C. Caraher, LPN

Chapter 10

NCLEX-PN® ANSWERS

1. (2) The client with a Paranoid Personality Disorder is suspicious of others. S/he has more confidence in a nurse who shows self-confidence and treats the client in a direct, matter-of-fact way. Other approach choices here would be more likely to enhance the client's suspiciousness rather than allay it.

2. (1) The client with a Schizoid Personality Disorder typically avoids relationships even with caregivers. Not having visitors or receiving phone calls would validate the lack of social relationships. A flat affect is common. The client is not lonely, as he prefers to be alone. Depression and shame would be highly unusual with the client with this personality disorder.

3. (3) As a client with Schizotypal Personality Disorder, she would prefer to be alone because of severe social anxiety. The stress of being made to interact with other residents could precipitate delusional thinking or perceptual alterations. Inviting her to one meal a day should be nonthreatening. Allow her to move at her own pace and praise her when she is able to comply.

4. (4) Clients with Antisocial Personality Disorder are often very charming and manipulative. They can wreak havoc on a unit by causing disagreements among staff members concerning the special treatment the clients feel they deserve. Staff members need to be consistent in care and in all unit rules. Unit rules should never be compromised to favor a specific client. Refusing to let him go out at all will increase the antisocial behavior and further disrupt the unit environment.

5. (2) Although some of the other choices might be appropriate, your first *priority* would be to prevent self-injury. A common response to stress for clients with Borderline Personality Disorder is to cut or burn themselves.

6. (4) This client is demonstrating classic symptoms of Histrionic Personality Disorder. She directs all attention to herself. She feels that her problems are more important than anyone else's, and everyone present in the group should be interested in assisting her in managing her life. The client with a Schizotypal Personality Disorder would not be open in a group such as this due to severe social anxiety. The client with Borderline Personality Disorder has an unstable self-image and would not be portraying herself as being more important than others. The client with an Avoidant Personality Disorder shows evidence of inadequacy and does not readily join in social activities such as this one for fear of being embarrassed.

7. (1) The client is demonstrating the thought distortions that are common with Narcissistic Personality Disorder. The nurse may briefly empathize with his stress, but must consistently lay down the limits with what is appropriate and what is not. The nurse must maintain a professional, no-nonsense approach and not respond to him in the same tones and with the same attitude he is using. Lying to a client and responding to him in a derogatory manner are not appropriate. Asking him how he can be made happier puts power into his hands, as he will see the nurse as weak and able to be manipulated; expectations and limits are blurred.

8. (2) Persons with this personality disorder often feel inadequate and have low self-esteem. This client might be more comfortable beginning therapy in her room rather than in front of other people. If this is possible and acceptable in the facility, this would be a nonthreatening way to begin. Praise her for any successes. Forcing her to go, giving glib or false assurances, or giving her permission to avoid compliance would not be acceptable.

9. (1) The obsessive-compulsive behavior seen in persons with this personality disorder is the result of anxiety. Although the client may also experience a disruption in sleep, the anxiolytic may help relieve those symptoms as well. Depression and psychotic ideation do not often accompany Obsessive-Compulsive Personality Disorder.

10. (1, 3, 5) When working with a client with Dependent Personality Disorder, the nurse should provide as many experiences as possible where the client can successfully make decisions and participate in care without forcing the issue. Give the client choices to make regarding care, such as the time s/he would like a bath. If asked what the nurse would do in a particular situation, refer the question back to the client, "Let's look at your options." Then have the client list those. Guide the client through the choices until s/he makes a decision. Participating in a support group is a helpful therapy for clients with this disorder if the client has not already been a part of a group. The nurse can refer the client to Social Services or the physician for that recommendation. Clients with this disorder are not prone to self-injury and do not require supervision for attempts. Including family members in decision making (unless the client absolutely cannot make a decision regarding posthospital care) only reinforces the client's dependency.

CARE PLAN HINTS

1. Although listening to music is an adaptive coping method and may help Brenda in the short term, it will not solve her coping problem. She has ineffective coping because of her personality disorder, which takes years and much motivation to change.

2. The nurse can suggest therapy to Brenda or can suggest a therapy referral to her physician, but nobody can force the client to go to therapy, even when it is a good idea.

3. It is best for Brenda to learn that angry outbursts do not achieve the desired outcome. The nurse should say, calmly and respectfully, that she will continue to be Brenda's nurse and will give her the medication as the doctor has ordered.

CRITICAL THINKING CARE MAP

Subjective data   Client states, "Yes, whatever you say." When asked if she needs pain medication, she states, "No, I don't want to bother you." When asked if she needs anything, she states, "I don't know." Client asks nurse, "What do you think I should do?"

Objective data   BP 158/90, P110, R24. Grimaces and sweats when ambulating or moving in bed. Awake on all 2-hour checks during the night.

Interventions   Ask the client, "Are you in pain?" Tell the client, "Most people have a lot of pain after surgery. You have signs of pain; does your incision hurt?" Tell the client, "It is no trouble to give you some pain medication. I will be glad to get some if you need it." Say to the client, "Sometimes people don't like to ask for help. While you are in the hospital, we want to help you, so please tell us what you need." Help the client practice identifying her needs. Encourage the client to take the ordered pain med. Include offering pain med regularly (every 4 hours) in the plan of care. Visit the client hourly to determine whether she needs help. Discuss outpatient referral for therapy with treatment team.

Report   Yes, to charge nurse.

Documentation   Client has signs of pain (elevated BP, P, R, grimacing with movement, sleeplessness) but is not asking for pain med. Will offer pain med. every 4 hours and encourage her to take it if indicated by noted pain behaviors. Will assist client in identifying any other needs.—Monica Arte, LPN

Chapter 11

NCLEX-PN® ANSWERS

1. (2) This is a response to a specific situation and may not be an anxiety disorder. Validate his feelings, then assess for the source of his anxiety. Does he need more information about the process? Does he fear the results? Is he concerned about being in a small, closed space? The other choices do not give the nurse the opportunity to address the root of the client's fears.

2. (4) A patient is rarely admitted for Generalized Anxiety Disorder unless the condition is severe or near panic. Therefore, she will have a difficult time focusing on what you are saying. Encourage her to discuss "where" she is at this point in time. Touching may be threatening, and you need to facilitate a trusting relationship with the patient so she will open up to you. Calling her family to come in might reinforce her fear that she is dying.

3. (3) It is possible that a person will have an isolated panic attack without developing panic disorder. You cannot assure a client that this is definite but a possibility. S/he will worry about it, and that concern should be validated.

4. (2) This phobia concerns open spaces and is often associated with Obsessive-Compulsive Disorder.

5. (2) Counting is often a ritual demonstrated by the person with Obsessive-Compulsive Disorder. It is not a component of the other disorders mentioned.

6. (1) The nursing student is reliving the trauma of seeing her mother die suddenly in this room. The room number has triggered the remembrance of this event for her. It is common that such episodes occur within 3 months of the actual event. None of the other choices are applicable. A panic attack may not have a trigger. A phobic attack will be triggered by a common phobia, which is not the case here. Because of its isolated occurrence, acute stress disorder is not a possibility either.

7. (3) The patient should be encouraged to recognize previous responses to anxiety-producing situations and objects. The goal here is for the patient to view the situation realistically and replace negative self-talk with positive thoughts that are supportive and calming. Avoiding the situation does not precipitate restructuring nor does focusing on the negative thoughts. Acceptance will not support the client in developing a more positive response but will cause him/her to also accept the status quo.

8. (3) Because these drugs are usually CNS depressants, the patient may develop tolerance quickly; therefore, they have a high abuse potential. Patients need to be assessed accurately to ensure that medications are appropriate and will not be used as a substitute for more adaptive problem-solving techniques. Suicidal ideation and depression are not common side effects of the anxiolytic drugs. Blood sugars are generally not affected.

9. (1) Persons dealing with anxiety disorders often need guidance in developing effective coping mechanisms that are right for them. Leaving them alone does not often work. Relaxation and deep breathing responses are effective for many different anxiety-producing events. It is not often effective for a client to be given reading material, as the nurse takes the chance that it will not be read or read and not understood. The client does not need to hear coping strategies, as it is an individual response.

10. (2, 3, 5) Persons in an anxious state often demonstrate the same responses one would find with any sympathetic nervous system stimulation. Thus, cool skin, increased heart rate, and piloerection, or "goose bumps," might be found. Contrary to the other choices, the pupils would appear dilated and the blood pressure would be increased.

CARE PLAN HINTS

1. A steady dosage schedule ensures that Mrs. M. will experience a steady analgesic effect. Her pain will not be allowed to rise to an intolerable and anxiety-producing level. Regular inquiring about her pain level reassures her that the nurses care and that they are monitoring her condition.

2. The stress of being in the hospital in unfamiliar surroundings and in pain has aggravated Mrs. M.'s anxiety. Providing staff who are increasingly familiar is a simple way to create an environment that feels safer.

3. Mrs. M.'s cognitive impairment (mild dementia) may have made it impossible for her to learn to do the self-relaxation exercises independently. This outcome was partially met. It was not a completely realistic goal for Mrs. M.

CRITICAL THINKING CARE MAP

Subjective data Client asks, "Am I going to die from this?" Client states, "I think my incision is going to tear open." Client complains of feeling dizzy. Nurse stated in report: Client slept approximately 3 hours last night.

Objective data   VS: T 99°, P108, R32, BP130/86. Skin is cool, diaphoretic. Client's hands are constantly moving, picking at the sheets. Oral membranes are dry. Eyes are glancing around the room, darting from one thing to another.

Interventions   Encourage the Client to talk about her feelings. Accept the client as she is. Acknowledge that client is anxious. Keep communication simple and concrete. Provide comfort measures. Be calm and confident with the client. Discuss healthy ways to talk about and relieve anxiety. Assess coping skills client has used successfully in past. Assess client's resources for support. Use progressive relaxation to assist client in relaxing.

Report   Yes, to physician.

Documentation   05/13/07 Client is demonstrating anxious behavior, e.g., asks if she is dying, c/o dizziness, hands constantly moving, picking at her sheets. Skin cool, diaphoretic; mucous membranes dry. P, R, BP elevated. Provided comfort measures, discussed client's feelings and coping techniques. Client participated in progressive relaxation exercise, responding with decreased anxiety as evidenced by vital signs within normal limits and quiet hands. Reported severe anxiety to physician.—Emma Charles, LPN

Chapter 12

NCLEX-PN® ANSWERS

1. (1) Clients who are tolerant to alcohol will have cross-tolerance to other CNS depressants. He will probably require a larger dose of narcotics to control his pain. He may seem manipulative, but the physical need for more narcotics is real. If he is in alcohol withdrawal, he might be uncooperative, but the scenario does not give this information. Do not read anything into a question that is not there. Pain assessment and pain control are two important aspects of nursing care. Do not withhold pain medications.

2. (3) Alcoholic encephalopathy is caused by a deficiency in vitamin B_1, which can be treated or prevented with a thiamine injection. Demerol (meperidine) is a narcotic pain medication; Valium (diazepam) might be used in alcohol withdrawal to treat the anxiety or prevent seizures but will not treat alcoholic encephalopathy; Dilantin (phenytoin) is an anticonvulsant and might be used but not for the vitamin deficiency.

3. (1) One of the cardinal characteristics of clients with schizophrenia is that they have difficulty relating to others. In the case of this dual diagnosis having this disorder makes it more difficult for this client to relate to other people to get help to quit drinking. This fact alone will make it difficult for the client to seek or benefit from treatment. Even being able to talk to the client about alcoholism will be a challenge for the nurse; he might understand if he is willing to listen.

4. (2) Alcohol when taken with antianxiety drugs causes added CNS depression, which can be life threatening. In most cases, it is unnecessary to take the drug every 4 hours; it is a p.r.n. medication. Antianxiety medications usually produce drowsiness when a client first begins the drug, so driving is not recommended. However, after the client has adjusted to the drug, driving might be permitted.

5. (4) The nursing supervisor must be notified when a nurse may be too impaired to protect the client and also the nurse him- or herself. This may be the impetus s/he needs to seek help. Confronting the nurse in your role as a peer might have no influence. Although the charge nurse might be included in the loop, it is the supervisor who has the most authority here.

6. (2) Some clients do not think of other alternatives to substance use for coping with stress or problems. A client may begin new problem-solving or coping behavior by making a list of healthy alternatives to drinking alcohol. Explaining signs and symptoms of alcohol withdrawal and teaching about his medications will not help the client change coping behavior. You cannot teach a client not to drink.

7. (2) The client who is abusing methamphetamines will most likely develop skin lesions from picking at the face or from an outbreak of acne. Depression, weight gain, and incontinence are not symptoms of methamphetamine use, rather euphoria, weight loss, and urinary retention might be observed in this client.

8. (4) Discussing the circumstances that lead her or him to drink suggests the meaning of alcohol for this client. If the client is in denial, s/he might not admit to being an alcoholic or will minimize the incidence of substance abuse. S/he might not recognize the behavior exhibited while under the influence.

9. (3) Cirrhosis causes esophageal varices (varicose veins of the esophagus), which can rupture and hemorrhage. In addition, the client is more at risk for stomach ulcers, which could also bleed. The client is not likely to develop pneumonia, encephalitis, and CHF related to his liver failure.

10. (2, 4, 5) The client is most likely to demonstrate irritability, elevated vital signs, and confusion. Depressed affect and hypotension would not be part of the clinical picture.

CARE PLAN HINTS

1. He will be at risk for relapse when someone offers him a drink, when he feels lonely, and when he has problems he does not know how to solve. He will also be at risk if he stops taking his antipsychotic medication.

2. He used alcohol for recreation and for coping with his problems.

3. He will have more difficulty working in a group such as AA to maintain sobriety because of reduced social skills. He probably has difficulty looking to the future and lives in the moment. Because of this, when he feels like drinking, he may not be able to think about the longer-term consequences. If it solves his problems in the moment, he may continue drinking.

CRITICAL THINKING CARE MAP

Subjective data   Client states, "Drinking helps me forget my problems"; states, "What else can I do besides drink? It is all I know anymore"; states, "I can quit when I want. I just don't want to quit"; states, "Maybe I should go home today. I can take care of myself."

Objective data   None pertinent to the diagnosis.

Report   Yes, because of the need for referral to social service on discharge.

Interventions   Discuss the consequences of the client's drinking when he is able. Help him develop a list of his resources for help. Help him develop a list of healthier things he could do when he feels like drinking, to prevent relapse. Encourage the client to spend time in the unit's living room where he can be with other people. Ask why he wants to go home. Spend time with the client each shift—talk with him or sit beside him. Encourage the client to take his antidepressant medication.

Documentation   7/17/07 The client is making statements about drinking as his only choice to solve his problems. Will work with him on new coping strategies. Will encourage him to take his antidepressant to help with thought processes and problem solving ability.—M. Wood, LPN

Chapter 13

NCLEX-PN® ANSWERS

1. (1) Dyslexia has all of these characteristics. Mathematics Disorder relates to math ability. Disorder of Written Expression relates to writing skills. Developmental Coordination Disorder is related to motor coordination.

2. (3) The child with dyslexia will have difficulty with any materials that require him to read. Diagrams and lists may be misinterpreted. The best teaching techniques will involve discussions, demonstrations, and verbal explanations.

3. (4) Expressive Language Disorder improves dramatically with age. It would be rare that it would remain the same or worsen.

4. (1) There is thought to be a genetic component to stuttering. Although females may also stutter, it is more common in males.

5. (3) Autistic children often relate better to objects than to people. Insisting that the child conform to standards for other children of her age would serve to increase her stress and decrease cooperation with staff. As long as no harm can come to the child as a result of the ritual, it should be allowed. Autistic children do not respond well to touching, and staff time in the room should be minimized.

6. (2) The child is following the regression seen in Rett's Syndrome. This disorder is seen only in females and occurs before the age of 4. The child will demonstrate normal functioning until the onset of the disorder.

7. (3) Insomnia is one of the most common side effects of the stimulant medications given for ADHD. Therefore, it should be given no later than 6 hours before bedtime and should be given with food. If drug holidays are recommended while the child is on the medication, they should be taken during school vacations and not on short weekends.

8. (2) Prevention of the anxious behavior or at least minimizing its effect would be a good approach. To do this, development of a trusting nurse-client relationship would be imperative. Setting limits on parental visitation would probably be anxiety-inducing. Ignoring the anxiety would also cause it to escalate. This client would probably be a good candidate for a mental health consult, and the nurse should advocate for one.

9. (1) This client is a high suicide risk. She has been the victim of abuse and has shown self-destructive behavior in the form of promiscuity. If she sees no way out of her current situation, to her, the next step would be to kill herself. The first thing the nurse should do is assess whether or not the client has a plan for suicide. Although her mother should be informed of the abuse and the father arrested, this is not the highest priority at this time. Giving false reassurances is never appropriate in caregiving.

10. (4) Children are more apt to act out any emotional problems they are having than to discuss them. Observing the child at play or having him draw pictures will probably tell you more about his mental health. Although you should always listen to the parents' assessment, you should

observe things on your own as well. Consider Erikson's developmental stages to see if the child is on track with his/her development, but that is not the first and best way to assess for mental health problems.

CARE PLAN HINTS

1. Mohammed's incorrect inhaler use put him in a position where his asthma attacks were not being prevented, but only treated as an emergency when they occurred. With correct use of medications he might have avoided the need for all these ED visits.

2. On this hospital visit the nurse used a teaching approach that was planned with the client's learning style in mind.

3. Besides his obvious ADHD, the child is also sick in the ED recovering from an asthma attack. He is probably tired also. As is often true in the hospital, this was not the ideal teaching situation, yet the nurse was able to probably improve the health care of this child.

CRITICAL THINKING CARE MAP

Subjective data   Client states, "I was just trying to do a good job on the school project." Client's mother states, "I'm afraid he's becoming a drug addict. This isn't the first time he has done this." Client states, "I feel up on some days and down on other days." Client states, "Everybody is always telling me what to do." Client's mother states, "I let him be responsible for taking his medications, but I wonder if I should take back the responsibility. He is not taking them safely." Client states, "I want to be in charge of myself."

Objective data   Physician's order: Ritalin 20 mg twice a day, PO

Report   Yes, to charge nurse and physician.

Interventions   Assess the client's knowledge about his medication, desired effects, side effects, and dosing schedule. Teach him what he does not know about his medication regimen (treatment plan). Reinforce teaching about the safe administration of Ritalin with the client and his mother. Explain that this client is not a drug addict. Let the family decide who takes responsibility for giving the medication. Tell the client that his injury (not taking the med., going on the roof impulsively, and then falling) is likely a result of not taking his medication as prescribed. Tell the client that he is responsible for his own behavior. Ask the client and his mother if they have any questions.

Documentation   8/20/07 1100 Discussed medication compliance with client and mother. Answered their questions about the effects of the med. and dosing schedule. They were receptive to planning to take the med. safely. They are deciding who will be responsible for giving his Ritalin at home—Brandon Samson, LPN

Chapter 14

NCLEX-PN® ANSWERS

1. (3) Persons with eating disorders are most likely to have bradycardia, hypotension, and dry, cracking skin. The other signs and symptoms choices are basically the opposite of what you might see in eating disorders.

2. (3) The daughter most likely is suffering from the restricting type of Anorexia Nervosa. It sounds as if the behavior is in its early stages and would be the appropriate time to begin interventions. It is not a normal phase of adolescence and does require attention. Waiting longer will allow the pattern of maladaptive behavior to become more ingrained and more difficult to treat. Laxative abuse and purging could occur later if the condition were allowed to continue.

3. (4) An individual with Anorexia Nervosa sees weight loss as a successful result of her ability to maintain control over her body. She is usually in denial over medical complications that can occur from the malnourished state that might result. There is no fear of death and no concern for her overall physical health. All that matters is losing weight.

4. (1) The Borderline Personality Disorder is more common with these eating disorders. This personality disorder presents as self-destructive behaviors. Individuals with the disorder are generally impulsive and manipulative. Chronic anxiety is common. Narcissistic and histrionic personality disorders are rarely found in eating disorders. Having passive-aggressive tendencies is not part of the disease either.

5. (2) Although all of these behaviors might be present in the client with Anorexia Nervosa and need to be addressed at some point, the expression of suicidal thoughts needs to be confronted first. Clients with eating disorders not only talk about suicide but also may act on their self-destructive thoughts. The nurse needs to be aware of this risk and protect the client from harm.

6. (2) By the time that an eating disorder has reached the point where the client must be hospitalized, it has become a consistent, maladaptive response to stress and anxiety. A habit that has become so ingrained will take a long time to unlearn. Learning healthy responses will

then take an equally long time to become part of the individual's behavior pattern. It does not benefit the family to give false hope of a quick recovery.

7. (1) Zyprexa, an antipsychotic drug, has been the one that effectively treats the body-image distortion associated with Anorexia Nervosa. It also helps the individual to gain weight. Prozac and Elavil are both antidepressants and may help with any depression associated with the disorder but are not effective on a long-term basis. The same could be true of Ativan, which is an antianxiety drug. It should be noted that drugs alone are not the answer in this disorder, and other therapies must accompany the use of medications.

8. (2) Using the calculations for figuring BMI, this individual has a BMI of 34.4, which puts this person in the obese range. Any BMI over 30 indicates the person is at risk for the complications of obesity. The formula calls for multiplying the weight in pounds by 705 and then dividing twice by the height in inches.

9. (4) By eating nutritious foods themselves, the parents are serving as healthy role models for children. Posting a photo on the refrigerator serves to focus the child in on the importance of a perfect body. This encourages the avoidance of food and weight loss as a means of becoming one of the "beautiful" people. On the other hand, insistence upon a clean plate makes the child see eating as a way to gain parental approval and love. Rewarding a child with food is a habit that can continue into adolescence where a person seeks food as a comfort measure.

10. (1, 2, 3, 5) Impaired liver function (indicated by abnormal liver enzyme lab studies), amenorrhea (absence of menstruation), constipation, and hypothermia (low body temperature) are all medical complications of Anorexia Nervosa. Renal impairment is not a medical complication of this eating disorder.

CARE PLAN HINTS

1. No. The aunt's name is mentioned, but she is not really involved. The problem is Katie's mechanism for coping with life stressors.

2. Whether Katie or her mother is right or wrong, in the nurse's opinion, is not important. Katie needs to change her behavior because she wants to be healthy, not to please the nurse.

3. They can truly understand her feelings and provide her with coping suggestions that come from personal experiences.

CRITICAL CARE THINKING MAP

Subjective data   Client states that she eats when she feels nervous. Client states that she frequently overeats in the evenings. Friends bring candy to hospital for client. Client asks, "Is there a pill that will make me lose weight?"

Objective data   5'5" tall, 190 lbs

Report   Yes, to physician who will follow up her outpatient care.

Interventions   Discuss with the client her reasons for wanting to lose weight. Work with dietitian to determine realistic goals and to plan an eating program based on the food guide pyramid. Teach the client about the relationship between dietary intake, calorie burning by exercise and metabolism, and weight. Encourage client to accept herself as a person, just as she is, and to lose weight for her health and well-being. Discuss strategies for dealing with feelings in other ways than overeating. Discuss cues for eating that are not related to hunger. Encourage increasing physical activity at the client's ability level. Set realistic goals for weight loss, including a discussion of the expected increases and decreases of weight due to hormonal changes and dietary and physical fluctuations. Encourage adequate fluid intake. Discuss the use of food as a comfort measure.

Documentation   08/20/07 Client expresses interest in weight loss. BMI is 31.7 Strategies for behavior change discussed. Will ask dietitian and physician to participate.—D. King, LPN

Chapter 15

NCLEX-PN® ANSWERS

1. (1) Your first action would be to notify the physician as soon as possible. Your second action would be to take vital signs on your client and assess for a source for the confusion, including the time of the last pain medication and recent lab results such as an elevated BUN. You would not withhold the pain medication, as the pain could be the source of the confusion. Sending a urine specimen to the lab requires a physician's order.

2. (4) Delirium is unpredictable and differs with each client. It is impossible to tell the client's family how long the confusion will last. Some cases clear up in days and some take weeks and months.

3. (3) The symptoms of delirium do fluctuate. This is one of the cardinal differences between delirium and

dementia. Both disorders have impaired memory problems and possible aphasia. Dementia develops gradually, and delirium develops suddenly.

4. (2) The best technique to protect your clients is to encourage a family member to stay in the room. Psychotropic medications and physical restraints often make the client more agitated and confused. Leaving the side rail down with no one in attendance would be a poor choice in this situation and may be against your facility's policy.

5. (1) Agnosia is a failure to recognize a familiar common object causing the client to misuse the object. Aphasia would indicate a problem with language. Apraxia is an impaired ability to perform a motor activity. Disturbance of executive function indicates an inability to use abstract thinking.

6. (3) Having a parent or sibling with AD is a definite risk, although there is no way of positively predicting the development of the disease. Even genetic testing cannot definitively predict AD. Being female is a possible risk factor.

7. (1) It takes time for the client with delirium or dementia to process what is being said. Therefore, it is critical that you repeat what you have said at least three times, using the exact same words. Changing the words makes the client go back and begin the processing all over. You need to be patient. Threatening the client will increase the client's anxiety and add to the processing time.

8. (3) By acknowledging the client's anxious condition and offering to help look for the lost item, you are validating her feelings and therefore her worth. It would be pointless to try to convince the client that you did not hide anything. Your offering to help her look makes her feel important. Shifting the suspicion on to someone else could be setting the client up for a catastrophic reaction.

9. (4) Let the client bring the doll. If the client with AD wished to do something that will result in no harm to self or others, it should be allowed. Leaving the doll in the room or with someone else might increase the client's anxiety. This could also be a source of refusal for the bath both now and in the future.

10. (3) By asking the client to recall events about her children, you are encouraging the client to return in her mind to a time when her children were small. This allows her to mentally "go home" when physically returning is impossible. Trying to orient the client to your reality would increase anxiety and possibly lead to a catastrophic reaction.

CARE PLAN HINTS

1. Peter feared for Blanche's safety. He was losing sleep and becoming exhausted. He found himself losing patience with her. If Blanche were to remain at home, Peter would have to hire help to assist in her care, especially at night. He would have to provide safety measures within the home to prevent her from getting outside.

2. These nursing diagnoses are high priority, because they relate to the primary human needs that serve as the basis for Maslow's hierarchy of needs (physiological needs, then safety and security needs).

3. Peter would need to know that Blanche would eventually lose all ability to use language and would not be able to express her needs. He would have to learn to manage total incontinence and how to provide all physical care, including feeding, bathing, and dressing her. He would need to be educated on ways to communicate and relate to Blanche and how to recognize caregiver stress in himself. He should be prepared to recognize ways to prevent catastrophic reactions and how to respond to them if they occur. The Alzheimer's Association would be a helpful resource, and he should arrange for respite care and become part of an Alzheimer's support group.

CRITICAL THINKING CARE MAP

Subjective data Wife states that client takes several over-the-counter medications for nasal congestion, GI upset, and occasional headaches. Client states, "I don't know what to do."

Objective data The neurologist prescribed several medications. The internist prescribed several medications. The urologist prescribed several medications. Client had sudden onset of change in mental status. His symptoms are inconsistent; sometimes he is oriented, sometimes not. Client is unable to bathe himself, which he could do before this episode.

Report Yes, to physician.

Interventions Orient client to reality. Make a list of all the medications the client is taking, both prescribed and over the counter. Assist the client with ADLs while he is acutely confused. Place frequently used personal items near the bed within easy reach. Use simple words and sentences. Introduce yourself each time you enter the room. Encourage a family member to stay with the client when possible.

Documentation 07/12/07 Client admitted with sudden onset of acute confusion. Is intermittently oriented to person. Consistently disoriented to time and place. Has prescriptions from three different physicians in addition to dosing himself with OTC meds. All meds listed and given to primary physician. Will assist client with ADLs as needed and provide safe environment. Family encouraged to stay with client when possible. Son at bedside this evening.—Melissa Presley, LPN

Chapter 16

NCLEX-PN® ANSWERS

1. (3) It is obvious from the wife's comments that her understanding of abuse is that it is physical. Until she realizes that abuse may also be emotional or psychological, she will not realize that she and her husband need to seek out help to improve their relationship.

2. (2) Violence is a complex problem related to a multitude of factors. It is not just one thing that causes a perpetrator to use violence as a response to a current life situation.

3. (1) It is important for clients to realize that abuse is no respecter of persons, culture, or socioeconomic levels. It is a problem at all levels. You want to find out why the man suspects his daughter is being abused after reassuring him that even professional people can be perpetrators of abuse.

4. (4) Because of the length of the abusive situation, it is possible that the client's son will be an abuser himself when he grows up. The mother should be aware that she may need to receive help for her child to resolve issues results from witnessing and experiencing abuse, so that the cycle is not repeated.

5. (1) The "honeymoon" phase after an abusive episode is common. What this woman is describing is a common response of the perpetrator when the abuse is a new behavior. Even though the wife may not accept what you are telling her, it is your responsibility to inform her of the odds that this behavior will be repeated. The more the abuse occurs, the fewer periods there will be of remorse and the more violent the behavior will become.

6. (2) All states have laws requiring that you report suspicions of child abuse to the proper authorities. In many cases, this is the child protection unit of the local social services department. The social worker will investigate and, if warranted, will involve the local police. The nurse should notify the supervisor as well, but it is the nurse's responsibility to report the abuse.

7. (3) The other behaviors described here are perfectly normal behaviors or questions for those age groups. For an infant to have recurrent herpes lesions in the mouth would be significant for sexual abuse. This could indicate that a perpetrator who had genital herpes was placing his penis in the child's mouth thereby infecting the infant with a sexually transmitted disease.

8. (4) The observations you have made indicate neglect, which is definitely a form of elder abuse. Most states have laws that would require the nurse to inform the appropriate authorities of the situation. This could be an ombudsman who is usually hired by an area agency on aging. The local social services office may have a division of adult protective services which has a caseworker assigned to only elderly clients. In this case, the report would be made to that social worker for follow-up.

9. (3) Beginning the process of grief resolution would be a good short-term outcome. Resuming usual social relationships and lifestyle would be more of a long-term outcome. The best answer here would be that the client will begin those steps that will allow her to recognize and begin the process for dealing with her grief. Grief is always associated with a loss, and rape certainly causes a sense of loss in the victim. Refusing to discuss it could be a form of denial and would not be beneficial to the grieving process.

10. (1, 3, 5) The nurse must consider his/her own safety during this situation. The nurse should never allow an aggressive or unpredictable client to block the escape route. In the meantime, the nurse would also want to be talking to the client calmly and in a quieter tone of voice than what the client is using to try to deescalate his behavior. The nurse should remain out of the client's personal space and should not walk toward the client but remain toward the side, giving the client concrete suggestions as to what to do. The client may be overwhelmed and need guidance for appropriate behavior. Although medication might be needed later, other means of defusing the aggressive behavior should be tried first.

CARE PLAN HINTS

1. It is challenging for nurses to care objectively for clients when the clients engage in behaviors that the nurse does not condone.

2. The husband is still not proven guilty. However, it can be easier if one nurse cares for the client and another is available to the husband.

3. The nurse is not able to legally initiate a criminal investigation of the husband without the client's consent.

CRITICAL THINKING CARE MAP

Subjective data   Client states, "They are trying to dry me to death." Client states, "I don't know what to do."

Objective data   Client is restless, first moving around in bed, then walking around his room. His fists are clenched. His voice is loud. The client has a history of pushing a caregiver in the group home where he lives. Client is looking around, as if he can see things that are not present in the room.

Report   Yes, to charge nurse (physician already knows).

Interventions   Act calmly and confidently. Talk in a quiet tone. Ask the client if he wants a drink of water. Stand near the door in the client's room. Stand out of the client's reach. Tell the client that the doctor is coming in about 15 minutes to see what she can do to help him. Reassure the client that he is safe in the hospital. Tell the client that you are the nurse, and you are here to help. Ask the client if he needs anything. Tell the client, "I think you should go back to bed until the doctor comes."

Documentation   08/17/07 0900 Client is agitated, talking loudly, fists clenched. Having delusional thinking about demons coming to get him. Physician notified. Will reassure client until physician arrives.—Suma Hegde, LPN

Chapter 17

NCLEX-PN® ANSWERS

1. (2) The most appropriate response would be to acknowledge the client's anxiety, and then encourage him to express his feelings. The first response does not deal with the source of his anxiety and allow the client to vent any concerns. If the anxiety is intense enough, medication may not be successful. Although it would be helpful to know what helps him sleep at home, he does not have the same type of situation at home. The last response minimizes his concerns, so the nurse does not have to deal with them.

2. (1) This client is reaching a severe anxiety state and needs to be protected from an escalating behavior where he could injure himself or others. Although his respiratory status is very important, indications are that this is stable at this point. This is a situation where the nurse needs to deal with the safety and security issues first as long as there are no signs or symptoms of acute respiratory distress. Reassuring that he is not going to die negates his feelings without addressing them. The client in an acute anxiety state should not be left alone. Medication may be appropriate but should not be your first response.

3. (4) A diagnosis of chronic disease can be devastating to any of these clients. However, the 55-year-old single female appears to be lacking a support system and has also witnessed first-hand the devastation of a chronic illness. At 55, she is approaching retirement and may feel a lack of fulfillment in her life anyway. The 25-year-old male has a wife and solid job. The 35-year-old has already demonstrated strong coping skills. The 70-year-old also has a supportive wife and may feel that at 70, chronic illness is to be expected, and he may have the experience to accept the diagnosis without too much stress.

4. (3) The nurse needs to identify ways of coping that have been successful for the client and see if any of these methods would be appropriate for the current situation. Support groups might be appropriate later on but not at this point in time. It is not up to the nurse to advise the client on what should be done. The nurse should provide choices and allow the client to make the decision. To do otherwise only increases his/her sense of powerlessness.

5. (2) The nurse needs to focus and encourage the client to focus on the present. Past and future are not important considerations at this time.

6. (3) The nurse should be at eye level with the client. Sitting indicates that the nurse has time to listen. The pulled curtain indicates a concern for client privacy. Standing indicates that the nurse has little time, and folded arms could give off the message of a closed mind. Moving around the unit communicates to the client that the nurse has other things to do than listen. Interpreting the client's statements does not really give the nurse time to listen to what the client is saying.

7. (1) The first response validates the client's anger. It also gives the client a suggestion as to how to deal with her feelings. This is the most critical element at this time. Although it might help her in the future to discuss her loss with someone who has undergone a similar procedure, now is not the time. The last two responses minimize the anger she is feeling.

8. (2) The goal for anger is that the client will acknowledge his/her feelings and begin to work on constructive problem solving to alleviate the source of the anger. By not showing anger, the client may be hiding the anger and keeping it inside only to manifest itself at a later date. Denying anger does not mean that it is no longer there. Being loud but not violent is still not dealing with the anger issue.

9. (3) Passive-aggressive clients will not state their feelings about ordered therapy. Therefore, the client will agree to go, but then procrastinate until it is too late to participate.

10. (1) Manipulative clients should always be held accountable for their behavior and comments. Rather than allowing

this client to split staff, the client should be encouraged to discuss complaints with the appropriate person. This would be the night supervisor or charge nurse, not the day supervisor. The nurse should never allow the client to flatter one shift or one nurse as opposed to others. Denying a client concern is never appropriate.

CARE PLAN HINTS

1. The American Cancer Society has volunteers who visit clients. Many other agencies that represent clients with life-threatening or difficult-to-manage disorders also have volunteers. Good sources of information about these resources are the phone book and physicians who specialize in the pertinent area. For example, an orthopedic surgeon may know someone who is coping well with an amputation who would visit a client.
2. Spending a lot of time and energy on blaming others for the illness can divert the client from a healthy recovery.
3. A support group includes people who all share a challenging experience. Members can share strategies that have helped them, ask questions about how to solve realistic problems, and share feelings that only affected people understand. See the Community Care Box 17-4 for more information about support groups.

CRITICAL THINKING CARE MAP

Subjective data   Client states, "You are the only person who really understands me"; states, "The other nurses never give me enough pain medicine. They don't seem to care"; states, "Will you do me a favor and give it early just this once?"; states, "I plan to give a dozen roses and $100 to every nurse who takes good care of me." Client told the physician that the nurses are not caring for him. Client told the nurses that the physician does not like him.

Objective data   Client requests pain medication every hour; BP 120/80, T 98.8°F (tympanic), P 80, R 12; responding well to physical therapy, ambulating with a walker; sleeps 8 hours per night in hospital; peripheral pulses palpable and strong, bilaterally.

Report   Yes, to physician and charge nurse.

Interventions   Assess the client's pain. Assign consistent staff to this client. Change his medication schedule from p.r.n. to a regular schedule of Demerol 75 mg IM every 4 hours. Tell the client that he will be given his pain medication on a schedule every 4 hours. He does not need to ask for it. The physician visits daily and can change the dose then if necessary. Offer nondrug pain relief interventions. Encourage the client to express his feelings. Tell the client, "I care about you. I will help you learn how to communicate with us directly. This is a skill you need to develop." Have a staff conference about the client and develop a plan of care that everyone follows consistently. Include the client in planning. If the client complains about staff members, take his concerns seriously and assess each situation objectively. Give the client positive reinforcement when he asks for help assertively, without manipulation.

Documentation   7/22/07 Client requests pain med. every hour. Ambulating without difficulty with walker, sleeping well, VSS. Peripheral pulses palpable and strong. Skin warm, dry. Incision well-approximated. No exudate. Good circulation, movement, and sensation in toes. Many complaints about staff. Offering gifts. Coping by attempting to manipulate staff. Case conference planned this evening.—Florence Wren, LPN

Appendix II

Global Assessment of Functioning (GAF) Scale

Consider psychological, social, and occupational functioning on a hypothetical continuum of mental health-illness. Do not include impairment in functioning due to physical (or environmental) limitations.

Code	(Note: Use intermediate codes when appropriate, e.g., 45, 68, 72.)

100	Superior functioning in a wide range of activities, life's problems never seem to get out of hand, is sought by others because of his or her many positive qualities. No
91	symptoms.
90	Absent or minimal symptoms (e.g., mild anxiety before an exam), good functioning in all areas, interested and involved in a wide range of activities, socially effective,
81	generally satisfied with life, no more than everyday problems or concerns (e.g., an occasional argument with family members).
80	If symptoms are present, they are transient and expectable reactions to psychosocial stressors (e.g., difficulty concentrating after family argument); no more than slight
71	impairment in social, occupational, or school functioning (e.g., temporarily falling behind in school work).
70	Some mild symptoms (e.g., depressed mood and mild insomnia) OR some difficulty in social, occupational, or school functioning (e.g., occasional truancy, or theft within the
61	household), but generally functioning pretty well, has some meaningful interpersonal relationships.
60	Moderate symptoms (e.g., flat affect and circumstantial speech, occasional panic attacks) OR moderate difficulty in social, occupational, or school functioning (e.g., few
51	friends, conflicts, unable to keep a job).
50	Serious symptoms (e.g., suicidal ideation, severe obsessional rituals, frequent shoplifting) OR any serious impairment in social, occupational, or school functioning
41	(e.g., no friends, unable to keep a job).
40	Some impairment in reality testing or communication (e.g., speech is at times illogical, obscure, or irrelevant) OR major impairment in several areas, such as work
31	or school, family relations, judgment, thinking, or mood (e.g., depressed man avoids friends, neglects family, and is unable to work; child frequently beats up younger children, is defiant at home, and is failing at school).
30	Behavior is considerably influenced by delusions or hallucinations OR serious impairment in communication or judgment (e.g., sometimes incoherent, acts grossly inappropriately,
21	suicidal preoccupation) OR inability to function in almost all areas (e.g., stays in bed all day; no job, home, or friends).
20	Some danger of hurting self or others (e.g., suicide attempts without clear expectation of death; frequently violent; manic excitement) OR occasionally fails to maintain minimal personal
11	hygiene (e.g., smears feces) OR gross impairment in communication (e.g., largely incoherent or mute).
10	Persistent danger of severely hurting self or others (e.g., recurrent violence) OR persistent inability
1	to maintain minimal personal hygiene OR serious suicidal act with clear expectation of death.
0	Inadequate information.

The rating of overall psychological functioning on a scale of 0–100 was operationalized by Luborsky in the Health-Sickness Rating Scale (Luborsky, L., "Clinicians' Judgment of Mental Health," *Archives of General Psychiatry, 7*, 407–417, 1962). Spitzer and colleagues developed a revision of the Health-Sickness Rating Scale called the Global Assessment Scale (GAS) (Endicott, J., Spitzer, R. L., Fleiss, J. L., Cohen, J., "The Global Assessment Scale: A Procedure for Measuring Overall Severity of Psychiatric Disturbance." *Archives of General Psychiatry, 33*, 766–771, 1976). A modified version of the GAS was included in *DSM-III* as the Global Assessment of Functioning (GAS) Scale. [used with permission—American Psychiatric Association]

Appendix III

NANDA-Approved Nursing Diagnoses

Note: The initial letter of the key word in each NANDA diagnosis is in boldface.

Activity
  Activity Intolerance
  Risk for Activity Intolerance

Adaptive Capacity
  Decreased Intracranial Adaptive Capacity

Airway Clearance
  Ineffective Airway Clearance

Allergy Response
  Latex Allergy Response
  Risk for Latex Allergy Response

Anxiety
  Death Anxiety

Aspiration
  Risk for Aspiration

Attachment
  Risk for Impaired Attachment, Parent
  Risk for Impaired Attachment, Infant
  Risk for Impaired Attachment, Child

Blood Glucose
  Risk for Unstable Blood Glucose

Body Image
  Disturbed Body Image

Body Temperature
  Risk for Imbalanced Body Temperature

Bowel
  Bowel Incontinence

Breastfeeding
  Effective Breastfeeding
  Ineffective Breastfeeding
  Interrupted Breastfeeding

Breathing Pattern
  Ineffective Breathing Pattern

Cardiac Output
  Decreased Cardiac Output

Caregiver Role Strain
  Risk for Caregiver Role Strain

Comfort
  Readiness for Enhanced Comfort

Communication
  Readiness for Enhanced Communication
  Impaired Verbal Communication

Confusion
  Acute Confusion
  Chronic Confusion
  Risk for Acute Confusion

Constipation
  Perceived Constipation
  Risk for Constipation

Contamination
  Risk for Contamination

Coping
  Ineffective Community Coping
  Readiness for Enhanced Community Coping
  Defensive Coping
  Compromised Family Coping
  Disabled Family Coping
  Readiness for Enhanced Family Coping
  Readiness for Enhanced Individual Coping
  Ineffective Coping

Decision Making
  Readiness for Enhanced Decision Making
  Decisional Conflict (Specify)

Denial
  Ineffective Denial

Dentition
  Impaired Dentition

Development
  Risk for Delayed Development

Diarrhea

Disuse Syndrome
  Risk for Disuse Syndrome

Diversional Activity
  Deficient Diversional Activity

Dysreflexia
  Autonomic Dysreflexia
  Risk for Autonomic Dysreflexia

Energy Field
  Disturbed Energy Field

Environmental Interpretation Syndrome
  Impaired Environmental Interpretation Syndrome

Failure to Thrive
  Adult Failure to Thrive

Falls
  Risk for Falls

Family Processes
  Dysfunctional Family Processes: Alcoholism
  Interrupted Family Processes
  Readiness for Enhanced Family Processes

Fatigue

Fear

Fluid Balance
  Readiness for Enhanced Fluid Balance

Fluid Volume
  Deficient Fluid Volume
  Risk for Deficient Fluid Volume
  Excess Fluid Volume
  Risk for Imbalanced Fluid Volume

Gas Exchange
  Impaired Gas Exchange

Grieving
  Complicated Grieving
  Risk for Complicated Grieving

Growth
  Risk for Disproportionate Growth

Growth and Development
  Delayed Growth and Development

Health Behavior
  Risk-Prone Health Behavior
  Health Seeking Behaviors (Specify)

Home Maintenance
  Impaired Home Maintenance

Hope
  Readiness for Enhanced Hope

Hopelessness

Human Dignity
  Risk for Compromised Human Dignity

Hyperthermia

Hypothermia

Identity
  Disturbed Personal Identity

Immunization Status
  Readiness for Enhanced Immunization Status

Infant Behavior
  Disorganized Infant Behavior
  Risk for Disorganized Infant Behavior
  Readiness for Enhanced Organized Infant Behavior

Infant Feeding Pattern
  Ineffective Infant Feeding Pattern

Infection
  Risk for Infection

Injury
  Risk for Injury

Insomnia

Knowledge
  Deficient Knowledge (Specify)
  Readiness for Enhanced Knowledge (Specify)

Lifestyle
  Sedentary Lifestyle

Liver Function
  Risk for Impaired Liver Function

Loneliness
  Risk for Loneliness

Memory
  Impaired Memory

Mobility
  Impaired Bed Mobility
  Impaired Physical Mobility
  Impaired Wheelchair Mobility

Moral
  Moral Distress

Nausea

Neglect
  Unilateral Neglect

Neurovascular Dysfunction
  Risk for Peripheral Neurovascular Dysfunction

Noncompliance (Specify)

Nutrition
  Imbalanced Nutrition: Less than Body Requirements
  Imbalanced Nutrition: More than Body Requirements
  Risk for Imbalanced Nutrition: More than Body
    Requirements
  Readiness for Enhanced Nutrition

Oral Mucous Membrane
  Impaired Oral Mucous Membrane

Pain
  Acute Pain
  Chronic Pain

Parenting
  Impaired Parenting
  Readiness for Enhanced Parenting
  Risk for Impaired Parenting

Perioperative Positioning Injury
  Risk for Perioperative Positioning Injury

Poisoning
  Risk for Poisoning

Post-Trauma Syndrome
  Risk for Post-Trauma Syndrome

Power
  Readiness for Enhanced Power

Powerlessness
  Risk for Powerlessness

Protection
  Ineffective Protection

Rape-Trauma Syndrome
  Rape-Trauma Syndrome: Compound Reaction
  Rape-Trauma Syndrome: Silent Reaction

Religiosity
  Impaired Religiosity
  Readiness for Enhanced Religiosity
  Risk for Impaired Religiosity

Relocation Stress Syndrome
  Risk for Relocation Stress Syndrome

Role Conflict
  Parental Role Conflict

Role Performance
  Ineffective Role Performance

Self-Care
  Readiness for Enhanced Self-Care

Self-Care Deficit
  Bathing/Hygiene Self-Care Deficit
  Dressing/Grooming Self-Care Deficit
  Feeding Self-Care Deficit
  Toileting Self-Care Deficit

Self-Concept
  Readiness for Enhanced Self-Concept

Self-Esteem
  Chronic Low Self-Esteem
  Situational Low Self-Esteem
  Risk for Situational Low Self-Esteem

Self-Mutilation
  Risk for Self-Mutilation

Sensory Perception
  Disturbed Visual Sensory Perception (Specify)
  Disturbed Auditory Sensory Perception (Specify)
  Disturbed Kinesthetic Sensory Perception (Specify)
  Disturbed Gustatory Sensory Perception (Specify)
  Disturbed Tactile Sensory Perception (Specify)
  Disturbed Olfactory Sensory Perception (Specify)

Sexual Dysfunction

Sexuality Pattern
  Ineffective Sexuality Pattern

Skin Integrity
  Impaired Skin Integrity
  Risk for Impaired Skin Integrity

Sleep Deprivation

Sleep
  Readiness for Enhanced Sleep

Social Interaction
  Impaired Social Interaction

Social Isolation

Sorrow
  Chronic Sorrow

Spiritual Distress
  Risk for Spiritual Distress

Spiritual Well-Being
  Readiness for Enhanced Spiritual Well-Being

Stress Overload

Sudden Infant Death Syndrome
  Risk for Sudden Infant Death Syndrome

Suffocation
  Risk for Suffocation

Suicide
  Risk for Suicide

Surgical Recovery
  Delayed Surgical Recovery

Swallowing
  Impaired Swallowing

Therapeutic Regimen Management
  Ineffective Community Therapeutic Regimen Management
  Effective Therapeutic Regimen Management
  Ineffective Family Therapeutic Regimen Management
  Ineffective Therapeutic Regimen Management
  Readiness for Enhanced Therapeutic Regimen Management

Thermoregulation
  Ineffective Thermoregulation
Thought Processes
  Disturbed Thought Processes
Tissue Integrity
  Impaired Tissue Integrity
Tissue Perfusion
  Ineffective Renal Tissue Perfusion (Specify)
  Ineffective Cerebral Tissue Perfusion (Specify)
  Ineffective Cardiopulmonary Tissue Perfusion (Specify)
  Ineffective Gastrointestinal Tissue Perfusion (Specify)
  Ineffective Peripheral Tissue Perfusion (Specify)
Transfer Ability
  Impaired Transfer Ability
Trauma
  Risk for Trauma
Urinary Elimination
  Impaired Urinary Elimination
  Readiness for Enhanced Urinary Elimination

Urinary Incontinence
  Functional Urinary Incontinence
  Overflow Urinary Incontinence
  Reflex Urinary Incontinence
  Stress Urinary Incontinence
  Total Urinary Incontinence
  Urge Urinary Incontinence
  Risk for Urge Urinary Incontinence
Urinary Retention
Ventilation
  Impaired Spontaneous Ventilation
Ventilatory Weaning Response
  Dysfunctional Ventilatory Weaning Response
Violence
  Risk for Other-Directed Violence
  Risk for Self-Directed Violence
Walking
  Impaired Walking
Wandering

References and Resources

CHAPTER 1

American Psychiatric Association. (2000). *Diagnostic and statistical manual of mental disorders* (4th ed., Text Revision). Washington, DC: American Psychiatric Press.

Carson, V. B. (2000). *Mental health nursing: The nurse patient journey* (2nd ed.). Philadelphia: Saunders.

Frisch, N. C., & Frisch, L. E. (2006). *Psychiatric mental health nursing* (3rd ed.). Albany: Delmar.

National Institute of Mental Health. (2006). *The numbers count: Mental disorders in America*. (NIMH Pub. No. 06-4584). Washington, DC: Author. Retrieved July 30, 2006, from http://www.nimh.nih.gov/healthinformation/

Substance Abuse and Mental Health Services Administration, National Mental Health Information Center. (2003). *Homelessness*. Washington, DC: Author. Retrieved July 30, 2006, from http://www.mentalhealth.samhsa.gov/cmhs/Homelessness/

Torrey, E. F. (1997). *Out of the shadows: Confronting America's mental illness crisis*. New York: John Wiley & Sons.

U.S. Department of Health and Human Services. (2000). *Healthy People 2010: National health promotion and disease prevention objectives*. Washington, DC: Author.

CHAPTER 2

Aiken, T. D., & Catalano, J. T. (1994). *Legal, ethical, and political issues in nursing*. Philadelphia: F. A. Davis.

American Nurses' Association. (2001). *Code for nurses with interpretive statements*. Washington, DC: Author.

Bill of Rights for Mental Health Patients. Mental Health Systems Act of 1980.Title II, Public Law 99-319.

Guido, G. W. (2006). *Legal and ethical issues in nursing* (4th ed.). Upper Saddle River, NJ: Prentice Hall.

Johnson, M. E. (1998). Being restrained: A study of power and powerlessness. *Issues in Mental Health Nursing, 19*(3), 191.

Joint Commission on Accreditation of Healthcare Organizations. (2005). *Restraint and seclusion standards for behavioral health*. Retrieved October 3, 2006, from http://www.jointcommission.org/accreditationprograms/hospitals/standards/FAQ

Meehan, T., Bergen, H., & Fjeldsoe, K. (2004). Staff and patient perceptions of seclusion: Has anything changed? *Journal of Advanced Nursing, 47*, 33–38.

National Federation of Licensed Practical Nurses. (2003). *Nursing practice standards for the licensed practical/vocational nurse*. Garner, NC: Author.

National Standards for Culturally and Linguistically Appropriate Services in Health Care. Final Report by Office of Minority Health. (2001). Washington, DC: Office of Public Health and Science, USDHSS.

Office of Minority Health. (2001). *National standards for culturally and linguistically appropriate services in health care. Final report*. Washington, DC: Office of Public Health and Science.

Sailas, E. A., Wahlbeck, K., & Lie, D. (2005). Restraint and seclusion in psychiatric inpatient wards. *Current Opinion in Psychiatry, 18*(5), 555–559.

Sheline, Y., & Nelson, T. (1993). Patient choice: Deciding between psychotropic medication and physical restraints in an emergency. *Bulletin of the American Academy of Psychiatric Law, 21*, 321–329.

Steele, S. M., & Harmon, V. M. (1979). *Values clarification in nursing*. New York: Appleton-Century-Crofts.

Stuart, G. W., & Laraia, M. T. (2005). *Principles and practice of psychiatric nursing* (8th ed.). St. Louis, Mosby.

Torrey, E. F. (1997). *Out of the shadows: Confronting America's mental illness crisis*. New York: John Wiley & Sons.

Townsend, M. C. (2006). *Essentials of psychiatric mental health nursing* (3rd ed.). Philadelphia: F. A. Davis.

CHAPTER 3

Bandura, A. (1977). *Social learning theory*. Englewood Cliffs, NJ: Prentice Hall.

Carson, V. B. (2000). *Mental health nursing: The nurse patient journey* (2nd ed.). Philadelphia: Saunders.

Erikson, E. H. (1963). *Childhood and society* (2nd ed.). New York: Norton.

Erikson, E. H. (1980). *The life cycle completed*. New York: Norton.

Frankl, V. E. (1963). *Man's search for meaning*. New York: Washington Square.

Friedman, H. S., & Schustack, M. W. (1999). *Personality: Classical theories and modern research*. Boston: Allyn and Bacon.

Gardner, H. (1999). *Intelligence reframed. Multiple intelligences for the 21st century*. New York: Basic Books.

Giger, J. N., & Davidhizar, R. E. (2004). *Transcultural nursing assessment and intervention* (4th ed.). St. Louis: Mosby.

Hockenberry, M. J. (2005). *Wong's essentials of pediatric nursing* (7th ed.). St. Louis: Mosby.

Maslow, A. H. (1968). *Toward a psychology of being* (2nd ed.). Princeton, NJ: Van Nostrand.

Maslow, A., & Lowery, R., Ed. (1998). *Toward a psychology of being* (3rd ed.). New York: Wiley & Sons.

Peplau, H. E. (1989). Future directions in psychiatric nursing from the perspective of history. *Journal of Psychosocial Nursing, 27*(2), 18–28.

CHAPTER 4

Aiken, L. H., Clarke, S. P., Sloane, D. M., Sochalski, J., & Silber, J. H. (2002). Hospital nurse staffing and patient mortality, nurse burnout, and job dissatisfaction. *Journal of the American Medical Association, 288*(16), 1987–1993.

Beattie, M. (1992). *Codependent no more. How to stop controlling others and start controlling yourself*. New York: MJF Books.

Bunner, K., & Yonge, O. (2006). Boundaries and adolescent residential treatment settings: What clinicians need to know. *Journal of Psychosocial Nursing and Mental Health Services, 44*(9), 38–40.

Frisch, N. C., & Frisch, L. E. (2006). *Psychiatric mental health nursing* (3rd ed.). Clifton Park, NY: Thomson Delmar Learning.

Hess, A. K. (2005). Ensure a long and safe career. *American Journal of Nursing, 105*(6), 96.

Leininger, M. (1985). Transcultural care: Diversity and universality. *Nursing & Health Care, 6*(4), 208–212.

Leininger, M., & McFarland, M. R. (2002). *Transcultural nursing concepts, theories, research, & practice* (3rd ed.). Andover, MA: McGraw-Hill.

Lopez, R. P. (2007). Suffering and dying nursing home residents: Nurses' perceptions of the role of family members. *Journal of Hospice and Palliative Nursing, 9*(3), 141–149.

Malach-Pines, A. (2000). Nurses' burnout: An existential psychodynamic perspective. *Journal of Psychosocial Nursing, 38*(2), 23–31.

Pines, A. M., & Aronson, E. (1988). *Career burnout: Causes and cures.* New York: Free Press.

Roach, M. (1987). *The human act of caring.* Ottawa: Canadian Hospital Association.

Snow, C., & Willard, D. (1989). *I'm dying to take care of you.* Redmond, CA: Professional Counselor Books.

Watson, J. (1979). *Nursing: The philosophy and science of caring.* Boston: Little, Brown.

Zerwekh, J., & Claborn, J. C. (2006). *Nursing today: Transitions and trends* (5th ed.). New York: Elsevier.

CHAPTER 5

Eckroth-Bucher, M. (2001). Philosophical basis and practice of self-awareness in psychiatric nursing. *Journal of Psychosocial Nursing, 39,* 32.

Fortinash, K. M., & Holoday Worret, P. A. (2004). *Psychiatric mental health nursing* (3rd ed.). St. Louis: Mosby-Elsevier.

Frisch, N. C., & Frisch, L. E. (2005). *Psychiatric mental health nursing: Understanding the client as well as the condition* (3rd ed.). Albany, NY: Delmar.

Jourard, S. (1971). *The transparent self* (Rev. ed.). New York: Litton.

Knapp, M. L. (1980). *Essentials of nonverbal communication.* New York: Holt, Rinehart, & Winston.

Peplau, H. (1952). *Interpersonal relations in nursing.* New York: Putnam.

Psychopathology Committee of the Group for the Advancement of Psychiatry. (2001). Reexamination of therapist self-disclosure. *Psychiatric Services, 52,* 1489–1493. Retrieved June 27, 2007, from http://ps.psychiatryonline.org/cgi/content/full/52/11/1489

Stuart, G. W., & Laraia, M. T. (2005). *Principles and practice of psychiatric nursing* (8th ed.). St. Louis: Mosby.

Travelbee, J. (1971). *Interpersonal aspects of nursing* (2nd ed.). Philadelphia: F. A. Davis.

Varcarolis, E. M., Carson, V. B., & Shoemaker, N. C. (2006). *Foundations of mental health nursing* (5th ed.). Philadelphia: W. B. Saunders-Elsevier.

Walker, K., & Alligood, M. (2001). Empathy from a nursing perspective: Moving beyond borrowed theory. *Archives of Psychiatric Nursing, 15,* 140.

CHAPTER 6

Allen, K., Shykoff, B., & Izzo, J. L. Jr. (2001). Pet ownership, but not ACE inhibitor therapy, blunts home blood pressure responses to mental stress. *Hypertension, 38,* 815.

Gonzales, C. A., Griffith, E. E. H., & Ruiz, P. (2001). Cross cultural issues in psychiatric treatment. In G. O. Gabbard (Ed.), *Treatment of psychiatric disorders* (3rd ed., pp. 47–70). Washington, DC: American Psychiatric Publishing.

Hertig, V. (2004). Stress, stress response, and health. *Nursing Clinics of North America, 39,* 1–17.

Kabat-Zinn, J. (1993). Meditation. In B. Moyers (Ed.), *Healing and the mind.* New York: Doubleday.

Lazarus, R. S., & Folkman, S. (1984). *Stress, appraisal, and coping.* New York: Springer.

Porth, C. M. (2007). *Essentials of pathophysiology: Concepts of altered health states* (2nd ed.). Philadelphia: Lippincott, Williams, & Wilkins.

Roy, C. (1976). *Introduction to nursing: An adaptation model.* Upper Saddle River, NJ: Prentice Hall.

Salmon, P. (2000). Effects of physical exercise on anxiety, depression, and sensitivity to stress: A unifying theory. *Clinical Psychological Review, 21*(1), 33–61.

Sapolsky, R. M. (2004). *Why zebras don't get ulcers* (3rd ed.). New York: Henry Holt.

Selye, H. (1976). *The stress of life.* Highstown, NJ: McGraw-Hill.

Townsend, M. C. (2005). *Psychiatric mental health nursing: Concepts of care* (4th ed.). Philadelphia: F. A. Davis.

Varcarolis, E. M., Carson, V. B., & Shoemaker, N. C. (2005). *Foundations of psychiatric mental health nursing: A clinical approach.* Philadelphia: W. B. Saunders.

CHAPTER 7

American Psychiatric Association. (2000). *Diagnostic and statistical manual of mental disorders* (4th ed., Text Revision). Washington, DC: American Psychiatric Press.

Caspi, A., Sugden, K., Moffitt, T., Taylor, A., Craig, I., Harrington, H., McClay, J., Mill, J., Martin, J., Braithwaite, A., & Poulton, R. (2003). Influence of life stress on depression: Moderation by a polymorphism in the 5-HTT gene. *Science, 301,* 386.

Collins, F. (1999). Medical and societal consequences of the Human Genome Project. *New England Journal of Medicine, 341,* 28–37.

Egan, M., Goldberg, T., Kolachana, B., Callicott, J., Mazzanti, Straub, R., Goldman, D., & Weinberger, D. (2001). The effect of COMT Val[108/158] met genotype on frontal lobe function and risk for schizophrenia. *Proceedings of the National Academy of Sciences, U.S.A., 98,* 6917.

Keltner, N. L. (2000). Neuroreceptor function and psychopharmacologic response. *Issues in Mental Health Nursing, 21,* 31.

Keltner, N. L., Schwecke, L. H., & Bostrom, C. E. (2007). *Psychiatric nursing* (5th ed.). St. Louis: Mosby.

Kneisl, C. R., Wilson, H. S., & Trigoboff, E. (2004). *Contemporary psychiatric–mental health nursing.* Upper Saddle River, NJ: Prentice Hall.

Stuart, G. W., & Laraia, M. T. (2005). *Principles and practice of psychiatric nursing* (8th ed.). St. Louis: Mosby.

Torrey, E. F. (2001). *Surviving schizophrenia: A manual for families, consumers, and providers* (4th ed.). New York: Quill, HarperCollins.

Trigoboff, E., Wilson, B. A., Shannon, M. T., & Stang, C. L. (2005). *Prentice Hall psychiatric drug guide.* Upper Saddle River, NJ: Prentice Hall.

CHAPTER 8

Allison, D. B., & Casey, D. E. (2001). Antipsychotic-induced weight gain: A review of the literature. *Journal of Clinical Psychiatry, 62* (suppl. 7), 22–31.

Amador, X. (2001). *I am not sick, I don't need help! Helping the seriously mentally ill accept treatment.* Peconic, NY: Vida Press.

American Psychiatric Association. (2000). *Diagnostic and statistical manual of mental disorders* (4th ed., Text Revision). Washington, DC: American Psychiatric Press.

Anthony, W., Cohen, M., Farkas, M., & Cagne, C. (2002). *Psychiatric rehabilitation* (2nd ed.). Boston: Center for Psychiatric Rehabilitation.

Beebe, L. H. (2003). Health promotion in persons with schizophrenia: Atypical medications. *Journal of the American Psychiatric Nurses Association, 9*(4), 115–122.

Brown, T., Cooper, M. C., Crimson, M. L., & Enderle, H. E. (2002). *Special report: Medication management considerations in schizophrenia* (pp. 1–21). Washington, DC: American Pharmaceutical Association.

Deegan, P. E. (1988). Recovery: The lived experience of rehabilitation. *Psychosocial Rehabilitation 11*(4), 11–19.

Goff, D. C., & Coyle, J. T. (2001). The emerging role of glutamate in the pathophysiology and treatment of schizophrenia. *American Journal of Psychiatry, 158*(9), 1367–1376.

Jacobson, N., & Greenley, D. (2001). What is recovery? A conceptual model and explication. *Psychiatric Services, 52*(4), 482–485.

Keltner, N. L., Schwecke, L. H., & Bostrom, C. E. (2007). *Psychiatric nursing* (5th ed.). St. Louis: Mosby.

Kneisl, C. R., Wilson, H. S., & Trigoboff, E. (2004). *Contemporary psychiatric–mental health nursing*. Upper Saddle River, NJ: Prentice Hall.

Mills, J. (2000). Dealing with voices and strange thoughts. In C. Gamble & G. Brennan (Eds.), *Working with serious mental illness: A manual for clinical practice*. London: Bailliere Tindall.

National Collaborating Centre for Mental Health. (2002). *Schizophrenia: Core interventions in the treatment and management of schizophrenia in primary and secondary care*. London: National Institute for Clinical Excellence. Retrieved November 26, 2006, from http://guideline.gov/summary/summary.aspx?view_id=1&doc_id=5070

O'Connor, F. W., & Delaney, K. R. (2007). The recovery movement: Defining evidence-based processes. *Archives of Psychiatric Nursing, 3*(21), 172–175.

Ollendorf, D. A., Joyce, A. T., & Rucker, M. (2004, Jan. 20). Rate of new-onset diabetes among patients treated with atypical or conventional antipsychotic medications for schizophrenia. *Medscape General Medicine*, ejournal. Retrieved January 29, 2004, from http://www.medscape.com/viewarticle/466800?mpid-23840

Rankin, E. A. (2000). *Quick reference for psychopharmacology*. Albany, NY: Delmar.

Stahl, S. M. (2001). Dopamine system stabilizers, aripiprazole, and the next generation of antipsychotics, Part II: Illustrating their mechanism of action. *Journal of Clinical Psychiatry, 62*(12), 923–924.

Stuart, G. W., & Laraia, M. T. (2005). *Principles and practice of psychiatric nursing* (8th ed.). St. Louis: Mosby.

Substance Abuse and Mental Health Services Administration. (2005). Transforming mental health care in America. The federal action agenda: First steps. Retrieved June 28, 2007, from http://www.samhsa.gov/federalactionagenda/NFC.intro.aspx

Torrey, E. F. (1997). *Out of the shadows: Confronting America's mental illness crisis*. New York: John Wiley.

Torrey, E. F. (2001). *Surviving schizophrenia: A manual for families, consumers, and providers* (4th ed.). New York: Harper Collins.

Townsend, M. C. (2006). *Nursing diagnoses in psychiatric nursing: Care plans and psychotropic medications* (5th ed.). Philadelphia: F. A. Davis.

Videbeck, S. L. (2004). *Psychiatric mental health nursing*. Philadelphia: Lippincott.

CHAPTER 9

American Psychiatric Association. (2000). *Diagnostic and statistical manual of mental disorders* (4th ed., Text Revision). Washington, DC: American Psychiatric Press.

Avery, D. H., Holtzheimer, P. E., III, Fawaz, W., Russo, J., Neumaier, J., Dunner, D. L., Haynor, D. R., Claypoole, K. H., Wajdik, C., & Roy-Byrne, P. (2006). The use of repeated transcranial magnetic stimulation for medication-resistant depression. *Biological Psychiatry, 59, 2*, 187–194.

Beck, A. T., & Rush, A. J. (2004). Cognitive therapy. In B. J. Sadock & V. A. Sadock (Eds.), *Comprehensive textbook of psychiatry* (8th ed., vol. 2). Philadelphia: Lippincott, Williams & Wilkins.

Bowden, C. L. (2003). *Improving bipolar outcomes across the life cycle*. Paper presented at American Psychiatric Association 156th Annual Meeting, Bipolar CME. Retrieved July 31, 2003, from http://www.medscape.com/viewprogram/2469_pnt

Caspi, A., Sugden, K., Moffitt, T., Taylor, A., Craig, I., Harrington, H., McClay, J., Mill, J., Martin, J., Braithwaite, A., & Poulton, R. (2003). Influence of life stress on depression: Moderation by a polymorphism in the 5-HTT gene. *Science, 301*, 386.

Keltner, N. L., Schwecke, L. H., & Bostrom, C. E. (2007). *Psychiatric nursing* (5th ed.). St. Louis: Mosby.

Lurie, S. J., Gawinski, B., Pierce, D., & Rousseau, S. J. (2006). Seasonal affective disorder. *American Family Physician, 74*(9). Retrieved March 13, 2007, from http://www.aafp.org/afp/20061101/1521.html

Mayo Clinic. (2007). Antidepressant patch Emsam approved by FDA. Retrieved February 24, 2007, from http://www.mayoclinic.com/health/antidepressant/DI00057

Mendelowitz, A. J., Dawkins, K., & Lieberman, J. A. (2000). Antidepressants. In J. A. Lieberman & A. Tasman (Eds.), *Psychiatric drugs*. Philadelphia: W. B. Saunders.

National Alliance for Mental Illness. (2006). Study confirms that stigma still a barrier to psychiatric care. *NAMI Connection*. Retrieved March 1, 2007, from http://www.nami.org/Content/NavigationMenu/Whats_New43/The_NAMI_Connection/20065/Study_on_Stigma.htm

National Institute of Mental Health. (2006). *Suicide in the U.S.: Statistics and prevention*. Washington, DC: Author.

Rihmer, Z. (2007). Suicide risk in mood disorders. *Current Opinions in Psychiatry, 20*(1), 17–22. Retrieved February 25, 2007, from http://www.medscapecom/viewarticle/550672_1

Roach, M. J., Connors, A., Dawson, N., Wenger, N., Wu, A., Tsevat, J., Desbiens, N., Covinsky, K., & Schubert, D. (1998). Depressed mood and survival in seriously ill hospitalized adults. *Archives of Internal Medicine 158*, 397–404.

Sheikh, J. I., & Yesavage, J. A. (1986). Geriatric depression scale: Recent evidence and development of a shorter form. *Clinical Gerontologist, 5*, 165–172.

Sonne, S. C., & Brady, K. T. (1999). Substance abuse and bipolar comorbidity. *The Psychiatric Clinics of North America, 22*(3), 609–628.

Spires, R. A. (2006). Depression in the elderly. *RNWeb*. Retrieved January 15, 2007, from http://www.rnweb.com/rnweb/article/articleDetail.jsp?id=329133&searchString=depression

Stahl, S. (2005). *Essential psychopharmacology: The prescriber's guide*. Cambridge, United Kingdom: University of Cambridge.

Stoner, S. C., & Dubisar, B. (2006). Psychotropics. *RN, 69*(7), 31–37.

Stuart, G. W., & Laraia, M. T. (2005). *Principles and practice of psychiatric nursing* (8th ed.). St. Louis: Mosby.

U.S. Public Health Service. (1999). *The Surgeon General's call to action to prevent suicide.* Washington, DC: Author.

World Health Organization. (2007). *Depression management.* Geneva: Author. Retrieved March 18, 2007, from http://www.WHO.int/mental_health/management/ depression

CHAPTER 10

American Psychiatric Association. (2000). *Diagnostic and statistical manual of mental disorders* (4th ed., Text Revision). Washington, DC: American Psychiatric Press.

Bohrer, G. J., & Haynes, L. (2005). Compulsive hoarding: Sign of a deeper disorder. *NurseWeek, 6*(15), 13–15.

Davidson, R. J., Jackson, D. C., & Kalin, N. H. (2000). Emotion, plasticity, context and regulation: Perspectives from affective neuroscience. *Psychological Bulletin, 126*(6), 873–889.

De Clercq, B., & De Fruyt, F. (2007). Childhood antecedents of personality disorder. *Current Opinion in Psychiatry, 20*(1), 57–61.

Limandri, B., & Boyd, M. A. (2005). Personality and impulse control disorders. In M. A. Boyd (Ed.), *Psychiatric nursing: Contemporary practice* (3rd ed.). Philadelphia: Lippincott.

Linehan, M. (1993). *Cognitive-behavioral treatment of borderline personality disorder.* New York: Guilford.

Miller, M. C. (Ed.). (2006). Borderline personality disorder: Treatment. *Harvard Mental Health Letter, 20*, 7.

Millon, T., & Davis, R. (1999). *Personality disorders in modern life.* New York: John Wiley & Sons.

Nathan, P., & Gorman, J. M. (2002). *A guide to treatments that work* (2nd ed.). Oxford: Oxford University Press.

Stern, A. (1938). Psychoanalytic investigation of and therapy in the borderline group of neuroses. *Psychoanalytic Quarterly, 7*, 467–489.

Swenson, C. R., Sanderson, C., Dulit, R. A., & Linehan, M. (2001). The application of dialectical behavioral therapy for patients with borderline personality disorder on inpatient units. *Psychiatric Quarterly, 72*(4), 307–324.

Zanarini, M. C. (2000). Childhood experiences associated with the development of borderline personality disorder. *Psychiatric Clinics of North America, 23*(1), 89–101.

CHAPTER 11

American Psychiatric Association. (2000). *Diagnostic and statistical manual of mental disorders* (4th ed., Text Revision). Washington, DC: American Psychiatric Press.

Antai-Otong, D. (2005). Current treatment of generalized anxiety disorder. *Journal of Psychosocial Nursing and Mental Health Services, 41*, 12.

Braun, C. A., & Anderson, C. M. (2007). *Pathophysiology: Functional alterations in human health.* Philadelphia: Lippincott Williams & Wilkins.

Carpenito-Moyet, L. J. (2006). *Handbook of nursing diagnosis* (11th ed.). Philadelphia: Lippincott Williams & Wilkins.

National Institute of Mental Health. (2006). *Anxiety disorders.* Retrieved May 13, 2007, from http://www.nimh.nih.gov/publicat/anxiety.cfm#anx1

O'Toole, A., & Welt, S. (Eds.). (1989). *Interpersonal theory in nursing practice. Selected works of Hildegard E. Peplau.* New York: Springer.

Rosenbaum, J. F., & Covino, J. W. (2005). Stress and resilience: Implications for depression and anxiety. Depression Expert Column Series. *Medscape Psychiatry & Mental Health, 10*(2). Retrieved May 21, 2007, from: http://www.medscape.com/viewarticle/518761

Satcher, D., Delgado, P. L., & Masand, S. (2005). A surgeon general's perspective on the unmet needs of patients with anxiety disorders. *psychCME.* Retrieved April 10, 2007, from http://www.medscape.com/viewprogram/4650

Schultz, J. M., & Videbeck, S. L. (2005). *Psychiatric nursing care plans* (7th ed.). Philadelphia: Lippincott.

Stahl, S. M. (2005). *Essential pharmacology: The prescriber's guide.* Cambridge, MA: Cambridge University Press.

Street, A., & Stafford, J. (2004). Military sexual trauma: Issues in caring for veterans. In E. B. Carlson et al., *The Iraq War clinician guide.* Washington, DC: United States Department of Veterans' Affairs, National Center for Posttraumatic Stress Disorder. Retrieved May 15, 2007, from http://www.ncptsd.va.gov/ncmain/ncdocs/manuals/iraq_clinician_guide_v2.pdf

Stuart, G. W. (2005). Anxiety responses and anxiety disorders. In G. W. Stuart & M. T. Laraia (Eds.), *Principles and practice of psychiatric nursing* (8th ed.). St. Louis: Mosby.

Yaeger, D., Himmelfarb, N., Cammack, A., & Mintz, J. (2006). DSM-IV diagnosed posttraumatic stress disorder in women veterans with and without military sexual trauma. *Journal of Internal Medicine, 21*(S3), S65–S69.

CHAPTER 12

American Psychiatric Association. (2000). *Diagnostic and statistical manual of mental disorders* (4th ed., Text Revision). Washington, DC: American Psychiatric Press.

Bailey, K. P. (2004). The brain's rewarding system and addiction. *Journal of Psychosocial Nursing and Mental Health Services, 42*, 6.

Centers for Disease Control and Prevention. (2007, March). *Smoking & tobacco use.* Retrieved September 21, 2007, from http://www.cdc.gov/tobacco/data_statistics/Factsheets/cessation2.htm

Deglin, J. H., & Vallerand, A. H. (2007). *Davis's drug guide for nurses* (10th ed.). Philadelphia: F. A. Davis.

El-Mallakh, P. (1998). Treatment models for clients with co-occurring addictive and mental disorders. *Archives of Psychiatric Nursing, 12*(2), 71.

Ewing, J. A. (1984). Detecting alcoholism: The CAGE questionnaire. *JAMA, 252*, 1902–1907.

Fontaine, K. L., & Fletcher, J. S. (2003). *Mental health nursing* (5th ed.). Upper Saddle River, NJ: Pearson.

Giger, J. N., & Davidhizar, R. E. (2004). *Transcultural nursing: Assessment and intervention* (4th ed.). St Louis: Mosby.

Gordon, C., Williams, B., & Lapin, P. (2001). New program to help seniors quit smoking. *Nursing Spectrum, 2*(10), 18–19.

Keltner, N. L., Schwecke, L. H., & Bostrom, C. E. (2007). *Psychiatric nursing* (5th ed.). St. Louis: Mosby.

Kneisl, C. R., Wilson, H. S., & Trigoboff, E. (2004). *Contemporary psychiatric–mental health nursing.* Upper Saddle River, NJ: Pearson Education.

McGuinness, T. (2006). Methamphetamine abuse. *American Journal of Nursing, 106* (12), 54–59.

Morrison, C. (2000). Fear of addiction. *American Journal of Nursing,* 100(7), 81.

National Institute on Drug Abuse. (2007). *Medical and health professionals: Resources for patients: Methamphetamines.* Washington DC: Author. Retrieved June 3, 2007, from http://www.drugabuse.gov/drugpages/methamphetamine.html

Simpson, C. A., & Tucker, J. A. (2002). Temporal sequencing of alcohol-related problems, problem recognition, and help-seeking episodes. *Addictive Behaviors, 27,* 659–674.

CHAPTER 13

American Psychiatric Association. (2000). *Diagnostic and statistical manual of mental disorders* (4th ed., Text Revision). Washington, DC: American Psychiatric Press.

Biederman, J. (2003). Pharmacotherapy for attention deficit/hyperactivity disorder (ADHD) decreases the risk for substance abuse: Findings from a longitudinal followup of youths with and without ADHD. *Journal of Clinical Psychiatry, 64* (suppl.11), 3–8. Retrieved August 27, 2007, from http://www.psychiatrist.com/pcc/pccpdf/v05s05/v64s1101.pdf

Driever, M. J. (1976). Theory of self-concept. In C. Roy (Ed.), *Introduction to nursing: An adaptation model.* Upper Saddle River, NJ: Prentice Hall.

Gutman, A. R., & Spollen, J. J. III (2002). A new nonstimulant treatment for ADHD. In conference coverage of the American Association of Child and Adolescent Psychiatry, December, 2002. Retrieved August 27, 2007, from http://www.medscape.com/viewarticle/445221

Hockenberry, M. J. (2005). *Wong's essentials of pediatric nursing* (7th ed.). St. Louis: Mosby.

Keltner, N. L., Schwecke, L. H., & Bostrom, C. E. (2007). *Psychiatric nursing* (5th ed.). St. Louis: Mosby.

McCracken, J. T. (2000). Attention deficit disorders. In B. J. Sadock & V. A. Sadock (Eds.), *Comprehensive textbook of psychiatry* (7th ed., pp. 2711–2719). Baltimore: Williams & Wilkins.

National Institute of Mental Health. (2006a). *Attention deficit hyperactivity disorder.* Rockville, MD: Author. Retrieved August 24, 2007, from http://www.nimh.nih.gov/publicat/adhd.cfm

National Institute of Mental Health. (2006b). *Suicide in the U.S.: Statistics and prevention.* Rockville, MD: author. Retrieved August 27, 2007, from http://www.nimh.nih.gov/publicat/harmsway.cfm

Russell, S., & Joyner, K. (2001). Adolescent sexual orientation and suicide risk: Evidence from a national study. *American Journal of Public Health, 91,* 1276–1281.

Selekman, J. (2002). Learning disabilities: A diagnosis ignored by nurses. *Pediatric Nursing* 28(6), 630–632.

Simon, G. E., & Savarino, J. (2007). Suicide attempt pattern is the same regardless of initial treatment of depression. *American Journal of Psychiatry, 164,* 1029–1034. Retrieved August 20, 2007, from http://www.medscape.com/viewarticle/559487

Stahl, S. M. (2005). *Essential psychopharmacology: The prescriber's guide.* Cambridge, UK: University of Cambridge.

Townsend, M. C. (2006). *Psychiatric mental health nursing concepts of care* (5th ed.). Philadelphia: F. A. Davis.

CHAPTER 14

American Psychiatric Association. (2000a). *Diagnostic and statistical manual of mental disorders* (4th ed., Text Revision). Washington, DC: American Psychiatric Press.

American Psychiatric Association. (2000b). Practice guidelines for the treatment of patients with eating disorders. *American Journal of Psychiatry 157,* 1.

Blackburn, G. L., & Bevis, L. C. (2003). *The obesity epidemic: Prevention and treatment of the metabolic syndrome.* American Diabetes Association 63rd Scientific Sessions. Retrieved August 6, 2003, from http://www.medscape.com

Greeno, C. G., Wing, R. R., & Shiffman, S. (2000). Binge antecedents in obese women with and without binge eating disorder. *Journal of Consulting Clinical Psychology, 68*(1), 95.

Johnson, J. G., Cohen, P., Kasen, S., & Brook, J. S. (2002). Childhood adversities associated with risk for eating disorders or weight problems during adolescence or early adulthood. *American Journal of Psychiatry, 159,* 394–400.

Levine, M., & Smolak, L. (2006). Ten things parents can do to prevent eating disorders. *National Eating Disorders Association.* Retrieved August 30, 2007, from http://www.nationaleatingdisorders.org/p.asp?WebPage_ID=286&Profile_ID=41171

National Eating Disorders Association. (2007). *Causes of eating disorders.* National Eating Disorders Association Website Retrieved August 30, 2007, from www.NationalEatingDisorders.org

Perez, M., Voelz, Z. R., Pettit, J. W., & Joiner, T. E. Jr. (2002). The role of acculturative stress and body dissatisfaction in predicting bulimic symptomatology across ethnic groups. *International Journal of Eating Disorders, 31*(4), 442–454.

Petrie, T. A., & Tripp, M. (2001). Sexual abuse and eating disorders: A test of a conceptual model. *Sex Roles: A Journal of Research.* Retrieved August 30, 2007, from http://findarticles.com/p/articles/mi_m2294/is_2001_Jan/ai_77384284/pg_1

Ricciardelli, L. A., Williams, J., & Kiernan, M. J. (1999). Bulimic symptoms in adolescent girls and boys. *International Journal of Eating Disorders, 26*(2), 217.

Spearing, M. (2001). Eating disorders: Facts about eating disorders and the search for solutions. National Institute of Mental Health Publication No. 01-4901. Retrieved August 30, 2007, from www.nimh.nih.gov/publicat/eatingdisorders.cfm

Woodside, D. B., Garfinkel, P. E., Lin, E., Goering, P., Kaplan, A. S., Goldbloom. D. S., & Kennedy, S. H. (2001). Comparisons of men with full or partial eating disorders, men without eating disorders, and women with eating disorders in the community. *American Journal of Psychiatry, 158,* 570–574.

Zhu, A. J., & Walsh, B. T. (2002). Pharmacologic treatment of eating disorders. *Canadian Journal of Psychiatry, 47*(3), 227–234.

CHAPTER 15

Alzheimer's Association. (2003). Relating to someone with Alzheimer's. *Rocky Mountain Chapter News, 23*(4), 4.

Alzheimer's Association. (2005). Mid-life heart risk factors raise chances of late-life dementia. *Colorado Chapter Newsletter,* Summer, pp. 5, 27.

Alzheimer's Association. (2006a). Alzheimer's may have a link to diabetes. *Colorado Chapter Newsletter,* Summer, p. 6.

Alzheimer's Association. (2006b). Be a healthy caregiver. *Colorado Chapter Newsletter,* Winter, p. 4.

Alzheimer's Association. (2007a). *Caring for Alzheimer's.* Retrieved July 3, 2007, from http://www.alz.org/living_with_Alzheimer's_caring_for_alzheimer's.asp

Alzheimer's Association. (2007b). *Diagnosing Alzheimer's.* Retrieved July 3, 2007, from http://www.alz.org/alzheimers_disease_diagnosis.asp

Alzheimer's Association. (2007c). *Diversity.* Retrieved July 15, 2007, from http://www.alz.org/Resources/Diversity/downloads/GEN_EDU-10steps.pdf

Alzheimer's Association. (2007d). *Symptoms of Alzheimer's.* Retrieved July 3, 2007, from http://www.alz.org/alzheimers_disease_symptoms_of_alzheimers.asp

Alzheimer's Association. (2007e). *Treatments.* Retrieved July 3, 2007, from http://alz.org/alzheimers_disease_treatments.asp

Alzheimer's Learning Institute. (2001). Alzheimer's: *The disease process.* Denver: Alzheimer's Association, Rocky Mountain chapter.

Alzheimer Research Forum. (2007). *Drugs in clinical trials.* Retrieved March 4, 2007, from http://www.alzforum.org/dis/tre/drc/detail.asp?id=84&print=y

American Psychiatric Association. (2000). *Diagnostic and statistical manual of mental disorders* (4th ed., Text Revision). Washington, DC: American Psychiatric Press.

Brindle, J. (2005). Meeting the challenges of Alzheimer's care. *RN, 68*(1), 29–34.

Buettner, L., & Kolanowski, A. (2003). Practice guidelines for recreation therapy in the care of people with dementia. *Geriatric Nursing, 24*(1), 18–23.

Conroy, M., & Nottoli, M. J. (1999). Memory lane: A path to compliance. *RN, 62*(8), 40–41.

Deglin, J., & Vallerand, A. (2007). *Davis's drug guide for nurses* (10th ed.). Philadelphia: F. A. Davis.

Doerflinger, D. (2007). *Mental status assessment of older adults: The mini-cog.* Retrieved July 25, 2007, from http://www.GeroNurseOnline.org

Fazio, S., Seman, D., & Stansell, J. (1999). *Rethinking Alzheimer's care.* East Peoria, IL: Health Professions Press.

Feil, N. (1993). The validation method, helping families and professionals communicate. *The Alzheimer's Caregiver, 7*(4), 1–2.

Gleason, O. (2003, March 1). Delirium. *American Family Physician.* Retrieved June 3, 2007, from http://www.afp.org/afp/20030301/1027.html

Gray-Vickrey, P. (2002). Advances in Alzheimer's disease, forget me not. *Nursing2002, 32*(11), 64.

Gruetzner, H. (2001). *Alzheimer's, A caregiver's guide & sourcebook* (3rd ed.). New York: John Wiley & Sons.

Kuhn, D. (1999). *Alzheimer's early stages.* Alameda, CA: Hunter House Publishers.

Mace, N., & Rabins, P. (1999). *The 36-hour day.* Baltimore: The Johns Hopkins University Press.

Napierkowski, D. (2002). Using restraints with restraint. *Nursing, 32*(11), 58–62.

National Institute on Aging. (2006, December 14). Alzheimer's disease medication fact sheet. Retrieved June 3, 2007, from http://www.nia.nih.gov/Alzheimer's/Publications/medicationsfs.htm

Naylor, M., Stephens, C., Bowles, K., & Bixby, B. (2005). Cognitively impaired older adults: From hospital to home. *American Journal of Nursing, 105*(2), 52–61.

Petersen, R. (Ed.). (2002). *Mayo Clinic on Alzheimer's disease.* Rochester, MN: Mayo Clinic Health Information.

Rathier, M., & McElhaney, J. (2005). Delirium in elderly patients: How you can help. *Applied Neurology.* Retrieved June 3, 2007, from http://appneurology.com/showArticle.jhtml?articleID=170100541

Resnick, B. (2003). Putting research into practice: Behavioral and pharmacologic management of dementia. *Geriatric Nursing, 24*(1), 58–59.

Rowe, M. (2003). People with dementia who become lost, preventing injuries and death. *American Journal of Nursing, 103*(7), 32–39.

Schweiger, J., & Huey, R. (1999). Alzheimer's disease, your role in the caregiving equation. *Nursing1999, 29*(6), 34–41.

Shankle, W., & Amen, D. (2004). *Preventing Alzheimer's.* New York: G.P. Putnam's Sons.

Valeo, T. (2006). How to treat ailing memory. *Neurology Now, 2*(2), 40–41.

Vogel, C. (2005). Clearing up the confusion about delirium. *NurseWeek, 6*(12), 17–19.

Waszynski, C. (2007). The confusion assessment method. *Best Practices in Nursing Care to Older Adults, 13.* Hartford Institute for Geriatric Nursing. Retrieved June 3, 2007, from http://www.GeroNurseOnline.org

CHAPTER 16

American Medical Association. (2000). *AMA data on violence between intimates (1–00).* Retrieved August 6, 2007, from http://www.ama-assn.org/ama/pub/category/13577.htm#violence_between_samesex_partners

Anbarghalami, R., Yang, L., Van Sell, S., & Miller-Anderson, M. (2007). When to suspect child abuse. *RN, 70*(4), 34–38.

Bavolek, S. J. (2000). The nurturing parenting programs. *Juvenile Justice Bulletin.* Retrieved August 6, 2007, from http://www.ncjrs.org/html/ojjdp/2000_11_1/contents.html

Berlinger, J. (2001). Domestic violence, how you can make a difference. *Nursing2001, 31*(8), 58–63.

Center for Substance Abuse Prevention. (2004). *It won't happen to me: Alcohol abuse and violence against women (for those who are concerned about the issue).* Substance Abuse and Mental Health Services Administration. Washington, DC: Author. Retrieved August 28, 2007, from http://pathwayscourses.samhsa.gov/vawc/vawc_intro_pg1.htm

Fishwick, N., Parker, B., & Campbell, J. C. (2001). Care of survivors of abuse and violence. In G. W. Stuart & M. T. Laraia (Eds.), *Principles and practice of psychiatric nursing* (7th ed.). St. Louis: Mosby.

Gray-Vickrey, P. (2004). Combating elder abuse. *Nursing2004, 34*(10), 47–51.

Hastings, D. P. (2001). The New Hampshire health initiative on domestic violence. *Nursing Forum, 36*(1), 31.

Hockenberry, M. J. (2005). *Wong's essentials of pediatric nursing* (7th ed.). St. Louis: Mosby.

Isaac, N., & Enos, V. (2001). Documenting domestic violence: How health care providers can help victims. *National Institute of Justice Research in Brief.* Retrieved August 6, 2007, from http://www.ncjrs.org/pdffiles/nij/188564.pdf

Kneisl, C. R., Wilson, H. S., & Trigoboff, E. (2004). Contemporary psychiatric–mental health nursing. Upper Saddle River, NJ: Prentice Hall.

Kovach, K. (2004). Intimate partner violence. *RN, 67*(8), 38–43.

McFarlane, J., Malecha, A., Gist, J., Watson, K., Batten, E., Hall, I., & Smith, S. (2004). Increasing the safety-promoting behaviors of abused women. *American Journal of Nursing, 104*(3), 40–50.

Moss, H. B., Lynch, K. G., Hardie, T. L., & Baron, D. A. (2002). Family functioning and peer affiliation in children of fathers with antisocial personality disorder and substance dependence: Association with problem behaviors. *American Journal of Psychiatry, 159,* 607–614.

Mulryan, K., Cathers, P., & Fagin, A. (2000). Combating abuse: Protecting the child. *Nursing2000, 30*(7), 39–43.

National Center on Elder Abuse. (2005). Elder abuse prevalence and incidence. *Fact Sheet.* Retrieved August 8, 2007, from http://www.elderabusecenter.org/pdf/publication/FinalStatistics050331.pdf

National Center on Elder Abuse. (2006). Abuse of adults aged 60+ 2004 survey of adult protective services. *Fact Sheet.* Retrieved August 8, 2007, from http://www.elderabusecenter.org/pdf/2-14-06%2060FACT%20SHEET.pdf

National Institute for Occupational Safety and Health (NIOSH). (2002). *Violence: Occupational hazards in hospitals.* Dept. of Health and Human Services (NIOSH) Pub. No. 2002-101. Retrieved August 30, 2007, from www.cdc.gov/niosh/2002-101.html

Pryor, J. (2006). What do nurses do in response to their predictions of aggression? *Journal of Neuroscience Nursing 38*(3), 177–182. Retrieved August 17, 2007, from http://www.medscape.com/viewarticle/548017?rss

Rape, Abuse & Incest National Network. (2005). *Key facts.* Retrieved August 5, 2007, from http://www.rainn.org/statistics/index.html

Rickelman, B. L. (2003). The client who displays angry, aggressive, or violent behavior. In Mohr, W. K. (Ed.), *Johnson's psychiatric–mental health nursing.* Philadelphia: Lippincott.

Smith, M. E., & Kelly, L. M. (2001). The journey of recovery after a rape. *Issues in Mental Health Nursing, 22,* 337–352.

Voice of America. (2004, March 4). Help for battered immigrant women. Retrieved August 13, 2007, from http://www.voanews.com/english/archive/2004-03/a-2004-03-04-43-1.cfm

Walton-Moss, B., & Campbell, J. (2002). Intimate partner violence: Implications for nursing. *Online Journal of Issues in Nursing, 7*(1), 1–15. Retrieved August 23, 2007, from http://www.nursingworld.org/MainMenuCategories/ANAMarketplace/ANAPeriodicals/OJIN/JournalTopics/DomesticViolence.aspx

Widom, C. S., & Maxfield, M. G. (2001). *An update on the cycle of violence. National Institute of Justice Research in Brief, Feb. 2001.* Retrieved August 23, 2007, from http://www.ncjrs.org/pdffiles1/nij/184894.pdf

Wilkinson, S. (2003). A recipe for violence. *Chemical and Engineering News, 81*(22), 33–37. Retrieved August 6, 2007, from http://pubs.acs.org/cen/science/8122/8122sci1page1.html

World Health Organization. (2002). *World report on violence and health.* Geneva: Author. Retrieved August 31, 2003, from http://www.who.int/violence_injury_prevention/violence/world_report/wrvh1/en/

World Health Organization. (2007). *Third milestones of a global campaign for violence prevention report 2007, scaling up.* Geneva: Author. Retrieved August 6, 2007, from http://whqlibdoc.who.int/publications/2007/9789241595476_eng.pdf

CHAPTER 17

Aguilera, D. C. (1998). *Crisis intervention: Theory and methodology* (8th ed.). St. Louis: Mosby.

AIDS Dementia Complex. (2005, June 12). *Alzheimer's disease.* Retrieved July 22, 2007, from http://www.alzheimers.about.com/od/typesof dementia/a/hiv_complex.htm

American Psychiatric Association. (2000). *Diagnostic and statistical manual of mental disorders* (4th ed., Text Revision). Washington, DC: American Psychiatric Press.

Andrews, M. M., & Boyle, J. S. (2003). *Transcultural concepts in nursing care* (4th ed.). Philadelphia: Lippincott.

Arnold, E., & Hallinan, K. (2000). Mind over matter: Helping a mentally ill patient in the acute care setting. *Nursing, 30*(10), 50–53.

Childers, L. (2003). Uncool customers. *NurseWeek, 4*(2), 22–23.

Cohan, C. L., & Cole, S. W. (2002). Life course transitions and natural disasters: Marriage, birth, and divorce following Hurricane Hugo. *Journal of Family Psychology, 16*(1), 14–25.

Doenges, M. E., Moorhouse, M. F., & Geissler-Murr, A. (2002). *Nurse's pocket guide: Diagnoses, interventions, and rationales* (8th ed.). Philadelphia: F. A. Davis.

Dunn, K. S., & Horgas, A. L. (2000). The prevalence of prayer as a spiritual self-care modality in elders. *Journal of Holistic Nursing, 18*(4), 337–351.

Gorman, L. M., Raines, M. L., & Sultan, D. F. (2002). *Psychosocial nursing for general client care* (2nd ed.). Philadelphia: F. A. Davis.

Hemmila, D. (2002). You gotta have faith. *NurseWeek, 3*(12), 11–12.

Hicks, T. J. (1999). Spirituality and the elderly. *Geriatric Nursing, 20*(3), 144–146.

Joint Commission. (2003). The expert connection: Five strategies for effective spiritual assessment. *The Source, 1*(8), 1–2. Retrieved July 22, 2007, from http://www.jcrinc.com/5408/. Used with permission.

Joint Commission. (2005). Evaluating your spiritual assessment process. *The Source, 3*(2), 6–7. Retrieved July 27, 2007, from http://www. pastoralreport.com/archives/spiritual.pdf

Kneisl, C. R., Wilson, H. S., & Trigoboff, E. (2004). *Contemporary psychiatric–mental health nursing.* Upper Saddle River, NJ: Prentice Hall.

Meisenhelder, J. B., & Chandler, E. N. (2000). Prayer and health outcomes in church members. *Alternative Therapies in Health and Medicine, 6*(4), 56–60.

Millon, T., & Davis, R. (1999). *Personality disorders in modern life.* New York: John Wiley & Sons.

Mohr, W. K. (2003). *Johnson's psychiatric mental health nursing.* Philadelphia: Lippincott.

North American Nursing Diagnosis Association International (NANDA I). (2005). *Nursing diagnosis definitions and classifications 2005–2006* (4th ed.). Philadelphia: Author.

Registered Nurses Association of Ontario. (2006). *Crisis intervention* (revised supplement). Toronto, Ontario: Author. Retrieved July 27, 2007, from www.guideline.gov/summary/summary.aspx?ss=15&doc_id=9192&nbr=4950

Schultz, J. M., & Videbeck, S. L. (2004). *Lippincott's manual of psychiatric nursing care plans* (7th ed.). Philadelphia: Lippincott.

Stuart, G. W., & Laraia, M. T. (2001). *Principles and practice of psychiatric nursing* (7th ed.). St. Louis: Mosby.

Townsend, M. (2002). *Essentials of psychiatric mental health nursing.* Philadelphia: F. A. Davis.

Varcarolis, E. M. (2000). *Psychiatric nursing clinical guide: Assessment tools and diagnoses.* Philadelphia: W. B. Saunders.

Weber, D. (2006). Balancing act: Where spirituality and healthcare meet. *RN, 69*(9), 53–54.

Glossary

(Note: Boldface numbers after the glossary term indicate the chapter in which the term is defined. Other words or terms that may require definitions are italicized in the text and are defined there.)

A

Abstinence: complete lack of drug use **(12)**

Acetylcholine: neurotransmitter chemical that controls sleep-wake cycle, and signals muscles to become active **(7)**

Acting out: using actions instead of thoughts or feelings to respond to stress or emotional distress **(3)**

Active listening: careful attention to the sender's whole verbal and the nonverbal message **(5)**

Adaptability: ability to compromise, plan, and be flexible **(1)**

Adaptation: behavior that maintains the integrity of the individual **(6)**

Adaptive behavior: positive, health-promoting problem-solving behavior **(3)**

Addiction: the compulsive and maladaptive use of a substance (drug or alcohol) as a coping mechanism or to relieve anxiety **(12)**

Adverse effects: undesired or toxic effects of a drug **(7)**

Affect: (a'fekt) nonverbal expression of emotion **(8)**

Aggression: forceful physical or verbal action, which can be dangerous or perceived as dangerous **(16)**

Agnosia: loss of comprehension of auditory or verbal stimuli although the sensory organs remain intact **(15)**

Agonists: drugs that stimulate cellular functions **(7)**

Akathisia: restlessness, intense need to move **(8)**

Alogia: decreased amount or richness of speech. Also called *poverty of speech.* Suggests a reduction in thinking. Associated with schizophrenia and depression **(8)**

Amenorrhea: absence of menstrual periods **(14)**

Anhedonia: lack of the ability to feel pleasure **(8)**

Antagonists: drugs that prevent or inhibit cell functions **(7)**

Antisocial Personality Disorder: pervasive pattern of disregarding and violating the rights of others, lack of conscience **(10)**

Anxiety: feeling of uneasiness and activation of the autonomic nervous system in response to a vague, nonspecific threat **(11)**

Aphasia: the inability to either understand received communication or to communicate verbally due to brain dysfunction **(15)**

Apraxia: impaired ability to perform purposeful movement even though motor abilities and sensory functions are intact **(15)**

Attending behaviors: actions that communicate the listener's attention and interest **(5)**

Attributions: the meaning a person places on (attributes to) an event **(16)**

Autonomy: self-determination and personal freedom; the right to choose what will happen to oneself **(2)**

Avoidant Personality Disorder: a pervasive pattern of social shyness, feelings of inadequacy, and hypersensitivity to negative evaluation **(10)**

Avolition: a lack of motivation **(8)**

B

Beneficence: promoting good for others **(2)**

Beta-amyloid plaques: buildup of fragments produced when certain enzymes in the body act on amyloid protein **(15)**

Binge: eating in a limited period of time (usually within 2 hours) an amount of food that is definitely larger than most individuals would eat under similar circumstances **(14)**

Blackouts: loss of memory of events that happened while intoxicated (happens late in the disease of alcoholism) **(12)**

Body image: the perception that people have about their own bodies, how they see themselves **(13)**

Body mass index (BMI): a calculation intended to determine how fat or lean a person is; the formula is body weight divided by the square of height; normal is 18.5–25; obese is greater than 30 **(14)**

Borderline Personality Disorder: pervasive pattern of unpredictable and impulsive behavior, irritability, sadness, fear, self-mutilation, and difficulty maintaining relationships **(10)**

Burnout: state of physical, emotional, and mental exhaustion caused by long-term involvement in situations that are emotionally demanding **(4)**

C

Cachexia: a state of malnutrition, illness, and body wasting **(14)**

Caring: concern for the well-being of another **(4)**

Catastrophic reactions: explosive responses that are totally out of proportion to the situation that caused them **(15)**

Catatonic behavior: associated with schizophrenia, a stupor in which the client is unable to move or talk **(8)**

Cholinesterase inhibitors: medications that prolong the time that the body has use of acetylcholine; useful in early and middle stages of AD **(15)**

Chronic illness: a disease of long duration, usually characterized by exacerbations and remissions **(17)**

Circadian: happening on a day/night cycle, as *circadian rhythm* **(13)**

Civil commitment: involuntary hospitalization **(2)**

Clarifying: restating the client's message in the nurse's own words, or asking about the client's message for the purpose of ensuring that sender and receiver understand the same message **(5)**

Codependency: letting another person's behavior affect you and becoming obsessed with controlling that person's behavior; also, reinforcing another person's addictive behavior by allowing that person to avoid consequences of behavior **(4)**

Cognition: mental process by which knowledge is acquired and processed, including reasoning, judgment, memory, awareness, and perception **(3)**

Cognitive reframing: restructuring irrational or self-defeating beliefs (6)

Commitment: personal pledge to some course of action (4)

Communication: the act of sending and receiving a message (5)

Compassion: sharing in the emotional state of another; includes empathy and acceptance (4)

Compensation: attempt (conscious or unconscious) to overcome perceived inadequacies (3)

Competence: proficiency in understanding important information and applying this knowledge to problem solving and decision making (4)

Competency: legal assessment that a person is able to make reasonable judgments and decisions (2)

Competency to stand trial: ability of a person to understand the significance and consequences of his/her actions, to understand what is right and wrong, to assist a lawyer in his/her defense (2)

Compulsions: repetitive behaviors or mental acts that the affected person feels driven to perform in response to obsessive thoughts (11)

Compulsive substance use: repetitive substance use behavior for the purpose of reducing distress; often unwanted and time-consuming (12)

Concreteness: the use of realistic language, rather than abstract terms, jargon, or medical terminology (5)

Conduct Disorder: cruelty to people or animals, deceitfulness or theft, destruction of property, and serious violations of rules (10)

Confabulation: created (made up) responses to conceal that the client does not remember what happened (12)

Confidence: belief in oneself (4)

Confidentiality: limits on access to information about a client (2)

Congruence: matching of verbal and nonverbal messages (5)

Conscience: having an ethical conviction or belief about what is right and wrong (4)

Consumers (of mental health services): as part of the advocacy movement for mentally ill people, some affected people came to prefer the term *consumer* to *client* (8)

Control issues: informal term that refers to how people behave when they experience the sense of their own loss of control (which is important to them) (14)

Coping: behaviors to help a person adapt to or manage stress or change (11)

Coping mechanism: pattern response in reaction to stress for purpose of handling stress (6)

Countertransference: situation in which the nurse has feelings toward the client based on the nurse's previous experiences (5)

Crisis: an acute, time-limited state of disequilibrium or imbalance (17)

Cross-tolerance: tolerance to several drugs in the same classification (12)

D

Dangerousness: actions that have a high risk of harming self or others (16)

Defense mechanisms: thoughts and behaviors that distort reality to protect the self (3)

Deinstitutionalization: the movement to discharge people from psychiatric institutions to treat them in the community (1)

Delirium: an acute, reversible state of mental confusion (15)

Delusions: fixed false beliefs, despite evidence that they are not true (8)

Dementia: a progressive, irreversible loss of cognitive functioning that impairs a person's ability to function in social or occupational situations (15)

Denial: refusal to acknowledge a painful reality (12)

Dependent Personality Disorder: pervasive pattern of submissive and clinging behavior and fears of separation and abandonment (10)

Depot injection: drug form injected intramuscularly for the purpose of slow release of the drug over several weeks (8)

Detoxification: the period of time during which all the drugs or alcohol the client has consumed are removed from the body (12)

Developmental tasks: activities required for mastery of each of the eight stages in Erikson's psychosocial development theory (3)

Disorganized behavior: sequence of behavior that does not make sense; disjointed, unconnected; suggests disorganized thinking (8)

Disorganized symptoms: purposeless behavior; evidence that the client's thoughts are disorganized (8)

Disorganized thinking: thinking, reflected in speech and behavior, that is not logically connected (8)

Displacement: transferring a feeling about one person or object to another usually safer one (3)

Dissociation: a disruption in the usually integrated functions of consciousness so that one feels detached from the self, as if an outside observer. This is a mechanism for coping with unendurable stress or psychological trauma (3)

Distractibility: inability to screen out excess sensory stimuli (9)

Disturbance of executive functioning: inability to think abstractly or to use critical thinking to plan, initiate, sequence, monitor, and stop complex behavior (15)

Dopamine: neurotransmitter chemical that controls complex movements, cognition, motivation, pleasure, and regulation of emotional responses (7)

Dual diagnosis: existence of both a substance use disorder and a serious mental illness (12)

Dyskinesia: abnormal involuntary movement (8)

Dyslexia: the central feature of Reading Disorder; includes decreased reading accuracy, speed, or comprehension (13)

Dysphoric mood: uncomfortable, dissatisfied, low mood but not as low as depression (9)

Dystonia: muscular rigidity, abnormal muscle contraction (8)

E

Elder abuse: physical or emotional abuse or neglect of an older adult by a spouse, a grown child, or a caregiver (16)

Electroconvulsive therapy (ECT): an effective treatment for depression in which electrical brain stimulation causes a controlled generalized seizure (9)

Elevated mood: an exaggerated sense of well-being (9)

Emaciated: excessively thin, muscle-wasted (14)

Emotional abuse: demeaning, devaluing, intimidating, instilling fear, or otherwise mistreatment of another by psychological means (16)

Emotionally labile: rapid change in moods for no apparent reason (15)

Empathy: ability to understand a situation from the client's point of view without losing objectivity or identity (5)

Encopresis: voluntary or (usually) involuntary passing of feces into inappropriate places (13)

Enuresis: repeated voiding of urine into bed or clothes (either involuntary or intentional), which occurs at least twice per week for at least 3 months (13)

Ethical dilemma: situation in which there are conflicting moral alternatives for action and each option includes positive and negative consequences (2)

Ethics: science relating to moral principles or standards governing conduct (2)

Euthymic mood: in the normal range (9)

Exacerbation: flare-ups of a chronic disease (17)

Executive function: abstract thinking and problem solving (8)

Extrapyramidal symptoms: abnormal involuntary movements (dyskinesia, akathisia, dystonia, pseudoparkinsonism, Tardive Dyskinesia), which are adverse effects of antipsychotic drugs (8)

F

Fidelity: faithfulness; keeping promises (2)

Fight or flight response: physiological reaction to stress (6)

Flight of ideas: state in which thoughts are moving so fast that the client's speech jumps from one subject to another frequently (9)

Focusing: making generalizations specific (5)

G

General leads: a brief statement intended to indicate that the nurse is listening and to encourage the client to continue talking on the same subject (5)

Genuineness: honesty, sincerity, openness, and congruence in verbal and nonverbal messages (5)

H

Hallucinations: sensory perceptions that seem real but are not related to external stimuli (8)

Histrionic Personality Disorder: pervasive pattern of excessive emotionality and attention-seeking behavior (10)

Holism: philosophy that considers the client a total being with psychosocial, spiritual, and physical needs (3)

Homeostasis: a state of balance necessary for many physiological functions (6)

Humanism: an approach to care that is person-centered. It assumes that the person (client) is the priority and that people have autonomy and the desire to participate in their own problem solving and personal growth (17)

Hyperorality: infantile behavior of putting everything into the mouth (15)

I

Ideas of reference: misinterpretation of clients with psychosis that everyday events have a personal meaning for them (10)

Illusion: a misinterpretation of environmental stimuli (15)

Impaired nursing: practicing nursing under the influence of intoxicants (12)

Incompetence: inability to make judgments and be responsible for one's own decisions or actions (2)

Informed consent: agreement by a client to a treatment after a physician has explained it in understandable terms including potential outcomes with and without the treatment (2)

Insight: self-understanding (1)

Insomnia: difficulty falling asleep, staying asleep, or awakening too early and not being able to go back to sleep (11)

Integrity: acting consistently on one's values (2)

Intoxication: a reversible set of physical, psychological, and behavioral symptoms caused by use of a substance (12)

Irritable mood: state of being easily annoyed, upset, or provoked to anger (9)

J

Justice: equal, fair treatment of people (2)

K

Kindling: a hypothesis suggesting that a series of stressful stimuli may alter neurotransmitter function such that it requires progressively less stimulation to cause future seizures or manic episodes (9)

L

Least restrictive alternative: treatment that restricts personal freedom as little as possible (2)

Limit setting: setting parameters for behavior and making the client aware of these (17)

M

Maladaptation: unhealthy behavior that disrupts the integrity of the individual (6)

Maladaptive behavior: behavior that is unhealthy and does not promote problem solving (3)

Malpractice: failure of a professional person to act in accordance with accepted professional standards, or failure to act as a reasonable member of the profession would act (2)

Manipulation: maladaptive social response in which a person attempts to meet self-needs by controlling the behavior of others (17)

Milieu: the therapeutic environment (8)

Mood: a pervasive and sustained emotion that influences how a person perceives the world (9)

N

Narcissistic Personality Disorder: a pervasive pattern of grandiosity, need for admiration, and lack of empathy for others (10)

Nature or nurture controversy: debate about whether personality is due to biology (genetics) or to environment and experiences **(3)**

Negative symptoms: symptoms of schizophrenia characterized by deficits or slowness of movement, speech, and thinking **(8)**

Neglect: failure to provide for the physical, emotional, or developmental needs of a child **(16)**

Neurofibrillary tangles: tangled pairs of tau proteins in nerve cells **(15)**

Neuroleptics: an older name of antipsychotic drugs **(8)**

Neurotransmitters: chemicals that transmit impulses from one neuron to the next **(3)**

Nonmaleficence: doing no harm **(2)**

Norepinephrine: neurotransmitter chemical that affects attention, learning, memory, and regulation of mood, sleep, and wakefulness **(7)**

O

Objectivity: freedom from bias and personal identification **(5)**

Obsessions: recurrent and intrusive thoughts that cause marked distress **(11)**

Obsessive-Compulsive Personality Disorder: a pervasive pattern of preoccupation with orderliness, perfectionism, and mental and personal control **(10)**

Open-ended question: a question that requires an explanation or extended response by the client **(5)**

Orientation phase: first phase of Peplau's three-phase nurse-client relationship in which introductions are made, goals for the interaction are set, and the time limit of the interaction is defined **(5)**

Outpatient commitment: court order requiring the mentally ill person to take medication and to comply with the individual's treatment plan as a condition of release from the hospital **(2)**

P

Panic attack: an episode of intense fear or discomfort accompanied by autonomic stimulation **(11)**

Paradoxical: contradictory, opposite **(11)**

Paranoid Personality Disorder: a pattern of distrust and suspiciousness that other people are acting maliciously toward the affected individual **(10)**

Paternalism: acting "in the best interest" of other people; making decisions for others **(2)**

Perpetrator: person who inflicts violence on another **(16)**

Perseveration: repetitive speech or behavior **(15)**

Personal boundaries: limits people set on their interactions with others **(4)**

Personal identity: the perception of people of their own characteristics, thoughts, feelings, sense of self **(13)**

Personality: relatively stable way that a person thinks, feels, and behaves **(3)**

Phobia: persistent and irrational fear **(11)**

Physical abuse: violence toward another or in some cases physical restraint **(16)**

Polydipsia: excessive thirst **(7)**

Polypharmacy: the use (or prescription) of many drugs **(15)**

Positive symptoms: symptoms of schizophrenia characterized by extra thought processes that people without the disorder do not have, such as hallucinations and delusions (psychosis) **(8)**

Posttraumatic Stress Disorder (PTSD): debilitating condition that follows an extreme traumatic stressor **(11)**

Pressured speech: speech that is so fast and determined that it is hard to interrupt **(9)**

Process recording: a written record of a therapeutic conversation between a nursing student and a client that is analyzed by the student for the purpose of developing the student's insight and communication skills **(5)**

Projection: attributing one's own unacceptable feelings or thoughts to another **(10)**

Pseudoparkinsonism: (dyskinesia) including or consisting of stiff, stooped posture; shuffling gait; tremor; slow movements; cogwheel rigidity; and mask-like facies **(8)**

Psychomotor agitation: increased activity as a result of mental processes **(9)**

Psychomotor retardation: reduced physical activity as a result of mental processes **(9)**

Psychosis: disorganization of the personality and impaired ability to interpret reality, to relate to self and others, and to function; may include hallucinations and delusional thinking **(8)**

Psychotropic drugs: drugs that affect thinking and treat mental illness **(1)**

Purging: self-induced vomiting or abuse of laxatives or diuretics **(14)**

R

Rape: sexual assault or sexual violence perpetrated against the will of the victim or against a victim who is too young to give consent **(16)**

Reaction formation: substituting behavior or feelings that are the opposite of what one actually feels **(3)**

Reality: what really is or exists **(1)**

Reality orientation: reminding the client of the real date, place, and the client's identity **(15)**

Redirection: changing the client's attention from an unacceptable behavior to one that is more acceptable **(17)**

Reflection: a therapeutic communication technique in which the nurse repeats back all or part of what the client said to encourage the client to expand on or explain the original statement **(5)**

Regression: return to an earlier, less stressful level of development **(3)**

Relapse: recurrent episode of a chronic disorder after a period free of symptoms **(12)**

Reminiscence therapy: therapy in which clients with dementia are encouraged to talk about long-term memories **(15)**

Remission: decrease or resolution of disease symptoms of chronic illness **(17)**

Repression: removing unacceptable thoughts or wishes from consciousness **(3)**

Resilience: the ability to return to normal after a stressful traumatic situation that would change most people or with which most people could not cope **(13)**

Respect: to hold in high regard; to honor **(5)**

Reuptake: is the process in which the neurotransmitter is taken back into the axon to be stored for later use **(7)**

S

Seasonal affective disorder (SAD): depression that is associated with shortened exposure to daylight **(9)**

Seclusion: confinement in a room alone **(2)**

Self-disclosure: in the context of mental health nursing, the relating of the nurse's feelings or personal experiences to the client **(5)**

Self-efficacy: the belief that a person is able to cause a desired outcome (reach a goal) by his or her own efforts **(3)**

Self-esteem: one's personal view or regard of the self **(13)**

Serotonin: neurotransmitter chemical that affects sleep, wakefulness, especially falling asleep, and affects mood and thought processes **(7)**

Sexual abuse: mistreatment of another by sexual means (rape, fondling, sexual molestation); perpetrator and victim can be of either gender **(16)**

Sexual assault: any forced sexual contact without consent, or sexual contact with a minor regardless of consent **(16)**

Sharing observations: expressing client behavior in words to call attention to implied meanings, or contradictions **(5)**

Side effects: a drug action that is other than the desired effect **(7)**

Somatic therapies: therapies involving the body, such as electroshock therapy **(1)**

Somatization: the experience of emotional stress as physical symptoms **(9)**

Splitting: tending to see people or situations as either all good or all bad **(17)**

Staff splitting: playing one staff member against another; using staff to obtain privileges or to avoid responsibilities **(17)**

Standards of nursing care: ethical and legal expectations for practice; they are the level of work quality considered adequate by the profession **(2)**

Stigma: mark of disgrace **(1)**

Stress response: the physiological response to stress; sympathetic nervous system stimulation **(6)**

Stressor: event that causes the stress response **(6)**

Sublimation: unacceptable feelings are diverted into socially acceptable behavior **(3)**

Substance abuse: a maladaptive pattern of substance use leading to significant impairment or distress **(12)**

Substance dependency: a maladaptive pattern of substance use despite continuing negative consequences of substance abuse; includes tolerance and withdrawal symptoms **(12)**

Substance-induced delirium: a reversible delirium caused by substances (drugs or alcohol) **(15)**

Suicidal ideation: suicidal thinking **(9)**

Sundowning: increased confusion noted in clients with Alzheimer's Disease in the late afternoon or evening **(15)**

Suppression: intentionally avoiding thinking about unacceptable or stressful feelings **(3)**

Synapse: space between the axon and its target cell's dendrite **(7)**

T

Tardive dyskinesia: late onset of abnormal involuntary movement; a side effect of antipsychotic drugs that may be permanent **(8)**

Target symptoms: specific symptoms that medications are expected to treat **(7)**

Termination phase: final phase of the nurse-client relationship that occurs after the work of the relationship is complete; the nurse and client summarize their progress toward the goals set in the orientation phase **(5)**

Therapeutic communication: intervention in which the nurse uses communication techniques to help the client achieve desired outcomes **(5)**

Therapeutic use of self: the ability to use the self consciously and in full awareness, to structure nursing interventions **(5)**

Tolerance: a need for increased amounts of the substance to achieve the same effect; a diminished effect with continued use of the same amount of the substance **(12)**

Toxic effects: a term usually used to describe adverse effects of drugs resulting from too high a dose or inability of the body to metabolize and excrete a drug fast enough **(7)**

Transference: situation in which a client feels emotions from the past and applies (or transfers) them to the therapeutic relationship **(5)**

Trustworthiness: behavior that is predictable, competent, and in the client's best interest **(5)**

U

Unconscious mind: the part of the mind that is not accessible to conscious thoughts **(3)**

V

Validation: verbal recognition and acknowledgment of the client's feelings **(5)**

Values: personal beliefs about the worth of an idea, object, or behavior **(2)**

Values clarification: a process of self-discovery in which people identify their own values and prioritize them **(2)**

Veracity: truth telling **(2)**

Vicious cycle of behavior: self-defeating, rigid behaviors that perpetuate problems; a hallmark of people with personality disorder **(10)**

Violence: intentional use of physical force or power, threatened or actual, against another person, against oneself, or against a group or community, that either results in or has a high likelihood of resulting in injury, death, psychological harm, abnormal development, or deprivation **(16)**

W

Withdrawal: the symptoms experienced when a person with substance dependency abstains from substance use; caused by imbalance during which the homeostatic mechanism in CNS that balances the effects of alcohol or other substances has not returned to normal **(12)**

Working phase: the second phase of the nurse-client relationship in which the nurse implements interventions designed to reach the goals set in the orientation phase; nurse and client work together to achieve the client's optimal level of functioning based on the client's strengths and challenges **(5)**

Index

(*Note:* Material presented in boxes, figures, and tables is indicated respectively with an italicized *b, f,* or *t* following the page number.)

F

Falling out, explained, 5*b*
Falls, protecting against, 317, 319
Familial disorders, 115–116, 304. *See also* Genetics
Families
  Alzheimer's disease, 316
  input from, for assessment, 134
  violence, 331–337, 332*f*, 334*b*, 334*f*, 336*b*
  violence, perpetrators of, 341–342, 341*b*
Fear, 200
Feedback, 65
Fetal alcohol syndrome, 232, 232*f*
Fidelity as ethical principle, 18
Fight or flight response, 83–84, 84*f*
Filipino heritage, clients with, 238*b*
Five-axis diagnosis system, 6
Five Cs of caring, 50, 50*f*
Five Senses Exercise, 192
Flat affect
  mental status assessment, 133*b*
  schizophrenia, 119
Flight of ideas
  mental status assessment, 133*b*
  mood disorder assessment, 166–167
Fluid and electrolyte balance, 163
Fluoxetine (Prozac)
  dementia, 314
  depression, 152*t*
  eating disorders, 284
  Symbyax for bipolar disorder, 164
  violence in the healthcare setting, 347
Fluphenazine (Prolixin)
  depot injection, 129
  schizophrenia, 123*t*
Flurazepam (Dalmane), 215*t*, 216*t*
Fluvoxamine (Luvox), 152*t*
Focusing as communication technique, 74*t*
Folstein Mini-Mental State Exam, 300
Foreseeability of injury, 25
Forgetting, 218
Formal operations stage of cognitive
  development, 41
Frankl, Victor, 43
Free radicals, 306
Freud, Sigmund, 31, 32, 34
Fun activities, 56–57, 57–58*b*, 57*f*

G

GABA (gamma-aminobutyric acid), 98*t*
Galactorrhea, 128
Galantamine (Razadyne), 312–313, 312*t*
Gamma-aminobutyric acid (GABA), 98*t*
Gardner, Howard, 41–42
Gastrointestinal system, 229, 231*f*
Gay, lesbian, bisexual, and transgender
  individuals, 269
Gender differences
  Anorexia Nervosa, 280
  Borderline Personality Disorder, 183
  Bulimia Nervosa, 281
  Childhood Disintegrative Disorder, 259
  Conduct Disorder, 265

  depression, 146
  family violence, 332
  Generalized Anxiety Disorder, 204
  Rett's Disorder, 259
  Specific Phobias, 211
General leads as communication technique, 74*t*
Generalized Anxiety Disorder, 203–204, 219–220
Generalized statements as barrier to
  communication, 70*t*, 71
Generativity *versus* stagnation stage of psychosocial
  development, 37*t*
Genetics
  ADHD, 259–260
  Alzheimer's disease, 304, 311
  bipolar disorder, 160
  depression, 145
  eating disorders, 282, 283*f*
  mental illness, 100
  Mental Retardation, 254*b*
  resilience, 253
  schizophrenia, 115–116
Genuineness in nurse-client relationship, 65*b*
Geodon (ziprasidone), 123*t*
Gephyrophobia, 211*t*
Geriatric Depression Scale, 148, 150, 150*b*, 164
Gestalt theory, 40–41
Gestalt therapy, 42–43
Gifts, accepting from clients, 76–77
Gingko biloba, 314*b*
Glaucoma, 155
Glutamate, 98*t*
Goal directed therapeutic relationships, 63
Goals, realistic, and self-esteem, 270
Grandiose delusions, 118*t*
Grandiosity, and mental status assessment, 133*b*
Group interventions, 181
Group therapy
  bipolar disorder, 164
  special populations, 368, 368*b*
  substance abuse, 239, 239*b*
Gynecomastia, 128

H

Halcion (triazolam), 215*t*, 216*t*
Haldol. *See* Haloperidol (Haldol)
Hallucinations
  mental status assessment, 133*b*
  schizophrenia, 117–118, 125*b*, 135, 136*t*
Hallucinogens, 234–235, 236*t*
Haloperidol (Haldol)
  delirium, 301
  dementia, 314
  depot injection, 129
  schizophrenia, 123*t*
  violence in the healthcare setting, 347
Harrell, Tom, 119, 119*f*
Health problem, substance abuse as, 225, 225*f*, 226*f*
Healthcare workplace, violence in, 344–347, 345*f*,
  346*t*, 347*b*
Healthy People 2010, 9*b*
Hematophobia, 211*t*
Hepatic encephalopathy, 231–232
Hepatitis, 229, 231*f*

Heroin, 230*t*
Hierarchy of needs theory, 44–45, 44*f*
Hippocampus, 200*t*
Hippocrates, 7
Historical perspectives of mental illness, 7–9, 8*f*, 9*b*
Histrionic Personality Disorder, 177*t*, 184–185,
  184*f*, 189*t*, 191*b*, 193
HIV (human immunodeficiency virus), 368
Hoarding, 188, 188*f*
Holism, defined, 31
Holistic nursing care, 355, 355*f*
Homelessness, 115, 120
Homeostasis, emotional, 83, 83*f*
HOPE (Hope, Organized religion, Personal
  spirituality, Effects on medical care or end-
  of-life issues) mnemonic to assess spiritual
  health, 369
Hopelessness
  adolescent suicide, 269
  mood disorders, 169
Hormones, 101*t*
Horney, Karen, 34–35, 35*f*
Hostility, 217
HPA (hypothalamus, pituitary, adrenal) axis, 145
Human Genome Project, 100
Human immunodeficiency virus (HIV), 368
Humanism, defined, 360
Humanistic theories of personality, 43–45, 44*f*, 45*bf*
Humor as defense mechanism, 33*t*
Humors, body, as cause of illness, 7
Huntington disease, 98*t*
Huperzine A, 314*b*
Hydrophobia, 211*t*
Hydroxyzine (Atarax, Vistaril), 216*t*
Hyperactive delirium, 298*t*
Hyperactivity with ADHD, 260, 260*b*, 260*f*
Hyperorality, 308
Hypertensive crises with MAOIs, 156, 156*b*
Hyperthyroidism, 211*b*
Hypnotics
  effects of, and overdosage, and withdrawal, 230*t*
  substance abuse, 233
Hypoactive delirium, 298*t*
Hypocrisy, defined, 16
Hypoglycemia, 211*b*
Hypothalamus
  anxiety disorders, 200*t*
  depression, 145

I

Iatrophobia, 211*t*
Ibuprofen (Motrin), 314
Id, 31
Ideas of reference
  mental status assessment, 133*b*
  Schizotypal Personality Disorder, 180
Identity *versus* role confusion stage of psychosocial
  development, 36*f*, 36*t*
Idiosyncratic reaction to drugs, 300
Illness. *See* Medical conditions and illnesses
Illusions, 307
Imidazopyridines, 215–216*t*
Imipramine (Tofranil), 153*t*

Immigrants, 341, 341*b*
Immune system, 116
Impaired nursing, defined, 240
Impressionistic speech, 184
Impulsive behavior
    ADHD, 260, 260*b*, 261*f*
    Antisocial Personality Disorder, 181
    Borderline Personality Disorder, 183
    personality disorders, 177
    suicide, 268
Inappropriate affect, 180
Inapsine (droperidol), 123*t*
Incompetence, legal, 23
Independence, 187
Inderal (propranolol), 214*t*, 215*t*
Individuals, cultural identity of, 5*b*
Indocin (indomethacin), 314
Indomethacin (Indocin), 314
Industry *versus* inferiority stage of psychosocial
        development, 36*t*
Inferiority complex, 34
Inflammatory response abnormalities, 116
Inflexibility of behavior, 177
Informed consent, 23
Inhalants, 235, 235*f*, 236*t*
Initiative *versus* guilt stage of psychosocial
        development, 36*t*
Injuries, and malpractice, 25
Insight, defined, 3
Insomnia, 213
Integrity, defined, 16
Intellectualization
    anxiety disorders, 218
    as defense mechanism, 33*t*
Intelligence, 41–42
Intention tremor, 96*t*
Internal standards of nursing care, 18
Interpersonal psychotherapy, 157
Interpersonal relationships, 178
Interpersonal theories of personality, 46
Interventions for workplace safety, 346–347, 347*b*
Intimacy *versus* isolation stage of psychosocial
        development, 36*t*
Intimate partner violence, 334–335, 334*f*
Intimate personal space, 67*f*, 68
Intoxication, defined, 227
Introverts, 38
Involuntary admission (commitment), 20–21
Ion channels into dendrites, 98
Irish heritage, clients with, 238*b*
Irresponsibility, 181
Irritable mood, 144
Isocarboxazid (Marplan), 153*t*
Isolation, 179, 179*f*

J

Japanese heritage, clients with, 238*b*
Jewish faith, 238*b*
Johns Hopkins Hospital School, 8
Joint Commission (formerly Joint Commission on
        Accreditation of Healthcare Organizations,
        or JCAHO), 300, 368, 369

Jung, Carl, 34
Justice, 18

K

Kemadrin (procyclidine), 126*t*
Kindling, described, 145
Klein, Melanie, 37
Klonopin (clonazepam), 214*t*, 216*t*
Korsakoff's syndrome, 95*t*, 232

L

Labile affect, 133*b*
Lactulose (Cephulac), 232
Lamictal (lamotrigine), 163*t*, 164
Lamotrigine (Lamictal), 163*t*, 164
Language, foreign
    Communication Disorders, assessing, 257*b*
    culturally appropriate care, 26, 26*b*
Language, using, with survivors of violence, 342
Language disturbances with Alzheimer's disease,
        309–310, 318–319*b*
Latino heritage, clients with
    cultural relativism, 133*b*
    depression, signs and symptoms of, 166*b*
Learning Disorders
    ADHD, 261
    developmental disorders, 254–256, 255*f*, 256*b*
Learning personality theories, 39–40
Least restrictive alternative, defined, 21
Legal issues. *See also* Ethical and legal issues
    advance care directives, 24
    Americans with Disabilities Act (1990), 24
    competency, 22–24, 24*f*, 28
    culturally appropriate care, standards of,
        25–26, 26*b*
    documentation, nurse's responsibility in, 24–25
    family violence, 340–342, 341*b*
    law, types of, 19, 20*f*
    legal rights for mental health clients, 21–22,
        21*b*, 22*f*
    malpractice, 25
    nurse practice acts, 19–20
    psychiatric hospitalization, 20–21
Lexapro (escitalopram), 152*t*
Libido, 126
Librium (chlordiazepoxide), 214*t*, 216*t*
Lifestyle changes, and obesity, 286
Limbic system
    anxiety disorders, 200, 200*f*, 200*t*
    brain anatomy and function, 95*t*
Limit setting
    angry client, 362
    workplace safety, 346
Liquid oral forms of medication, 130
Lithium (Eskalith, Lithobid)
    bipolar disorder, 161, 162*t*, 163
    discovery of use as psychotropic drug, 8
    lithium levels, 161
    metabolic rate, ethnic variations in, 102*b*
    SSRIs, interaction with, 155
    toxicity, 161, 162*t*, 163
    violence in the healthcare setting, 347
Lithobid. *See* Lithium (Eskalith, Lithobid)

Logotherapy, 43
Long-term care facilities
    elder abuse, 340, 340*f*
    legal issues, 340
Loose association, 133*b*
Lorazepam (Ativan)
    anxiety disorders, 214*t*, 216*t*
    dementia, 314
    violence in the healthcare setting, 347
Love, unconditional, 270
Loxapine (Loxitane)
    delirium, 301
    schizophrenia, 123*t*
Loxitane. *See* Loxapine (Loxitane)
LSD (lysergic acid diethylamide), 234, 236*t*
Ludiomil (maprotiline), 153*t*
Lunatic, described, 7
Lunesta (eszopiclone), 215*t*
Luvox (fluvoxamine), 152*t*
Lysergic acid diethylamide (LSD), 234, 236*t*

M

Maclobemide (Manerix), 154*t*, 156
Magnetic resonance imaging (MRI), 99, 99*t*,
        100, 100*f*
Mahler, Margaret, 37
Maintenance phase of medication treatment, 103
Major Depressive Disorder
    anxiety disorders, 203
    common mental disorders, 6*b*
    depression, 144–149, 145*f*, 146*b*, 146*f*, 147*b*,
        147*f*, 148*f*
    diagnostic criteria, 144*b*
    electroconvulsive therapy, 157–158, 157*f*
    exercise, 157
    medications, 151–156, 152–154*t*, 152*f*, 154*b*,
        154*f*, 155*f*, 156*b*
    Military Sexual Trauma, 209
    psychotherapy, 156–157
    suicide, 149–151, 149*b*, 149*f*, 150*b*, 151*f*
    transcranial magnetic stimulation, 158, 158*f*
Mal de ojo, 5*b*
Maladaptation, explained, 85–86
Maladaptive behavior as defense mechanism, 34
Maladaptive (negative) stress responses, 86
Maladaptive problem solving, 202, 203
Males and eating disorders, 282
Malnutrition, 281
Malpractice, 25
Mandatory reporting of child abuse, 340
Manerix (maclobemide), 154*t*, 156
Mania
    neurotransmitters, 98*t*
    psychobiology of mental disorders, 101*t*
Manic-depressive disorder, 158. *See also* Bipolar
        disorder
Manipulation
    Antisocial Personality Disorder, 181
    critical thinking care map, 374
    general client care, 365
    nursing care, 366
MAOIs. *See* Monoamine oxidase inhibitors
        (MAOIs)

Guide to Special Features

CASE EXAMPLES

CRITICAL THINKING CARE MAPS

CULTURAL PULSE POINTS

LEARNING ABOUT YOU !

NURSING CARE CHECKLISTS

Guide to Special Features

 ## NURSING PROCESS CARE PLANS